MANUAL OF COMMUNITY HEALTH NURSING

MANUAL OF COMMUNITY HEALTH NURSING

As per the Nursing Syllabus

Second Edition

I Clement

PhD (Nursing) Doctor of Science (DSc) MSc (N) Medical Surgical Nursing MBA (Education) (Madras University) MA (Sociology)
MSc (Psychology) MA (Child Care and Education) MSW (Master of Social Work)

Presently
Professor and Head, Department of Research and Development
RV College of Nursing
Bengaluru, Karnataka, India

Former, Professor and Principal
Columbia College of Nursing
VSS College of Nursing
Bengaluru, Karnataka, India

Professional Assignment
PhD (N) Guide
INC PhD (N) Guide
Chief Editor for Nursing Journals
Rajiv Gandhi University of Health Sciences
Bengaluru, Karnataka, India

Professional Life Member
PhD Society of India, Chennai, Tamil Nadu, India
Nursing Research Society of India, New Delhi, India
Trained Nurses Association of India, New Delhi
Christian Medical Association of India, New Delhi
Indian Society of Psychiatric Nursing, Bengaluru
Medical Surgical Nursing Society of India, Chennai
Indian Society of Neuroscience Nursing, New Delhi
Asian Association of Cardiac Nurses, Kolkata, West Bengal, India

Health Organization Member
Indian Red Cross Society, Bengaluru
St. Johns Ambulance Association, Bengaluru
General Secretary, Indian Society of Medical Surgical Nurses

Assignments and Examiner
Faculty of Nursing, RGUHS, Bengaluru, Karnataka, India
LIC Inspector, Chief Squad, Observer
PhD Research Guide, RGUHS, Bengaluru
UG and PG Examiner, Paper-setter, Valuator other Universities in India

Professional Activity and Editorial
MAT Nursing Journal Chief Editor and PUB Journals
Indian Journal of Practical Nursing
National Editorial Advisory Board, New Delhi
Nurses of India (Former) Bengaluru
Chairman-Souvenir Committee, Florence Nightingale Awards-2012

Winner
Florence Nightingale Awards-2013
Rajiv Gandhi Education Excellence Award
National Mahila Rattan Gold Medal Award, New Delhi

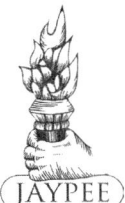

JAYPEE BROTHERS MEDICAL PUBLISHERS

The Health Sciences Publisher

New Delhi | London

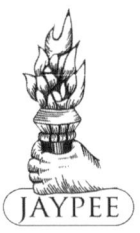

Jaypee Brothers Medical Publishers (P) Ltd

Headquarters
Jaypee Brothers Medical Publishers (P) Ltd
EMCA House, 23/23-B
Ansari Road, Daryaganj
New Delhi 110 002, India
Landline: +91-11-23272143, +91-11-23272703
+91-11-23282021, +91-11-23245672
Email: jaypee@jaypeebrothers.com

Corporate Office
Jaypee Brothers Medical Publishers (P) Ltd
4838/24, Ansari Road, Daryaganj
New Delhi 110 002, India
Phone: +91-11-43574357
Fax: +91-11-43574314
Email: jaypee@jaypeebrothers.com

Overseas Office
J.P. Medical Ltd
83 Victoria Street, London
SW1H 0HW (UK)
Phone: +44 20 3170 8910
Fax: +44 (0)20 3008 6180
Email: info@jpmedpub.com

Website: www.jaypeebrothers.com
Website: www.jaypeedigital.com

© 2024, Jaypee Brothers Medical Publishers

The views and opinions expressed in this book are solely those of the original contributor(s)/author(s) and do not necessarily represent those of editor(s) and publishers of the book.

All rights reserved. No part of this publication may be reproduced, stored or transmitted in any form or by any means, electronic, mechanical, photocopying, recording or otherwise, without the prior permission in writing of the publishers.

All brand names and product names used in this book are trade names, service marks, trademarks or registered trademarks of their respective owners. The publisher is not associated with any product or vendor mentioned in this book.

Medical knowledge and practice change constantly. This book is designed to provide accurate, authoritative information about the subject matter in question. However, readers are advised to check the most current information available on procedures included and check information from the manufacturer of each product to be administered, to verify the recommended dose, formula, method and duration of administration, adverse effects and contraindications. It is the responsibility of the practitioner to take all appropriate safety precautions. Neither the publisher nor the author(s)/editor(s) assume any liability for any injury and/or damage to persons or property arising from or related to use of material in this book.

This book is sold on the understanding that the publisher is not engaged in providing professional medical services. If such advice or services are required, the services of a competent medical professional should be sought.

Every effort has been made where necessary to contact holders of copyright to obtain permission to reproduce copyright material. If any have been inadvertently overlooked, the publisher will be pleased to make the necessary arrangements at the first opportunity.

Inquiries for bulk sales may be solicited at: jaypee@jaypeebrothers.com

Manual of Community Health Nursing

First Edition: 2012

Second Edition: **2024**

ISBN: 978-93-5696-800-4

Printed in India at Sterling Graphics Pvt. Ltd.

Preface to the Second Edition

It gives me immense pleasure and privilege to draft this 2nd edition of *Manual of Community Health Nursing* dedicated to all nursing students. First and foremost, I thank my lord almighty for his wonderful blessing who has strengthened me to complete this book in time. Community health nursing is essential particularly at this point in time because it maximizes the health status of individuals, families, groups and the community through direct approach to them. Today, community participation and involvement is getting due attention before the occurrence of illnesses as life-style changes continue to play a significant role in morbidity and mortality. Community health nurses use their nursing skills to provide care and guidance to patients, especially those with limited resources or access. They provide assistance to pregnant women, the elderly, homeless or disabled by directing them to social services. This book has 19 chapters drafted based on revised nursing syllabus. Each chapter includes a glossary, valid diagrams, tables, and suitable illustrations of the topic that are in line with the syllabus and were created with exams in mind. Every section of the subject has been explained in clear, simple lucid English, making it easier for each student to get ready for the exam according to the new syllabus.

I wish the entire nursing community cherish this book.

I Clement

Preface to the First Edition

Community health nursing is a specialized branch in nursing as it holds major responsibilities of health sector, i.e. through it the health status of people can safeguarded and improved. Community health nursing has its own theoretical and conceptual underpinnings. Many of these are drawn from public health sciences. These include concepts of community health, nutrition, environmental health, health planning, health reports, health education and communication skills, epidemiology, behavioral sciences, personal hygiene, and biomedical waste management.

Community health nursing has goal to help the individuals, families and community in attaining highest standard of health by means of prevention of illnesses and promotion of health. Community health nurse's special concerns are looking after healthy families, treatment of patients who are not hospitalized and health problems of the community.

Manual of Community Health Nursing textbook designed to assist students in developing expertise and in-depth understanding in the field of community health nursing. It would help students to appreciate holistic lifestyle of individual, families, groups and develop skills to function as community health nursing specialist/practitioner. It would further enable the students to function as an educator, manager and researcher in the field of community health nursing.

Manual of Community Health Nursing textbook to fulfill the need of community health nurses holistically. The community health administration and management has been discussed in detail, which fulfills the need of INC syllabus.

I Clement

Acknowledgments

I am thankful to the lord almighty, who strengthened me with his abundant blessings through innumerable means, helping me in all my accomplishments. Firstly, thanks to all the contributors and reviewers for their active participation. My heartfelt thanks to Shri V Somanna, Ex-housing Minister of Karnataka and Chairman of VSS Group of Institutions for his constant support and encouragement.

My sincere gratitude to Dr Sharan Shivraj Patil, Chairman of Sparsh Hospitals and Chief Orthopedic Surgeon MBBS, MS, Mch (Orth), Liverpool, FRCS (England), also my sincere thanks to my Guru BT Basavanthappa, Former Principal, Rajarajeshwari College of Nursing, Bengaluru and PV Ramachandran, Former Chairman, College of Nursing, Sri Ramachandra University, Porur, Chennai, India. A great philosopher and an internationally renowned teacher of nursing who helped me in discovering the world of knowledge. I am also grateful to Dr BC Bhagavan, Professor, Department of Surgery, Kempegowda Institute of Medical Sciences, Bengaluru.

Special thanks to Dr TV Ramakrishnan, Professor of Anesthesiology and Head of Clinical Services, Department of Accident and Emergency Medicine, Sri Ramachandra University, Porur, Chennai. Dr Jeyaseelan Manickam Devadason, Dean, Dr Tamilmani, Principal, Prof (Mrs) Jessie Sudarsanam, Head of Department of Medical Surgical Nursing, Annai JKK Sampoorani Ammal College of Nursing, Komarapalayam and all my teachers and students. I convey my sincere thanks to my beloved parents, brothers and sisters, and my wife Dr Nisha Clement for her continuous support and constant encouragement in each step of my life. I take this opportunity to thank my children's, Cibin John, Cynthia Elizabeth and Cavin Jacob.

I am very grateful to the whole team of M/s Jaypee Brothers Medical Publishers (P) Ltd, New Delhi, India, who helped and guided me, Shri Jitendar P Vij (Group Chairman), Mr Ankit Vij (Managing Director), Mr MS Mani (Group President), Dr Madhu Choudhary (Director-Educational Publishing), Ms Pooja Bhandari [Director-Production (Books and Journals)], Ms Sunita Katla (Executive Assistant to Group Chairman and Publishing Manager), Mr Ajay Kumar Sharma (Deputy General Manager), Ms Samina Khan (Executive Assistant to Director-Educational Publishing), Ms Jitika Royal (Content Strategist), Mr Rajesh Sharma (Production Coordinator), Ms Seema Dogra (Cover Visualizer) and their team members, for all their support to work in this project and make it a success. Without their cooperation, I could not have completed this project.

Contents

1. **Introduction to Community Health............... 1**
   - Concepts of health and disease 2
   - Meaning of disease/illness 2
   - History and development of community health in India and its present concept 3
   - History and development of community health nursing 3
   - Dimensions of health 5
   - Health determinants 6
   - Indicators of health 7
   - Health–illness continuum 9
   - Models of health and illness 9
   - Stages of illness behavior 10
   - Impact of illness on family 11
   - Levels of health care 11
   - Levels of illness prevention 12
   - Primary health care: elements and principles nurses role in primary health care 12
   - Health for all 14
   - Millennium development goals 15
   - Promotion and maintenance of health 16

2. **Community Health Nursing 19**
   - Concept of community health nursing 20
   - Philosophy of community health nursing 20
   - Objectives of community health nursing 20
   - Goals of community health nursing 21
   - Principles of community health nursing 21
   - Skills of community health nurse 22
   - Community health team 22
   - Qualities and functions of a community health nurse 23
   - Scope of community health nursing 24
   - Community health nursing process 25
   - Community assessment/problem identification 26
   - Community health diagnosis 28
   - Components of nursing process 28
   - Establishing interpersonal relationship 30
   - Community healthcare plan 31
   - Comprehensive community health nursing 32

3. **Health Assessment 34**
   - Concept of health assessment 34
   - Purposes and factors affecting health assessment 35
   - Principles of health assessment 35
   - Responsibilities of nurse in health assessment 36
   - Characteristics of a healthy individual 36
   - Approach to physical assessment 38
   - Health assessment of infant 38
   - Health assessment of toddler and preschool child 41
   - Health assessment of school going child 42
   - Health assessment of adolescent 42
   - Comprehensive health assessment 44
   - Health assessment of antenatal woman 45
   - Health assessment of postnatal woman 48
   - Health assessment of elderly 50
   - Role of nurse in health assessment 51
   - Recording of health assessment 51

4. **Principles of Epidemiology and Epidemiological Methods 53**
   - History of epidemiology and population health 53
   - Concept of epidemiology 54
   - Aims of epidemiology 55
   - Functions/uses of epidemiology 55
   - Objectives of epidemiology 55
   - Components of epidemiology 55
   - Types of epidemiology 56
   - Basic tools of measurement in epidemiology 56
   - Principles of epidemiology 57
   - Scope of epidemiology 57
   - Dichotomies in epidemiological studies 58
   - Epidemiology in community nursing 58
   - Uses of epidemiology 58
   - Advantages of epidemiology 59
   - Epidemiological approaches 59
   - Preventive epidemiology 61
   - Importance of epidemiology 61
   - Disease cycle 61
   - Modes of disease transmission 62
   - Spectrum of disease 62
   - Disease causation 62
   - Epidemiological triad 62
   - Natural history of diseases 63
   - Levels of disease prevention 65
   - Control of infectious diseases 66
   - Disinfection 67
   - Role of community health nurse in epidemics 67

5. **Family Health Nursing Care 69**
   - Family 70
   - Family as a unit of community health services 71
   - Family health care 71
   - Family health nursing 72
   - Family-centered nursing approach 72
   - Family health nursing process 73
   - Family health assessment 74
   - Methods of data collection 74
   - Assessment of health problems 75
   - Assessment of families 75
   - Planning for nursing action 75
   - Implementing the program 76

- Evaluation of program action 76
- Nursing care plan 76
- Nursing care 76
- Core competencies family health nurse 76
- Family health services—maternal, child care and family welfare services 77
- Responsibilities of community health nurse in MCH services 78
- Roles and function of a community health nurse in family health service 79
- Family health records 79

6. Family Healthcare Settings 82
- Concept of healthcare setting 83
- Healthcare settings 83
- Scope of practice for registered nurses 84
- Types of home healthcare services 84
- Home visit 85
- Bag techniques 86
- Home health nursing procedures 87
- Handwashing 87
- Cleaning, disinfecting and sterilization 87
- Thermometer techniques 88
- Measurement of weight and height 88
- Records and reports pertaining to family health care 89
- Nursing clinic 89

7. Referral System 93
- Referral in health systems 94
- Purposes of health systems 94
- Levels of health care and healthcare settings 94
- Concept of referral system 96
- Components of a referral system 96
- Principles of a referral system 96
- Rationale, benefits and objectives 96
- Need of referral system 97
- Importance of referral 97
- Advantages of referral cases 97
- Levels of health care: referral system 97
- Immediate referral 98
- Referral form 98
- Benefits of referral system 99
- Barrier to referral process 99
- Nurse's role in referral system 99

8. Records and Reports in Community Health Nursing 101
- Concept of record and report 101
- Definitions of records and reports 102
- Meaning of records and reports 102
- Characteristics of good recording and reporting 102
- Importance of reports and records 102
- Purposes of recording and reporting 103
- Values and uses of records 103
- Principles of recording and reporting 104
- Care of the records 104
- Types of records, reports and registers in community health nursing 104
- Legal implications of records and reports 105
- Role of community health nurse in recording and reporting 105
- Nurses responsibility for record keeping and reporting 106
- Community health nursing registers 106

9. Minor Ailments 109
- Basic principles of care during minor ailments and accidents ailments 109
- Management of minor ailments 110
- Minor ailments in respiratory tract 110
- Minor ailments in eyes and ears 110
- Minor ailments in cardiovascular system 111
- Minor ailments in digestive system 111
- Minor ailments in urinary system 111
- Minor ailments in neuromuscular system 112
- Minor ailments in reproductive system 112
- Standing orders 112
- Care of patient with fever 113
- Care of patient with sore throat 114
- Care of patient with sore eye 114
- Care of patient with convulsions 115
- Care of patient with diarrhea 115
- Care of patients with constipation 117
- Care of patients with animal bite—dog bite 117
- Care of patient with snake bite 118
- Care of patient with fracture 118
- Care of patient with anemia 119
- Care of patient with epitasis (nose bleeding) 120
- Care of patient with heat stroke 120
- Care of patient with edema 121
- Care of patient with scabies 121
- Care of patient with wounds 122
- Care of patient with toothache 122
- Care of patient with shock 122
- Care of patient with unconscious 124

10. Health System in India 127
- Health system 128
- Aims and goals of health system 128
- Determinants of health system 128
- Forces influence the health system 129
- Health administration 129
- Model of healthcare delivery system 130
- Organization and administration of health system in India 131
- Central level healthcare administration 131
- Directorate general of health services 132
- Central council of health 133
- State level healthcare administration 133
- District level healthcare administration 134
- Community level healthcare administration 135
- Health organization at district level 136
- Health organization at block level 137
- Health organization at subcenter 137

- Health organization at urban 137
- Panchayat Raj 137

11. Healthcare Delivery System 141
- Types of healthcare delivery 141
- Infrastructure and health sectors 144
- Delivery of health services at subcenter (SC) 146
- Delivery of health services at PHC 147
- Delivery of health services at CHC 148
- Administration of nursing personnel 148
- Community development program 150
- Integrated rural development 151
- Sustainable development goals (SDGs) 151
- Reduce inequality within and among countries 155
- Make cities and human settlement inclusive safe, resilient and sustainable 155
- Ensure sustainable consumption and production patterns 156
- Take urgent action to combat climate change and its impacts 156
- Conserve and sustainably use the oceans, seas and marine resources for sustainable development 156
- Protect, restore and promote sustainable use of terrestrial ecosystem, sustainably manage forest, combat desertification and halt and reverse land degradation and halt biodiversity loss 157
- Promote peaceful and inclusive societies for sustainable development; provide access to justice for all and build effective, accountable and inclusive institutions at all levels 157
- Strengthen the means of implementation and revitality the global partnership for sustainable development 158

12. Health Planning in India 160
- Health planning 160
- Specific quantitative goals and objectives 161
- Health systems performance 161
- Health systems strengthening 161
- Health planning steps 162
- Planning cycle 163
- Health planning in India 164
- Planning commission 164
- National health committees 165
- Bhore committee (1946) 165
- Mudaliar committee (1962) 165
- Chadah committee (1963) 166
- Mukherjee committee (1965) 166
- Mukerji committee (1966) 166
- Jungalwala committee 166
- Kartar Singh committee (1973) 167
- Shrivastav committee (1975) 167
- Rural health scheme (1977) 167
- Bajaj committee (1986–87) 168
- National health policies 168
- Planning commission of India 168
- National development council and health (NDC) 169
- Five year plan and health 169
- First five year plan (1951–56) 170
- Second five year plan (1956–61) 170
- Third five year plan 171
- Fourth five year plan 171
- Fifth five year plan 171
- Sixth five year plan 172
- Seventh five year plan 172
- Eighth five year plan 172
- Ninth five year plan (1977–2002) 172
- Tenth five year plan (2002–2007) 173
- Eleventh five year plan (2007–2012) 173
- Community development and health 174
- Planning process in community health nursing 174

13. Specialized Community Health Services and Nurse's Role 178
- Reproductive and child health (RCH) 179
- National health mission (Rural/Urban) 201
- Janani Suraksha Yojana 205
- Emergency ambulance services 207
- Government health insurance schemes 208
- School health services 211
- Maintenance of school health records 223
- Occupational health nursing (including healthcare providers) 224
- Geriatric nursing 236
- Care of differently abled physical and mental 245

14. National Health Problems 264
- Communicable diseases 264
- Non-communicable diseases 264
- Environmental sanitation problems 266
- Medical care problems 266
- Population problem 266
- Sanitation 268
- Man–environment relationship 268
- Importance of environmental science 269
- Components of environmental science 270
- Renewable and nonrenewable resources 271
- Problems associated with natural resources 271
- Natural resources and associated problems 271
- Forest resources 273
- Water resources 274
- Water pollution 274
- Mineral resources 275
- Food resources 278
- Energy resources 279
- Land resources 279
- Role of individuals in conservation of natural resources 280
- Equitable use of resources for sustainable lifestyles 281
- Ecosystem 281
- Forest ecosystem 282

- Ecosystem—scope and importance 282
- Importance of ecosystem 283
- Ecological pyramid 283
- Energy flow in ecosystem 284
- Biodiversity 285
- Significance of biodiversity 286
- Productive use value of biodiversity 287
- Threats to biodiversity 287
- Conversation of biodiversity 288
- National Biodiversity Act 288
- Environmental pollution 288
- Air pollution 289
- Water pollution 290
- Noise pollution 290
- Soil or land pollution 291
- Marine pollution 292
- Thermal pollution 293
- Nuclear hazards and their impact on health 293
- Global environmental problems 294
- Global warming 295
- Hazardous waste management 297
- Wastewater management 297
- Population explosion and its pressure on environment 297
- Ozone depletion 298
- Policy and legislation 299
- Towards sustainable future 300
- 17 New undevelopment goals for 2030 301
- Environmental education 301
- Concept of environmental health and sanitation 302
- Concept of safe water 304
- Water-borne diseases 305
- Water purification processes 305
- Household purification of water 307
- Physical and chemical standards of drinking water 307
- Bacteriological quality of water 308
- Concepts of water conservation 309
- Rainwater harvesting 310
- Watershed management 310
- Concept of pollution prevention: air and noise pollution, role of nurse in prevention of pollution 312
- Lighting 314
- Ventilation 315
- Radiation 316
- Meteorological environment 317
- Housing 318
- Town planning 319
- Disposal of solid waste 319
- Commonly used insecticides and pesticides 322

15. National Health Programs 325
- National ARI Control Programme 325
- Revised National Tuberculosis Control Programme (RNTCP) 326
- National Antimalaria Programme 327
- National Filaria Control Programme 328
- National Guinea Worm Eradication Programme 329
- National Leprosy Eradication Programme 330
- STD Control Program 333
- National Programme for Control of Blindness 334
- Iodine deficiency control program 335
- Expanded programme of immunization 336
- National Family Welfare Programme 336
- Role of community health nurse in family welfare services 337
- National water supply and sanitation programme 338
- Minimum needs program 339
- National Diabetes Control Programme 339
- Polio eradication: Pulse Programme 339
- National Cancer Control Programme 340
- Yaws eradication program 341
- National Nutritional Anemia Prophylaxis Programme 342
- 20 Point Program 343
- ICDS Program 344
- Mid-day Meal Program 344
- National Mental Health Programme 345
- Adolescent Health Program 346
- Role of nurse in the National Health Programme 346

16. Demography and Family Welfare 349
- Concept of demography 349
- Importance of demography 350
- Demographic cycle 351
- World population trends 352
- Concept of fertility and infertility 353
- Small family norm 354
- Family planning 356
- Family planning programme 359
- Birth control pills 360
- Barrier methods 361
- Long-term contraceptive methods 361
- Natural family planning (NFP) 361
- Natural methods of space methods 362
- Calendar or rhythm method 363
- Basal body temperature (BBT) method 363
- Cervical mucus method (CMM) 363
- Lactational amenorrhea method 364
- Coitus interruptus (withdrawal or pulling out) method 365
- Condom 365
- Biological, chemical and mechanical methods 365
- Terminal methods (tubectomy, vasectomy) 367
- Counseling in reproductive, sexual health including problems of adolescents 369
- Medical termination of pregnancy and MTP Act 370
- National family welfare programme 372
- Role of a nurse in family welfare program 375

17. Health Team 378
- Building up of a team   378
- Characteristics of an effective team   379
- Advantages and disadvantages of team functioning   379
- Aims of health team   379
- Role of nurse in team functioning   380
- Roles and responsibilities of community health nursing personnel in family health services   380
- District public health nurse   380
- Community health nurse   381
- Health assistant supervisor (female)   382
- Health worker (female and male health worker)   382
- Community health volunteers   383
- Traditional birth attendants (TBAs)   383
- Principles and techniques of counseling   383

18. Health Information System/Health Management Information System 386
- Concept of HMIS   386
- Types of healthcare information systems   388
- Health information system (HIS)   388
- Nursing management information system (NIMS)   390
- Vital statistics   390
- Vital statistics measurements   392
- Sources of vital statistics   392
- Civil registration system   393
- Ad-hoc survey   394
- Vital registration   395
- Common sampling techniques   396
- Frequency distribution   398
- Collection of data   400
- Data collection process   400
- Data collection methods and instruments   401
- Selection criteria for data collection method   401
- Questionnaires   402
- Interviews   402
- Observation methods   403
- Other observational methods   404
- Psychological tests   404
- Likert scales   404
- Data presentation   405
- Diagrammatic/graphical presentation of data   405
- Qualitative data presentation   408
- Analysis of data   411
- Interpretation of data   412
- Communication of nursing research findings   415

19. Health Agencies 417
- Types of international health agencies   417
- World Health Organization   418
- United Nations Fund for Population Activities   420
- United Nations Development Programme   421
- World Bank   421
- Food and Agriculture Organization   422
- United Nations International Children's Emergency Fund   424
- European Commission   425
- International Red Cross   428
- United States Agency for International Development   431
- United Nations Educational Scientific and Cultural Organization   432
- International Labor Organization   435
- Cooperative for American Relief Everywhere   436
- Canadian International Development Agency   437
- JHPIEGO   437
- Rockefeller foundation   438
- Ford foundation   438
- Colombo plan   439
- Voluntary association   439
- Indian Red Cross Society   441
- Indian Council of Child Welfare   443
- Family Planning Association of India   443
- Tuberculosis Association of India   444
- Central Social Welfare Board   445
- All India Women's Conference   446
- All India Blind Relief Societies   446
- Activities   446
- Hind Kusht Nivaran Sangh   447
- Child Relief and You   447
- Bharat Sevak Samaj   448
- Kasturba Memorial Funds   448

Index.. *451*

Nursing Syllabus

Placement: First Year

Time—180 hours
CHN-I – 80 hours Environmental Hygiene—30 hours
Health Education and Communication Skills—40 hours
Nutrition—30 hours

COMMUNITY HEALTH NURSING – I

Course Description

This course is designed to help students gain an understanding of the concept of community health in order to introduce them to the wider horizons of rendering nursing services in a community set-up, both in urban and rural areas.

General Objectives

Upon completion of this course, the students shall be able to:
- Describe the concept of health, community health and community health nursing.
- State the principles of epidemiology and epidemiological methods in community health nursing practice.
- Explain the various services provided to the community and role of the nurse.
- Demonstrate skills to practice effective nursing care of the individuals and families in the clinics as well as in their homes, using scientific principles.

Total Hours: 80

Unit No.	Learning objectives	Content	Hr	Teaching learning activities	Method of assessment
I.	Describe the concept of health and disease and community health	**Introduction to Community Health** ➢ **Definitions:** Community, community health, community health nursing ➢ Concept of health and disease, dimensions and indicators of health, health determinants ➢ History and development of community health in India and its present concept ➢ Primary health care, Millennium Development Goals ➢ Promotion and maintenance of health	10	Lecture cum discussions	Short answers
II.	Explain various aspects of community health nursing. Demonstrate skills in applying nursing process in community health nursing settings	**Community Health Nursing** ➢ Philosophy, goals, objectives and principles, concept and importance of community health nursing ➢ Qualities and functions of community health Nurse ➢ Steps of nursing process; community identification, population composition, health and allied resources, community assessment, planning and conducting community nursing care services	14	➢ Lecture cum discussions	➢ Short answers ➢ Essay type
III.	Demonstrate skill in assessing the health status and identify deviations from normal parameters in different age groups	**Health Assessment** ➢ Characteristics of a healthy individual ➢ Health assessment of infant, preschool, school going, adolescent, adult, antenatal woman, postnatal woman, and elderly	10	➢ Lecture cum discussions ➢ Demonstration ➢ Role play ➢ Videos	➢ Short answers ➢ Objective type ➢ Essay type ➢ Return demonstration

Unit No.	Learning objectives	Content	Hr	Teaching learning activities	Method of assessment
IV.	Describe the principles of epidemiology and epidemiological methods in community health nursing practice	**Principles of Epidemiology and Epidemiological Methods** ➢ Definition and aims of epidemiology, communicable and non-communicable diseases ➢ Basic tools of measurement in epidemiology ➢ Uses of epidemiology ➢ Disease cycle ➢ Spectrum of disease ➢ Levels of prevention of disease ➢ Disease transmission—direct and indirect ➢ Immunizing agents, immunization and national immunization schedule ➢ Control of infectious diseases ➢ Disinfection	10	➢ Lecture cum discussions. ➢ Non-communicable disease module of government of India ➢ Field visit	➢ Short answers ➢ Objective type ➢ Essay type
V.	Demonstrate, skill in providing comprehensive nursing care to the family	**Family Health Nursing Care** ➢ Family as a unit of health ➢ Concept, goals, objectives ➢ Family health care services ➢ Family health care plan and nursing process ➢ Family health services—Maternal, child care and family welfare services ➢ Roles and function of a community health nurse in family health service ➢ Family health records	12	➢ Lecture cum discussions ➢ Role play ➢ Family visit	Short answers Essay type
VI.	Describe the principles and techniques of family health care services at home and in clinics	**Family Health Care Settings Home Visit** ➢ Purposes, principles ➢ Planning and evaluation ➢ Bag technique ➢ Clinic: Purposes, type of clinics and their functions ➢ Function of health personnel in clinics	10	➢ Lecture cum discussions. ➢ Demonstration ➢ Visits – Home, health center	➢ Short answers ➢ Return demonstration
VII.	Describe the referral system and community resources for referral	**Referral System** ➢ Levels of health care and health care settings. ➢ Referral services available ➢ Steps in referral ➢ Role of a nurse in referral	6	➢ Lecture cum discussions ➢ Mock drill	➢ Short answers ➢ Objective type
VIII.	List the records and reports used in community health nursing practice	**Records and Reports** ➢ Types and uses ➢ Essential requirements of records and reports ➢ Preparation and maintenance	3	➢ Lecture cum discussions ➢ Exhibit the records.	➢ Short answers ➢ Objective type
IX.	Explain the management of minor ailments	**Minor Ailments** ➢ Principles of management ➢ Management as per standing instructions/orders	5	Lecture cum discussions	➢ Short answers ➢ Objective type

CHAPTER 1

Introduction to Community Health

LEARNING OBJECTIVES

1. **Definitions:** Community, community health, community health nursing
2. Concept of health and disease, dimensions and indicators of health, health determinants
3. History and development of community health in India and its present concept
4. Primary healthcare, millennium development goals
5. Promotion and maintenance of health

INTRODUCTION

Health in its broadest sense is a dynamic state in which the individual adapts to changes in internal and external environments to maintain a state of well-being. The internal environment includes many factors that influence health, including genetic and psychological variables, intellectual and spiritual dimensions and disease processes.

The external environment includes factors outside the person that may influence health, the physical environment, social relationships, and economic variables because both environments continuously change, the person must maintain a state of well-being. Health and illness therefore must be defined in terms of individual. Health can include conditions that the client or nurse may have previously considered to be illness. Health is also closely related to an individual's work place and home life and stressors can be the result of those environments.

DEFINITIONS

Community

- Community can be defined in numerous ways, depending on the application. The variety of individuals, families and cultural groups represented in a community contribute to the overall character of the community.
- Community-based nursing needs to understand the community within which they practice. Knowledge of the community helps nurses to maintain quality of care.

Community Health

- Community health is defined more broadly and encompasses the entire gamut of community organized efforts for maintaining protection and improves the health of the people.
- Community health postulates a unified and balanced integration of curative, preventive and promotive health services. The primary motto is promotion of well-being (physical, mental and social).
- According to WHO, community health refers to the health status of the members of the community to the problems affecting their health and to the totality of healthcare provided for the community.
- Community health implies, in a broad sense, integration of curative, preventive and promotive health services. The traditional and important responsibilities of public health are now included in the concept of community health **(Fig. 1.1)**.
- Community health refers to the health status of the members of the community, the problems affecting their health and the totality of healthcare provided for the community—*Blum*.
- Community health or public health is defined as "the art and science of maintaining, protecting and improving health of people through organized effects."—*American Association of Public Health*.

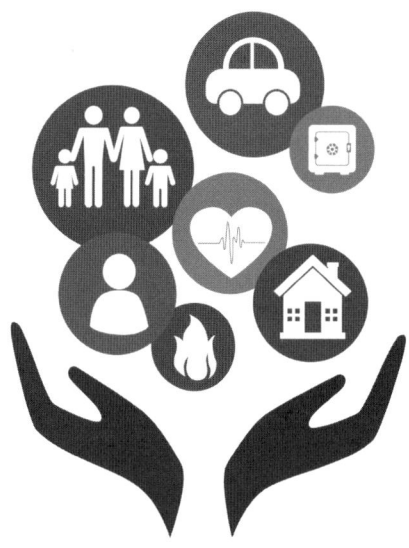

Fig. 1.1: Concept of community health.

Community Health Nursing

Nurses in community health provide an interpretative bridge between the acute sector and community services. They embrace a social model of health to advocate and give a voice to the community accessing care. In a system which is often complex and hard to navigate, nurses in community health are able to simplify the health systems, referral pathways, and access to care.

CONCEPTS OF HEALTH AND DISEASE (TABLE 1.1)

- It is useful for the nurse to be aware of the behavioral components of health, illness and sick role behavior.
- Every person develops a system of health belief and attitudes, and these tend to fall within the framework provided by society or cultural heritage.
- Health behavior activities of a person engage in, when feeling well, to take measures to prevent disease and illness to detect them before symptoms occur.
- Illness behavior activities of a person change when feeling ill that will lead to the defining of the state of health and illness.
- Sick-role behavior activities of a person engage in believing himself ill. For any individual the level of health behavior is determined by the significance of symptoms—danger value, visibility, ambiguity, fear of unknown, the expectations of those from whom help is sought, feeling about dependence and fear of loss of control, the expectations of the illness position, including past experiences with illness.

MEANING OF DISEASE/ILLNESS

Disease can be considered as something more than mere deviation from health, each disease being a distinct entity, with distinguishing qualities in its pathologic process, its typical clinical appearance and often its characteristic epidemiologic pattern of distribution in terms of time, place and person. The concept of disease also may vary from one society to another society. The classification of disease is depicted in **Figure 1.2**.

Causes and Risk Factors for Developing Illness

An illness is the response the person has to disease. It is an abnormal process in which the person's level of functioning is changed compared with a previous level **(Fig. 1.3)**.

Internal Variables

- **Developmental stage:** A person's thought and behavior patterns change throughout life.
- **Intellectual background:** Knowledge about body functions and illnesses, educational background and past experiences, all influence the health beliefs and practice of patients.
- **Emotional and spiritual factors:** The patient's degree of calm or stress can influence health beliefs and practices. Spiritual beliefs also influence whether and how a patient seeks or avoids healthy behavior.

External Variables

- **Family practices:** The way that patient's families use healthcare services, their perceptions of the seriousness of diseases and their preventive care behaviors can influence the health beliefs and practice.

TABLE 1.1: Concept of health.	
Being healthy	*Being disease-free*
It is a state of being well enough to function well physically, mentally and socially	It is a state of absence from diseases
It refers to the individual, physical and social environment	It refers only to the individual
The individual has good health	The individual may have good health or poor health

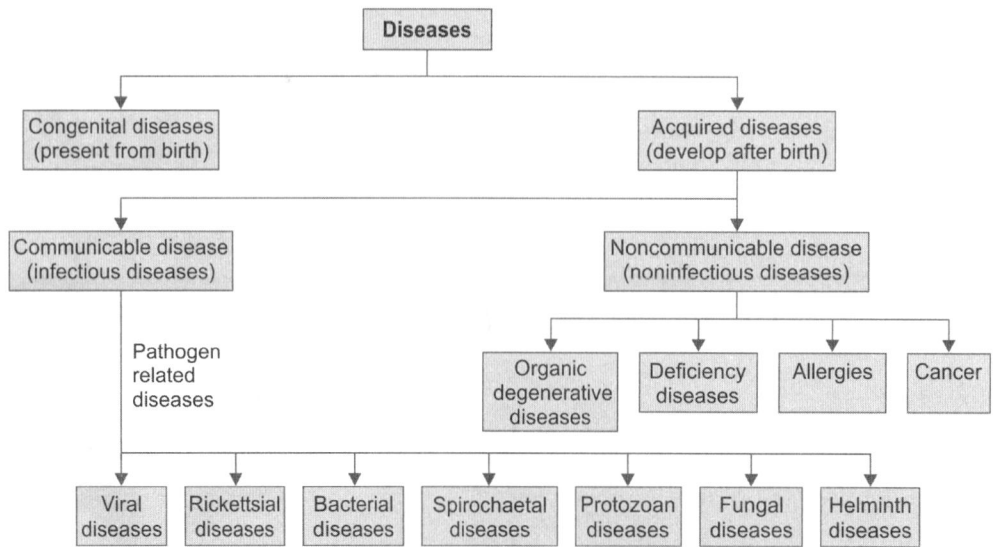

Fig. 1.2: Classification of disease.

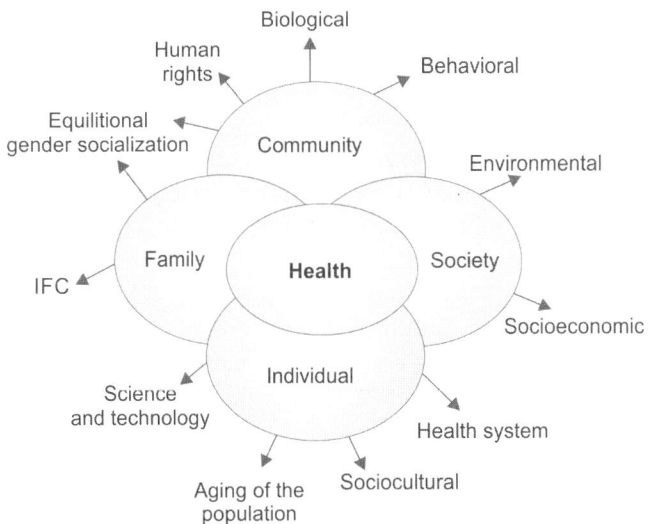

Fig. 1.3: Factors affecting a patient's health status.

- **Socioeconomic factors:** Social relationships, economic level and psychosocial factors influence health beliefs and practice.
- **Cultural background:** It influences beliefs, values and customs. It influences the approach to the healthcare system, personal health practices and nurse-patient relationship.

Factors Affecting a Patient's Health Status
- Smoking
- Nutrition
- Alcohol use
- Habituating drug use
- Driving
- Exercise
- Sexuality and contraceptive use
- Family relationships
- Risk factor modification
- Coping and adaptation.

HISTORY AND DEVELOPMENT OF COMMUNITY HEALTH IN INDIA AND ITS PRESENT CONCEPT

- The medical systems that are truly of Indian origin and development are the Ayurveda and Siddha System. Ayurveda by definition implies "Knowledge of Life". Its origin is traced far back to the Vedic times, about 5000 BC. During this period, medical history was associated with mythological figures, sages and seers.
- Dhanvantari the Hindu god of medicine is said to have been born as a result of the churning of ocean during a tug war between gods and demons. According to some authorities medical knowledge in the Atharvaveda gradually developed into the science.
- The experience and concern in health development and public healthcare dates back to this Vedic period. In the Indus Valley Civilization (3000 BC) itself, one funds evidence of well-developed environmental sanitation program, such as arrangements of good water supply, underground drainages, public baths in cities, etc.
- In ancient India, the celebrated authorities in Ayurveda Medicine were Atreya, Charaka, Sushtra and Vagbhata. Atreya (about 800 BC) is acknowledged as the first great Indian Physician and Teacher. Charaka a famous Ayurvedic Medicine contributor and Sushtra the Father of Indian Surgery. From this early writings other authors wrote books, from these writings we learnt that surgery had advanced to a high level, also that doctors and the attendants (Nurse) must be the people of high character. Hospitals were large and well equipped.
- Medical education was introduced in the ancient Universities of Taxila and Nalanda. During Buddha period hospital system was developed for men and women and for animals. This was expanded during king Ashoka, Mughal Period (1000 AD). Yunani Medicine which (Arabic system) was introduced through Greek medicine has become a part of Indian medicine. Nursing and medicine are closely linked together.
- Nursing was regarded on the "Science of Care" and medicine as the "Science of Cure". As the science of cure, medicine is concerned with the diagnosis and treatment of illness. As the science of care, nursing is concerned with the care of people who are ill. The care and cure functions are complementary; both are necessary and important aspects of healthcare for the people.
- Community health has now entered an era of individual responsibilities and community participation. The traditional role of medical persons has been shifted from diagnosis and treatment of individual illness to treatment of all health hazards of community. Community diagnosis is based on collection and interpretation of relevant data related to distribution of population according to age, sex, educational status, marital status, religion, caste, birth rate, death rate, prevalence of disease, etc.

Development in the broader sense is not only the improvement or progress in the community health resources but also individual progress in the professional aspect of as community health nurse.

HISTORY AND DEVELOPMENT OF COMMUNITY HEALTH NURSING

In early history (Vedic period) Indus valley civilizations 3000 BC there were planned cities, houses built with public baths with drainage. People practiced proper environmental sanitation In 1400 BC Ayurveda and Siddha Systems of medicine came into existence which suggested development of comprehensive concept of health.

British India (18th Century to 1947)

1859—Royal commission came to India to study the problem.

1864—Sanitary commissioners were appointed in Bombay, Madras and Bengal.

1869—Sanitary Commissioner and a statistical officer were appointed with the Government of India.

1873—Birth and Death Registration Act was promulgated

1880—Vaccination Act was passed.

1881—First Indian Factories Act was passed and First All India Census Act was taken.

1869—The plague commission was appointed subsequent to an outbreak of plague.

1897—The Epidemic Disease Act was promulgated.

1907—Central Malaria Bureau at Kasauli was established for the purpose of research.

1917—Government of India sanctioned the appointment of deputy sanitary commissioners and health officers.

1918—Lady Reading Health School in Delhi was established. The nutrition Research laboratory at Coonoor was established.

1930—All India Institute of Hygiene and Public Health was established at Calcutta with aid from the Rockefeller Foundation.

1931—A maternal and Child Welfare Bureau was established by the Indian Red Cross society.

1935—All the health activities in the country were grouped as under the control of Central, Central-cum-Provincial or provincial Government.

1937—A Central Advisory Board of Health was setup.

1939—Madras Public Health Act was passed.

A rural health training center at Singur near Calcutta was started with assistance from the Rockefeller Foundation.

Indian Tuberculosis Association was established.

1940—The Drug Act was passed and for the first time was brought under control.

1943—A Health Survey and Development Committee (Bhore committee) was appointed by the Government of India.

1946—Bhore Committee report was submitted.

Post-independence Era—In 1947, India obtained its Independence. The National Government took up the responsibility of improving the health of the people, with the Bhore committee report and its recommendations forming a basis for planning and steps to be adopted.

1947—Ministries of Health were established both at the central and at the state government level.

1948—India joined as a member State of the World Health Organization. Employees State Insurance Act was passed. Report of the Environment Hygiene committee was published.

1949—The Constitution of India was adopted by the constituent assembly.

1950—Planning Commission was set up by government of India. Central Food Technological Research Institute was established in Mysore.

1951—BCG vaccination program launched in the country Central Drug Research Institute, first of its kind was opened at Lucknow. This year saw the beginning of first Five-Year plan.

1952—Community Development Program on rural areas was launched on October 2, 1952. A virus research center was established at Pune with joint help from ICMR and the Rockefeller Foundation. Indian Cancer Research Center at Bombay was inaugurated.

1953—National Malaria Control Programme, was initiated. National Smallpox Eradication Programme was started. National wide family planning Research and Programme Committee was set up.

1954—Contributory health services scheme was initiated in Delhi Central Social Welfare Board was set up. National water supply and sanitation scheme was inaugurated. National Leprosy Control Programme was started established at Chengalpattu in Tamil Nadu. National Tuberculosis Survey commenced.

1955—National Filaria Control Programme was started. Central Leprosy Training and Research Center was established at Chengalpattu in Tamil Nadu.

1956—Second Five-Year plan began. Central Health Education Bureau was established. Director for family planning was appointed at the Union Ministry of Health. Chemotherapy center at Madras was started.

1958—National Malaria Control Programme was changed to National Malaria Eradication Programme. National Tuberculosis survey was completed.

1959—Rajasthan was the first state to introduce Panchayat Raj. The National Tuberculosis Institute at Bangalore was established. The nutrition research laboratories at Coonoor were shifted to Hyderabad.

1960—School Health Committee was formed.

1961—Third five year plan was launched. Mudaliar committee's report published.

1962—National Smallpox Eradication Programme, National Goiter Control Programme, National School Health Programme and District Tuberculosis Control Programme was Established. Central Family Planning institute were established in Delhi.

1963—National Institute for Communicable Diseases (NICD) was established in Delhi. National Trachoma Control Programme was begun. Applied Nutrition Program started. The family planning program was changed to an extension approach scheme rather than one with a clinic approach.

1964—National Institute for Health Administration and Education (NIHAE) was established in Delhi.

1965—IVCD was introduced. Direct BCG vaccination programme without tuberculin test was introduced.

1966—Minister for Family Planning was appointed under the Ministry of Health.

1968—Medical Education Committee was appointed by government of India.

1969—Fourth Five-Year plan was launched.

1970—The Birth and Death Registration Act came into force. All India Hospital Family Planning Program was started.

1971—Medical Termination of Pregnancy Bill comes in force. National service Bill passed.

1973—The national program of minimum needs was incorporated with the health services. A new cadre of health worker called multipurpose health workers was formed on the basis of the recommendations for the Karter Singh committee report who will eventually replace auxiliary Nurse – Midwives, family planning workers and basic health workers.

1974—The fifth Five-Year plan comes into operation.

1975—On July 5th of this year. India was declared free from smallpox. Integrated child development scheme was launched in India. National Children's Welfare Board was set up.

1976—Indian Factories Act of 1948 was amended. National Programme for Prevention of Blindness was formulated.

1977—International commission declared India has eradicated smallpox. National Institute of Health and Family Planning was formed. Community health worker scheme was begun by the Union Minister of Health.

1978—The Slogan "Health for All by 2000 AD" came to light at the ALMA-ATA declaration in USSR.

1979—The year was observed as the year of the child all over the world.

1981—The theme of this year was year of the disabled around the world.

1982—Government of India announced "The New 20-point program as national health policy.

1983—National Leprosy Control Programme to be called National Leprosy Eradication Programme.

Guinea worm eradication program was launched.

1984—The Workmen's Compensation Act, 1984 came into effect form July 1. Juvenile Justice Act, 1986 came into force. Bhopal gas tragedy happened.

1985—Seventh Five-Year plan launched. Universal Immunization Program was launched. A separate development of women and child development was set up under Ministry of Human Resource Development.

1986—The Environment Act, 1986 was promulgated.

1987—National Diabetes Control Programme and National AIDS Control Programme was initiated.

1989—Blood Safety Programme was launched.

1990—Control of acute respiratory infections (ARI) program was initiated.

1992—Eight five-year plan was launched.

Child survival and Safe Motherhood program was launched.

1993—Revised National TB Programme with DOTS was introduced.

1995—ICDS was renamed as Integrated Mother and Child Development Services (IMCD).

1996—Pulse polio immunization was initiated.

1997—Reproductive and child health program was launched.

1998-1999—National Malaria Eradication Programme was renamed as National Anti-malaria Programme. National family health survey was undertaken.

2000—Government of India Announced National Population policy.

2002—National Health Policy 2002 was announced.

2002—Government announces National AIDS Prevention Control Policy.

2003—Launching of ART centers at Metro Centers, e.g., Sassoon

2004—NTCP inculcated DOTS

2007—Revision of National Population

2008—Revised in 2009 Swine Flu Awareness Program and Control Program.

DIMENSIONS OF HEALTH (FIG. 1.4)

The WHO definition envisages three dimensions—the physical, the mental and the social. Many more may be cited viz. spiritual, emotional, vocational and political dimensions.

- **Physical dimension:** The state of physical health implies the notion of 'perfect functioning" of the body. It conceptualizes health biologically as a state in which the every cell and every organ is functioning at optimum capacity and in perfect harmony with the rest of the body.
- **Mental dimension:** Mental health is the ability to respond to the many varied experiences of life with flexibility and a sense of purpose. More recently, mental health has been defined as, "A state of balance between individual and surrounding world, a state of harmony between oneself and others, a co-existence between realities of self and other people of the environment". Mind and body were considered independent entities.

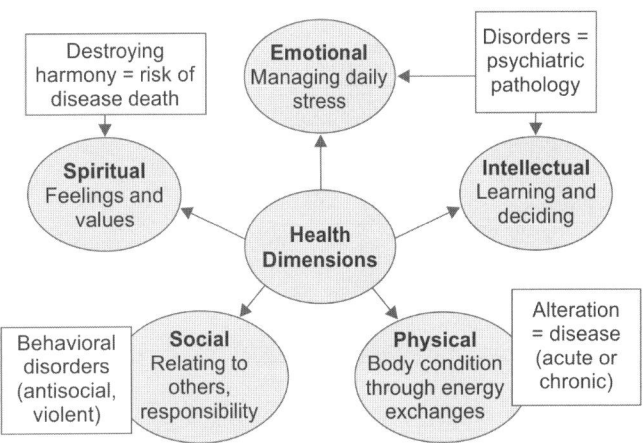

Fig. 1.4: Dimensions of health.

- **Social dimension:** It has been defined as the "quantity and quality of an individual's interpersonal ties and extent of involvement with the community".
  Social health takes into account that every individual is a part of a family; and of wider community, and focuses on social and economic conditions and well-being of the "whole person" in context of his social network.
- **Spiritual dimension:** It refers to that part of individual which reaches out and strives of meaning and purpose in life. It is intangible "something that transcends physiology and psychology. It includes integrity, principles of ethics, the purpose in life, commitment to some higher being and belief in concepts that are not subject to "state-of-the-art "explanation".
- **Emotional dimension:** Emotional health relates to "feeling". Experts in psychology have been relatively successful in isolating these two separate dimensions. With this new data, mental and emotional aspects of humanness may have to be viewed as two separate dimensions of human' health.
- **Vocational dimension:** It is a part of human of existence. When work is fully adapted to human goals, capacities and limitations, work often plays a role in promoting both physical and mental health. Physical work is usually associated with an improvement in physical capacity, while goal achievement and self-realization in work are a source of satisfaction and enhanced self-esteem.

HEALTH DETERMINANTS

Community health influenced by various factors which interact with each other and determine the health status of many individual, family and community at large at any given point of time (**Fig. 1.5**).

Human Biology

- **Genetic inheritance:** Hereditary or genetic predisposition to specific illness is a major physical risk factor. For example, a person with a family history of diabetes mellitus is at risk for developing the disease later in life. Other documented genetic risk factors include family history of cancer, coronary disease and renal disease.
- **Age:** Age increases susceptibility to certain illness. For example, the risk of cardiovascular disease increases with age for both sexes. The risk of birth defects and complications of pregnancy increase in women bearing children after age 35. Age risk factors are often closely associated with other risk factors such as family history and personal habits.
- **Race:** Race increases susceptibility to certain illness. For example, the risk of sickle cell anemia is more common in Africans and Mediterranean people.
- **Self-concept:** Self-concept implies individual's perception of his or physical, intellectual and social abilities.

Environment

Physical environment: The physical environment includes atmospheric pressures, gravity, light and sound waves, temperature, humidity, wind velocity, solar radiation, electromagnetic fields and seasonal variations, etc. The variety of pollutants is found to pollute air, water, food and soil and is the cause of various acute and chronic diseases, e.g., gastrointestinal, respiratory, skin cancer, cardiovascular diseases, etc.

Biological environment: Most of the plants and animals are useful to human being to promote health but are the same time, they produce diseases like malaria, insect bites and allergic reactions.

Social environment: The social environments include other people and social institutions, sociocultural events, religious beliefs, moral and ethical values and social rules and regulations, pertaining to living society, socioeconomic support system.

Lifestyle: Many activities, habits and practices involve risk factors, the stress of life crisis and frequent life changes also risk factors. Health practices and behaviors can have positive or negative effects in health. Practices with potential negative effects are risk factor these include overeating or poor nutrition, insufficient rest and sleep and poor personal hygiene. Other habits that put a person at risk for illness include smoking, alcohol or drug abuse, and activities involving a threat of injury such as skydiving or mountain climbing. Prolonged emotional stress may increase the chance of illness. Emotional stress may occur with events such as divorce, pregnancy and arguments. Job-related stresses, for example, many overtax a person's cognitive skills and decision-making ability leading to mental overload or burnout.

Health and Health Allied Resources

- **Health services:** Health services are directly concerned with improvement of health status of people. Health

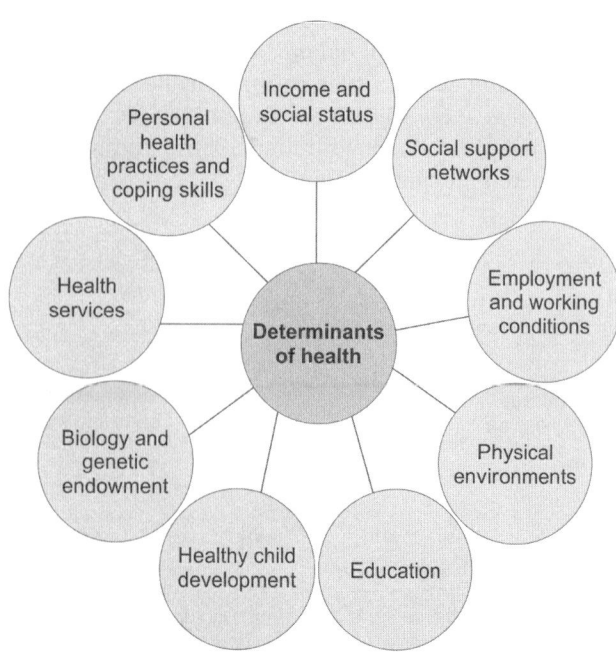

Fig. 1.5: Determinants of health.

services can also contribute on socioeconomic development of people because sound health can improve and increase the physical, intellectual and emotional capacity of people to get educated, work and earn for their livelihood improve their lifestyle which will further reinforce their health.
- **Socioeconomic conditions:** Socioeconomic conditions have significant influence on community health. In developed countries like America, UK and Canada, there has been significant reduction in the morbidity and mortality rates and increases in longevity at birth because of socioeconomic developments. Socio-economic conditions include economic status, education, occupation and living standards.
- **Political system:** The political system has a very strong role in health promotion of people in the country. The healthcare delivery system is determined by the political system though there is constitutional control. Decisions pertaining to health policy, allocation of funds, programs, manpower development, infrastructure, health technology and delivery of health services are made by the ruling party within the Parliament system.
- **Health-related services:** The health-related services include education governmental policies; social welfare developmental programs, food and agriculture, industry, communication and broadcasting rural and urban development and transportation facilities. The health-related services need to have balanced approach between National Health Policy and voluntary health promotes active participation.

INDICATORS OF HEALTH

Indicators help to measure the extent to which the objectives and targets of a program are being attained. Types of health indicators are depicted in **Figure 1.6**.

Characteristics of Indicators

- It should be **valid:** They are actually measures what they are supposed to measure.
- It should be **reliable** and objective: The answer should be the same if measured by different people in similar circumstances.
- It should be **sensitive:** They should be sensitive to changes in the situation concerned.

TYPES OF HEALTH INDICATORS
1. Mortality indicators
2. Morbidity indicators
3. Disability indicators
4. Indicators about social development
5. Healthcare delivery indicators
6. Environmental indicators
7. Health policy indicators
8. Quality of life
9. Specific issues, e.g. mental health, nutrition status, reproductive health

Fig. 1.6: Types of health indicators.

- It should be **specific:** They should reflect changes only in the situation concerned.
- It should be **feasible:** They should have the ability to obtain data need.
- It should be **relevant:** They should contribute to the understanding of the phenomenon of interest.

Uses

- To measure the health status of a country.
- To compare the health status of one country with that of another country.
- To assess the healthcare needs.
- To plan and implement healthcare services.
- To evaluate the health care services.

Since health is not defined in measurable terms and since health is multidimensional and is never static, health is measured multidimensionally, indirectly.

These indicators are classified as follows:
1. Crude death rate
2. Expectation of life
3. Maternal mortality rate
4. Infant mortality rate
5. Child mortality rate
6. Under 5 proportionate mortality rate
7. Disease specific mortality
8. Proportional mortality rate.

Mortality Indicators

S. No.	Indicators	Description
1.1	Crude death rate	It is defined as the number of deaths per 1,000 population per year in a given community. It indicates the rate at which people are dying
1.2	Expectation of life	Life expectancy at birth is the average number of years that will be lived by those born alive into population if the current age-specific mortality rates persist. Life expectancy is a good indicator of socio-economic development
1.3	Infant mortality rate	Infant mortality rate is the ratio of deaths under 1 year of age in a given year to the total number of live births in the same year; usually expressed as a rate per 1,000 live births
1.4	Child mortality rate	It is defined as the number of deaths at ages 1–4 years in a given year, per 1,000 children in that age-group at the mid-point of the year concerned
1.5	Under-5 proportionate mortality rate	It is the proportion of total deaths occurring under-5 age group. This rate can be used to reflect both infant and child mortality rates
1.6	Maternal mortality rate	Maternal mortality (puerperal) accounts for the greatest proportion of deaths among women of reproductive age in most of the developing world

Contd...

Contd...

S. No.	Indicators	Description
1.7	Disease-specific mortality	Mortality rates can be computed for specific disease as countries begin to extricate themselves from the burden of communicable diseases a number of other indicators such as deaths from cancer, cardiovascular diseases, accidents, diabetes, etc. have emerged as measures of specific disease problems.
1.8	Proportional mortality rate	The propositional mortality rate of communicable diseases means the percentage of total deaths due to communicable diseases is a useful indicator because it indicates the magnitude of preventable mortality.

Morbidity Indicators

S. No.	Indicators	Description
2.1	Incidence rate	It is the number of new cases occurring per 1,000 population in a year
2.2	Prevalence rate	It is the total number of both old and new cases existing in the population during a given period or time
2.3	Disability rate	It is the percentage of the population, unable to perform the routine expected, daily activities due to injury or illness
2.4	Sullivan's index	This is computed by subtracting the duration of bed disability (during life) from the expectation of life at birth
2.5	Health-adjusted life expectancy (HALA)	It is the number of years a newborn is expected to live in full health, based on current morbidity and mortality
2.6	Disability-adjusted life year (DALY)	It is the number of years lost in the healthy life of an individual due to disability

Other Indicators

S. No.	Indicators	Description
3.	Nutritional status indicators	Nutritional status is a positive health indicator. Three nutritional status indicators are considered important as indicators of health status. They are: ➤ Anthropometric measurements of preschool children, e.g., weight and height, mid-arm circumference; ➤ Heights (and sometimes weights) of children at school entry; and ➤ Prevalence of low birth weight (less than 2.5 kg).

Contd...

Contd...

S. No.	Indicators	Description
4.	Healthcare delivery indicators	The frequently used indicators of healthcare delivery are: ➤ Doctor—population ratio ➤ Doctor—nurse ratio ➤ Population—bed ratio ➤ Population per health/subcenter ➤ Population per traditional birth attendant These indicators reflect the equity of distribution of health. Resources in different parts of the country, and of the provision of healthcare.
5.	Indicators of social and mental health	These include the rates of crimes, assault, murder, theft, suicides, homicides, accidents, juvenile delinquency, prostitution, gambling, drug-abuse, lock-out of industries, etc. To these may be added divorces, family violence, battered baby syndrome, battered wife syndrome, etc. These indicators provide a guide to implement social action for improving the social and mental health of the people
6.	Socio-economic indicators	Socioeconomic indicators: ➤ Growth rate of the population ➤ Per capita income; Gross National Product (GNP) ➤ Percentage of people below poverty line ➤ Level of unemployment ➤ Dependency ratio ➤ Literacy rate ➤ Family size ➤ Per capita calorie availability ➤ Percentage of overcrowded houses Even though these do not directly measure the health status of a country, these are helpful in assessing the socioeconomic status of the country, which has got an impact on the health of the country
7.	Health policy indicators	These are the proportion of the budget (NGP) spent on health services and health-related services such as water supply, sanitation, nutrition, housing, community development, etc.
8.	Environmental indicators	These reflect the quality of physical and biological environment. These include the indicators relating to pollution of air, water, noise, radiation, solid waste, etc. Important ones are: ➤ Percentage of houses receiving safe water supply ➤ Percentage of houses having adequate sanitary facilities, etc.
9.	Indicator of quality of life	This is "Physical Quality of Life Index" (PQLI)—explained under "well-being" of health.'

Contd...

HEALTH–ILLNESS CONTINUUM

- According to Neuman (1990), health on a continuum is the degree of client wellness that exists at any point in time ranging from an optimal wellness condition, with available energy at its maximum, to death, which represents total energy depletion (**Fig. 1.7**).
- According to health–illness continuum model, health is a dynamic state that continuously alters as a person adapts to changes in the internal and external environments to maintain a state of physical, emotional, intellectual, social, developmental and spiritual well-being.
- The continuum is thought of a complex, dynamic process that includes physical, psychological and social components. There are adoptive or maladaptive behavioral responses to internal and external stimuli.
- Health and illness tend to merge but may represent pattern of adoptive change along the continuum. The direction of change may be reversible, depending on the quality of the individual's adoptive efforts.
- The individual at the illness end of the continuum is characterized by feeling of uncertainty, helplessness, loss of control, loss of identity and incapacity for problem solving.
- As the patient is in the sick role, there is incapacity to meet other social roles, the person has sought diagnosis and get treatment.
- Less far along the illness end of the continuum, as illness behaviors are brought into play, the person may be tired, rundown and irritable with complaints of loss of sleep, appetite, dependence, self-absorption, minor illnesses such as colds, infections, headaches and backaches.
- Between illness and wellness, there is the ambiguous area where no symptoms are present and the person is neither especially well nor especially ill.
- At the health end of the continuum, as health behaviors are utilized, the person is not only unaware of disease and without pain, fatigue or somatic complications but also tends to be resistant to infections, industrious, vigorous and physically able, with a strong sense of identity and autonomy, carrying out usual social roles and needing no healthcare.
- The goal in preventive healthcare is to maintain equilibrium between health and illness, with balance in favor of maximum wellness for the individual.

MODELS OF HEALTH AND ILLNESS

Health–Wellness Model

- It was developed by Dunn (1997), the high-level wellness model is oriented toward maximizing the health potential of an individual.
- This model requires the individual to maintain a continuum of balance and purposeful direction within the environment.
- It involves progress toward a higher level of functioning open-ended and expanding challenges to live at the fullest potential.

Agent-host-environmental Model (Fig. 1.8)

- The agent-host-environmental model of health and illness originated in the community health work of level, etc.
- According to this approach the health or illness of an individual or group depends on the dynamic relationship of the agent, host and environment.
- The agent is any internal or external factors that its presence or absence can lead to disease or illness or disease.
- The host is the person or persons who may be susceptible to a particular illness or diseases.
- The environment consists of all factors outside of the host. It includes physical environment, social environment and biological environment.

Health Belief Model (Fig. 1.9)

- Rosenstoch's (1794) and Bakerand Maiman's (1975) health belief model addresses the relationship between a person's belief and behavior.
- It provides a way of understanding and predicating how clients will behave in relation to their health and how they will comply with healthcare therapies.
- The first component in this model involves the individual's perception of susceptibility to an illness.
- The second component is the individual's perception of the seriousness of the illness. This perception is influenced and modified by demographic and sociopsychological variables, perceived threats of the illnesses, and cues to action.
- The third component: The likelihood that a person will take preventive action—is the person's perception of the benefits of taking action.

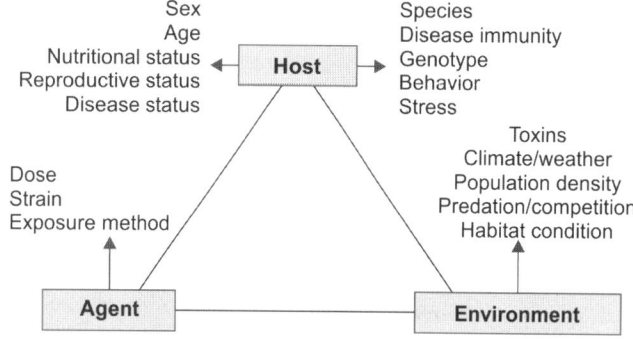

Fig. 1.8: Agent-host-environmental model.

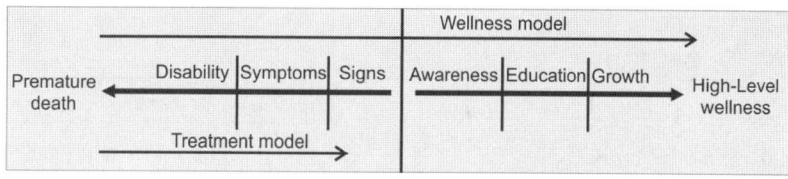

Fig. 1.7: Health–illness continuum.

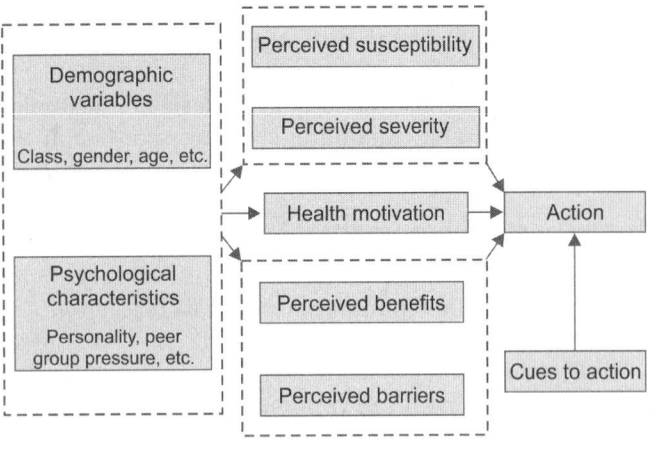

Fig. 1.9: Health belief model.

Health Promotion Model

- The health promotion model proposed by Pender (1996). It was designed to be a complementary counterpart to models of health protection (Fig. 1.10).
- Health promotion is directed at increasing a client's level of well-being. The model focuses on three functions.
- The model also organizes cues into a pattern to explain the likelihood of a client's participation in health-promotion behavior.
- The focus of this model is to explain the reasons that individuals engage in health activities. It is not designed for use with families or communities.

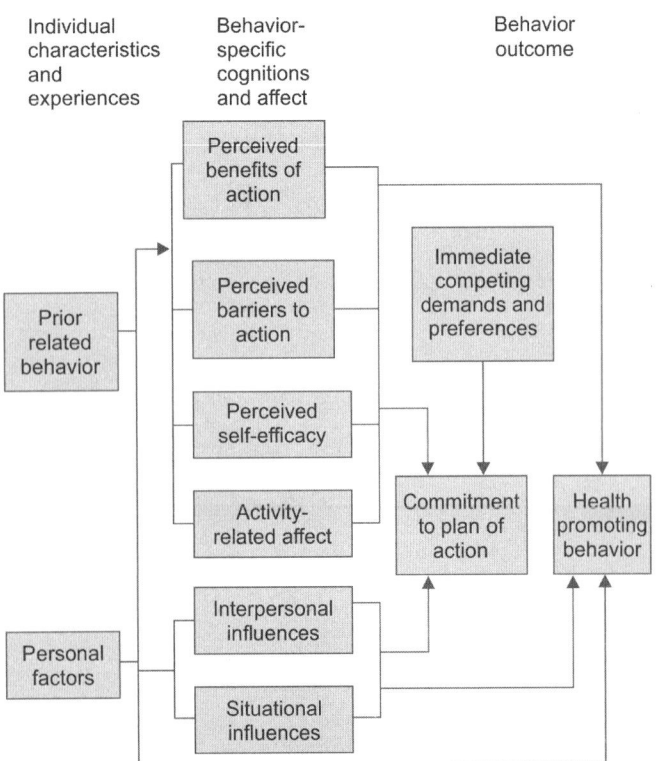

Fig. 1.10: Health promotion model.

STAGES OF ILLNESS BEHAVIOR (FIG. 1.11)

Symptom Experience

- During the initial stage, a person is aware that something is wrong. A person usually recognizes a physical sensation or a limitation in functioning but does not suspect a specific diagnosis.
- The person's perception of symptoms includes awareness of a physical change such as pain, a rash, or a lump.

Assumption of the Sick Role

- The assumption of the sick role results in emotional changes, such as withdrawal or depression, and physical changes.
- Emotional changes may be simple or complex, depending on the severity of the illness, the degree of disability and anticipated length of the illness.

Medical Care Contact

- If symptoms persist despite home remedies, become severe or require emergency care, the person is motivated to seek professional health services.
- In this stage the client seeks acknowledgment of the illness, as well as treatment. In addition, the client seeks an explanation of the symptoms, the cause of the symptoms and the course of the illness for future health.
- Client's illness can be validated at any point on the health illness continuum. A health professional may determine that they do not have an illness or that illnesses are present and may be life-threatening.

Dependent Client Role

- After accepting the illness and seeking treatment, the client enters the fourth stage of illness behavior.
- In this stage, the client depends on healthcare professionals for relief of symptoms. The client accepts care, sympathy and protection from the demands and stresses of life.

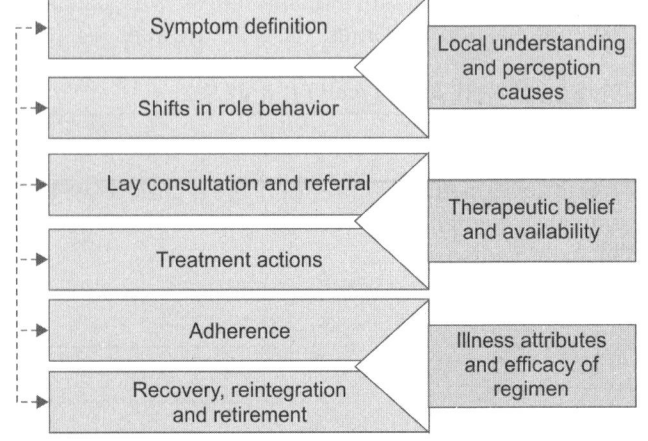

Fig. 1.11: Stages of illness behavior.

- It is socially permissible for clients in the dependent role to be relieved of normal obligations and tasks.

Recovery Stage
- The final stage of illness behavior—recovery and rehabilitation can arrive suddenly, such as a fever subsides.
- The recovery is not prompt; long-term care may be required before the client is able to resume an optimal level of functioning.
- In the case of chronic illness, the final stage may involve an adjustment to a prolonged reduction in health and functioning.

IMPACT OF ILLNESS ON FAMILY (TABLE 1.2)

Behavioral and Emotional Changes
- People react differently to illness. Individual behavioral and emotional reactions depend on the nature of the illness, the client's attitude towards it, the reaction of others to it, and the variables of illness behavior.
- Severe illness, particularly one that is life-threatening, can lead to more extensive emotional and behavioral change, such as anxiety, shock, denial, anger and withdrawal.

Impact of Family Roles
- When an illness occurs, the roles of client and family may change. Such a change may be suitable and short-term or drastic and long-term.
- An individual and family generally adjust more easily to suitable, short-term changes. In most cases they know that the role change is only temporary.
- Long-term changes, however, require an adjustment process similar to the grief process. The client and family often require specific counseling and guidance to assist them in coping with role changes.

Impact on Body Changes
- Some illnesses result in changes in physical appearance, and clients and families react differently to these changes.
- When changes in body image occur, such as results from a leg amputation, the client generally adjusts in the following phases: shock, withdrawal, acknowledgment, acceptance and rehabilitation.
- Withdrawal is an adaptive coping mechanism that can assist the client in making the adjustments.

Impact of Self-concepts
- Self-concept is individual's mental image of themselves, including how they view their strength and weaknesses in all aspects of their personalities.
- Self-concepts depend in part of body image and roles but also include other aspects of the psychological and spiritual self.
- Self-concept changes because of illness may no longer meet the expectations of the family, leading to tension or conflict.

Impact of Family Dynamics
- Family dynamics is the process by which the family functions, makes decisions, give support to individual members, and copes with everyday changes and challenges.
- If a parent in a family becomes ill, family activities and decision-making often come to a habit as the other family members wait for the illness to pass, or they delay action because they are reluctant to assume the ill person's roles or responsibilities.

LEVELS OF HEALTH CARE

Health services are usually organized at three levels, each level supported by a higher level to which the patient is referred. These levels are:

TABLE 1.2: Impact of illness on family.		
Impact	Main categories	Subcategories
Illness affects on family	Disease onset crisis	Confusion
		Disease-related tension
		Distress
	Disease burden	Finance problems
		Treatment problems
		Patient's physical and mental state
		Caregiver exhaustion
		Knowledge deficit
		Family issues
		Lack of support
	Living in the shadow of death	Disease progress and disabilities
		Fear of patient's death
		Waiting for patients death

S. No.	Levels of health care	Description
1.	Primary health care	➢ This is the first level of contact between the individual and the health system where essential healthcare (primary health care) is provided. ➢ A majority of prevailing health complaints and problems can be satisfactorily dealt with at this level. ➢ This level of care is provided by the primary health centers and their subcenters, with community participation.
2.	Secondary health prevention	➢ At this level, more complex problems are dealt with. ➢ This care comprises essentially curative services and provided by the district hospitals and community health centers. ➢ This level serves as the first referral level in the health system.
3.	Tertiary health care	➢ This level offers super specialty care. ➢ This care is provided by the regional/central level institutions.

LEVELS OF ILLNESS PREVENTION

The disease process, in many instances' is susceptible to interruption in order to limit its further progress or the speed of its progression. As disease involves interaction of host, agent and environment prevention can be achieved by altering one or more of these three elements so that interaction does not take place or is interrupted in favor of the host.

Effective preventive measure requires that the disease process be interrupted as early in its course as possible. The interaction between the agent and the host can be avoided either by the elimination of the agent in the environment or by converting the human host susceptible or immune to the attack of the agent. Those attempts to bring about changes in the three elements before the disease stimulus is produced are grouped under one type of prevention namely primary prevention. When the disease stimulus has already been practiced and the disease process has crossed over to the period of pathogenesis two types of prevention, namely secondary and tertiary prevention **(Table 1.3)**.

- **Primary prevention**: Primary prevention can be defined as "action taken prior to the onset of disease which removes the possibility that a disease will ever occur". It signifies intervention in the prepathogenesis phase of a disease or health problem or other departure from health. Primary prevention is applied at the prepathogenic period; it includes health promotion and specific protection.
    - *Health promotion:* The first level of prevention is by promoting and maintaining the health of the host by nutrition, health education, good heredity and other health promotion activities.
    - *Specific protection:* It may be directed towards the agent like disinfection of contaminated particles, materials, water, food, and other particles on the assumption that the agent has escaped into these vehicles or environment. Specific protection can also be achieved by immunizations to increase the resistance of the host so that the host will be able to withstand the onslaught of the agent. This is done by the active and passive immunizations.
- **Secondary prevention**: Secondary prevention can be defined as "action" which halts the progress of a disease at its incipient stage and prevents complications. The specific interventions are early diagnosis, e.g., screening tests, case finding programs and adequate treatment. The secondary prevention done by early diagnosis and treatment. Early diagnosis and prompt treatment comes under secondary prevention. If primary prevention fails or when suitable measures are not available (as in cancer) the disease stimulus is bound to be produced. Early detection of the disease is possible by periodic examinations of population groups who are at special risks like antenatal mothers, growing children, industrial worker, etc.

    Monitoring of persons middle age and above is one of the modern methods of early detection of cancer. In many instances, this detection of the diseases condition is possible only after the onset of the signs and symptoms. Early detection of the disease ensures prompt treatment so that the disease will not progress further.
- **Tertiary prevention:** When the disease process has advance beyond its early stages, it is still possible to accomplish prevention by what might be called "Tertiary prevention". It signifies intervention in the late pathogenesis phase. Tertiary prevention can be defined as "all measures available to reduce or limit impairment and disabilities, minimize suffering caused by existing departures and disabilities, minimize suffering caused by existing departures from good health and to promote the patient's adjustments to irremediable conditions". Tertiary prevention includes disability limitation and rehabilitation.
    - *Disability limitation:* It is necessary that the disability that is caused by limited by active medical or surgical treatment so that there is no further deterioration of the disease process.
    - *Rehabilitation:* Those with permanent disability as in the case of leprosy, tuberculosis, polio, mental retardation, etc. will not be able to lead an independent life unless they are rehabilitated. This level will be needed only when have failed in the application of previous levels of prevention.

PRIMARY HEALTH CARE: ELEMENTS AND PRINCIPLES, NURSES ROLE IN PRIMARY HEALTH CARE

Definition

Primary health care is essential healthcare made universally accessible to individuals and families in the community, by means acceptable to them, through their full participation and at a cost that the community and country can afford. It forms an integral part both of the country's health system of

TABLE 1.3: Levels of prevention.

	Primary prevention	*Secondary prevention*	*Tertiary prevention*
Definition	An intervention implemented before there is evidence of a disease or injury	An intervention implemented after a disease has begun, but before it is symptomatic	An intervention implemented after a disease or injury is established
Intent	Reduce or eliminate causative risk factors (risk reduction)	Early identification (through screening) and treatment	Prevent sequelae (stop bad things from getting worse)
Example	Encourage exercise and healthy eating to prevent individuals from becoming overweight	Check body mass index (BMI) at every well checkup to identify individuals who are overweight or obese	Help obese individuals lose weight to prevent progression to more severe consequences

Chapter 1: Introduction to Community Health

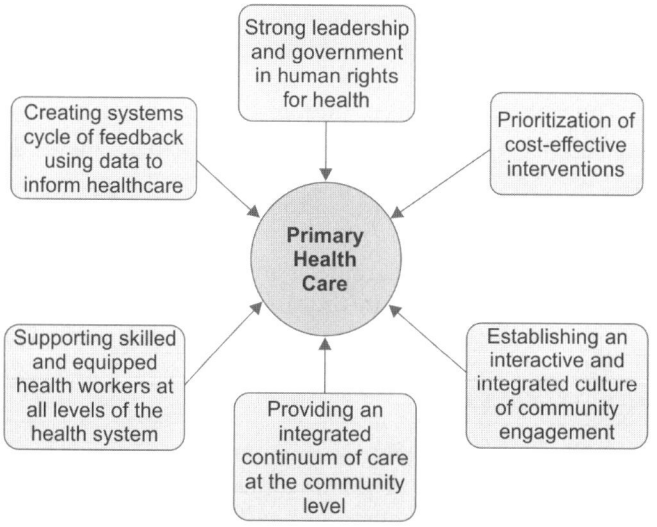

Fig. 1.12: Concept of primary health care.

which it is the nucleus and the overall social and economic development of the community (**Fig. 1.12**).

Highlights of this Definition

This definition highlights several attributes of primary health care. It stresses on:

- Its essentiality by observing that primary health is essential healthcare.
- Its '**accessibility**' by observing "made universally accessible to individuals and families in the community".
- Its '**acceptability**' by observing by means acceptable to them.
- Its '**patricianly**' by observing "acts a cost that the community and country can afford".
- Its '**affordability**' by observing "it forms an integral part both of the country's health system of which it is the nucleus and the overall social and economic development of the community".
- Its integrality by observing "it forms an integral part both of the country's health system of which it is the nucleus and the overall social and economic development of the community". Levels of care at community depicted in **Figure 1.13**.

```
                    ▲
         ┌──────────────────────────┐
         │       Acute Care         │
         │ Abrupt and/or severe alteration of bodily function │
         │ Unstable clinical signs (would include vital signs) │
         │ Closely supervised and monitored medical intervention │
         ├──────────────────────────┤
         │    Primary Health Care   │
         │ Unstable control of clinical conditions but vital signs and general condition fairly stable │
         │ Atypical clinical presentation of underlying health problems │
         │ Medical treatment under guidance and instruction │
         ├──────────────────────────┤
         │  Home/Work Environment   │
         │ Abnormal clinical parameters with no obvious signs and symptoms │
         │ Bodily signs and symptoms but might not seek help and/or not sure where and when to seek help │
         │ Barrier in compliance to medical treatment and advice │
         └──────────────────────────┘
```

Fig. 1.13: Levels of care at community.

Attributes of Primary Health Care

- **Accessibility:** Primary health care permeates uniformly to reach equitably to all segments of population.
- **Acceptability:** Primary health care achieves acceptability through cultural assimilation of its policies and programs.
- **Adaptability:** Primary health care system is highly flexible and adaptable. It believes in "adaptation" rather than "adoption".
- **Affordability:** Primary health care is affordable to consumer as well as providers.
- **Availability:** Primary health care is always ready to respond to any demand at any time.
- **Appropriateness:** Primary health care system evolves from the socioeconomic conditions, social values and health situation of a community, it is quite appropriate from all angles.
- **Closeness:** Primary health center is close at hand to people at their doorsteps.
- **Continuity:** Primary health service is a continuous service which extends from "womb" to tomb and addresses the changing needs of an individual in all situations of health and disease.
- **Comprehensiveness:** Primary health care is comprehensive and the curative needs of the community.
- **Coordinativeness:** Primary healthcare is dependent on inner-sectoral coordination and community participation.

Elements of Primary Health Care (Fig. 1.14)

As per Alma-Ata declaration primary health care includes:

- Education concerning prevailing health problems and methods of identifying, preventing and controlling them.
- Promotion of food supply and proper nutrition.
- An adequate supply of water and basic sanitation.
- Maternal and child healthcare including family planning.
- Immunization against the major infectious disease.
- Prevention and control of locally endemic diseases.
- Appropriate treatment of common diseases and injuries.
- Promotion of mental health.
- Provision of essential drugs.

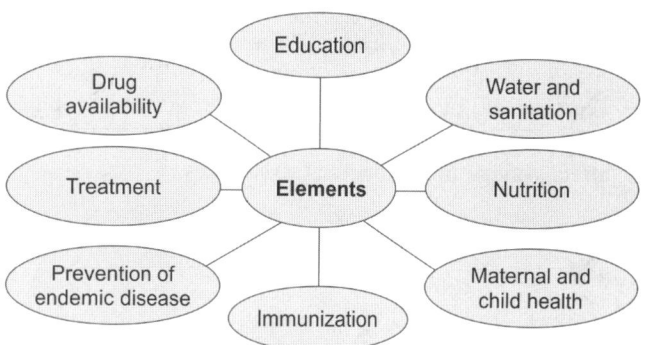

Fig. 1.14: Elements of primary health care.

TABLE 1.4: Principles of primary health care.

➢ Promote equity and human rights in healthcare
➢ Display biopsychosocial and cultural sensitivity towards the patient
➢ Practice health promotion at the individual and population level
➢ Promote evidence-based healthcare
➢ Treat patients at the appropriate level of care
➢ Promote multiprofessional healthcare
➢ Promote broad intersectoral collaboration
➢ Encourage communities to assert their rights and interests
➢ Monitor and evaluate the efficacy, efficiency and equity of health services

Principles of Primary Health Care (Table 1.4)

- **Equitable distribution:** Primary healthcare services must be shared equally by all people irrespective of their ability to pay (rich, poor, urban or rural).
- **Community participation:** Primary health care must be a continuing effort to secure meaningful involvement of the community in the planning, implementation and maintenance of health services.
- **Coverage and accessibility:** Primary healthcare implies providing healthcare services to all which are required by them. The care has to be appropriate and adequate in content and in amount to satisfy the essential health needs of the people and has to be provided by methods acceptable to them.
- **Intersectoral coordination:** Primary health care requires joint efforts of other health-related sectors such as agriculture, animal husbandry, food, industry, housing, social welfare, public works, communication and other sectors.
- **Appropriate health technology:** The technology that is scientific, adaptable to local need and socially acceptable instead of costly methods, equipment and technology.
- **Human resource:** Health resource is very essential to make full use of all the available resources including the human potential of the entire community.
- **Referral system:** Referral system would be desirable to develop referring from one level to another with laid down procedures and policies.
- **Logistics of supply:** The logistic of supply includes planning and budgeting for the supplies required procurement or manufacture, storage distribution and control.
- **Physical facilities:** The physical facilities for primary healthcare need to be simple and clean. It should have a specious waiting area with toilet facility.
- **Control and evaluation:** A process of evaluation has to be built in to assess the relevance, progress, efficiency, effectiveness and impact of the services.

Role of Community Health Nurse in Primary Health Care

An extent committee on community health nursing was concerned by WHO executive board in July 1974 to recommend way in which nursing could have critical impact on the urgent health problems throughout the world. Functions of primary health care are depicted in **Figure 1.15**. The committee made specific recommendations.

- The development of community health nursing services, responsive to community health needs that would assure primary healthcare coverage for all.
- The reformulation of basic and post-basic nursing education as to prepare all nurses for community health nursing.
- The inclusion of nursing in national development plans in a way that would ensure the rational distribution and the appropriate utilization and support of nursing personnel.

HEALTH FOR ALL

- Health for all, it means that resources for health are evenly distributed and that essential health care is accessible to everyone. It means that health begins at home, in schools, and at the workplace, and that people use better approaches for preventing illness and alleviating unavoidable disease and disability.
- Attainment of a level of health that will enable every individual to lead a socially and economically productive life. Role of CHN are depicted in **Figure 1.16**.

Goals

- Realization of highest possible of health which includes physical, mental and social well-being.
- Attainment of minimum level of health that would enable to the economically productive and participate actively in social life of community in which they live.
- Removal of obstacles to health such as unemployment, ignorance, poor living conditions, standards and malnutrition, etc.
- Healthcare services are within the reach of all in the country.

Strategies for Health for All

The Alma-Ata declaration called for global strategy to provide guidelines for member countries to refer. In 1981,

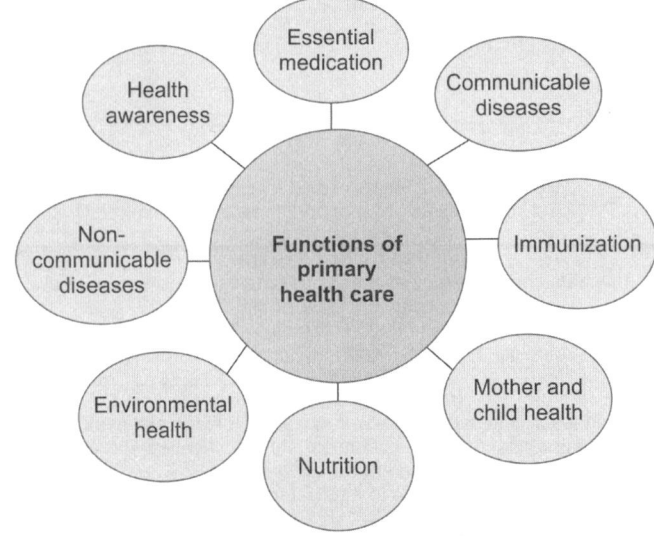

Fig. 1.15: Functions of primary health care.

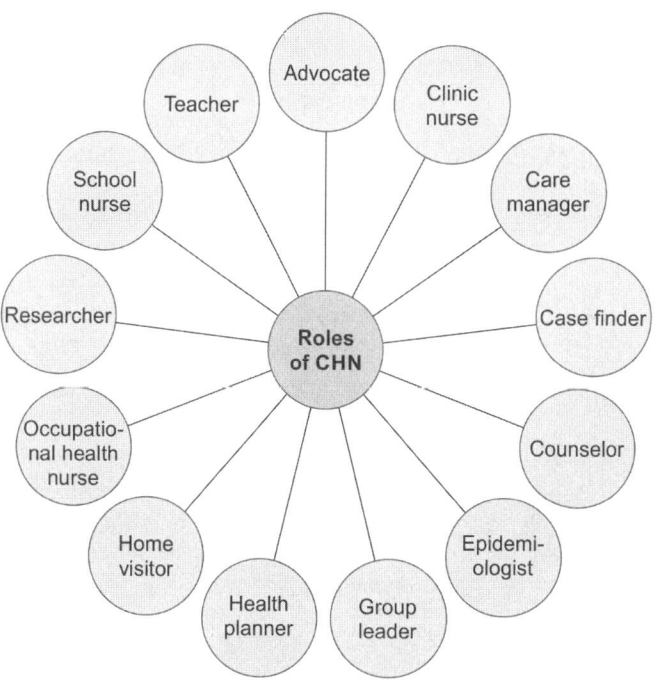

Fig. 1.16: Role of CHN.

the WHO after consultations with member countries developed a global strategy for health for all. The global strategy provides common broad framework which can be modified and adopted by countries according to their needs. The global strategy for HFA is based on the following principles **(Fig. 1.17)**:

- Health is a fundamental human right and a worldwide social goal and an integral part of social and economic development of the communities.
- People have right and the duty of participate individually and collectively in the planning and implementation of their healthcare.
- The existing gross inequality in the health strategies is of common concern of all countries and must be drastically reduced.
- Government has responsibility for the health of their people.
- Countries and people must become self-reliant in health matters.
- Governments and health professionals have the responsibility of providing health information to people.
- There should be equitable distribution of resources within and among the countries but should be allocated most to those who need most.
- Primary healthcare would be the key to the success of HPA and it has to be the integral part of the country's health system.
- Development and application of appropriate technology according to healthcare system of the nation.
- Research in the field of biomedical and health services must be conducted and findings should been applied soon.
- Reduction of infant mortality from the level of 125 (1978) to below 60.
- To raise the expectation of life at birth from the level of 523 years to 64.
- To reduce the crude death rate from the level of 14 per 1,000 population to 21.
- To reduce the crude birth rate from the level of 33 per 1,000 population to 21.
- To achieve a net reproduction rate of one rural population.

MILLENNIUM DEVELOPMENT GOALS

The United Nations Millennium Development Goals (MDGs) are 8 goals that UN Member States have agreed to try to achieve by the year 2015. The United Nations Millennium Declaration, signed in September 2000, commits world leaders to combat poverty, hunger, disease, illiteracy, environmental degradation, and discrimination against women. The MDGs are derived from this Declaration. Each MDG has targets set for 2015 and indicators to monitor progress from 1990 levels. Several of these relate directly to health are depicted in **Figure 1.18**.

Eradicate Extreme Poverty and Hunger

- Reduce by half the proportion of people whose income is less than $1 a day.
- Achieve full and productive employment and decent work for all, including women and young people.
- Reduce by half the proportion of people who suffer from hunger.

Achieve Universal Primary Education

Ensure that all boys and girls complete a full course of primary schooling.

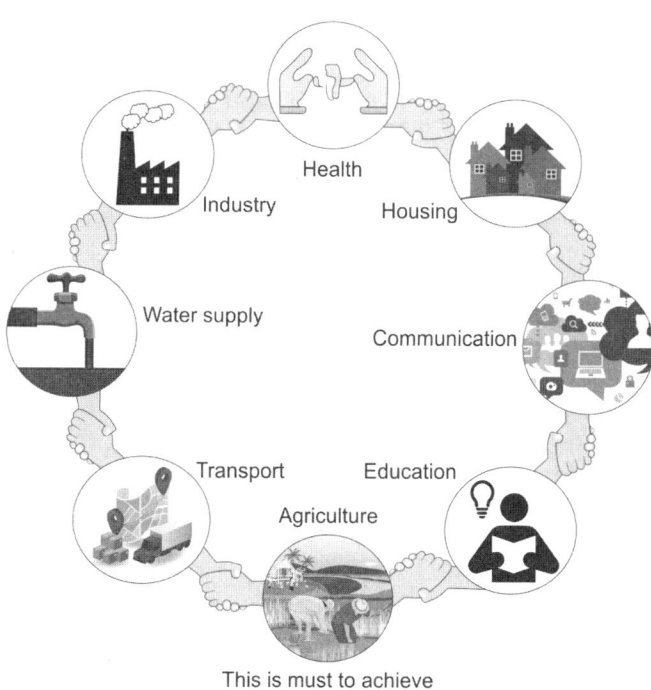

Fig. 1.17: Concept of health for all.

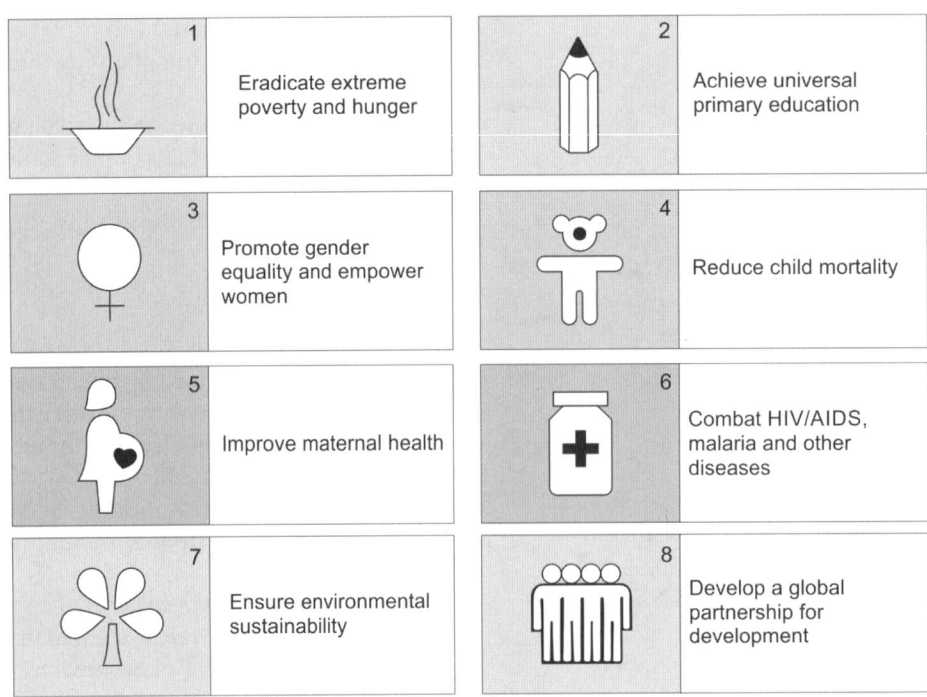

Fig. 1.18: Millennium development goals (MDGs).

Promote Gender Equality and Empower Women

Eliminate gender disparity in primary and secondary education preferably by 2005, and in all levels of education no later than 2015.

Reduce Child Mortality

Reduce by two thirds the mortality of children under five.

Improve Maternal Health

- Reduce maternal mortality by three quarters.
- Achieve universal access to reproductive health.

Combat HIV/AIDS, Malaria and Other Diseases

- Halt and reverse the spread of HIV/AIDS.
- Achieve, by 2010, universal access to treatment for HIV/AIDS for all those who need it.
- Halt and reverse the incidence of malaria and other major diseases.

Ensure Environmental Sustainability

- Integrate principles of sustainable development into country policies and programs; reverse the loss of environmental resources.
- Reduce biodiversity loss, a significant reduction in the rate of loss.
- Halve the proportion of people without access to safe drinking water and basic sanitation.
- Improve the lives of at least 100 million slum dwellers by 2020.

Develop a Global Partnership for Development

- Develop further an open, rule-based, predictable, non-discriminatory trading and financial system.
- Address special needs of the least developed countries, landlocked countries and small island developing states.
- Deal comprehensively with developing countries' debt.
- In cooperation with pharmaceutical companies, provide access to affordable essential drugs in developing countries.
- In cooperation with the private sector, make available the benefits of new technologies, especially information and communications technologies.

PROMOTION AND MAINTENANCE OF HEALTH

Health promotion refers to activities that increase well-being and enhance wellness or health. These activities lead to actualization of positive health potential for all individuals, even those with chronic or acute conditions. Examples include providing information and resources in order to:

- Enhance nutrition at each developmental stage
- Integrate physical activity into the child's daily events
- Provide adequate housing
- Promote oral health
- Foster positive personality development

Health promotion is concerned with developing sets of strategies that seek to foster conditions that allow populations to be healthy and to make healthy choices (World Health Organization, 2001). Health promotion strategies are depicted in **Figure 1.19**. and choices in health promotion are depicted in **Figure 1.20**.

Health maintenance (or health protection) refers to activities that preserve an individual's present state of health

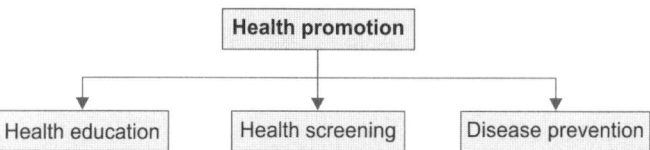

Fig. 1.19: Health promotion strategies.

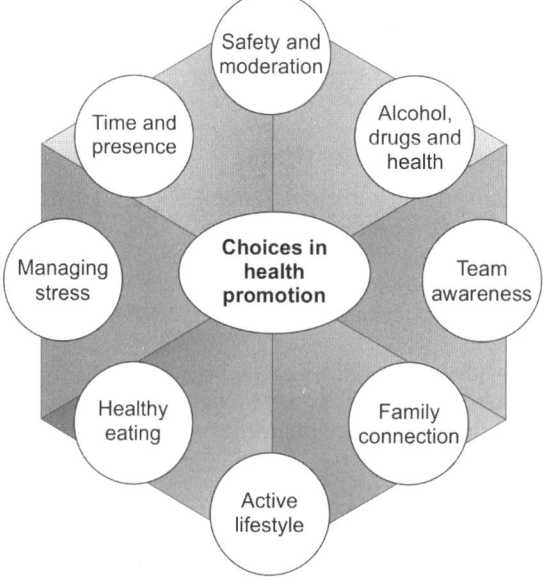

Fig. 1.20: Choices in health promotion.

and that prevent disease or injury occurrence. Examples of these activities include developmental screening or surveillance to identify early deviations from normal development, providing immunizations to prevent illnesses, and teaching about common childhood safety hazards.

Health promotion and health maintenance activities are closely linked and often overlap, but there are some differences. Health maintenance focuses on known potential health risks and seeks to prevent them, or identify them early so that intervention can occur. Health promotion looks at the strengths and goals of individuals, families, and populations, and seeks to use them to assist in reaching higher levels of wellness.

Components of Health Promotion/Health Maintenance

- **Growth and developmental surveillance in schools:** Growth and developmental surveillance provide important clues about the child's condition and environment. Evaluation of growth, child height, weight, and body mass index should be calculated at each health supervision visit. Parents should be given the information in written form and interpreted for them. Physical assessment is performed to be sure the child is growing as expected and has no abnormal or unexplained physical findings.
- **Nutrition:** Nutrition is a vital part of each health supervision visit. It makes important contributions to general health and fosters growth and development. Include observations and screening relevant to nutritional intake at each health supervision visit.
- **Physical activity:** Physical activity provides many physical and psychological health benefits. However, there is growing disparity between recommendations and reality among most of our children.
- **Oral health:** While oral health may seem to require the knowledge of a specialist, many implications relate to general healthcare. Oral health is important because teeth assist in language development, impacted or infected teeth lead to systemic illness, and teeth are related to positive self-image formation.
- **Eye and vision:** Eye exams for children are extremely important, because 5–10 percent of preschoolers and 25 percent of school-aged children have vision problems. Early identification of a child's vision problem can be crucial because children often are more responsive to treatment when problems are diagnosed early.
- **Mental and spiritual health:** Mental and spiritual health is important concepts to address in health promotion and health maintenance visits. Parents can be encouraged to keep a record of mental health issues to bring to health supervision visits. This helps them understand that the healthcare professional is willing to partner with them to assist in dealing with mental health.

Disease Prevention Strategies

Disease prevention strategies focus mainly on health maintenance, or prevention of disease. Some health disruptions can be detected early and treatment for the condition can begin. Screening is a procedure used to detect the possible presence of a health condition before symptoms are apparent. It is usually conducted on large groups of individuals at risk for a condition and represents the secondary level of prevention.

Vaccination

Like eating well and exercising, immunization is a foundation for a healthy life. Getting vaccinated is a safe and necessary part of keeping you and your family healthy. Vaccinations are incredibly important, because immunization does not just protect you; it also protects everyone around you.

Encourage Health Promotion Activities

Families often need health education and counseling to promote healthy behaviors in their own child. Examples of focused health education and counseling may be information about environmental control to limit sedentary behaviors, dietary changes to increase fruit and vegetable intake, and switching to low-fat dairy products. Patient education and counseling are most effective when the family understands the relationship between a behavior change and the resulting health outcome.

Steps in promoting patient education and counseling include:
- Clarifying learning needs of child and family
- Setting a limited agenda
- Prioritizing needs with family
- Selecting teaching strategy (explaining, showing, providing resources, questioning, practicing, giving feedback)
- Evaluating effectiveness

Periodic health check-up: Periodic health check-ups and screenings with healthcare provider are key to maximizing the chance of living a longer and healthier life. Not only can they help prevent health problems before they start, but regular check-ups may also help discover health problems early enough to increase chances of successful treatment and recovery.

CONCLUSION

One of the two major goals of healthy people is to help individuals of all ages increase life expectancy and improve their quality of life. The concepts of health promotion and health maintenance provide interventions that contribute to meeting this goal. Many students in health professions begin their studies with a strong interest in care of ill individuals. Healthcare management is a holistic profession that examines and works with all aspects of individuals' lives, and has a strong focus on family and community as well. Therefore, it should be uniquely positioned to provide health promotion and health maintenance activities. In fact, these activities should be a part of each encounter with families.

REVIEW QUESTIONS

Long Essays

1. Explain the concept of health and disease in detail.
2. Describe the history and development of community health in India and its present concept.
3. Define primary health care. Explain the elements, principles and nurse's role in primary health care.

Short Essays

1. Causes and risk factors for developing illness.
2. Dimensions of health.
3. Health determinants.
4. Mortality and morbidity indicators.
5. Describe health–illness continuum.
6. Enumerate the stages of illness behavior.
7. Discuss the levels of health care.
8. Impact of illness on family.
9. Levels of illness prevention.
10. Principles of primary health care.
11. Promotion and maintenance of health.

Short Answers

1. Define community health.
2. Define community health nursing.
3. Genetic inheritance.
4. Types of indicators of health.
5. Agent-host-environmental model.
6. Tertiary prevention.
7. Disability limitation.
8. Rehabilitation.
9. Health belief model.
10. Health promotion model.
11. Attributes of primary health care.
12. Elements of primary health care.
13. Health for all goals.
14. Vaccination.

Multiple Choice Questions

1. The term 'health' is defined in many ways. The most accurate definition of the health would be:
    a. Health is the state of body and mind in a balanced condition
    b. Health is the reflection of a smiling face
    c. Health is a state of complete physical, mental and social well-being
    d. Health is the symbol of economic prosperity
2. Community health influenced by various factors which interact with each other and determine the health status of:
    a. Individual
    b. Family
    c. Community
    d. All of the above
3. Health–Wellness Model was developed by Dunn in the year:
    a. 1996 b. 1997
    c. 1998 d. 1999
4. Principles of primary health care include all, *except*:
    a. Community leadership
    b. Equitable distribution
    c. Community participation
    d. Coverage and accessibility.
5. Disease prevention strategies focus mainly on:
    a. Health maintenance
    b. Prevention of disease
    c. All of the above
    d. None of the above
6. A Central Advisory Board of Health was setup in:
    a. 1936 b. 1937
    c. 1938 d. 1939
7. National Institute for Communicable Diseases (NICD) was established in Delhi:
    a. 1959
    b. 1961
    c. 1963
    d. 1966
8. Pulse polio immunization was initiated in the year:
    a. 1994 b. 1995
    c. 1996 d. 1997

ANSWERS

| 1. c | 2. a | 3. b | 4. a | 5. c | 6. b | 7. c | 8. c | | | |

2. Community Health Nursing

LEARNING OBJECTIVES
1. Philosophy, goals, objectives and principles, concept and importance of community health nursing
2. Qualities and functions of community health nurse
3. Steps of nursing process; community identification, population composition, health and allied resources, community assessment, planning and conducting community nursing care services

TERMINOLOGY

Nursing process: Nursing process is an orderly, systematic manner of determining the patient's problems, making plans to solve them, initiating the plan or assigning others to implement it, and evaluating the extent to which the plan was effective in resolving the problems identified.

Nursing diagnosis: Nursing diagnosis is a clinical judgment about individual, family or community responses to actual or potential health problems or life process. Nursing diagnosis provides the basis for selection of nursing interventions to achieve outcomes for which the nurse is accountable.

Nursing care plan: It is a structure which provides clear picture about the problem, reason, objectives, methods and action and evaluation for nurses to render prompt services to the patients.

Implementation: It is a process of implementing the interventions to ensure continuity of effective care to prevent, correct or reduce identified risks and to return the patient to the highest level of wellness attainable.

Evaluation: It is essential to permit the nurse to modify the plan of care and develop new interventions and patient education activities.

Functional nursing: It is a method of providing patient care where each licensed and unlicensed staff members provide a specific task for a longer group of patients.

Validating: Validating is an ongoing process that occurs during the data collection phase and on its completion when the data are reviewed and compared.

Objectives: Objectives or goals are stated in terms of anticipated patient outcomes. The goals must be realistic in terms of patients' potentials and nursing ability. They should be as specific as possible for a particular patient.

Community health nursing process: It is a systematic, rational method and providing nursing care for the prevention of disease and promotion of health of the community.

Planning: It involves the development of strategies designed to prevent, minimize or correct the problems identified in the nursing diagnosis. It sets the priorities for nursing action.

INTRODUCTION

The community is responsible for providing all facilities and total care to all. Such changes have led to the placement of the term public health with community health. Hence, "Community Health" encompasses all those processes of prevention of disease, promotion and protection of health of all people.

Community health nursing implies making systematic assessment and diagnosis of health status of people and their problems, planning and implementing comprehensive health care services **(Fig. 2.1)** for the entire community with their active co-operation and participation. In community health nursing, the major emphasis is laid on primary level prevention through community approaches.

DEFINITIONS

- It is a synthesis of nursing and public health practice applied to promoting and preserving the health of the people.

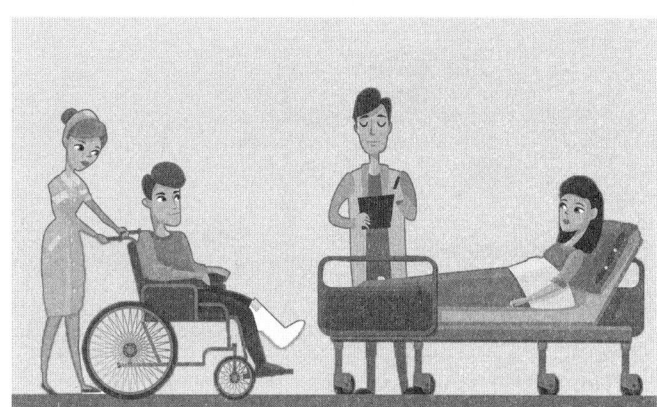

Fig. 2.1: Community health services.

- Community health nursing defined as "Community health refers to the health status of the members of the community, to the problem affecting their health and to the totality of healthcare provided to the community".
- Community health nursing is defined as nursing services organized by a community or agency to carry out nursing aspects of community health program in the homes, schools, industries or in the health centers.

CONCEPT OF COMMUNITY HEALTH NURSING

The community health nursing implies sound preparation of community health personnel so that they are knowledgeable and skillful. They need to acquire knowledge about community's structure, community dynamics, community approaches, population statistics, and community health indicators, epidemiological aspects of health problems, health planning, administration and delivery system. The Community health demands are placed on the nurse and the nursing profession as a result of changes in society, especially changes in modern technology. Social consciousness and the quality, type and financing of health care. Emphasis has shifted from acute hospital, based care to preventive community health care. All changes that affect the healthcare delivery system affect nursing.

PHILOSOPHY OF COMMUNITY HEALTH NURSING (FIG. 2.2)

Nursing contributes to the health services in a vital and significant way in the healthcare delivery system. It recognizes national health goals and is committed to participate in the implementation of National Health Policies and Programmes. It aims at identifying health needs of the people, planning and providing quality care in collaboration with other health professional and community groups.
- The essential dignity and worth of the individual.
- The right of an individual for basic necessities.
- The right of the individual to help in times of need and crisis.
- The great capacity for growth within all social beings.
- The possession by individuals of potentialities and resources for managing their own lives.
- The need for individuals to struggle and strive to improve their life and environment.
- The importance of freedom to express one's individuality.

OBJECTIVES OF COMMUNITY HEALTH NURSING

Nursing seeks to help people understand the importance of all segments of their life and the environment to their well-being. Nursing uses scientific knowledge to perform activities to prevent illness and to help those with health problems to regain vigor and joy of living. Social change taking place in the community must be considered in planning health care (Fig. 2.3).

The objectives of community health nursing are:
- Provide antenatal, intranatal and postnatal care to ensure safe pregnancy and delivery
- Immunization
- Provide under five children care
- Health education
- To improve the ability of the community to deal with their own health problems
- To strengthen the community resources
- To prevent and control communicable and non-communicable diseases
- To provide specialized services
- To conduct research

Nurses are key persons in providing healthcare in our changing society. Health education has for a long time been considered a major nursing responsibility. That responsibility is increasing with our social trends. Because nurses live in the community and have their own families, they are accessible to the people of the community. They are often called for help in emergencies or to give advice.

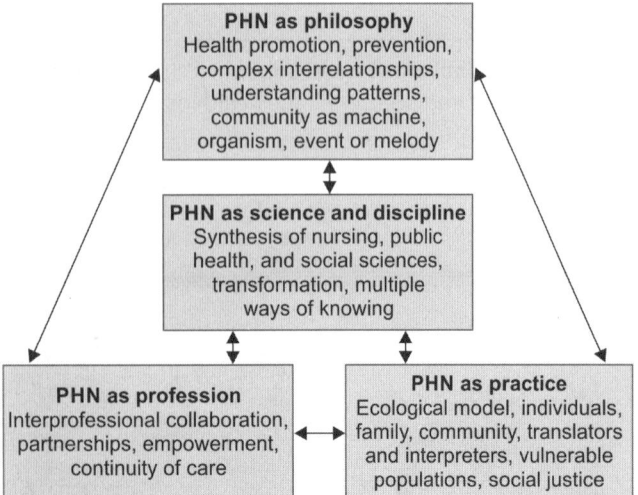

Fig. 2.2: Philosophical application in community practice.

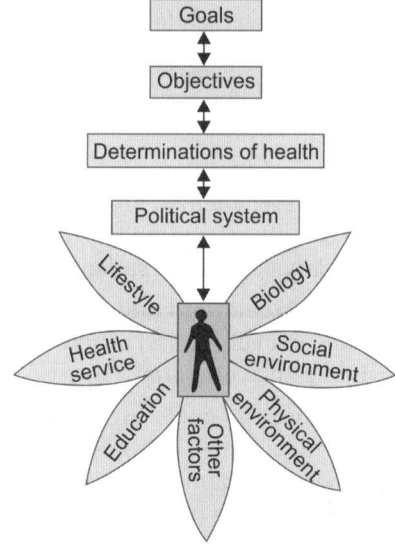

Fig. 2.3: Goals and objectives of community health nursing.

GOALS OF COMMUNITY HEALTH NURSING

- To increase the capacity of families, groups and communities to cope with health and illness problems.
- To support and supplement the efforts of other professional restoration and preservation of health.
- To control or counteract as much as possible physical and social environmental conditions that threaten health or decrease the enjoyment of life.
- To contribute to the reinforcement and improvement of nursing practice and public health practice and service.

PRINCIPLES OF COMMUNITY HEALTH NURSING (FIG. 2.4)

The following are some main principles which may be used to guide for the community health nurse:

- Effective health workers, irrespective of position or place of work, function as a team.
- The community nurse should be a qualified person by a recognized school or college.
- Health services should be based on the felt need of an individual family and community.
- Health services should be made available to all people, irrespective of their stage, sex and status.
- Community health nurses are accountable/responsible authorized health authority for her services.
- Health services should be realistic in terms of available personnel and facilities.
- Professional relationship and etiquette are essential in community health services.
- Community health nurse must be a nonpolitical and non-sectarian in her relationship with people.
- Evaluation and follow-up services is an important aspect in community health programs.
- Facilities for further training and continuing education should be provided by the health authority.
- Community health nurse should organize a periodical in-service education programs.

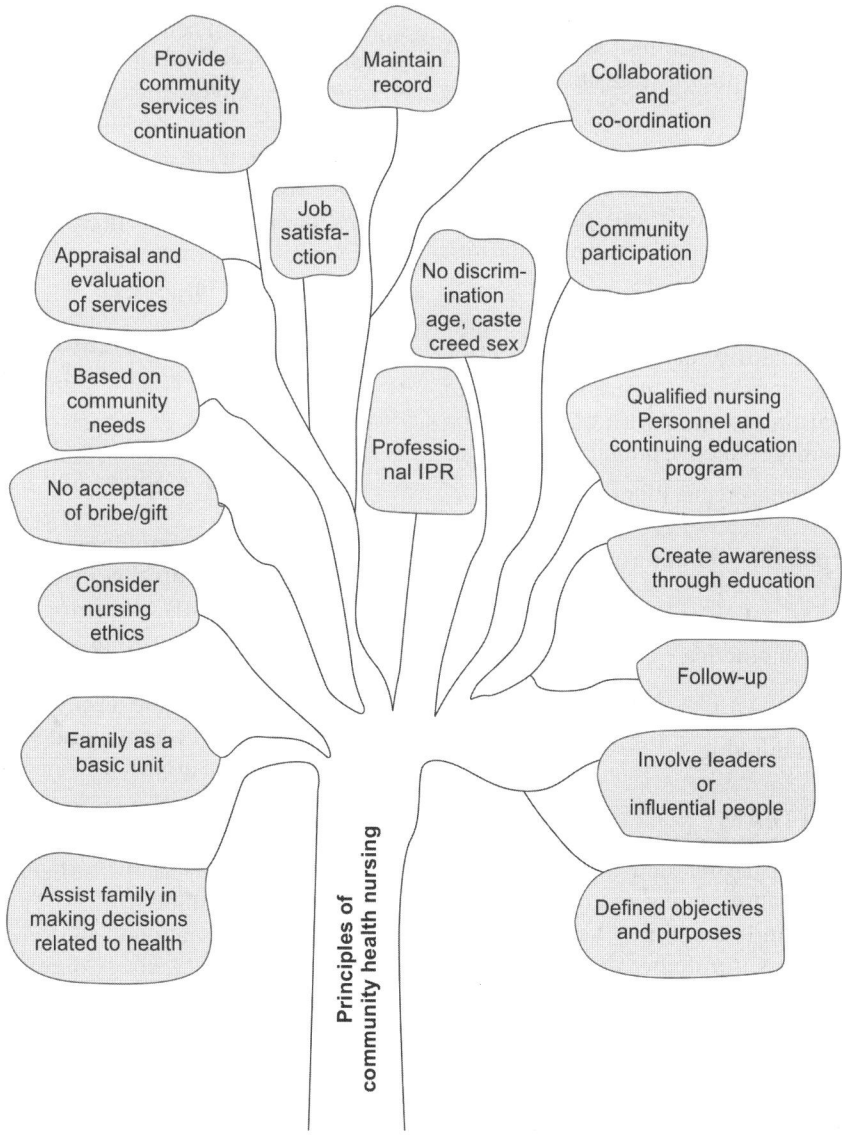

Fig. 2.4: Principles of community health nursing.

- Community health nurse should organize and lead a team effectively and efficiently to provide best service to the community.
- The family and community are the units of work. There should be adequate and accurate baseline data of the community essentially.
- Supervision and guidance are needed to help the worker to produce a high quality of work.
- Records and reports are essential in community health services.
- The community health nurse should prepare updated records and reports and sent to their higher level promptly.
- The public health worker must never accept gifts or bribes.
- Professional interest should be developed and maintained.
- Job condition should be conductive to optimum satisfaction.

SKILLS OF COMMUNITY HEALTH NURSE

Adaptability: Nurses must be able to adapt quickly to their surroundings and think on their feet. The day-to-day activities can vary greatly—one day you may be providing vaccinations to schoolchildren and the next day leading a seminar about malnutrition—so being able to smoothly transition between different tasks is key.

Ability to travel: Depending on the community, there can be significant travel involved to reach area residents. In particular, travel to rural, isolated or underserved areas may be common. You may also need to arrange visits with organizations in surrounding communities.

Focus on teamwork: While public health nurses may work independently, the majority of their work involves other healthcare entities, community organizations and government leaders. Learning to work with others for the greater good makes you a more effective public health nurse.

Other essential skills of community health nursing:
- Analysis/assessment
- Policy development/program planning
- Communication
- Cultural competency
- Community dimension of practice
- Public health sciences
- Financial planning and management
- Leadership and systems thinking

COMMUNITY HEALTH TEAM

Community health nursing is concerned with the people who are sick as well as the healthy, young and old, male and female. Community health and community health nursing draw knowledge and practices from other disciplines such as medicine, surgery, pediatrics, obstetrics, gynecology, dentistry, health education and vital statistics.

The community center may refer a patient directly to the state level hospital or the nearest medical college hospital. The community health center has the following staffs and collectively called community health team **(Fig. 2.5)**.

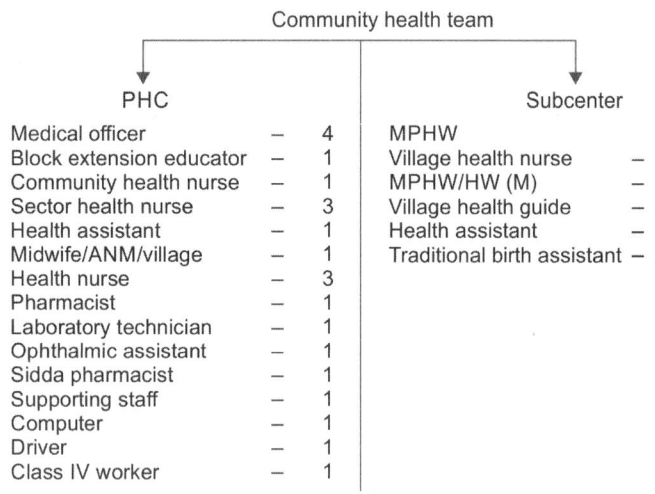

Fig. 2.5: Staffing pattern of community health center.

Functions of Community Health Team Members

Medical Officer

- Medical officer is planner, promoters, organizer, supervisor, co-ordinator and evaluator of all functions in primary health center (PHC).
- Medical officer monitors the OP patients in the morning and afternoon he does field visits.
- Visits subcenter on fixed days and hours. He gives guidance to team.
- He conducts staff meeting every month once and discusses problems, reviews the progress of health activities.
- He ensures that national health programs are implemented properly.

Functions of Female Health Worker

- Registration and care of prenatal and postnatal mothers at home.
- Registration and follow-up of all eligible couples.
- Provide nutrition advice and immunization to mother and children.
- Refer mothers and children at the time of need to hospitals and follow them up after discharge.
- Carry out family planning services including the distribution of contraceptives.
- Provide treatment for minor ailments.
- Notify communicable diseases.
- Maintenance of records and register of all the services provided and also of vital events such as births and deaths.

Functions of Male Health Workers

- Conduct survey of the subcenter area and maintain record of all families.
- Maintain information of all vital events.
- Participation in Malaria Control Program.
- Participate in family planning services by keeping a list of all eligible couples; provide information on the family planning acceptors.
- Participate in nutritional program.
- Promote health education activities.
- Identifying and reporting about communicable diseases.

- Coordinating the activities with female health worker and block staff
- Maintaining records

A qualified community health nurse is prepared to give a generalized or multipurpose service in home, school and in industry. She functions in the field of administration and supervision, education, training personnel, health services and research.

QUALITIES AND FUNCTIONS OF A COMMUNITY HEALTH NURSE

Community health nurse is a personnel, serving at the community level provides basic promotive, preventive, curative and rehabilitative services directly to the community. The specific nursing activities which are performed by the nurse will vary according to community needs and the structure of the primary healthcare system. Important role of community health nurse is depicted in **Figure 2.6**.

Qualities of Community Health Nurse

- A qualified community health nurse is one who has undergone basic general nursing, midwifery training and post-basic education in community health nursing.
- A community health nurse must have interest in people and in understanding human behavior.
- Sincerity and ability to empathize are basic qualities required of a nurse.
- A well-poised nurse has a friendly disposition, honest, charitable, resourceful, and cooperative and takes responsibilities with initiative.
- Minimum essential skills of a nurse are observation, communication, interviewing, and bedsides supportive and technical skills.
- She must have abilities to make interpretations, make judgments and take decisions.

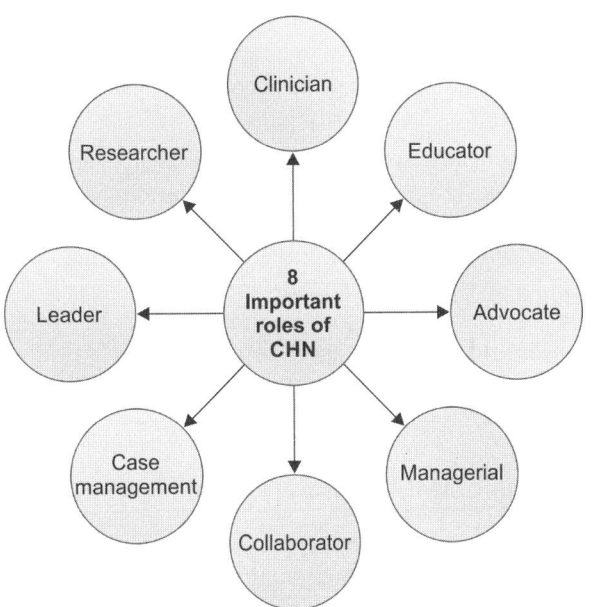

Fig. 2.6: Important roles of community health nurse.

Functions of Community Health Nurse

Community health nursing functions vary according to the designation for which the nurse is employed and according to her education and experience. Some community health nurses function on the staff level, while others serve in the capacity of administrator, supervisor or instructor in health organizations.

- Community health nurse provides comprehensive health care to individuals, families and groups by teaching, counseling and providing guidance.
- Community health nurse develops goals to meet the need. She develops an action program, evaluates progress and plans again as needed.
- Assistance to the family in improving environmental conditions that affect health, she helps to plan a safe environment in the home, school and industry.
- Providing supportive services to doctor such as early symptom detection and giving technical help.
- Demonstration and teaching of skilled nursing care of the sick in the home.
- Supervision of work of midwives, *dais* and other nursing personnel.
- Helping in the adjustment of social and emotional conditions that affect health.
- Coordination of her work with other members of the health team working in the community.
- Revising and revitalizing plan and programs.
- Epidemiologic investigation in the field of communicable diseases such as tuberculosis, sexually transmitted diseases, leprosy, etc.
- Organizing planned group classes in health with emphasis on applied nutrition, sanitation, child care and parent craft and family welfare services.
- Development and utilization of facilities such as other branches of health and welfare services for making referrals and for promotion of sound and adequate health programs.
- She is responsible for planning, implementation and evaluation of a practical plan of nursing administration within the primary center and its associated subcenters.
- The community health nurse involves in nursing research and collection of vital statistics.

Special Community Health Nursing Services

The aim of occupational health nurse is to keep the people at work healthy and to prevent them from illness and injury due to the working environment **(Fig. 2.7)**.

Industrial nursing: The aim of occupational health nurse is to keep the people at work healthy and to prevent them from illness and injury due to the working environment. The following are the basic functions of occupational or industrial nurse:

- Identify the occupational hazards.
- Educate them about the control of the occupational hazards.
- Initial treatment for the emergencies such as injuries and illnesses.

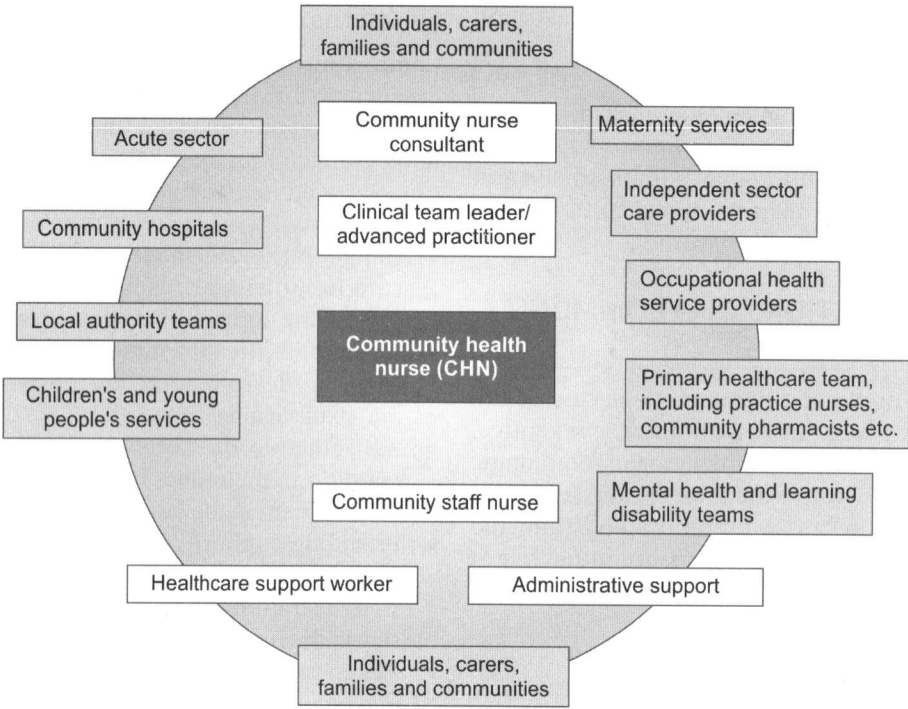

Fig. 2.7: Special community health nursing services.

- Early diagnosis of the occupational or other illnesses and to screen the people at risk.
- Assist the management in placement of the people in suitable work.
- Provide advice and supervision of conditions at work which may affect the health such as environmental sanitation.
- Health education.

Role of Nurses in Occupational Health Services

- Assist the doctor for the examination of the employees
- Protect and improve the physical and mental health of the workers
- Provision of first aid and treatment for minor illnesses and injuries
- Assess, identify and notify the management regarding the hazards affecting the workers
- Conduct health education
- Home visit to the employees to educate regarding the health and family welfare
- Nutrition
- Communicable disease prevention
- Environmental sanitation
- Protective measures for the employees
- Medical check-up and immunization.

Tuberculosis nursing: In the control of communicable diseases, nurses play a vital role in the community level. The following are the nurses role in control of tuberculosis which is an airborne infectious disease affecting the people living in poor living standards and with low immunity. Pulmonary tuberculosis is responsible for the majority 85% of TB infections.
- Case finding
- Health supervision (DOTS)
- Domiciliary care–Isolation
- Prevention of the spread of infection
- Drug compliance
- Nutrition
- Health education

Leprosy nursing: Leprosy is one of the major health and socioeconomic problems in the country. Nurse's responsibility in the care of leprosy patients is divided into the following categories:
- **Nurse–patient relationship:** An effective Nurse-patient relationship enhances the appropriate management of leprosy cases.
- **Recorder and observer of facts:** Accurate observation and correct recording of facts are vital role of a nurse and she has to provide accurate account of health.
- Health education regarding.

Leprosy is curable and the deformities are preventable and must be educated about the drug compliance.
- Family education about the preventive measures, isolation of under 15 years children, especially infants from active patients who are infective.
- Need for assistance and support during the course of illness and recovery stage.
- Family education–Educate the family regarding the misconceptions regarding leprosy.

SCOPE OF COMMUNITY HEALTH NURSING

Community health nursing is concerned with the people who are sick as well as the healthy, young and old, male and female. At the same time community health nurse is responsible for family-centered care rather than an individual oriented one. The community health nurse job is not only limited to the sick but has equal responsibility to prevent the disease and to preserve and promote the health of the people.

- **Home care:** Nursing practice is applied in meeting the health needs of communities, families and individuals in their normal environment such as at home.
- **Nursing homes:** The community health team who provides nursing care, treatment to the sick and health counseling given in nursing homes.
- **MCH and family planning:** The public health nurse plays a major role in the MCH and family planning services. It comprises antenatal, postnatal and child care services.
- **School health nursing:** The school health nurse provides services to promote and protect the health of the school children. She provides services like early detection of diseases, immunization, first-aid, dental health, school sanitation, maintenance of health records, health education, follow-up and referral services **(Fig. 2.8)**.
- **Healthcare services:** The purpose of healthcare services to improve the health status of the population. It aims at mortality and morbidity reduction, increase in expectation of life, decreased in population growth rate, improvements in nutritional status, provision of basic sanitation, health manpower requirements and resource development and certain other parameters such as food production, literacy rate, levels of poverty, etc.
- **Industrial nursing services:** The nursing service at industrial area includes periodic health check-up, care of the sick, first aid, health counseling, industrial sanitation and safety, organization of services to women and children, rehabilitation of the ill and disabled workers and administration.
- **Domiciliary nursing service:** Community health nurse focused at domiciliary nursing services includes maternity services health supervision, and disease prevention services and service for illness and accidents.
- **Geriatric nursing services:** Community health nurse should take care of old people in the community. The need of the geriatric nursing care is different and they need more care than the younger age-groups **(Fig. 2.9)**.
- **Mental health nursing service:** Mental health nursing services of a community health nurse includes early diagnosis and treatment, rehabilitation, psychotherapy, use of modern psychotropic drugs and after-care services
- **Rehabilitation centers:** The community health nurse provides care in rehabilitation units. Nursing is an important component in the rehabilitation of the disabled.

COMMUNITY HEALTH NURSING PROCESS (FIG. 2.10)

- Nursing process provides framework for the practice of nursing. It involves both art and science.
- Nursing process refers to a series of planned steps and actions directed at meeting the needs and solving the problems of patients.
- Nursing process is a deliberative problem-solving approach that requires cognitive, technical and interpersonal skills and is directed to meeting the needs of the patient.
- Nursing process is a goal-oriented humanistic and systematic plan of individualized care that is both effective and efficient.
- Nursing process is problem, solving process that addresses community health problems at all aggregate levels and aims to prevent illness and to promote the public health.
- Nursing process is deliberate intellectual activity whereby the practice of nursing is approached in an orderly, systematic manner to patient care in a dynamic, continuous method to assist the patient to achieve and maintain health.
- Nursing process is dynamic and continuous. It provides a blue print care and responds the client needs in a timely and reasonable manner to improve or maintain the client's level of health.

Definitions of Nursing Process

- Nursing process is a series of planned steps and actions directed toward meeting the needs and solving the problems of patients and their families in a systematic way.
- Nursing process provides the active driving force for change that is the first and most important tool employed by the community health nurse.
- Nursing process is a series of steps or components leading to achievement of goal. The three characteristics of a process are purpose, organization and creativity.
- Nursing process is a method for organizing and delivering nursing care to understand its functions, components and

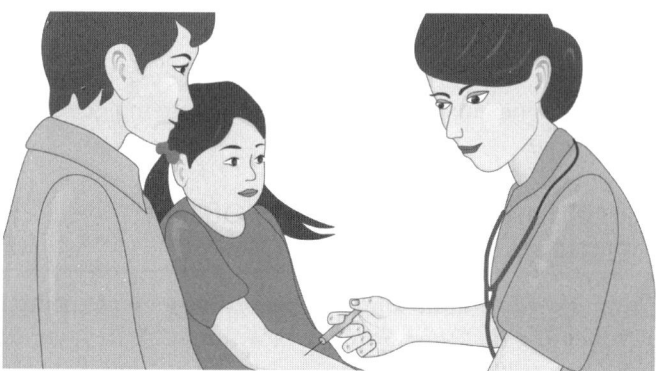

Fig. 2.8: School health nursing.

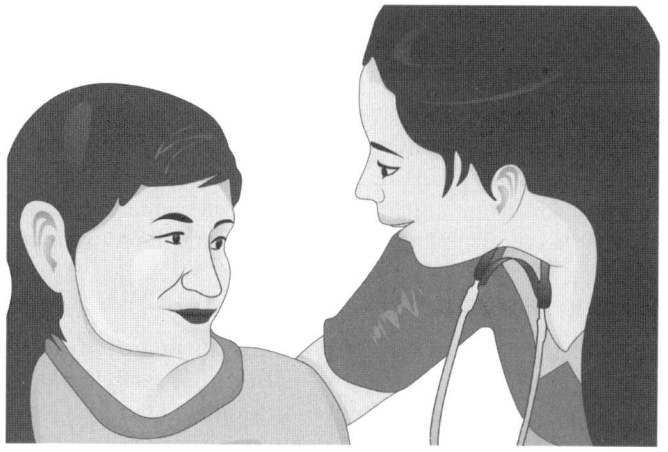

Fig. 2.9: Geriatric nursing services.

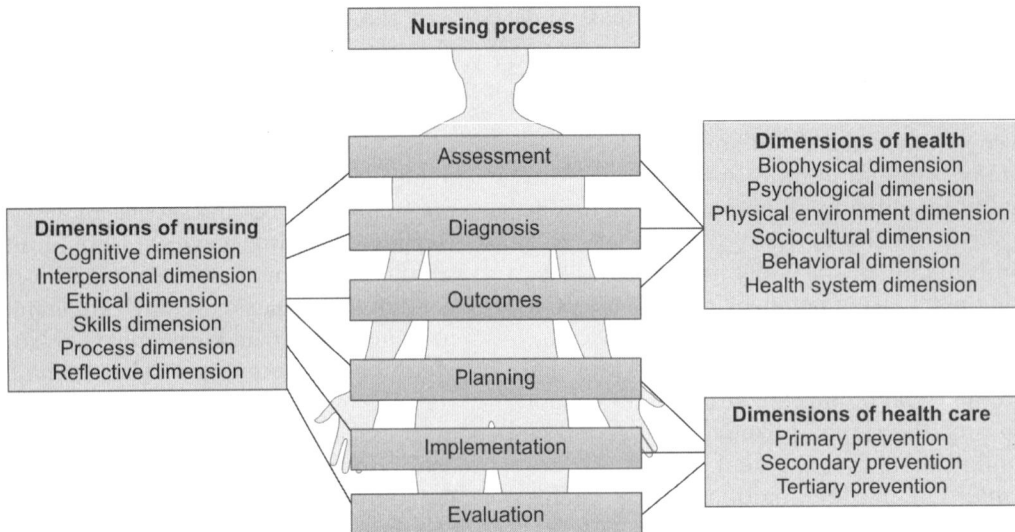

Fig. 2.10: Community health process.

interactions, the nurse should have a working knowledge of the nature of the process.
- Nursing process defined as a systematic purposeful set of interpersonal actions (White 1982).
- Nursing process is a systematic method of collecting data and formulating a nursing care plan in order to provide the most appropriate nursing intervention.
- Nursing process is the core and essence of nursing, it is central to all nursing actions, it is applicable in all setting. There is a basic theme that underlies the process; it is organized, systematic and deliberated.

Steps in Community Nursing Process

The nursing process is goal-oriented method of caring that provides a framework to nursing care. The steps are:
- **A:** Assess (what data is collected?)
- **D:** Diagnose (what is the problem?)
- **O:** Outcome Identification–(Was originally a part of the planning phase, but has recently been added as a new step in the complete process).
- **P:** Plan (how to manage the problem)?
- **I:** Implement (putting plan into action)
- **R:** Rationale (scientific reason of the implementations)
- **E:** Evaluate (did the plan work)?

Implications of Nursing Process

- Nursing process helps to identify the client's healthcare needs, determine priorities, establish goals and expected outcomes of care, establish and communicate a client-centered plan of care, provide nursing interventions designed to meet client needs and evaluate the effectiveness of nursing care in achieving expected client outcomes and goals.
- Nursing process involves scientific reasoning. The nurse makes inferences about the meaning of a client's functional state of health. The nursing process is simply one variation of scientific reasoning that allows nurses to organize, systemize and conceptualize nursing practice. It is a general approach to client system of individuals, families, groups or communities.
- Nursing process approach that allows nurses to differentiate their practice from that of physicians and other healthcare professionals. When nurses think critically, the client becomes an active participant and the ultimate outcome is a comprehensive, individualized approach to care.
- Nursing process forms the basis for nursing judgments in the form of diagnosis, nursing plans, implementation and evaluation. Conceptual frameworks such as pain management or theoretical models give basis for determining the information to be collected, diagnostic areas to be considered and attaining nursing goals and therapies.

COMMUNITY ASSESSMENT/PROBLEM IDENTIFICATION

Community health nursing process is a systematic method of collecting data for formulating a nursing care plan in order to provide the most appropriate nursing intervention. The community nursing process consists of the following major components assessment—data collection, planning, implementation and evaluation. Prevention of illness and maintenance of health care common goals in all areas of community health. The nursing process is which otherwise known as the problem-solving approach is a tool or guide for the provision of quality nursing care. A community health nurse provides of quality nursing care. A community health nurse provides skilled nursing care by making professional judgments and renders good nursing care to the family and the community.

Nursing Assessment

- Nursing assessment in community health nursing is a systematic process of gathering, verifying, and communicating data about individual and family.
- The community health nursing assessment has to be multidimensional.

- The assessment procedure therefore varies according to the age groups involved, it includes both physical and nutritional assessment.

Data Collection

- Data are collected from the individual and family for the purpose of the assessment to establish a database about the individuals' perceived needs, health problems, related experiences, health practices, goals, values and lifestyle particular health problem.
- Assessment data must be relevant. It is important for a nurse to learn to critically think about what to assess.
- The independent judgment of when a question or measurement is appropriate is influenced by the nurse's critical knowledge and experience.
- Data collected from an individual includes both objective and subjective data.

Objective data are detectable by an observer. Example of objective data are blood pressure recording, checking the temperature. *Subjective data* are apparent only to the individual concerned. Examples of subjective data are feeling of pain, vomiting, etc. Data collection requires professional skills such as making judgments, effective communication and investigations and measurements.

Sources of Data Collection (Fig. 2.11)

- The first level of data collection, the community health nurse has to establish productive working relationship and gain acceptance of the family.
- The community health nurse has to work together, know each other, develop faith and confidence and communicate their contribution in dealing with their needs and health problems.
- The community health nurse obtains relevant data collected from different sources like individual family members, friends, relatives, neighbors, local community, leader, primary health center, subcenters, member of health team, and medical and related records.

Data Collection Methods

- The community health nurse uses different methods to collect data from the individual and family.
- The nurse interviews the individual and his significant others to obtain data by asking relevant questions.
- The community nurse has to observe the home environment interaction and communication among family members.
- The community health nurse observes family characteristics, dynamics, socioeconomic level and resources, ability to cope within resource, health status of members and environmental health, etc.
- The community members nurse has to observe the family values, beliefs norms, and cultural practices.
- The community health nurse also uses other methods like active listening with eye contact can give meaningful cues, family information can be obtained by review of family health record.
- Examination and investigations are other very important methods of getting in formations about physiological and psychosocial aspects of family members.

Data Interpretation

- The collected data are examined, organized into revised categories for comparing with norms and standards of family health and development.
- The analysis includes interfering of health status of family members and the factors which might be associated with/contributing to their health status.
- Once the community has collected data about the individual/family, she must analyze the data to find out the actual and potential problems present in the family.
- Once the problem is detected, the community health nurse has to formulate appropriate nursing diagnosis.

Community Assessment (Table 2.1)

- Data collection technique/skills
  - Making appropriate judgments
  - Effective communication
  - Investigation and measurements
- Data collection methods
  - Interview
  - Observation
  - Listening
  - Review of family health record
  - Examination and investigations
- Data interpretation
  - Critical examination
  - Organization and comparison
  - Priorities the problem (actual /potential)
- Nursing diagnosis.

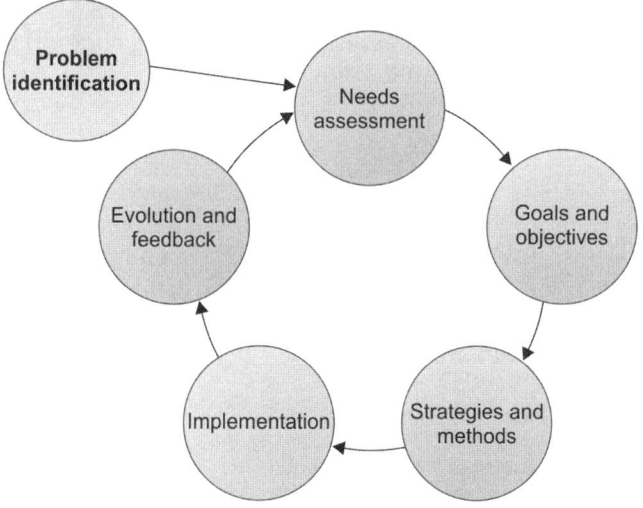

Fig. 2.11: Sources of data collection.

TABLE 2.1: Community assessment and diagnosis.

Procedures	Clinical diagnosis	Community diagnosis
Assessment	Patient/Family	Formal and informal leaders, other community members
To detect signs of illness	Examine patient	Observation in community, topographical features, leadership patterns, conflicting power groups
Investigations	Laboratory tests	Data collection primary sources, secondary sources
Preliminary diagnosis	Doctor's initial evaluation	Data processing and analysis
Explain diagnosis	To patient	Data presentation to/with community
Start treatment	Medications, surgery, etc.	Action plan
Expected and ensured	Patient follows doctor's orders	Community cooperation and collaboration enlisted
Behavior change	May/may not be needed	Lasting improvement in community health status, not possible without it
Who controls	Doctor	Community
Follow-up	Assess progress, confirm diagnosis, change diagnosis and treatment	Monitor, evaluate and plan new health actions

COMMUNITY HEALTH DIAGNOSIS

The community health nurse formulates nursing diagnosis based on data collection and interpretation of the relevant data. The community health nursing diagnosis can focus and highlight wide range of factors which influence health and wellness status of family members. The community health nursing diagnosis has five steps in the diagnostic process, such as analyze database, derive conclusions, assign diagnostic for conclusion, determining sustaining factors and formulate objectives.

Steps in Community Diagnosis

- Identification of problems, needs and resource
- Establishment of priorities
- Definition of objectives for action
- Establishment of a plan of action
- Choice of activities
- Mobilization and coordination of resources
- Evaluation

Stages of Community Diagnosis

- **Stage 1**—It involves the identification of the factors which may influence community health, includes knowledge relative to the concerned program.
- **Stage 2**—Identification and classification of data which includes quantitative and qualitative data.
- **Stage 3**—It involves data collecting, i.e. source of data and methodology of collection.

The community health nurse before coming to final diagnosis, she must have general knowledge of the community, and specific knowledge such as dietary pattern deficiencies syndrome, resources, etc.

COMPONENTS OF NURSING PROCESS (FIG. 2.12)

Nursing Assessment

Nursing assessment is the organized systematic and ongoing process of collecting data or information from a variety of sources. The data collection must pertain to a particular health problem. In other words, assessment data must be relevant.

Health assessment has no single measure of health; health measurement has to be multidimensional. Assessment is an independent nursing function that depends upon the investigating skills and all the sense in order to get relevant data about families and communities. Components of geriatric community health assessment are depicted in **Figure 2.13**.

Steps of Assessment

- **Health assessment:** It varies according to the age groups also, it includes both physical and nutritional assessment.
- **Nonphysical assessment:** Family coping index is basis for estimating the nursing needs of a particular family.

Principles of Data Collection

- Be systematic
- Explain the reason for seeking information
- Ensure confidentially
- Be polite and factual
- Make them comfortable
- Sympathize, listen attentively and record the data

Professional skills of assessment: 1. Making appropriate judgments, 2. Observation/interview.

Nursing Diagnosis

Nursing diagnosis is defined as "the statement that describes the client's actual and potential response to health problem that the nurse is competent to treat". ANA supported nursing diagnosis, a social policy statement which defined nursing as "the diagnosis a treatment of human responses to actual or potential health problems".

Steps of Nursing Diagnosis

- Analysis and interpretation of data
- Making and validating conclusions
- Comparing clues and clusters of cues with defining characteristics
- Identifying related factors
- Documenting the nursing diagnosis

Chapter 2: Community Health Nursing

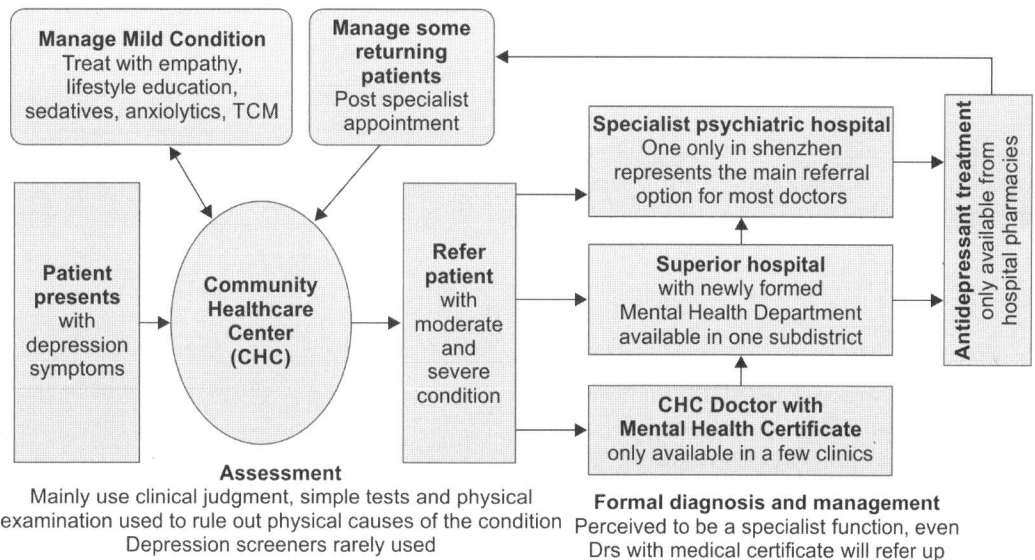

Fig. 2.12: Components of nursing process.

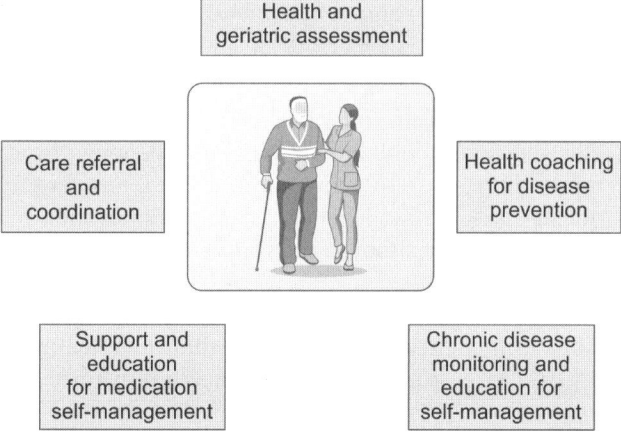

Fig. 2.13: Components of geriatric community health assessment.

Types of Nursing Diagnosis

- **Actual problem:** The actual problems are those present in the patient at the time of assessment, e.g., pain.
- **Potential problem:** A potential problem is one for which a patient has a high risk or that may occur in the future, e.g., decubitus ulcer.

Community Health Nursing Diagnosis

- The age and sex distribution of a population
- The distribution of population by social groups
- Birth rate and death rates
- Incidence and prevalence of the important diseases

Planning

Nursing assessment and the formulation of nursing diagnosis initiate the planning step of the nursing process. Planning is a category of nursing behavior in which client-centered goals and expected outcomes are established and nursing interventions are selected to achieve goals.

During planning, priorities are set. In addition to collaborating with individual and family the nurse consults with other members of healthcare team, reviews pertinent literature modifies care and records relevant information about the client's health care and community management.

Steps in Planning

- Setting priorities
- Establishing goals
- Determining resource personnel
- Written plan of action includes problems

Types of Nursing Care Plans

- Student nursing care plan
- Individualized nursing care plan
- Standardized nursing care plan
- Care management nursing care plan

Nursing Implementations

Implementation of a component of the nursing process is a category of nursing behavior in which the actions necessary for achieving the goals and expected outcomes of nursing care are initiated and completed. Implementation in nursing process is to translate the planning into practice according to the principles of nursing.

Implementation consists of activities aimed at achieving goals and objectives. It can be shaped by the nurses' chosen roles, the type of health problem selected, the family's readiness to participate in the care and the characteristics of social change process.

Implementation includes performing assisting or directing the performance of activities of daily living, counseling and teaching client's family, giving direct care to achieve client-centered goals, supervising, evaluating the work of staff members and recording and exchanging information relevant to the client's continued healthcare.

Implementation is continuous and interactive with other components of the nursing process. During implementation the nurses reassess the client, modify the care plan and rewrite expected outcomes as necessary. For effective implementation, the nurse must be knowledgeable about types of interventions, the implementation process and specific implementation methods.

Evaluation

Evaluation refers to judgments or appraisal. It is examining the outcome of the nursing action or extent to which the expected outcomes or goals were achieved. Evaluation is an ongoing process. Critical evaluation and revising therapies continues until problems are appropriately resolved.

Steps of Evaluation

- Identifying the outcome criteria and standards
- Compare the actual outcome with expected outcomes
- Summarizing the results of evaluation
- Making corrections and modifying care plans
- Documenting the evaluation process

Methods and Tools for Evaluation

- Direct observation
- Questioning/interview
- Record review

Types of Evaluation

- **Formative evaluation:** It determines the strength and weakness at each stage of the program.
- **Summative evaluation:** It determines the strength and weakness at the end of the program.

Criteria of Evaluation

- Outcomes must be realistic and adjusted on the basis of the clients' prognosis and condition.
- The nurse must realize that evaluation is dynamic and ever-changing, depending on the client's nursing diagnosis and condition.
- A client whose health status continuously changes, more frequent evaluation.

ESTABLISHING INTERPERSONAL RELATIONSHIP

Interpersonal communication is both a science and an art. As a science, it requires a disciplined study of concepts and practice of techniques to gain certain skills. As an art, it requires the fusion of the nurse self with creativity, insight and practice to achieve style. Human communication is a complex process in which two or more persons exchange message and derive meaning.

Effective communication occurs when persons exchange message and derive a mutual understanding of intended

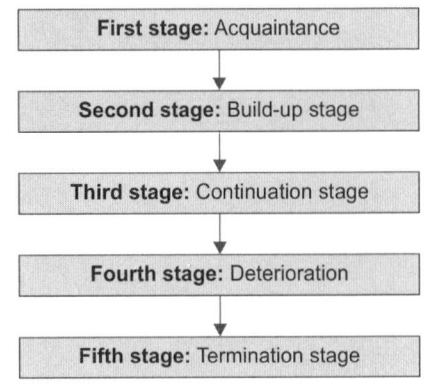

Fig. 2.14: Stages of interpersonal relationships.

meaning. A general classic principle of communication is applicable to nurse—client interactions as well as to all other interactions, both people are perceived by another. The community health nurse is an important member of the healthcare team work in cooperation and harmony for the care of the individual, family and community. Stages of interpersonal relationship are depicted in **Figure 2.14**.

Characteristic of Helping Relationships

- **Awareness of self and values:** The nurse needs to be able to answer "who am I"? What do I believe? What is important to me? To help another person answer those questions. A certain level of insight precedes the use of a most important tool in nursing, the "use of self" as a caretaker.
- **Ability to analyze own feeling:** Nurses as helper gradually learn to recognize and cope with their own feelings of joy and grief, power and anger, accomplishment and frustration.
- **Ability to serve as a model:** To show another person the route to health a nurse necessarily maintains a certain level of health in mind, body, spirit and lifestyle.
- **Altruism:** Nurses characteristically convey a sense of altruism that is they receive self-satisfaction from helping people in a humanistic way.
- **Strong sense of ethics:** Nurses strive to make the best possible judgments based on high principles of human welfare.
- **Responsibility:** Two dimensions of responsibility are inherent in nursing, taking responsibility for your actions and sharing responsibility with others.

Principles of Interpersonal Relationship

- Respect every one's individuality
- Keep emotion under control
- Develop habits of listening and focus attention on problem
- Be impartial to others and practice justice.
- There should be "team spirit" or "we feeling" among the members.

- There should be mutual understanding between the members.
- Delegation of responsibility in a group and every member should carry out responsibility to the satisfaction of the group.
- Establish a good rapport among the members in order to achieve the aim.
- Every member should be familiar with the organization plan and the policies of the group.
- Avoid arguments in the group.
- Praise the slightest improvement made by others, use words of encouragement.
- Prepare yourself mentally to accept the worst if necessary.

Phase of Nurse–Client Relationship

- **Initial/opening phase:** Introduction and preparation of personal growth conditions occur in this phase. In the opening phase of the relationship, the underlying goal of both persons is to adapt to each other and to establish trust.
- **Working/developmental phase:** In this phase relationship fosters growth and change, problem-solving and decision-making. Throughout the working phase, both nurse and client strive to maintain trust during stressful.
- **Terminating/closing phase:** The closing of a successful relationship between nurse and client. The closing phase requires to another caregiver or by agreements that the client is self–sufficient again.

Relationship of Nurse and Health Team

- **Nurse and physician:** The nurse must be loyal, honest dependable and willing to carry out the doctor's order in the matter of treatment and care of the patient.
- **Nurse and head nurse:** The attitude of the nurse to her head nurse should be respected, enthusiastic support intelligent and cooperative.
- **Nurse and hospital personal:** Good relationship between the personnel of different departments must be maintained satisfactorily. She should understand that the nursing department is coordinated with other departments of the hospital for its smooth functioning.
- **Nurse and non-professional workers:** The nurse must be decent and considerate in her behavior with the non-professional works. She should maintain a good relationship with them and should give them necessary guidance to carry out their functions.
- **Nurse and the patient:** The patient is the most important person in the hospital. The responsibility of the nurse to see that the patient feels homely. Treat him as an individual, understand him and help him to overcome his fear and anxiety. The nurse should be sympathetic and of understanding of nature. She should not accept any gifts or personal favors from patients.

COMMUNITY HEALTHCARE PLAN

The nursing care plan serves as the organizational framework for the practice of nursing. The nursing care plan involves a problem-solving approach that enables the nurse to identify patient problems and potential at-risk needs (problems) and to plan deliver and evaluate nursing care in an orderly, scientific manner. The process of community healthcare plan is depicted in **Figure 2.15**.

Definitions

- The nursing care plan is the method by which nursing practiced systematically and provides the means by which nurse demonstrates accountability and responsibility to clients and families.
- A nursing care plan is a blueprint for supporting patients adaptive responses to health or illness (NANDA).
- A nursing care plan is a document that reflects collaborative changes and patient's informed consent.

Principles for Constructing Care Plan

- Care plan should embody both 'patients and nurses' of health concerns.
- The nursing care plan should be drawn from patient's primary concerns.
- Nursing care plan should be drawn from patient's resources and capabilities.
- Nursing care plan should be the outcome of a shared decision-making process that empowers patients and communicates nurses respect for patient's individuality.
- Care plan should consider patient's individual characteristics such as nationality, age, education, personal habits and interest social status and family relationship.

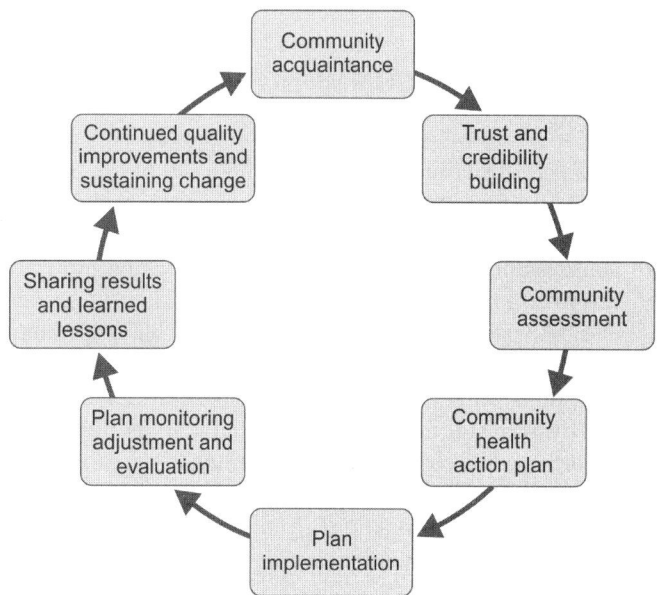

Fig. 2.15: Process of community healthcare plan.

- Nursing-care plan should be in brief and compact statements.
- Nursing care plan prepared and used by nurses in caring for a patient it is necessary to take into account diagnosis, physical and mental condition.

Advantages of Nursing Care Plan

- It is a summative structure where at a glance all the information of the patient is received.
- It portrays about the patients as a person, a little about his home background, his interests, his known worries and fears.
- It involves a collaborative team work head nurse, shift nurses, patient and his family members.
- Enables students to plan the care according to priority.
- Students can correlate all the steps of nursing process read in theory and can directly apply it practically.
- Students can prioritize the nursing care plans based on scientific principles.
- Writing patient care plans not only assists students to assimilate information, but also provides a vehicle for communicating students knowledge to faculty.

Common Problems in Writing Care Plans

- Incomplete database—leads to many errors in writing a care plan.
- Selecting patient behaviors that are not observable and measurable.
- Stating outcomes as nursing behavior rather than patient behaviors.

Disadvantages of Care Plan

- It is time-consuming.
- It cannot be formulated during emergency condition.
- All plans cannot be implemented because of unavailability of resource.

COMPREHENSIVE COMMUNITY HEALTH NURSING

- **General information:** Name of the head of the family, House no. family type and size, religion, caste and mother tongue.
- **Demographic characteristics:** Decision-making authority
- **Environmental conditions:** Housing, ventilation, source of light, water supply, and kitchen condition, disposal of waste, presence of domestic animals, insects, rodents, stray dogs, and accidental hazards observed.
- **Nutritional status:** Food habits and dietary patterns
- **Maternal and child health:** Eligibility status, antenatal services, immunization status of under-fives, health status of children, relationship of family members, vital signs and general health of family members.

CONCLUSION

Community health nursing is essential particularly at this point in time because it maximizes the health status of individuals, families, groups and the community through direct approach with them. Today community participation and involvement is getting a due attention before the occurrence of illnesses as lifestyle changes to continue to play a significant role in morbidity and mortality. Chronic illnesses, tobacco smoking, road traffic accident (RTA) etc, and environmental changes that affect health are steadily becoming the major concerns influencing human health in our country. As nurses of 21st century we have duties and responsibilities to keep a dynamic balance with the ever-changing needs of the health of our society. To maintain abreast with this societal needs we professional nurses must understand concepts and models of the community health nursing, the importance of health promotion and disease prevention and healthcare planning.

REVIEW QUESTIONS

Long Essays

1. Define community health nursing. Discuss the objectives and philosophy of community health nursing.
2. Enumerate the principles of community health nursing.
3. Discuss the qualities and functions of a community health nurse.
4. Define community health nursing process. Describe the steps of community health nursing process.

Short Essays

1. Skills of community health nurse.
2. Functions of community health team members.
3. Special community health nursing services.
4. Role of nurses in occupational health services.
5. Scope of community health nursing.
6. Implications of nursing process in community health nursing.
7. Community assessment/problem identification.
8. Components of nursing process.
9. Characteristic of helping relationships.
10. Phase of nurse–client relationship.
11. Community healthcare plan.
12. Principles for constructing care plan.

Short Answers

1. Nursing diagnosis.
2. Nursing care plan.
3. Community health nursing process.
4. Goals of community health nursing.
5. Functions of female health worker.
6. Industrial nursing.
7. Healthcare services.
8. Home care.
9. Domiciliary nursing service.
10. Geriatric nursing services.
11. Definition of nursing process.

Chapter 2: Community Health Nursing

12. Sources of data collection.
13. Stages of community diagnosis.
14. Principles of data collection.
15. Principles of interpersonal relationship.
16. Advantages of nursing care plan.
17. Comprehensive community health nursing.

Multiple Choice Questions

1. Which is the primary goal of community health nursing?
    a. To contribute to national development through promotion of family welfare, focusing particularly on mothers and children
    b. To support and supplement the efforts of the medical profession in the promotion of health and prevention of illness
    c. To increase the productivity of the people by providing them with services that will increase their level of health
    d. To enhance the capacity of individuals, families and communities to cope with their health needs.
2. PHC based on the following principles, *except:*
    a. Nation-wide coverage
    b. Inter-sectoral coordination
    c. Self-reliance
    d. Self-actualization
3. Which of the one the following is characteristics of community health nursing?
    a. Increase the average life expectancy
    b. Emphasizes wellness rather than illness
    c. Decreasing the morbidity rate
    d. Providing total health care to improve quality of life
4. _____ is barrier to community/ public participation.
    a. Lack of education or information
    b. Poverty/socioeconomic status
    c. Cultural minorities
    d. Negligence from government
5. Safe food supply and proper nutrition is:
    a. Essentials/Elements of primary health care
    b. Goal and objective of primary health care
    c. Basic requirement of primary health care
    d. Basic principle of primary health care

ANSWERS

| 1. d | 2. d | 3. d | 4. a | 5. a | | | | | | |

3 CHAPTER

Health Assessment

LEARNING OBJECTIVES
1. Concept of health assessment
2. Characteristics of a healthy individual
3. Health assessment of infant, preschool, school going, adolescent, adult, antenatal woman, postnatal woman, adult and elderly

TERMINOLOGY

Diagnosis: It is the determination of the nature and extent of a disease.

Prognosis: It is the forecast of the course and duration of a disease.

Etiology: It is the science of the cause of a disease.

Signs: The presence of a disease that can be seen or elicited, e.g., fever.

Symptoms: Any evidence as to the nature and location of a diseases noted by the client.

Subjective symptoms: When the symptoms are note by the client himself, e.g., pain.

Objective symptoms: When the symptoms are noted by the observer as well as by the client, e.g., jaundice.

Affect: Temporary expression of feeling of state of mind.

Delirium: Acute confusional change or LOC.

Dysmenorrhea: Painful menstruation.

Dysphagia: Difficult or discomfort swallowing.

Dyspnea: Difficult or labored breathing.

Dysuria: Difficult or painful urination.

Mood: Durable prolonged display of feelings that color whole emotional life, less focused cause.

Nocturia: Waking frequent at night to urinate.

Organic (disorder): Decreased mental function due to medical or physical disease.

Orthopnea: Shortness of breath when lying flat.

INTRODUCTION

A health assessment is a plan of care that identifies the specific needs of a person and how those needs will be addressed by the healthcare system or skilled nursing facility. Health assessment is the evaluation of the health status by performing a physical exam after taking a health history. Health assessments are usually structured screening and assessment tools used in primary care practices to help the healthcare team and patient develop a plan of care. Health assessment information can also help the healthcare team understand the needs of its overall population of patients. Health assessments can vary in length and scope. They can be completed during office visits or between office visits, either on paper or computers. Health assessment questions may be asked about patients of all ages, including children and adolescents.

DEFINITIONS

- **A health assessment** is a set of questions, answered by patients, that asks about personal behaviors, risks, life-changing events, health goals and priorities, and overall health.
- **A community health assessment (CHA),** as defined by the Public Health Accreditation Board (PHAB), is a systematic examination of health status indicators for a population, conducted for the purpose of identifying key problems and assets in a community and assisting with the development of strategies to address the community's health issues.
- **Admission assessment:** Comprehensive nursing assessment including patient history, general appearance, physical examination and vital signs.
- **Shift assessment:** Concise nursing assessment completed at the commencement of each shift or if patient condition changes at any other time.
- **Focused assessment:** Detailed nursing assessment of specific body system(s) relating to the presenting problem or current concern(s) of the patient. This may involve one or more body system.

CONCEPT OF HEALTH ASSESSMENT

A community health assessment is a process that uses quantitative and qualitative methods to systematically collect and analyze data to understand health within a specific community. An ideal assessment includes information on risk factors, quality of life, mortality, morbidity, community assets, force for changes, social determinants of health and health inequity, and information on how well the public health system provides essential services. Community health assessment data inform community decision-making, the prioritization of health problems, and the development, implementation, and evaluation of community health improvement plans. Community health assessment is a fundamental tool of public health practice. Its aim is to describe the health of the community, by presenting information on health status, community health needs, resources, and epidemiologic and other studies of current local health problems.

Some common health assessment questions are:
- Tobacco use
- Stress
- Healthy eating
- Physical activity
- Sexual practices
- Sedentary behaviors such as sitting and watching TV or playing computer games
- Alcohol usage
- Addictive behaviors such as gambling or drug use
- Violence, bullying or physical abuse
- Depression or anxiety
- Emotional and social support
- Safety issues such as wearing a seat belt while driving
- Overall health or well-being

Pre-requisites to Assessment

- **Beliefs:** The nurse's belief encompasses a caring philosophy about the client's, responsibilities and health and illness and the role of nursing in health care. These philosophies do not blossom overnight but are molded during the course of nursing education by nurses, other students, instructors and clients.
- **Knowledge:** The knowledge base for nurses is extensive and nurses are required to use information from sciences such as nursing, anatomy, physiology, microbiology, pharmacology, chemistry and nutrition using all of these sciences is guidelines, the nurse can analyze data collected about the client.
- **Skills:** A variety of skills are required to perform a complete assessment of the client. They include psychomotor and interpersonal.
  - Psychomotor skills are the technical skills required in many phases and nursing process. During the assessment phase, the most common skills are those of physical assessment such as inspection, palpation and auscultation.
  - Interpersonal skills are important in all phases of nursing process **(Fig. 3.1)** but are a critical component of the assessment phase. The term therapeutic relationship is often used to describe the communication techniques that allow the client and family to share views and telling openly.

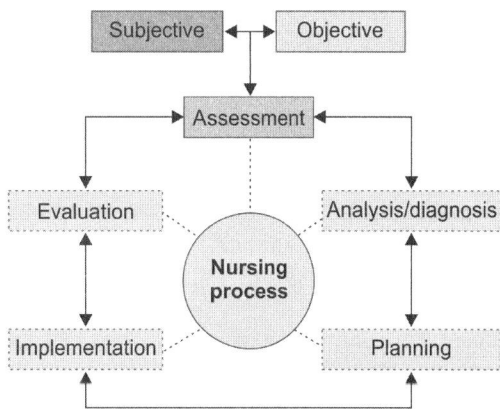

Fig. 3.1: Steps of nursing process application in health assessment.

PURPOSES AND FACTORS AFFECTING HEALTH ASSESSMENT

- To understand the physical and mental well-being of the patient.
- To detect disease in its early stage.
- To determine the cause and the extent of disease.
- To understand any changes in the condition of diseases, any improvement or regression.
- To determine the nature of the treatment or nursing care needed for the patient.
- To safeguard the patient and his family by noting the early signs especially in case of a communicable disease.
- To contribute to the medical research.
- To find out whether the person is medically fit or not for a particular task.

Purposes of Assessment

- To gather information regarding client's health.
- To determine client's normal function.
- To organize the collected information.
- To confirm hypothesis growing out of the nurse's interview.
- To enhance investigation of nursing problems.
- To frame nursing diagnosis.
- It increases greater managing skill of handling patient's problem.
- To identify the health problems.
- To identify client's strengths.
- To identify need for health teaching.

Factors Affecting Health Assessment

- Physical setting
- Clients personality and behavior
- Communication skill
- Problem
- Nurses personality and behavior
- Nurses knowledge and skill

PRINCIPLES OF HEALTH ASSESSMENT

In planning and performing health assessment, the nurse needs to consider the following:

- An accurate and timely health assessment provides foundation for nursing care and intervention.
- A comprehensive assessment incorporates information about a client's physiologic, psychosocial, spiritual health, cultural and environmental factors as well as client's developmental status.
- The health assessment process should include data collection, documentation and evaluation of the client's health status and responses to health problems and intervention.
- All documentation should be objective, accurate, clear, concise, specific and current.
- Health assessment is practiced in all healthcare settings whenever there is nurse-client interaction.
- Information gathered from health assessment should be communicated to other healthcare professionals in order to facilitate collaborative management of clients and for continuity of care.
- Client's confidentiality should be kept.

RESPONSIBILITIES OF NURSE IN HEALTH ASSESSMENT

- The nurse has the responsibility to carry out health assessment on every person under his/her care.
- The nurse should regularly perform focused assessments in response to client needs.
- The nurse needs to obtain client's consent prior to health assessment.
- The nurse should demonstrate a caring attitude, respect and concern for each client when doing a health assessment.
- The nurse has the responsibility in keeping confidentiality about the data being collected from his/her client.
- The nurse obtains information on a client using various techniques and tools, such as history taking, physical examination, reviewing clients' records and results of diagnostic tests. He/She has to draw inferences from data collected in order to make appropriate and sound clinical judgment.
- The nurse has to acquire specialized skills and competence in collecting accurate and relevant information on the patient's health in performing health assessment in order to make sound clinical decisions.
- The nurse should document the results of health assessment, analyze the data collected, evaluate the client's response to health problems and interventions, and provide feedback to the client as appropriate.
- The nurse should continuously advance their competence in health assessment throughout one's nursing career.
- The nurse who takes up an advanced practice role has the responsibility to prepare himself/herself in order to perform advanced and focused health assessment.

CHARACTERISTICS OF A HEALTHY INDIVIDUAL

Characteristics of a physically healthy individual like normal weight, blood pressure, blood glucose level, flawless healthy skin, healthy hair, good eye health, etc. **(Box 3.1)**. These

> **Box 3.1:** Characteristics of a healthy individual.
> - Clear skin
> - Steady heartbeat that is neither too fast nor too slow
> - Blood pressure in range
> - Symmetrical features
> - Clear eyes with even pupils that track together
> - Appropriate flexibility in the joints
> - Expected reflex responses
> - Weight in the expected ranges, neither too high nor too low
> - A reasonable amount of endurance and strength

are the key traits reflecting his physical fitness. A healthy person exhibits certain characteristics which are the key traits reflecting sound health of that person. No microscopic examination is essential to identify most of them as these characteristics can be seen very clear as external features with our naked eyes. The following are the characteristics of a physically healthy individual:

> - **Realistic self-concept:** Well adjusted person sees himself as he is, not as he would like to be. The gap between real and the ideal self-concept is very much smaller among the well adjusted.
> - **Realistic appraisal of situations:** He approaches situations with a realistic attitude, accepting the bad with the good.
> - **Realistic evaluation of achievements:** A well adjusted person is able to evaluate his achievements realistically and to react to them in a rational way.
> - **Acceptance of reality:** He is willing to accept reality instead of running away from it.

Physically Healthy Person Maintains Normal Weight

The characteristics of a mentally healthy individual is depicted in **Figure 3.2**.
- Healthy individual always maintains adequate weight. He is neither underweight nor overweight or obese.
- Weight plays a very important role in maintaining health. Body of underweight or overweight individuals do not work efficiently and as a result deficiencies and disorders make a room in body which is a calling bell for sickness.
- A healthy individual maintains normal weight which is ideal for his height.

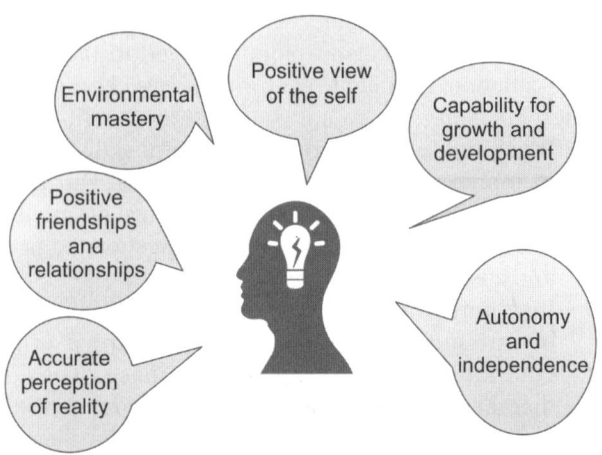

Fig. 3.2: Characteristics of a mentally healthy individual.

Posture is Always Right

- Another important characteristic of a physically healthy person is that he always maintains correct posture. He does not stoop while standing or while he walks.
- He walks with right pace which is neither very slow nor very fast, i.e., he walks with easy quick long steps and more importantly do not drag his feet while walking.
- His back always remains straight and he never hunches. Shoulder of a healthy person always remains in alignment with his heels.

Flawless Skin

- Skin reflexes inner health of an individual. If a person is healthy then definitely his skin will appear to be clear, blemish free and firm.
- No sort of rashes or indentations can be seen on skin. Healthy skin does not store up excess water leading to swelling on face.
- Pimples, stretch marks, blemishes, excessive oily or dry skin, indentations, swelling, rashes, and redness are all signs of unhealthy skin and improper functioning of internal organs.

Healthy Eyes

- Eyes of a physically healthy individual appears to be clear. No redness or yellowish discoloration can be seen.
- Skin around eyes remains blemish free and there will be no signs of dark under eye circles.
- Also, skin around eyes does not show signs of puffiness or sogginess. Pupils remain of their normal size and do not show signs of dilation or constriction.
- Blinking count is normal along with eye movements. There will be no erratic movements and wild stares.

Healthy Hair

- Like skin, hair health too reflects inner health of a person. Recurrence of dandruff, hair fall, brittle hair, too oily or too much dryness in hair, split ends are all signs of underlying diseases or deficiencies in body.
- Not only physical sickness causes hair problems but mental ill-health like too much stress and tension too result in hair-related problems.
- A person who is healthy always enjoys shine and luster in hair and never faces hair loss, dandruff or other hair related problems.
- Texture of hair remains fine along with normal oil secretion preventing hair from becoming too oily or dry.

Features are Symmetrical

- Right side and left side of a physically healthy person are symmetrical. No portion in either of the sides come protruded outside.
- Both the sides are well balanced. No cyst or any sort of swelling anatomically creates asymmetry.
- There is no sign of pain in any of the portion on either sides. Muscles, bone, skin, organs, etc., are in no way larger or smaller than the other side.

Good Grip and Flexibility

- A physically healthy individual always displays firm grip. There is quite firmness or tightness in his grip unlike diseased person whose grip is very loose.
- Healthy person has good palm control and good flexibility. Day to day functions can be performed by him without any difficulty.
- No pain or spasm is experienced by him while bending, walking or lifting anything from floor.
- No muscle or joint pain makes him suffer and delays his regular work. Normal body movements can be performed by him very smoothly.

Low Resting Heart Rate

- If resting heart rate is below 60 beats every minute then this is a sign of physical fitness and it promotes long life span.
- A physically healthy individual always displays low resting heart rate. Before completely shutting down, heart beats for certain number of times.
- Heart is nothing but more of a machine which pumps blood and oxygen to all the vital organs. This is the reason that resting heart rate should be low. If resting heart rate is low then an individual's chance of longevity increases.

Blood Pressure is within Normal Range

- Blood pressure of a physically healthy individual always remains within normal range. It neither lowers causing hypotension nor exceeds the normal range leading to hypertension.
- Increase or decrease in the normal blood pressure is considered to be an abnormality.
- Normal blood pressure should be in the range of 120/80 to 140/90. However, in elderly individuals, range increases to higher level and it is considered absolutely normal for their age.

Blood Glucose is within Normal Range

- A physically fit person always displays blood glucose level within normal range. Healthy lifestyle keeps glucose level in his blood within normal range which is 100 mg/dL on fasting and 140 mg/dL after 2 hours of eating.
- This ensures proper functioning of liver as insulin secretion is efficient. Too much or too little blood glucose level will cause severe damage to the body.
- Also, diabetes can cause many problems such as kidney diseases, heart attack, blindness, atherosclerosis, etc.

Response Time is Normal

- Response time of a physically fit individual is real quick, i.e., he displays quick reflexes.
- If reflex time is prolonged then this indicates underlying causes which are delaying reflexes and this definitely is not a good sign.

High Level of HDL Cholesterol

- A healthy individual always displays high level of high-density cholesterol, i.e., above 90 mg/dL of HDL cholesterol.
- This reduces risk of heart-related diseases. Importance of HDL cholesterol is that it prevents blockages from forming in the arteries of heart. Any blockage formed increase the risk of heart attacks and other heart-related diseases.

Respiration is Normal

- Respiration process, i.e., inhalation of oxygen and exhalation of carbon dioxide of a physically healthy person is stable.
- It is neither increased nor decreased abnormally. His respiration cycles are regular and within normal range which is 12 to 20 breaths/minute.
- This ensures that his lungs and his overall respiratory system is working efficiently and this is because there is an even flow of oxygen inside the body.

Possess Balanced Muscle Strength

- A physically healthy individual always displays balanced muscular strength. Opposing muscles should acquire balanced strength.
- For example, strength ratio of opposing muscles like biceps and triceps should be 1:1. Similarly, strength ratio of quadriceps and hamstrings should be 3:2. This is a characteristic of physically fit body.

Disease-free Body

- Most important characteristic of a healthy person or a healthy body is that it is free of diseases.
- Health and sickness contrast each other. Even if slight sickness is present in the body then it cannot be called or termed as healthy.
- An individual who shows no signs of any sickness or diseases present in him along with no signs of even slightest form of disorder will be called as physically fit.
- Even slight sickness or disorder takes away that tag called as physically healthy.

Healthy Signs of a Physically Healthy Person

- A physically fit individual always follows healthy habits which are signs of physical fitness. He eats properly, i.e., his appetite is good.
- He neither overeats or undereats his meals and always enjoys a well-balanced, healthy nutritious meal, avoiding too much of fats and complex carbohydrates.
- He gets his adequate sleep daily and shows no signs of disturbed sleep or insomnia. He hydrates his body well by drinking required amount of water and shows no signs of dehydration.
- He has high level of cardiovascular fitness and always follows an exercise regime and do not believe in sedentary lifestyle.
- He avoids drinking coffee, tea, alcohol and stays away from smoking, drug addiction and other such sorts of harmful addictions.

APPROACH TO PHYSICAL ASSESSMENT

- Consider the age and developmental stage of the child.
- Implement behaviors that show respect for child's age, gender, cultural values and personal preferences.
- Modify language and communicate style to be consistent with child's needs.
- Introduce yourself to the child and family and establish rapport. Use play techniques for infants and young children.
- Gather as much information as possible by observation first.
- Use systematic approach; but be flexible to accommodate child's behavior.
- Examine least intrusive areas first (i.e., hands, arms) and painful and sensitive assessment last (i.e., ears, nose, mouth).
- Determine what parts of the exam is to be completed before possible crying which may be seen in some children (i.e., heart, lungs and abdomen).
- Encourage the child and family to ask questions and voice any concerns.
- Where possible assessments should be clustered with other cares at a time when the child is relaxed and compliant. However, the clinical need of the assessment should also be considered against the need for the child to rest. For a stable child it may be appropriate to delay assessments until the child is awake.
- Throughout the assessment process, the nurse should refer any serious concerns to the ANM and to medical team.

HEALTH ASSESSMENT OF INFANT

The infant's first visit to the hospital may be as early as 2–3 days of age. Healthy babies are discharged from the nursery after 24 to 48 hours. This is a critical time for establishment of breastfeeding and assessment of problems such as jaundice. If the child is only a few days old, review the physical examination of the newborn and familiarize yourself with some of the common neonatal medical problems before you begin the infant health maintenance exam.

Assessments for Newborn Babies (Fig. 3.3)

- After birth, newborn babies are carefully checked for problems or complications.
- Throughout the hospital stay, physicians, nurses, and other care providers continually assess each infant for changes in health and signs of illness.
- One of the first assessments is a baby's Apgar score. At one minute and five minutes after birth, infants are checked for heart and respiratory rates, muscle tone, reflexes, and color.
- This helps identify babies that have difficulty breathing or have other problems that need further care.

Complete Family Medical and Social History

- Information about the family history can best be obtained by beginning with open-ended questions such as, "Tell me about any medical problems of your family members may have had"? You should inquire about the immediate family and grandparents.

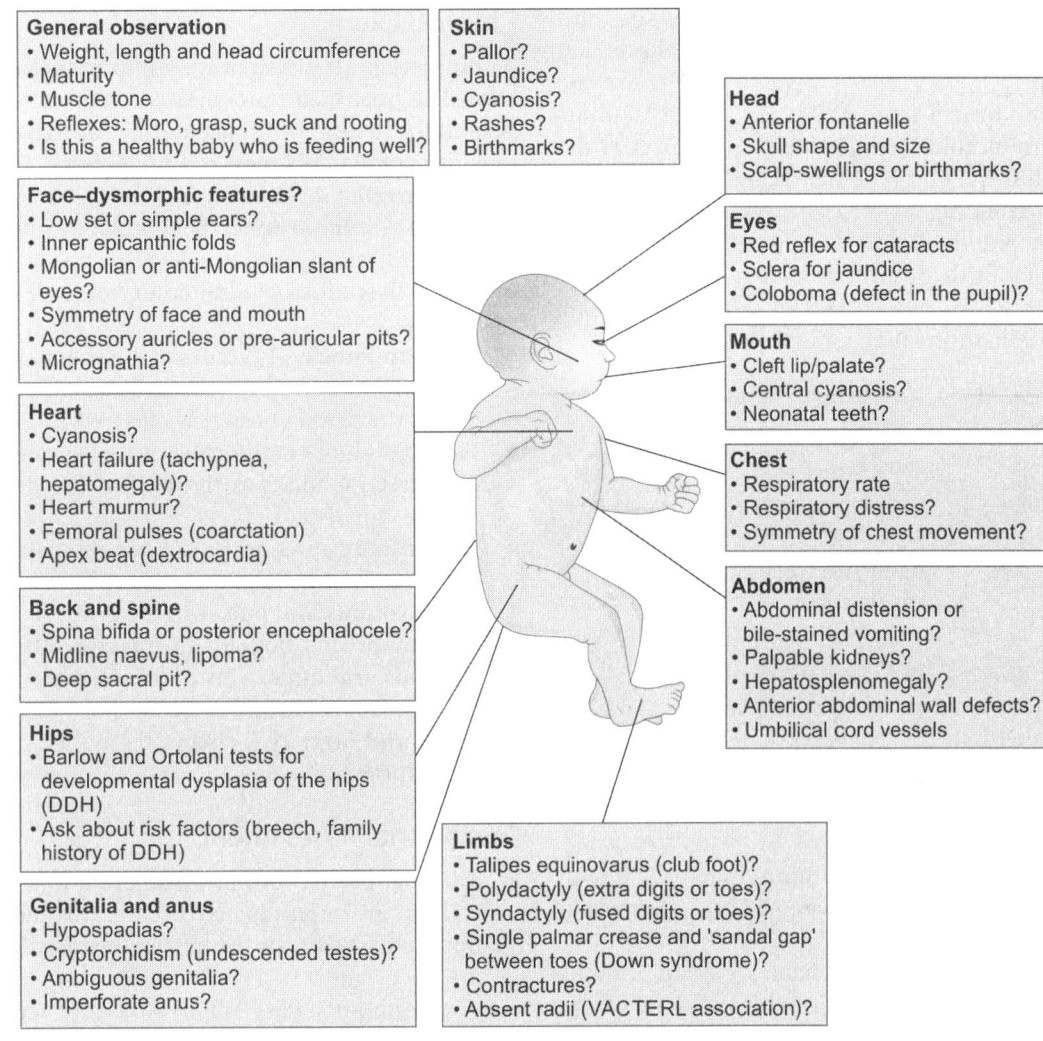

Fig. 3.3: Newborn health assessment.

- Extend the pedigree if the family has a history of hereditary diseases, or if other family members play an important role in the child's life.

Immunization Record

- The basic series of immunizations recommended by United States public health experts can be found here, but many clinics vary the recommended schedule, depending on their sources of funding, whether they have access to new multiple antigen vaccines, and if they are experiencing shortages.
- Ask your preceptor for a copy of the currently recommended schedule at your clinic site.

Complete Physical Exam

- Because birth weight is an important indicator of health, babies are weighed daily in the nursery.
- This indicates their growth, as well as their fluid and nutritional needs.
- Newborn babies may lose as much as 10% of their birth weight.
  In addition, each newborn undergoes a complete physical examination.
- Care providers evaluate vital signs including temperature, pulse, and breathing rate.
- They also check the infant's general appearance from head to toe, looking at everything from soft spots on the skull to breathing patterns to skin rashes to limb movement.
- The baby's head circumference, abdominal circumference, and length will also be measured.

Vital Signs

- **Temperature:** Able to maintain stable body temperature of 97.0°F to 98.6°F (36.1°C to 37°C) in normal room environment.
- **Heartbeat:** Normally 120 to 160 beats per minute. It may be much slower when an infant sleeps.
- **Breathing rate:** Normally 40 to 60 breaths per minute.
- **Blood pressure:** Normally an upper number (systolic) between 60 and 80, and a lower number (diastolic) between 30 and 45.
- **Oxygen saturation:** Normally 95% to 100% on room air.

Apgar Scoring

- The Apgar score helps find breathing problems and other health issues. It is part of the special attention given to a baby in the first few minutes after birth.

- The baby is checked at 1 minute and 5 minutes after birth for heart and respiratory rates, muscle tone, reflexes, and color.
- Each area can have a score of 0, 1, or 2, with 10 points as the maximum total. Most babies score 8 or 9, with 1 or 2 points taken off for blue hands and feet because of immature circulation.
- If a baby has a difficult time during delivery and needs extra help after birth, this will be shown in a lower Apgar score. Apgar scores of 6 or less usually mean a baby needed immediate attention and care.

Sign	Score = 0	Score = 1	Score = 2
Heart rate	Absent	Below 100 per minute	Above 100 per minute
Breathing effort	Absent	Weak, irregular, or gasping	Good, crying
Muscle tone	Flaccid	Some flexing of arms and legs	Well-flexed, or active movements of arms and legs
Reflex or irritability	No response	Grimace or weak, cry	Good cry
Color	Blue all over, or pale	Body pink, hands and feet blue	Pink all over

Birth Weight

- A baby's birth weight is an important marker of health. Full-term babies are born between 37 and 41 weeks of pregnancy.
- The average weight for full-term babies is about 7 pounds (3.2 kg). In general, very small babies and very large babies are at greater risk for problems. Babies are weighed every day in the nursery to look at growth, and the baby's need for fluids and nutrition.
- Newborn babies may often lose 5% to 7% of their birth weight. This means that a baby weighing 7 pounds, 3 ounces at birth might lose as much as 8 ounces in the first few days.
- Babies will usually gain this weight back within the first 2 weeks after birth. Premature and sick babies may not begin to gain weight right away.

Measurements

The hospital staff takes other measurements of each baby. These include:
- **Head circumference:** This is the distance around the baby's head.
- **Abdominal circumference:** This is the distance around the belly (abdomen).
- **Length:** This is the measurement from top of head to the heel.

The staff also checks these vital signs:
- **Temperature:** This checks that the baby is able to have a stable body temperature in a normal room environment.
- **Pulse:** A newborn's pulse is normally 120 to 160 beats per minute.
- **Breathing rate:** A newborn's breathing rate is normally 40 to 60 breaths per minute.

Physical Exam

A complete physical exam is an important part of newborn care. The healthcare provider carefully checks each body system for health and normal function. The provider also looks for any sign of illness or birth defects. Physical exam of a newborn often includes:
- **General appearance:** This looks at physical activity, muscle tone, posture, and level of consciousness.
- **Skin:** This looks at skin color, texture, nails, and any rashes.
- **Head and neck:** This looks at the shape of head, the soft spots (fontanelles) on the baby's skull, and the bones across the upper chest (clavicles).
- **Face:** This looks at the eyes, ears, nose, and cheeks.
- **Mouth:** This looks at the roof of the mouth (palate), tongue, and throat.
- **Lungs:** This looks at the sounds the baby makes when they breathe. This also looks at the breathing pattern.
- **Heart sounds and pulses in the groin (femoral)**
- **Abdomen:** This looks for any masses or hernias.
- **Genitals and anus:** This checks that the baby has open passages for urine and stool.
- **Arms and legs:** This checks the baby's movement and development.

Gestational Assessment

- The healthcare provider will check how mature the baby is. This is an important part of care. This check helps figure out the best care for the baby if the dates of a pregnancy are uncertain.
- For example, a very small baby may actually be more mature than they appear by size and may need different care than a premature baby needs.
- Healthcare providers often use an exam called the Dubowitz/Ballard examination for gestational age. This exam can closely estimate a baby's gestational age.
- The exam looks at a baby's skin and other physical features, plus the baby's movement and reflexes.
- The physical maturity part of the exam is done in the first 2 hours of birth.
- The movement and reflexes part of the exam is done within 24 hours after birth. The provider often uses the information from this exam to help with other maturity estimates.

Physical Maturity

The physical maturity part of the Dubowitz/Ballard exam looks at physical features that look different at different stages of a baby's gestational age. Babies who are physically mature usually have higher scores than premature babies. Points are given for each area of assessment. A low of 1 or 2 means that the baby is very immature. A score of 4 or 5 means that the baby is very mature (postmature). These are the areas looked at:
- **Skin textures:** Is the skin sticky, smooth, or peeling?
- **Soft, downy hair on the baby's body (lanugo):** This hair is not found on immature babies. It shows up on a mature infant but goes away for a postmature infant.

- **Plantar creases:** These are creases on the soles of the feet. They can range from absent to covering the entire foot.
- **Breast:** The provider looks at the thickness and size of breast tissue and the darker ring around each nipple (areola).
- **Eyes and ears:** The provider checks to see if the eyes are fused or open. They also check the amount of cartilage and stiffness of the ears.
- **Genitals, male:** The provider checks for the testes and how the scrotum looks. It may be smooth or wrinkled.
- **Genitals, female:** The provider checks the size of the clitoris and the labia and how they look.

Maturity of Nerves and Muscles

The healthcare provider does 6 checks of the baby's nerves and muscles.

A score is given for each area. Typically, the more mature the baby is, the higher the score. These are the areas checked.

1. **Posture:** This looks at how the baby holds their arms and legs.
2. **Square window:** This looks at how far the baby's hands can be flexed toward the wrist.
3. **Arm recoil.** This looks at how much the baby's arms "spring back" to a flexed position.
4. **Popliteal angle:** This looks at how far the baby's knees extend.
5. **Scarf sign:** This looks at how far the baby's elbows can be moved across the baby's chest.
6. **Heel to ear:** This looks at how near the baby's feet can be moved to the ears.

When the physical assessment score and the nerves and muscles score are added together, the healthcare provider can estimate the baby's gestational age. Scores range from very low for immature babies to very high scores for mature and postmature babies.

HEALTH ASSESSMENT OF TODDLER AND PRESCHOOL CHILD

The preschool child rapidly develops complex social and neurobehavioral capabilities, and the parents often have questions about the child's behavior and social functioning. Knowledge and experience are needed to differentiate normal variations from abnormal behavior. Use this opportunity to observe normal and abnormal growth and development in preschool children, and observe how experienced pediatricians approach these problems.

Weigh, height, head and chest circumference	Toddlers: Gain 4–6 lbs and grow 3 inches in height yearly. Head and chest circumferences are equal at 2 years old. Preschoolers: Gain 5 lbs and grow 2½ to 3 inches in height yearly
Vital signs	Gradual and slight increase in blood pressure and slight decrease in temperature, pulse and respirations

Contd..

Contd..

General Health Survey: Inspect overall appearance Noting: Appropriate growth and development for the child's age	Toddler's general Appearance: "Pot belly" and wide base of support are normal. Preschooler: Loses pot belly and becomes taller and leaner. Detect any delays or premature maturation. Note any obvious weight problems
Integumentary: Inspect skin for lesions	Lesions, such as tinea capitis or (ringworm), need treatment
Inspect hair and scalp for lice	Pediculosis common among preschoolers
Head and face: Inspect head and face	Size of head slows to 1 inch yearly until age 2, and then slows to ½ inch yearly until age 5
Head and face: Palpate anterior fontanel	Closes by 18 months
Eyes: Test visual acuity	Visual acuity is 20/40 during toddler years. Vision screening between 3 to 4 years old. Visual deficits warrant follow-up
Eyes: Test for "lazy eye" (Strabismus) with corneal light reflex or cover-uncover test	Referral needed for strabismus to prevent amblyopia (reduction or dimness in vision)
Ears: Test hearing with pure tone audiometer	Hearing deficits warrant follow-up
Ears: Inspect external ear canal and tympanic membrane	Hearing should be tested between 3 to 4-years-old
Ears: Otoscopic exam (leave until last part of the physical assessment)	High incidence of otitis media
Nose: Inspect the nasal septum and mucosa	Chronic rhinorrhea can result from allergic rhinitis (boggy, bluish-purple, or gray turbinates)
When inspecting the nares or the external ear canal	Foreign objects
Mouth: Inspect oral mucosa and pharynx	Tonsils are generally large
Mouth: Inspect number and condition of teeth	Eruption of primary teeth completed by 2½ years old. Note: Any nursing/baby-bottle caries. Review dental hygiene with parent and child
Neck: Palpate the neck for lymph nodes	Enlarged Lymph nodes may be associated with an infection or lymphoma
Respiratory: Inspect and measure size and shape of chest	Anteroposterior: lateral diameter 1:2 by end of 2nd year
Cardiovascular: Auscultate heart; Note: Rate and rhythm	Children often have a sinus arrhythmia and a split second heart sound. Both the arrhythmia and the split second sound change with respiration. This is a normal variation. Systolic innocent murmurs and venous hum are common findings. If murmur is detected, refer for follow-up to rule out pathology

Contd..

Contd..

Gastrointestinal: Inspect, auscultate and palpate abdomen	A pot belly is normal for a toddler; the condition disappears as the abdominal muscles strengthen
Musculoskeletal: Inspect gait	Toddlers walk alone by 12 to 13 months. Balance is unsteady with wide base of support. Genu valgus or varus may be present. Preschool's gait more balanced, smaller base of support; walks, jumps, climbs by 3-years-old
Musculoskeletal: Test muscle strength	Strength increases during preschool years

HEALTH ASSESSMENT OF SCHOOL GOING CHILD

The goals of the well-child examination in school-aged children (kindergarten through early adolescence) are promoting health, detecting disease, and counseling to prevent injury and future health problems. A complete history should address any concerns from the patient and family, and screen for lifestyle habits, including diet, physical activity, daily screen time (e.g., television, computer, and video games), hours of sleep per night, dental care, and safety habits. School performance can be used for developmental surveillance. A full physical examination should be performed.

Components of School Health Program

Screening, healthcare and referral:
- Screening of general health, assessment of anemia/nutritional status, visual acuity, hearing problems and dental check up.
- Skin conditions, heart defects, physical disabilities, learning disorders, behavior problems.
- Basic medicine kit to be provided to take care of common ailments prevalent among young school going children.
- Referral cards for priority services at district or sub-district hospitals.

History

- During a well-child examination of a school-aged child, the history should include screening questions and address any concerns raised by the child or parents.
- The patient's medical and surgical history, medications, allergies, and family history should be briefly reviewed.
- Social history can be particularly important in this age group. Living situation and lifestyle habits, including diet, physical activity, daily screen time (e.g., television, computer, and video games), hours of sleep per night, and dental care practices should be assessed.
- Physicians should also inquire about safety habits, such as use of protective sports equipment (e.g., helmets), seat belt use, and the presence of firearms in the home.

Physical Examination

A full physical examination should be performed during any health maintenance visit, and is required in a well-child examination for insurance billing. However, one study has shown that physical examination in an asymptomatic, school-aged child will find a new abnormality in less than 4% of patients, and most of these abnormalities are not clinically significant.

HEALTH ASSESSMENT OF ADOLESCENT

Adolescence is a unique time of rapid physical, psychologic, sexual, social, and cognitive growth and development that distinguishes the adolescent and his or her health care needs and expectations from those of the child or adult. Although puberty cannot be precisely defined by chronologic age, the process usually has its onset and completion during the second and the early part of the third decade of life, spanning approximately 10 to 24 years of age. Serious health problems, risky behavior, and poor health habits persist among adolescents despite access to medical care.

Home	Connected, caring parents or family members, acceptance of responsibility, chores, care of siblings or other relatives
Education and employment	Better than average school performance, feelings of connection to school, limited employment (<20 hour/week) Strong participation in extracurricular, school-related activities, including sports
Activities	Leadership among peers Religious affiliation
Drugs	Pledge to abstain Refusal skills
Sexuality	Pledge to abstain Refusal skills Consistently responsible sexual behavior
Suicidality	No personal history of attempted suicide No family history of attempted or accomplished suicide Access to a confidant Successful coping skills Substance free
Safety	Seat belt and helmet use Conflict resolution skills Substance free Refusal to ride in cars with potentially intoxicated driver

Comprehensive History

- An initial health history includes the adolescent's family medical history, the adolescent's own physical and behavioral or mental health and developmental history, immunization history, review of previous and current eating habits or nutrition issues, and a complete review of the adolescent's body systems, and may include menstrual history for females.
- The HEADDSSS (Home, Education/Employment, Eating, Activities, Drugs, Sexuality, Suicide/Depression, and Safety) psychosocial screening tool described later in this section offers one possible way to sequence your questions for adolescents and parents/guardians.

Physical Examination

A complete physical examination is required at each checkup with adolescents undressed and suitably draped. This physical exam includes a review of all body systems. Providers are encouraged to record the patient's pubertal development according to the Tanner Sexual Maturity Rating (SMR) scale (**Tables 3.1 and 3.2** for female and male). Height, weight, and Body Mass Index (BMI), for adolescents must be determined and compared to identify significant deviations from age norms. Due to rising weights in the general population, it is difficult to "eyeball" if a patient is actually overweight. The normal range of BMIs varies significantly. Calculating the patient's BMI and determining his or her percentile depends on age, sex, height, and weight variables.

Nutritional Screening

Dietary practices should be assessed to identify eating habits or possible eating disorders. It is helpful to make a qualitative and quantitative determination of the adolescent's diet. Providers can assess if there is adequate calcium, vitamin D, and iron intake, as well as the amount of "junk food" and "sweet drinks" consumed.

Sensory Screening

Vision and hearing screening must be completed at every checkup. Results of school sensory screenings or results from other providers may be used in place of adolescent vision or hearing screening by a healthcare provider if the school screening occurred within one year of the routine check-up. Results of the screening must be included in the patient record.

Vision screening in adolescence includes screening for visual acuity using an eye chart, such as the Snellen eye chart, at the specific ages required on the Texas Health Steps Periodicity Schedule. Screening is still required at all other visits, but may consist of history and observation.

Hearing screening uses audiometric screening at the specific ages required on the Texas Health Steps Periodicity Schedule. Screening is still required at all other visits, but may consist of history and observation.

Laboratory Screening

Adolescent check-ups can include a variety of laboratory screening procedures, depending on risk.

Anemia: A hemoglobin or hematocrit test should be performed at ages 12 and 16, or if the adolescent is thought to be at risk for anemia.

Hemoglobin type: If the hemoglobin type was performed as a part of newborn screening (NBS) and results are documented on the chart, the test does not need to be repeated. NBS results from dates of service on or after July 12, 2002, are available from the DSHS Laboratory.

Diabetes: A fasting blood glucose (FBG) test of 100–125 mg/dL indicates prediabetes. A reading of 126 mg/dL or higher on two separate occasions indicates diabetes. Also, a random glucose of greater than 200 with symptoms indicates diabetes.

Hyperlipidemia: The most current recommendation is to screen adolescents with a positive family history of dyslipidemia or premature (55 years of age for men and 65 years of age for women), cardiovascular disease (CVD) or dyslipidemia.

TABLE 3.1: Tanner sexual maturity rating (SMR) scale for female.

Tanner stage	Breasts	Pubic hair	Growth	Other
1.	Elevation of papilla only	Villus hair only	2–2.4 inches per year	Adrenarche and ovarian growth
2.	Breast bud under the areola, areola enlargement	Sparse hair along the labia	2.8–3.2 inches per year	Clitoral enlargement, labia pigmentation, growth of uterus
3.	Breast tissue grows but has no contour or separation	Coarser hair curled pigmented covers the pubes	3.2 inches per year	Axillary hair, acne
4.	Projection of areola and papilla, secondary mound formation	Adult hair, does not spread to the thigh	2.8 inches per year	Menarche and development of menses
5.	Adult type contour, projection of papilla only	Adult hair, spreads to the medial thigh	Cessation of linear growth	Adult genitalia

TABLE 3.2: Tanner sexual maturity rating (SMR) scale for male.

Tanner stage	Genitalia	Pubic hair	Growth	Other
1.	Testes <2.5 cm	Villus hair only	2.0–2.4 inches per year	Adrenarche
2.	Testes 2.5–3.2 cm, thinning and reddening of the scrotum	Sparse hair at penis base	2.0–2.4 inches per year	Decreases in body fat
3.	Testes 3.3–4.0 cm, increase of penis length	Thicker curly hair spreads to the pubis	2.8–3.2 inches per year	Gynecomastia, voice break, increased muscle mass
4.	Testes 4.1–4.5 cm, penis growth darkening of scrotum	Adult hair does not spread to thighs	4.0 inches per year	Axillary hair, voice change, acne
5.	Testes >4.5 cm, adult genitalia	Adult hair spreads to medial thigh	Deceleration, cessation	Facial hair, muscle mass increases

COMPREHENSIVE HEALTH ASSESSMENT

A comprehensive health assessment gives nurses insight into a patient's physical status through observation, the measurement of vital signs and self-reported symptoms. It includes a medical history, a general survey and a complete physical examination.

The general survey consists of a patient's age, weight, height, build, posture, gait and hygiene. Nurses use health assessments to obtain baseline data about patients and to build a rapport with them that can ease anxiety and lead to a trusting relationship.

A comprehensive health assessment is generally conducted at the time of admission into an acute care facility or during the first visit to an outpatient clinic. When nurses perform an assessment, they may use techniques as described in below box:

ADULT HEALTH ASSESSMENT

Review of systems
Height, weight, vital signs, and temperature

Pulmonary System
- Upper or lower respiratory disease or infections (acute or chronic)
- Dyspnea (at rest or exertional), pain in sinus, nose, throat, or chest; congestion or discharge from nose (rhinorrhea, epistaxis, snoring); hemoptysis; cough (productive or nonproductive with sputum characteristics); hoarseness; olfactory perception; wheezing; abnormal breath sounds

Cardiovascular System
- Heart disease (chronic, acute, congenital), vascular disease (hypertension, arterial or venous circulatory disorders)
- Chest, arm, throat or jaw pain; leg pain or claudication; paresthesias; edema; varicosities or ulcer; dyspnea (exertion, nocturnal); palpitations; orthopnea; murmur; abnormal heart sounds

Neurologic System
- Neuromuscular or neurosensory conditions; head or spinal trauma; seizure activity; vertigo or syncope; headache; tremors or spasms; paralysis; paresis; paresthesias
- Mentation changes (memory, orientation, level of consciousness); motor changes (gait, coordination)
- Sensory perception changes (touch, taste, smell, vision, hearing); presbycusis; presbyopia; tinnitus; eye or ear pain or drainage; pruritus; photophobia; blurring; diplopia; floaters
- Use of glasses, contact lenses, hearing aid; sleep and rest pattern (rested, fatigue, muscle cramps); speech pattern (aphasia, slurred, alternate speech method)

Inspection: This is the most frequently used method for assessment. Nurses look for indications of a health problem by using their eyes, ears and nose. They may inspect skin color, lesions, bruises or rashes as well as pay attention to abnormal sounds and odors.

Auscultation: Nurses listen to the sounds of the abdomen by placing the diaphragm or bell of a stethoscope on the bare skin of a patient.

Palpation: Nurses apply varying degrees of pressure on the patient with different parts of their hands. Palpation allows nurses to assess for texture, tenderness, temperature, moisture, pulsations and the presence of masses.

Percussion: Nurses firmly press on sections of a patient's body with the distal part the middle finger on their non-dominant hand. The technique is used directly over suspected areas of tenderness to check a patient's level of discomfort.

Head to Toe Examination

After the health history data is recorded, a physical is conducted which covers a review of the patient's body systems. A head to toe examination includes assessments of the following:
- Skin
- Neurological function
- Ears, eyes, nose and throat
- Respiratory function
- Cardiopulmonary system
- Abdomen
- Muscles and joints
- Limbs, shoulders, hips, ankles and feet
- Reproductive system
- Nutrition

A thorough and accurate assessment is important because it helps differentiate the normal condition of the patient from the abnormal. And, a comprehensive health assessment establishes if a patient needs diagnostic testing or additional medical care.

ADULT HEALTH ASSESSMENT

Musculoskeletal System
- Bone or joint disease; fracture; pain or stiffness in joints and muscles; redness; swelling, or heat at joint sites; deformity
- Limited range of motion (ROM) and movement; fatigue; weakness; energy and endurance; ability to perform activities of daily living (ADL) (total, assisted), deficits and use of assistive devices; limb prosthesis; exercise or activity pattern review; rehabilitation services; reaction to disability; Katz index of ADL independence

Integumentary System
Skin color; eruptions; elasticity; turgor; texture; scarring; dryness or moisture; pruritis; alopecia; hair and nails characteristics and changes; corns; calluses; infection; pattern of daily skin, hair, nail care review

Renal/Urinary System
Upper or lower renal tract disorders, urinary pattern review, difficulty in urination (dysuria, dribbling, urgency, frequency, oliguria, nocturia, retention, incontinence), hematuria, calculi, dialysis, urinary tract infection, presence of catheter, 24-hour fluid intake and output, dialysis.

Reproductive System
- Breast male and female genital or organ disorders, sexually transmitted diseases, infection, lesions, discharges, bleeding, pain (testicular, pelvic, dyspareunia)
- Infertility, impotence, pattern of sexual activity and changes, menstrual information (menarche, last period, abnormal bleeding or irregularities, menopause), pregnancies (live births, abortions, complications).

Holistic health assessment of adults and older adults with a focus on physical assessment:
- Comprehensive assessment
- Focused systems assessment

- Ongoing, continuous, and episodic assessment (introduction)
- Vital sign measurement
- Integumentary assessment
- Rest and sleep
- Nursing health history
- Reporting and documenting assessments and nursing care

Psychomotor skills commonly used in nursing practice with adult and older adult clients:
- Hygiene
- Toileting
- Occupied bed making
- Range of motion
- Medication administration
- Specimen collection
- Prevention of complications

Safety
- Safe work practices
  - Falls risk assessment
  - Transfers
  - Positioning
  - Body mechanics
  - Mechanical assists
  - Mobility aids
- Infection transmission precautions
- Handling biohazardous materials
- Cultural safety

Nurse's Role

Consolidation, integration, and application of course and other nursing knowledge in simulated nursing practice experiences.

Concepts relative to health assessment to be explored include:
- Purpose
- Principles
- Engaging with clients
- Planning
- Rationale
- Implementation
- Evaluation
- Preventing complications

Evaluation of Pain

Present health status obtaining information about a patient's present health status allows the nurse to investigate current complaints. The mnemonic, PQRST, utilizes a structured format for information gathering, including evaluation of pain, and provides an efficient methodology to communicate with other healthcare providers. Use PQRST to assess each symptom and after any intervention to evaluate any changes or responses to treatment.

- **P** = Provocative or Palliative: What makes the symptom(s) better or worse?
- **Q** = Quality: Describe the symptom(s).
- **R** = Region or Radiation: Where in the body does the symptom occur? Is there radiation or extension of the symptom(s) to another area of the body?
- **S** = Severity: On a scale of 1-10 (10 being the worst) how bad is the symptom(s)? Another visual scale may be appropriate for patients that are unable to identify with this scale.
- **T** = Timing: Does it occur in association with something else (i.e., eating, exertion, movement)?

HEALTH ASSESSMENT OF ANTENATAL WOMAN

In India, one woman dies every five minutes from pregnancy related causes. Most of these deaths can be prevented or can be avoided if preventive measures are taken and adequate care is available. Maternal death is a tragedy for the individual woman, family and community. In developed countries, the maternal mortality is 27 maternal deaths per 1 lakh live births and in developing countries the ratio is nearly 20 times, i.e., 480 maternal deaths per lakh live births. To reduce the maternal mortality antenatal care can play a very important role. In this practical unit, we will tell you about antenatal examination and how you will perform antenatal examination. Perinatal health assessment is depicted in **Figure 3.4**.

Aims of Antenatal Care

- Ensure normal pregnancy with healthy baby and mother.
- Monitor the progress of pregnancy by conducting regular examination.
- Prepare and encourage the pregnant woman and her family to have a healthy psychological adjustment to child bearing.
- Prevent and detect any complication at the earliest and provide care as required.
- Provide need based health education an all aspects of antenatal care and importance of planned parenthood.
- Prepare the mother for confinement and postnatal care and child rearing.

History-taking

A detailed history of the woman needs to be taken to:
- Confirm the pregnancy (first visit only).
- Identify whether there were complications during any previous pregnancy/confinement that may have a bearing on the present one.
- Identify any current medical/surgical or obstetric condition(s) that may complicate the present pregnancy.
- Menstrual history to calculate the Expected Date of Delivery (EDD)
- Ask her about the nausea and vomiting/heartburn/constipation/increased frequency of urination

Ask about symptoms indicating complications:
- Fever
- Persistent vomiting
- Abnormal vaginal discharge/itching
- Palpitations, easy fatigability
- Breathlessness at rest/on mild exertion

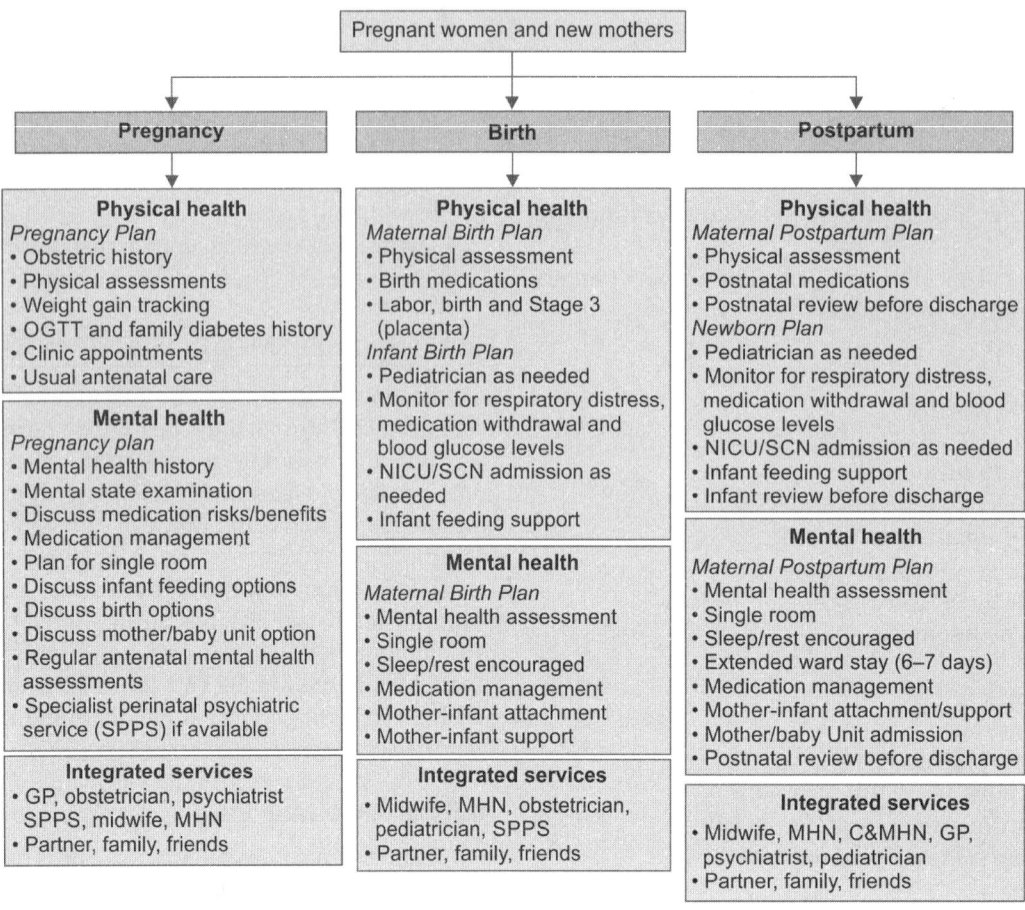

Fig. 3.4: Perinatal health assessment.

- Generalized swelling of the body, puffiness of the face
- Severe headache and blurring of vision
- Passing smaller amounts of urine and burning sensation during micturition
- Vaginal bleeding
- Decreased or absent fetal movement
- Leaking of watery fluid per vaginum (P/V)

Ask about her previous pregnancies or obstetric history:
- Ask about the number of previous pregnancies. Confirm whether they were all live births, and if there was any stillbirth, abortion or any child who died.
- Ascertain the date and outcome of each event, along with the birth weight, if known. Find out if there was any adverse perinatal (period between 7 days before birth and 28 days after birth) outcome.
- Obtain information about any obstetric complications and events in the previous pregnancies—Recurrent early abortion/postabortion complications/hypertension, pre-eclampsia or eclampsia/antepartum hemorrhage (APH)/breech or transverse presentation/obstructed labor, including dystocia/perineal injuries/tears/excessive bleeding after delivery/puerperal sepsis.
- Ascertain whether the woman has had any obstetrical operations (cesarean sections/instrumental delivery/vaginal or breech delivery/manual removal of the placenta).
- Ask for a history of blood transfusions.

History of any current systemic illness/past history of illness:
- High blood pressure (hypertension)
- Diabetes
- Breathlessness on exertion, palpitations (heart disease)
- Chronic cough, blood in the sputum, prolonged fever (tuberculosis)
- Renal disease
- Convulsions (epilepsy)
- Attacks of breathlessness or asthma
- Jaundice
- Malaria
- Other illnesses, e.g., reproductive tract infection (RTI), sexually transmitted infection (STI) and HIV/AIDS. Family history of systemic illness
- History of intake of habit-forming or harmful substances. chews or smokes tobacco and/or takes alcohol.

General Examination

- Pallor
- Pulse
- Respiratory rate
- Jaundice
- Edema
- Blood pressure
- Weight
- Breast examination

Physical Examination

This includes complete systematic examination of each system and assessing its function. Physical measurements include:
- **Height:** Make the woman stand against the wall and measure the height. Average height of an Indian woman is 145–150 cm. Height indicates the pelvic size.
- **Weight:** Weight checking should be done at each visit. Obesity can lead to risk of gestational diabetes. Average weight of an Indian woman in the age group of 25–30 years is 60 kg. During pregnancy the weight increase in the:
    - First trimester: 1 kg.
    - Second trimester and third trimester: 5 kg (2 kg/month)
    - Total weight gain during pregnancy is approximately 11 kg.

  The total weight gain during pregnancy indicates the birth weight of the child a higher than normal increase in weight indicates early manifestation of toxemia. Stationary weight for some period of pregnancy suggests intrauterine growth retardation or intrauterine death. Poor weight gain also indicates fetal abnormality.
- **Blood pressure:** Blood pressure should be recorded during each visit. Any reading above 140/90 should be reported.
- **Vital signs:** Temperature, pulse, respiration to be recorded in each visit.

Components of Antenatal Care

Setting up antenatal clinic with all essential facilities
- Registration
- History taking
- Investigations
- Antenatal examination
- Abdominal examination (obstetric examination)
- Vaginal examination
- Health education on various aspects (family centered maternity care)

Abdominal Examination

- Measurement of fundal height
- Determination of fetal lie and presentation by fundal palpation, lateral palpation and pelvic grips
- Auscultation of the fetal heart sounds
- Inspection of scars/any other relevant abdominal findings

Fundal Height Examination

- 12 weeks—uterus is just about the symphysis pubis
- 18 weeks—uterus half way between the symphysis pubis and umbilicus 20 weeks—above the half way but 2.5 cm below the umbilicus
- 24 weeks—fundus will be present at the upper margin of the umbilicus about 20 cm from the symphysis pubis or 3 finger breadth above 20 weeks.
- 28 weeks—fundus is 1/3rd from the umbilicus to the xiphisternum or 30 cm from the symphysis pubis approximately.
- 32 weeks—2/3rd distance from the umbilicus and xiphisternum, 6 finger above the umbilicus
- 36 weeks—3/3rd distance, which means at the level of xiphisternum approximately 35 cm or 13-14 inches
- 40 weeks—mostly lightening takes place and uterus descends down to the level of 32 weeks

Breast Changes

Normal changes during pregnancy:
- 3–4 weeks—pricking and tingling sensation
- 6 weeks—enlarged, tense, painful
- 8 weeks—Bluish surface, veins visible
- 8–12 weeks—Montgomery glands become prominent on the areola
- 16 weeks—Colostrum can be expressed

Back and Spine

- Observe the back and spine for any deformity
- Observe the symmetry of the rhomboids of Michaelis which is a diamond shaped area formed anteriorly by the fifth lumbar vertebra laterally by the dimples, of the superior iliac spine and posteriorly by the gluteal cleft.

Laboratory Investigations

- Urine pregnancy test
- Blood investigations for hemoglobin estimation and blood grouping including Rh factor
- Urine test to assess the presence of sugar and proteins
- Rapid test for malaria and syphilis.

Nurse's Role

- At every antenatal visit you should assess all pregnant women for signs and symptoms of poor nutrition or iodine deficiency, including pallor, lack of energy and goiter.
- Most women gain 9–12 kg during a normal pregnancy, but weight gain is not a reliable indicator of pregnancy outcome. Sudden weight gain near the end of pregnancy is a warning of possible pre-eclampsia and the woman should be referred to a health center.
- Fever (a temperature of above 37.5°C) should be treated initially with fluids, paracetamol and cold sponging. Refer a pregnant woman to a health center if her temperature stays high. She needs to be screened for infections such as malaria.
- If the pulse rate rises above 100 beats per minute, it is a sign of ill health and the woman needs referral to a health center.
- Signs and symptoms of anemia include pallor, tiredness, fast pulse and shortness of breath.
- Shortness of breath is usual near the end of pregnancy as the growing baby crowds the mother's lungs. Refer her if it causes major discomfort.

- If the blood pressure of a pregnant woman reaches 140/90 mm Hg or higher, she has hypertension. All hypertension in pregnancy is a serious illness, which requires immediate referral to a health center.
- Abnormal vaginal discharge, itching or swelling of the external genitalia, and burning or pain when urinating or during sex, are symptoms of vaginal infection, and the woman should be referred.

Micro-Birth Planning and Counseling

- Registration of pregnant woman and filling up of the Maternal and Child Protection Card and JSY card/below poverty line (BPL) certificates/necessary proofs or certificates for the purpose of keeping a record.
- Informing the woman about the dates of antenatal visits, schedule for TT injections and the Expected Date of Delivery.
- Identifying the place of delivery and the person who would conduct the delivery.
- Identifying a referral facility and the mode of referral.

HEALTH ASSESSMENT OF POSTNATAL WOMAN

Conventionally, the first 42 days (six weeks) after delivery are considered the postpartum period. The first 48 hours of the postpartum period, followed by the first one week, are the most crucial period for the health and survival both of the mother and her newborn. Most of the fatal and near-fatal maternal and neonatal complications occur during this period. Evidence has shown that more than 60% of maternal deaths take place during the postpartum period. Ensuring postnatal care during this period is hence important for identification and management of emergencies occurring during postnatal period.

Postnatal Check-up Schedule

- First visit—If the delivery has not happened in the health center, the first visit is to be within 24 hours of delivery.
- Second visit - 3rd day after delivery
- Third visit - 7th day after delivery
- Fourth visit - 6 weeks after delivery

First Visit for Mother

- **History-taking:**
  - Place of delivery
  - Person who conducted the delivery
  - History of any complications during the delivery/bleeding per vaginum/convulsions or loss of consciousness
  - Pain in the legs/abdominal pain/fever/dribbling or retention of urine/any breast tenderness, etc.
  - Initiation of breastfeeding the baby
  - Has she started her regular diet?
  - Are there any other complaints?
- **Examination:**
  - Pulse, blood pressure, temperature and respiratory rate
  - Presence of pallor
  - Abdominal examination
  - Examine vulva and perineum for the presence of any tear, swelling or discharge of pus
  - Examine the pad for bleeding to assess if the bleeding is heavy, and also see if the lochia is healthy and does not smell foul
  - Examine the breasts for any lumps or tenderness, check the condition of the nipples and observe breastfeeding
- **Management/Counseling:**
  - Postpartum care and hygiene
  - Nutrition
  - Contraception
  - Registration of birth
  - Iron and folic acid (IFA) supplementation
  - Breastfeeding

First Visit for Baby

- **History-taking:**
  - When did the child pass urine and meconium?
  - Has the mother started breastfeeding the baby and are there any difficulties in breastfeeding?
  - Fever
  - Not suckling well
  - Difficulty in breathing
  - Umbilical cord is red or swollen, or is discharging pus
  - Movements of the newborn are less than normal
  - Skin infection (pustules)—red spots which contain pus or a big boil
  - Convulsions.
- **Examination:**
  - Count the respiratory rate for one minute
  - Look for severe chest indrawing
  - Check the baby's color for pallor/jaundice/central cyanosis (blue tongue and lips)
  - Check the baby's body temperature
  - Examine the umbilicus for any bleeding, redness or pus
  - Examine for skin infection
  - Examine the newborn for cry and activity
  - Examine the eyes for discharge
  - Examine for congenital malformations and any birth injury.
- **Management/Counseling:**
  - Maintain hygiene while handling the baby
  - Delay the baby's first bath to beyond 24 hours after birth.
  - Maintain body temperature.
  - Should not apply anything on the cord, and must keep the umbilicus and cord dry.
  - Should observe the baby while breastfeeding and try to ensure proper/good attachment.

Second and Third Visits for Mother

- **History-taking:** Apart from the questions asked during the first visit, also ask about the following:

- Continued bleeding P/V - occurring 24 hours or more after delivery
- Foul-smelling vaginal discharge
- Fever
- Swelling (engorgement) and/or tenderness of the breast
- Any pain or problem while passing urine (dribbling or leaking)
- Fatigue/'not feeling well'
- Unhappiness/cry easily - postpartum depression
- **Examination:**
  - Pulse, blood pressure and temperature
  - Check for pallor
  - Conduct an abdominal examination to see if the uterus is well-contracted
  - Examine the vulva and perineum for the presence of any swelling or pus
  - Examine the pad for bleeding and lochia
  - Examine the breasts for the presence of lumps or tenderness
  - Check the condition of the nipples.
- **Management/Counseling:**
  - Diet and rest
  - Contraception

Second and Third Visits for Baby

- **History-taking:** Same questions as during the first postpartum visit
- **Examination:** Observe the baby for the following:
  - Whether he/she is sucking well
  - If there is difficulty in breathing (fast or slow breathing and chest indrawing)
  - If there is fever or the baby is cold to the touch.
  - If there is jaundice (yellow palms and soles)
  - Whether the cord is swollen or there is discharge from it
  - If the baby has diarrhea with blood in the stool
  - If there are convulsions or arching of the baby's body.
- **Management/Counseling:** In addition to what was provided during the first visit counsel:
  - Exclusively breastfeed the baby for six months.
  - Should feed the baby on demand or every 2 hours
  - Supplementary foods should be introduced at 6 months of age, while breastfeeding can continue simultaneously.
  - Baby's weight loss
  - Hygiene of the baby
  - When and where to seek help in case of signs of illness
  - Immunization.

Fourth Visit for Mother

- **History-taking:** Ask the mother the following:
  - Has the vaginal bleeding stopped
  - Has her menstrual cycle resumed
  - Is there any foul-smelling vaginal discharge
  - Does she have any pain or problem while passing urine (dribbling or leaking)
  - Does she get easily fatigued and/or 'does not feel well'
  - Is she having any problems with breastfeeding
- **Examination:** It includes the following:
  - Check the woman's blood pressure.
  - Check for pallor.
  - Examine the vulva and perineum for the presence of any swelling or pus.
  - Examine the breasts for the presence of lumps or tenderness.
- **Management/Counseling:**
  - Diet and rest
  - As in the second and third visits, emphasize the importance of nutrition/contraception.

Fourth Visit for Baby

- **History-taking:** Ask the mother the following:
  - Has the baby received all the vaccines recommended so far
  - Is the baby taking breastfeeds well
  - How much weight has the baby gained
  - Does the baby have any kind of problem?
- **Examination:**
  - Check the weight of the baby
  - Check if the baby is active/lethargic.
- **Management/Counseling:**
  - Emphasize the importance of exclusive breastfeeding.
  - Tell the mother that if the baby is having any of the following problems, he/she should be taken immediately to the MO (medical officer) and FRU (First referral unit). The baby is not accepting breastfeeds/The baby looks sick (lethargic or irritable)/The baby has fever or feels cold to the touch/The baby has convulsions/Breathing is fast or difficult/There is blood in the stools/The baby has diarrhea.
  - Counsel the mother on where and when to take the baby for further immunization.

Postpartum Danger Signs in the Woman

She should go to the hospital or health center immediately, day or night. She should not wait if she has any of the following danger signs:
- Vaginal bleeding has increased
- Fits
- Fast or difficult breathing
- Fever and too weak to get out of bed
- Severe headaches with blurred vision
- Calf pain, redness or swelling; shortness of breath or chest pain.

She should go to the health center as soon as possible if she has any of the following signs:
- Swollen, red or tender breasts or nipples
- Problems urinating, or leaking
- Increased pain or infection in the perineum
- Infection in the area of the wound (redness, swelling, pain, or pus in wound site)

- Smelly vaginal discharge
- Severe depression or suicidal behavior (ideas, plan or attempt).

Danger Signs for the Newborn

Advise the mother and family to seek care immediately, day or night. They should not wait if the baby has any of these signs:
- Difficulty in breathing or indrawing
- Fits
- Fever
- Feels cold
- Bleeding
- Not feeding
- Yellow palms and soles of feet
- Diarrhea

The mother and family should go to the health center as soon as possible if a baby has any of the following signs:
- Difficulty feeding (poor attachment, not suckling well)
- Is taking less than 8 feeds in 24 hours
- Pus coming from the eyes or skin pustules
- Irritated cord with pus or blood
- Yellow eyes or skin
- Ulcers or thrush (white patches) in the mouth (explain that this is different from normal breast milk in the mouth)

HEALTH ASSESSMENT OF ELDERLY

A health assessment of an older person is an in-depth assessment of a patient aged 75 years and over. It provides a structured way of identifying health issues and conditions that are potentially preventable or amenable to interventions in order to improve health and/or quality of life.

Components of a health assessment for a person aged 75 years and older

The health assessment must include:
- Information collection, including taking a patient history and undertaking or arranging examinations and investigations as required
- Making an overall assessment of the patient
- Recommending appropriate interventions
- Providing advice and information to the patient
- Keeping a record of the health assessment, and offering the patient a written report about the health assessment, with recommendations about matters covered by the health assessment

Specific components of the health assessment for older people include:
- Measurement of the patient's blood pressure, pulse rate and rhythm
- An assessment of the patient's medication
- An assessment of the patient's continence
- An assessment of the patient's immunization status for influenza, tetanus and Pneumococcus
- An assessment of the patient's physical function, including the patient's activities of daily living, and whether or not the patient has had a fall in the last 3 months
- An assessment of the patient's psychological function, including the patient's cognition and mood, and
- An assessment of the patient's social function, including the availability and adequacy of paid and unpaid help, and whether the patient is responsible for caring for another person.

Major Components

Core components of comprehensive geriatric assessment (CGA) **(Fig. 3.5)** that should be evaluated during the assessment process are as follows:
- Functional capacity
- Fall risk
- Cognition
- Mood
- Polypharmacy
- Social support
- Financial concerns
- Goals of care
- Advance care preferences

Additional components may also include evaluation of the following:
- Nutrition/weight change
- Urinary continence
- Sexual function
- Vision/hearing
- Dentition
- Living situation
- Spirituality

Functional Status

- Functional status refers to the ability to perform activities necessary or desirable in daily life.
- Functional status is directly influenced by health conditions, particularly in the context of an elder's environment and social support network.
- Changes in functional status (e.g., not being able to bathe independently) should prompt further diagnostic evaluation and intervention.
- Measurement of functional status can be valuable in monitoring response to treatment and can provide prognostic information that assists in long-term care planning.

Activities of daily living: An older adult's functional status can be assessed at three levels: basic activities of daily livings (BADLs), instrumental or intermediate activities of daily livings (IADLs), and advanced activities of daily living (AADLs). BADLs refer to self-care tasks which include:
- Bathing
- Dressing
- Toileting
- Maintaining continence
- Grooming
- Feeding
- Transferring

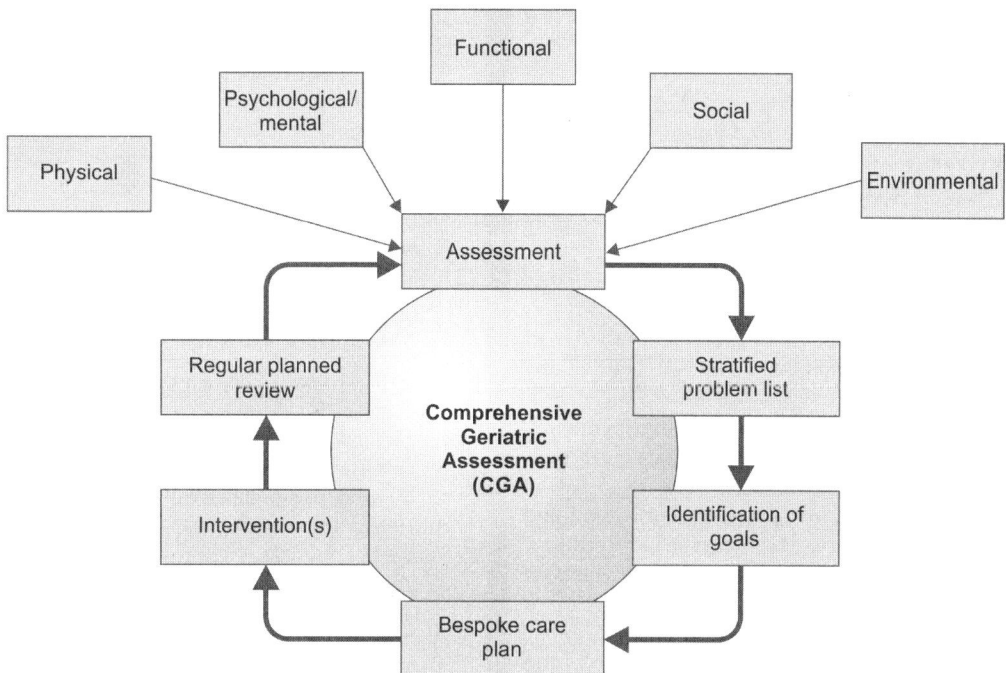

Fig. 3.5: Comprehensive geriatric assessment: Gold standard.

IADLs refer to the ability to maintain an independent household which include:
- Shopping for groceries
- Driving or using public transportation
- Using the telephone
- Performing housework
- Doing home repair
- Preparing meals
- Doing laundry
- Taking medications
- Handling finances

Other possible IADLs that reflect the increased reliance on technology, which have not been validated, include:
- Ability to use a cellphone or smartphone
- Ability to use the internet
- Ability to keep a schedule of activities

AADLs vary considerably from individual to individual. These advanced activities include the ability to fulfill societal, community, and family roles as well as participate in recreational or occupational tasks.

ROLE OF NURSE IN HEALTH ASSESSMENT

The professional nurse plays a vital role in the assessment of patient problems. Educational preparation and the clinical setting in part determine the extent to which the nurse participates in the assessment process. For example, a nurse in primary care may perform a comprehensive physical assessment of patients, while a critical care nurse may conduct selected patient assessments to monitor and evaluate current health problems. In either case, nurses are expected to be familiar with and comfortable using physical assessment skills. Today's nurses are sophisticated professionals who require information in order to make clinical decisions.

RECORDING OF HEALTH ASSESSMENT

Assessment is the first step is the nursing process. In this step, nurse systematically collects verifies, analysis and communicates data about the client's health status. It focuses on gathering the data about a client's state of well-being, functional ability, physical status, strengths and responses to actual and potential health problems. Recording of collected data should be done systematically. It saves time, energy and manpower by helping the nurse to make right diagnosis and treatment.

CONCLUSION

A physically healthy person has certain special characteristics which will help us to understand the reason behind his good physical health and wellness. He displays normal weight and no signs of any sickness or illness. His respiration cycles are normal and health easily gets reflected through his skin, hair and eyes. His flexibility is good and grip is not loosened. He displays symmetrical features and other bodily functions are very normal as all the organs function efficiently. These key traits or special characteristics are only present in a physically healthy individual.

BIBLIOGRAPHY

1. Ardel SB. Assessing the Needs in "The Health Planner's Toolkit. Ontario: System Intelligence Project, Ministry of Health and Long-Term Care.
2. Barnes HV. Disorders of adolescent growth and development. In: Stein JH, ed, Internal medicine. 2nd ed. Boston: Little, Brown, 1987.
3. Brady MA, Starr NB, Blosser CG. Pediatric primary care. 4th ed. St. Louis, MO: Saunders Elsevier; 2009.
4. Chiocca EM. Advanced pediatric assessment/Ellen M. Chiocca (1st ed.): Philadelphia, Lippincott William and Wilkins; 2011.
5. Cibula DA, Novick LF, Morrow CB, Sutphen SM. Community health assessment. Am J Prev Med. 2003;24(4 Suppl):118-23.

3. Shift assessment.
4. Focused assessment.
5. Purposes of assessment.
6. Characteristics of healthy personalities.
7. Apgar scoring.
8. Nutritional screening.
9. Vision and hearing screening.
10. Aims of antenatal care.
11. Components of antenatal care.
12. Postpartum danger signs in the woman.

Multiple Choice Questions

1. The process in which diseases detect early in people that may look and feel well is called:
   a. Medical assessment
   b. Disease assessment
   c. Investigation of disease
   d. Health assessment
2. Nurses use physical assessment skills to:
   a. To identify and manage a variety of patient problems
   b. To discharge the patient from hospital
   c. To collect the health history
   d. To realize the patient importance to relatives
3. When a client have a complain of sever headache a nurse assess that it is:
   a. Objective data   b. Subjective data
   c. Client history   d. Chief complain
4. A patient admit in general ward and have a complain of vertigo a nurse check blood pressure and inform to doctor it is called:
   a. Subjective data   b. Take vital sign of client
   c. Health history   d. Objective data
5. The normal range for body temperature is:
   a. 96°F to 98°F   b. 97°F to 99°F
   c. 98°F to 99°F   d. 97°F to 100.4°F
6. A temperature of 103°F is classified as:
   a. Normal   b. Hypopyrexia
   c. Hyperpyrexia   d. Low-grade fever
7. One respiration consists of:
   a. One inhalation
   b. One exhalation
   c. One inhalation and one exhalation
   d. The opening and closing of the valves of the heart
8. The normal respiratory rate of an adult ranges from:
   a. 8 to 16 respirations per minute
   b. 10 to 18 respirations per minute
   c. 12 to 20 respirations per minute
   d. 16 to 22 respirations per minute
9. The abbreviation used to record oxygen saturation as measured by a pulse oximeter is:
   a. SaO_2 b. PCO_2
   c. SpO_2 d. SpO_4
10. Blood pressure is measured in:
    a. Units   b. Degrees
    c. Beats/min   d. Millimeters of mercury
11. Over which artery is the stethoscope placed when taking blood pressure:
    a. Radial   b. Brachial
    c. Apical   d. Femoral

REVIEW QUESTIONS

Long Essays

1. Enumerate the purposes and factors affecting health assessment.
2. Describe the principles of health assessment.
3. Explain in detail about health assessment of infant.
4. Health assessment of toddler and preschool child.
5. Head to toe examination.

Short Essays

1. Pre-requisites to assessment.
2. Responsibilities of nurse in health assessment.
3. Characteristics of a healthy individual.
4. Assessments for newborn babies.
5. Health assessment of school going child.
6. Health assessment of adolescent.
7. Comprehensive health assessment.
8. Health assessment of antenatal woman.
9. Health assessment of postnatal woman.
10. Health assessment of elderly.
11. Role of nurse in health assessment.
12. Recording of health assessment.

Short Answers

1. Community health assessment (CHA).
2. Admission assessment.

ANSWERS

| 1. d | 2. a | 3. b | 4. d | 5. c | 6. c | 7. c | 8. c | 9. c | 10. d | 11. b |

4 Principles of Epidemiology and Epidemiological Methods

> **LEARNING OBJECTIVES**
> 1. Definition and aims of epidemiology, communicable and noncommunicable diseases
> 2. Basic tools of measurement in epidemiology
> 3. Uses of epidemiology
> 4. Disease cycle
> 5. Spectrum of disease
> 6. Levels of prevention of disease
> 7. Disease transmission—direct and indirect
> 8. Immunizing agents, immunization and national immunization schedule
> 9. Control of infectious diseases
> 10. Disinfection

TERMINOLOGY

Incidence: Number of people developing the disease during a defined time period per 1000 population.

Prevalence: Number of people having disease at a given point of time (point prevalence) or during a defined time period (period prevalence) per 1000 population. The number consists of all cases including new and old ones.

Rate: Number of occurrences of an event per unit time. It is the time fraction in which all cases contributing to numerator are also counted in denominator. Denominator is the entire population at risk. Rates are generally expressed as per 1000.

Case: A person identified as having a particular disease, behavior or condition. Cases may be divided into possible, probable and definite depending on how well a set of specific criteria is satisfied.

Carrier: Presence of a specific infectious agent in the absence of clinical disease. A carrier serves as potential source for further transmission of disease in the community. Temporary carrier state lasts for less than six months. Chronic carrier state may last lifelong.

Contact: Exposure to a source of an infection. Transmission due to direct contact may occur when skin or mucous membranes touch, as in body contact, kissing and sexual intercourse. Disease transmitted by contact is also known as contagious disease.

Reservoir: Reservoir of infection means the natural habit of an infectious agent where the infectious agent may survive or multiply. It may be human, animal or inanimate environment such as soil.

Pathogen: A microorganism capable of causing disease is a pathogen; those that do not cause disease and are part of the normal flora are known as nonpathogens. Opportunistic pathogens are microbes, which are capable of causing disease only when the host resistance is compromised.

Epidemic: Occurrence of a disease in a community area, clearly in excess of what is expected. This is also referred to as an outbreak. A worldwide epidemic is known as pandemic.

Eradication: Extermination of an infectious agent resulting in cessation of transmission of infection altogether from given area.

INTRODUCTION

Epidemiology is the study of the distribution and determinants of disease frequency in human populations. Interest in frequency or occurrence of disease derives largely from a basic tenet of epidemiology, namely that disease does not develop at random. In essence, all persons are not equally likely to develop a particular disease. The level of risk for different individuals typically is a function of their personal characteristics and environment. The epidemiologist's perspective of the relationship between exposure to risk factors and the development of disease in human populations may appear rather crude in comparison to exacting research performed at the molecular level. Indeed, epidemiology is not particularly useful for characterizing the precise biologic mechanisms of disease development.

HISTORY OF EPIDEMIOLOGY AND POPULATION HEALTH

- 1849–54: John Snow formed and tested the hypothesis on the origin of cholera in London—one of the first studies in analytic epidemiology
- 1910: Flu pandemic

- 1920: Goldberger published a descriptive field study showing the dietary origin of pellagra
- 1940s: Fluoride supplements added to public water supplies in randomized community trials
- 1949: Initiation of the Framingham study of risk factors for cardiovascular disease
- 1950: Epidemiological studies link cigarette smoking and lung cancer, demonstrating the power of case-control study design
- 1954: Field trial of the Salk polio vaccine—the largest formal human experiment
- 1959: Mantel and Haenszel develop a statistical procedure for stratified analysis of case-control studies
- 1960: McMahon published the first epidemiologic text with a systematic focus on study design
- 1964: US Surgeon General's report on smoking and health establish criteria for evaluation of causality
- 1970: Large community-based trials implemented, such as North Karelia and Stanford Three Communities; worldwide eradication of smallpox
- 1980: Chronic disease, injury and occupational epidemiology; HIV epidemic
- 1990: Behavioral risk factor epidemiology; prevention of adverse health outcomes through policies and regulations; national programs in breast and cervical cancer prevention; tobacco epidemiology; emerging infectious diseases; criticism of epidemiology for being inconsequential ('small' risk ratios); standardization of surveillance methods; bovine spongiform encephalopathy (BSE), also known as mad cow disease in England and Europe; variant Creutzfeldt-Jacob disease (vCJD); aging of USA; disaster epidemiology
- 2000: Genetic and molecular epidemiology; health disparities; racialism; HIPAA in the USA; West Nile Virus - bioterrorism; anthrax and smallpox threat and vaccinations
- 2003: SARS, quarantines and public health law; and worldwide epidemiology; BSE in Canada—SARS recurrence; BSE in the USA; the flu epidemic
- 2009: H1N1 pandemic

CONCEPT OF EPIDEMIOLOGY (FIG. 4.1)

Epidemiology is a compound of three Greek words 'epi' meaning upon, 'demos' meaning people, and 'logos', meaning science. Thus on etymological basis, epidemiology is a science that deals with mass phenomena. This "definition" though not precise, is sufficiently broad-based to suit the expanding scope of epidemiology.

- Epidemiologists are concerned not only with death, illness, and disability, but also with more positive health status and, most importantly, with the means to improve health.
- The term "disease" encompasses all unfavorable health changes, including injuries and mental health.
- In simple terms, epidemiology is the study of how the disease is distributed in populations and the factors that influence or determine this distribution.
- Epidemiology is the study of the distribution and determinants of diseases within human populations. Research in this field is based primarily upon observing people directly in their natural environments.
- Epidemiology can be used for descriptive purposes, such as surveillance of the occurrence (incidence) of a particular illness.
- Epidemiology can be used for analytic purposes, such as studying risk factors for disease development.
- Epidemiologic methods can be used to assess the performance of diagnostic tests.
- Epidemiology can be used to study the progression or natural history of a disease.
- Epidemiologic methods can be used to study prognostic factors, which are determinants of the progression of a disease.
- Epidemiology can be used to evaluate treatments for a disease.

DEFINITIONS

Epidemiology has no single definition to which all epidemiologists subscribe; three components are common

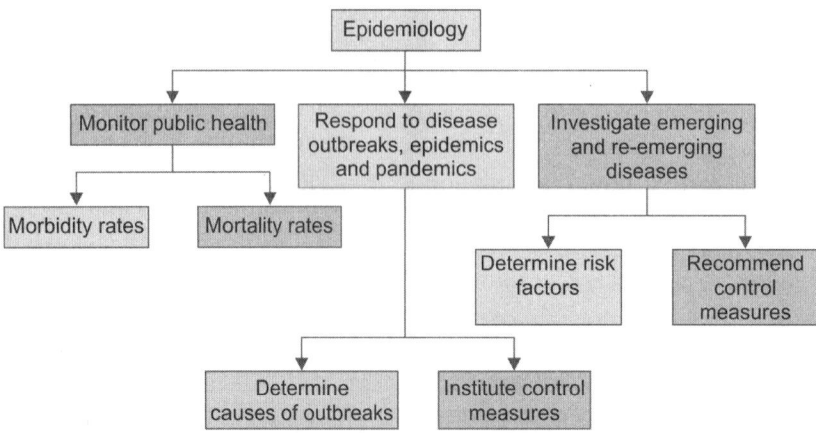

Fig. 4.1: Concept of epidemiology.

to most of them. First, studies of disease frequency; second, studies of the distribution and third, studies of the determinants.
- Epidemiology is a branch of medical science which treats of epidemics—Park, 1873.
- Epidemiology is the branch of science which deals with the mass phenomena of infectious diseases—Frost, 1927.
- Epidemiology is the study of the disease, any disease as a mass phenomenon—Greenwood, 1934.
- Epidemiology is the study of the distribution and determinants of disease frequency in man—McMahon, 1960.
- Epidemiology is defined as the study of the distribution and determinants of health-related states of events in specified populations and the application of this study to the control of health problems—John M Last, 1988.
- Epidemiology is the study of various factors and conditions that determine the occurrence and distribution of health, disease, defect, disability and death among groups of individuals—Clark, 1965.
- Epidemiology is the study of the distribution of a disease or a physiological condition in human population and of the factors that influence this distribution—Lilienfeld, 1980.

AIMS OF EPIDEMIOLOGY

According to the International Epidemiological Association, Epidemiology has three main aims.
1. To describe the distribution and size of disease problems in human populations.
2. To identify etiological factors in the pathogenesis of disease.
3. To provide the data essential to the planning, implementation, and evaluation of services for the prevention, control and treatment of disease and to the setting up of priorities among these services. The ultimate aim of epidemiology is to lead to effective action to eliminate or reduce the health problems or its consequences and to prevent its occurrence in future.

In brief, epidemiology is said to be concerned with all health and illness in population groups and with the factors including health services that affect them. The aims of epidemiology include knowledge of distribution of disease in order to elucidate causal mechanisms, explain local disease occurrence, describe the natural history of a disease, and provide guidance in the administration of health services. The following are human characteristics that are of concern to epidemiologists:
- Biological characteristics such as biochemical level of blood, including antibodies and enzymes; cellular constituents of the blood; and measurement of physiological functions of different organ systems of the body.
- Demographic characteristics such as age, sex, race, and ethnic group.
- Social and socioeconomic characteristics such as status, education, occupation and nativity.
- Personal living habits such as tobacco use, diet and exercises.

Factors other than personal characteristics useful in epidemiology for administrative purposes for the study of the etiology of disease include place or geography of the existence of an illness and its time or secularity. The interaction between person, place and time are also important in studying the causes of disease.

FUNCTIONS/USES OF EPIDEMIOLOGY

- To find causation of the disease
- To describe natural history
- Description of health status of populations
- Evaluation of intervention
- Community diagnosis
- Planning and evaluation
- Syndrome identification

OBJECTIVES OF EPIDEMIOLOGY

- To identify the etiology, or cause, of a disease and its relevant risk factors (i.e., factors that increase a person's risk for a disease)
- To intervene to reduce morbidity and mortality from the disease.
- To develop a rational basis for prevention programs based on identified etiologic or causal factors.
- To work on to reduce or eliminate exposure to those factors.
- To develop appropriate vaccines and treatments, that can prevent the transmission of the disease to others?
- To determine the extent of disease found in the community
- To help plan health services and facilities for effective healthcare facilities.
- To study the natural history and prognosis of the disease
- To define the baseline natural history of a disease in quantitative terms so that as we develop new modes of intervention, either through treatments or through new ways of preventing complications.
- To help compare the results of using new modalities with the baseline data to determine whether new approaches have truly been effective.
- To evaluate both existing and newly developed preventive and therapeutic measures and modes of healthcare delivery.
- To help provide the foundation for developing public policy relating to environmental problems, genetic issues, and other social and behavioral considerations regarding disease prevention and health promotion.

COMPONENTS OF EPIDEMIOLOGY

- **Population:** The main focus of epidemiology is on the effect of disease on the population rather than individuals. For example malaria affects many people in Ethiopia but lung cancer is rare. If an individual develops lung cancer, it is more likely that he/she will die. Even though lung cancer is more killer, epidemiology gives more emphasis to malaria since it affects many people.

- **Frequency:** This shows that epidemiology is mainly a quantitative science. Epidemiology is concerned with the frequency (occurrence) of diseases and other health related conditions. Frequency of diseases is measured by morbidity and mortality rates.
- **Health-related conditions:** Epidemiology is concerned not only with disease but also with other health-related conditions because everything around us and what we do also affects our health. Health-related conditions are conditions which directly or indirectly affect or influence health. These may be injuries, births, health related behaviors like smoking, unemployment, poverty, etc.
- **Distribution:** It refers to the geographical distribution of diseases, the distribution in time, and distribution by type of persons affected.
- **Determinants:** Determinants are factors which determine whether or not a person will get a disease.
- **Application of the studies to the promotion of health and to the prevention and control of health problems:** This means the whole aim in studying the frequency, distribution, and determinants of disease is to identify effective disease prevention and control strategies.

TYPES OF EPIDEMIOLOGY

- **Descriptive epidemiology:** Examining the distribution of disease in a population, and observing the basic features of its distribution.
- **Analytic epidemiology:** Investigating a hypothesis about the cause of disease by studying how exposures relate to disease.
- **Experimental epidemiology:** It deals with experimental confirmation of the cause-effect associations upheld by observational studies of analytical epidemiology.
- **Applied epidemiology:** It deals with the use and application of information collected through descriptive, observation and experimental studies.
- **Constructive epidemiology:** It deals with the application of epidemiological methodology in the investigation of epidemics and their management during epidemic and interepidemic phases.

BASIC TOOLS OF MEASUREMENT IN EPIDEMIOLOGY

Incidence

It is number of *NEW* cases occurring in a defined population during a specified period of time.
Formula of incidence: (No. of NEW cases in a defined population during a specified time period)/(Population at risk during the same time period) × 1000

Prevalence

It refers to ALL the cases (old and new) present in a population at a given period of time.
Formula of prevalence: (No. of All cases in a defined population during a specified time period)/(Mid-interval population at risk) × 1000

Uses of 'Incidence'

Incidence can be used:
- As the indicator of health services as it usually responds earlier than prevalence
- In research for 'risk factors' or cause
- For checking the efficacy of therapeutic of preventive measures, e.g., comparing the incidence of disease among the vaccinated and the unvaccinated.

Uses of 'Prevalence'

Prevalence can be used for:
- Measuring the disease burden in the community
- For prioritizing the health problems of the population, e.g., the amounts of TB, leprosy, etc. Indian have made the government give them a higher priority
- It is needed for planning health services, e.g., number of beds needed for the particular disease, amount of medicines needed in the store.

Measurements of Mortality

- Crude death rate (CDR)
- Specific death rates
- Case fatality ratio (CFR)
- Proportional mortality rate (PMR)
- Survival rates
- Standardized death rate (SDR)
- Standardized mortality ratio (SMR)

Formulas for the Above Death Rates

Crude death rate: Number of deaths from any cause, per 1000 population in one year, in a defined population (No. of deaths in one year in a specified area)/(Mid-year population of the specified area during the same year) × 1000

Specific Death Rates

- **Cause specific death rate,** e.g., tuberculosis death rate (No. of deaths due to the cause in one calendar year in a specified area)/(Mid-year population of the specified area during the same calendar year) × 1000
- **Age specific death rate,** e.g., death rate in the reproductive age group (No. of deaths in the age group 15–44 years, in one year in a specified area)/(Mid-year population of the 15–44 years old, during the same year)) × 1000
- **Death rate for a month, e.g., in January** (No. of deaths in January × 12)/(Mid-year population) × 1000
- **Weekly death rate** (No. of deaths in the given week × 52)/(Mid-year population) × 1000
- **Proportional mortality ratio:** [No. of deaths due to the cause (or in a particular group)]/(total no. of deaths during the same year in the same population) × 1000
- **Case fatality ratio (CFR):** (No. of deaths due to the particular disease in one year in a specified area)/(No. of cases diagnosed with the disease in the same year and area) × 1000

PRINCIPLES OF EPIDEMIOLOGY

- Epidemiology is the study of occurrence distribution and causes of disease of mankind. It is mainly concerned with the preventive and social science, an important aspect of community medicine. Epidemiology focuses on population or community to measure the distribution and determinants of disease for the purpose of preventing disease and promoting health.
- Epidemiology approach offers the community health nurses a theoretical basis or framework implementing and evaluating health care at community level.
- Primary purpose epidemiology is disease prevention and early intervention for the maintenance and promotion of health by which the ultimate aim that is the well-being of the society can be achieved.
- Epidemiological difference between infectious and non-infectious diseases mainly depends on the element of time. In comparison to infectious disease, noninfectious diseases have long incubation period and a lower frequency of occurrence.
- Epidemiological process (**Fig. 4.2**) in which the epidemiological investigation takes place in six steps:
    1. Establishing the occurrence of a problem
    2. Verifying the diagnosis
    3. Collecting related data
    4. Describing the occurrence in terms of person, place and time
    5. Formulating a hypothesis
    6. Testing the hypothesis
- Epidemiological study methods can be classified in different ways and there is no strict limitation about any classification.
- Epidemiological measurements are so many criteria or standards are set also used for these measurements. The main measurements have concern with mortality and morbidity.

SCOPE OF EPIDEMIOLOGY

- Epidemiology has very wide scope, wider than what is normally conceived. Besides communicable and noncommunicable diseases, the field of epidemiology covers all other health related states and events such as alcoholism, drug abuse, accidents, divorces, migrations, etc.
- Epidemiology studies the distribution of health-related states and events. The distribution is viewed in three epidemiological dimensions of time, place and person.
- Epidemiology studies the determinants of health-related states and event. These determinants are identified by observing the distribution pattern of diseases and verifying cause-effect relationships.
- Epidemiology finds application in the control of health problems. Having identified the determinants and their cause-effect relationships, epidemiological principles guide the formulation of appropriate interventional strategies for the prevention and control of health problems.

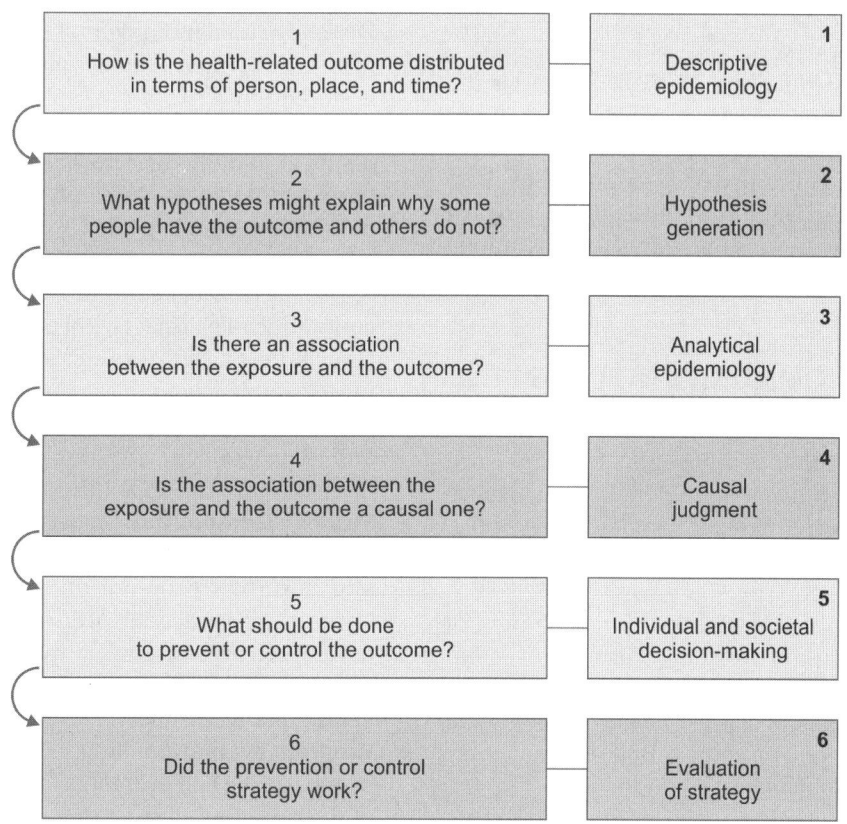

Fig. 4.2: Epidemiological process.

DICHOTOMIES IN EPIDEMIOLOGICAL STUDIES

When designing epidemiologic studies, choices must be made about the role of the investigator, the purpose of the study, the hypothesis regarding exposure, and the unit of analysis. Here are some examples:

Role of Investigator

- **Observational:** The investigator does not manipulate the exposure of participants to risk factors. Most epidemiological studies are observational.
- **Experimental:** According to the study design, the investigator manipulates the exposure of participants to some factor. Clinical trials and intervention studies are examples of such experiments. If the study participants themselves act to change their exposure to an influence, a *natural experiment* may occur. For example, a study of persons who have migrated from one environment to another could constitute a natural experiment.

Purposes of the Study

- **Descriptive:** Describes the distribution of disease by time, place, person; used to generate hypotheses of disease causation or for health planning
- **Analytic:** Measures and tests the association between a hypothesized risk factor and a disease.

Hypothesized Effect of Exposure

- **Harmful:** Exposure increases risk or presence of disease
- **Beneficial:** Exposure reduces risk or presence of disease.

Unit of Analysis

- **Individual:** The individual (e.g., person, animal) is the unit of analysis; potential to ignore the impact of the community or group effect on individual risk
- **Community:** The community (e.g., county, hospital) is the unit of analysis. There is potential for ecological fallacy in such studies. Lacking individual data, assuming that individuals perform similarly to the average of the group may not be true.

EPIDEMIOLOGY IN COMMUNITY NURSING

Epidemiology and nursing are important for the attainment of optimal health of the individuals, families and communities. But the approach may be different to achieve this goal. Nursing is as old as mankind. Epidemiology is also an older concept that is found in the health field since third century BC.

Epidemiology aims at describing the occurrence of disease, risk identification and providing data for prevention and control. Community health nursing has the greater concern with the occurrence of disease, health problems and risk factor prevalent in the community. Both epidemiology and nursing needs community participation.

The recent nursing is more inclined to community's healthcare setting, as it is necessary to raise the health status of the individual and the nation. Thus, both epidemiology and nursing are utmost essential in the field of health science. Nursing and epidemiology are closely related, mutually helpful, and inseparable and have coexistence. Epidemiology describes the future trends of disease and recommends the specific control measures, which are based upon the epidemiological studies. Nursing researches also provide the clues and steps for prevention of the diseases. Community health nurse is a key person in the health information system as well as in health management.

USES OF EPIDEMIOLOGY

Epidemiology process is bound to continue in future adding new challenges to the practice of public health. In these circumstances, epidemiology is designed to play an increasingly important role in defining the magnitude of the problems, forecasting their long-term consequences and deriving appropriate strategies for their promotion and control. Presently the use of epidemiology is mainly confined to following areas:

- **Disease antecedents:** Epidemiology has always stressed the importance of exploring the natural history of disease, entirely, with special stress on the identification of disease antecedents rather than disease consequents.
- **Disease correlates:** Epidemiology has revolutionized the concept of etiology and etiogenesis. Epidemiological studies identified a variety of disease correlates not all of which are casually associated diseases and some of which behave as risk factors. The risk factors increase the probability of contracting a particular disease.
- **Disease behavior:** Epidemiological surveillance is applied to disease of international significance. Disease behavior is studied by a process of epidemiological surveillance whereby diseases are kept under constant observation; firstly, to identify their normal distribution patterns and normal temporal fluctuations, and secondly, to detect any deviation in their expected behavior patterns.
- **Disease causation:** Epidemiological studies not only establish cause-effect association of many non-communicable diseases, but also estimate the strength of associations in terms of relative and absolute risks. The most notable example are the cause-effect associations established by epidemiological studies between smoking and lung cancer, and smoking and coronary heart diseases, etc.
- **Strategy formulation:** Epidemiology plays an important role in strategy formulation for disease control programs and improves program efficiency and effectiveness. Control and eradication of disease is much more complex than their prevention or treatment. A sound control strategy is one that is epidemiologically relevant and operationally feasible.
- **Program evaluation:** Program performance is evaluated by measuring achievements in various operational areas of the program. Evaluation of public health program is both managerial and an epidemiological process.

ADVANTAGES OF EPIDEMIOLOGY

- Epidemiology provides framework within which basic science and behavioral science can be used for community nursing practice.
- Epidemiology provides an interdisciplinary language to promote interprofessional communication and trust.
- Public health principle of family is the unit of society. Prevention and control of disease and health promotion are activated and quantifies through epidemiological approach.
- The epidemiologic model promotes understanding the relationship between the environment and agents that expose susceptible populations at risk of impediments to health.
- The epidemiology helps to plan effective need-based healthcare services on the basis of epidemiological information regarding frequencies and distribution of disease and disabilities, their associated factors and causes.
- The epidemiology helps to determine the effectiveness of healthcare services planned and implemented on the basis of predetermined criteria regarding its relevance, effectiveness, efficiency and impact on community health. This can helps to plan better services in future.
- Nursing process is extended through application of epidemiological methods to describe community needs and evaluate nursing services.
- An epidemiological perspective provides a method of extending the relationship of family problems to community welfare.
- The epidemiology helps to identify syndrome by describing the distribution and association of clinical phenomena in the population.
- The epidemiology helps to determine the usefulness and effectiveness of new innovative techniques, measures and programs.

Studies	Advantages	Disadvantages
Qualitative research	Generates hypotheses and initial exploration of issues in participants' own language without bias of investigator	Cannot test study hypotheses Can explore only what is presented or stated Has potential for bias
Cross-sectional surveys	Are fairly quick and easy to perform Are useful for hypothesis generation	Do not offer evidence of a temporal relationship between risk factors and disease Are subject to late-look bias Are not good for hypothesis testing
Ecological studies	Are fairly quick and easy to perform Are useful for hypothesis generation	Do not allow for causal conclusions to be drawn because the data are not associated with individual persons Are subject to ecological fallacy Are not good for hypothesis testing

Contd...

Contd...

Cohort studies	Can be performed retrospectively or prospectively Can be used to obtain a true (absolute) measure of risk Can study many disease outcomes and are good for studying rare risk factors	Are time-consuming and costly (especially prospective studies) Can study only the risk factors measured at the beginning Can be used only for common diseases May have losses to follow-up
Case-control studies	Are fairly quick and easy to perform Can study many risk factors Are good for studying rare diseases	Can obtain only a relative measure of risk Are subject to recall bias Selection of controls may be difficult Temporal relationships may be unclear Can study only one disease outcome at a time
Randomized controlled trials	Are the "gold standard" for evaluating treatment interventions (clinical trials) or preventive interventions (field trials) Allow investigator to have extensive control over research process	Are time-consuming and usually costly Can study only interventions or exposures that are controlled by investigator May have problems related to therapy changes and dropouts May be limited in generalizability Are often unethical to perform at all
Systematic reviews and meta-analysis	Decrease subjective element of literature review Increase statistical power Allow exploration of subgroups Provide quantitative estimates of effect	Mixing poor quality studies together in a review or meta-analysis does not improve the underlying quality of studies
Cost-effectiveness analysis	Clinically important	Difficult to identify costs and payments in many healthcare systems

EPIDEMIOLOGICAL APPROACHES

The epidemiological approach to problems of health and disease is based on two major foundations:
1. Asking questions
2. Making comparisons. The community health nurse or any health worker need to bear in mind always to use what is known as epidemiological approach in the control of communicable diseases, which includes finding out the source of infection. For this, community health nurse needs to have a guide in the following manner of questioning:
   - When did the disease occur?
   - Where did the disease occur?
   - Who were the people affected?
   - Why should it appear?
   - What should be done to prevent the spread?

Asking questions and making observations: Epidemiological studies are done to know the incidence and prevalence of disease in the various subgroups of population by time, place and person.

Epidemiologist asks variety of questions and makes observation related to nature and extend (magnitude) of the problem, geographical distribution (where?) time trends (when?) and personal characteristics of people who get the disease (who?). Answer to these questions would help in finding clues to the determinants of disease, which are further evaluated.

Making comparisons: The basic approach in epidemiology is to make comparisons and draw inferences. This may be comparison of two or more groups—one group having the disease (or exposed to risk factor) and the other groups not having the disease (or not exposed to risk factors), or comparison between individuals. Making comparison is another approach which is very important in epidemiological studies, especially analytical and experimental studies to test etiological hypothesis of various disease and evaluate the effectiveness of preventive and therapeutic measures. The similar group for comparison can be obtained either by random selection method or by matching selected characteristics, which might affect the results and interpretation.

Epidemiological Methods

Epidemiological methods are applied to know the disease etiology. Various epidemiological studies can be conducted to find out the occurrence of disease in people or persons, which may be involved in process of spreading the disease. Epidemiological study methods can be classified in different ways and there are no strict limitations about any complements.

Descriptive Method

This method of epidemiological study is concern with the study of frequency and distribution of disease and health related events in population I terms of person, place and time. Descriptive method is the first phase of an epidemiological investigation. It concerned with observing the distribution of disease or health related characteristics with which the disease in question seems to be associated.

Descriptive epidemiology deals with the distribution of health-related states and events by time, place and person. Distribution of cases by time of their appearance gives the time trend of disease.

The time trends commonly observed are epidemic, seasonal, cyclical and secular.

Objectives of Descriptive Method
- To provide a database for planning, providing and evaluating health services.
- To evaluate the trends in health sector and provide a basis for comparisons among groups.
- To identify problems for further analysis.

Data Collection in Descriptive Method
- Personal characteristics such as age, sex, race, marital status, occupation, education, income, social class, dietary pattern, habits, etc.
- Place distribution of cases, i.e., areas of high concentration, low concentration and spotting cases in the map
- Time distribution trends such as year, season, month, week, day and hour of onset of the disease.

Analytical Method

Analytical studies are more specific in focus, test hypothesis and attempt to determine casual factors of disease. Analytical method is contrast to descriptive studies that look at entire population, in analytical studies the subject of interest is the individuals within the population.

Analytical method is carried out to test the hypothesis. These hypotheses are formulated on the information gathered from the descriptive method.

Approaches of Analytical Method

Case control study: It is often called retrospective study which is the common and first approach to test casual hypothesis. A case control study is a longitudinal, observational enquiry undertaken to verify the existence as well as the strength of cause-effect associations in disease phenomena.

Case control studies are used for:
- Estimating the risk of exposure to various factors associated with disease phenomena.
- Identify the modifiable causal factors that can be arrested in the interest of public health.
- Evolving risk intervention strategies for prevention and control of public health problems.

Cohort study: Cohort study is another type of analytical study, which is usually undertaken to obtain additional evidence to refuse or support the existence of an association between suspected cause and disease. Cohort study is known by variety of names—prospective study, longitudinal study, incidence study and forward-looking study.

Cohort study is useful for:
- Estimating directly the risk of exposure to various factors associated with disease phenomena.
- Exploring the natural history of disease in entirely and identifying additional pathological events to complete the natural history.
- Identifying appropriate outcome events in the natural history of diseases for appropriate intervention for disability limitation.
- Identifying modifiable causal factors for evolving appropriate risk intervention strategies.

Experimental Method

It involves some action intervention or manipulation such as deliberate application or withdrawal of the suspected cause or changing one variable the causative chain in the experimental group while making no change in the control group observing and comparing the outcome of the experiment in both the groups.

An experimental method is a longitudinal interventional process of trial or verification, undertaken to confirm cause-effect relationship of disease phenomena or to evaluate the efficiency of various preventive or curative procedures or programs applicable in hospital or community settings.

Experimental studies are used for:
- Confirming cause effect associations or judging the validity of hypotheses established by observational studies.
- Evaluating various treatment modalities and interventional procedures applicable in hospital situations.
- Evaluating the feasibility, efficacy and relevance of various preventive programs of public health significance.
- Evaluating the feasibility, efficacy and relevance of various risks, intervention approaches of public health importance.

PREVENTIVE EPIDEMIOLOGY

- **Health surveys** are investigation to identify frequency, distribution and the determinants of health-related events or states in the community. Health survey helps in knowing the community and making diagnosis. The health survey can be collected by using questioning, health examination and laboratory investigation, record review and observation.
- **Screening** is testing for infection or disease in population or in individuals who are not seeking healthcare for example serological testing for AIDS virus in blood donors. The screening is used in case detection, control of disease research purposes and provide opportunities for creating public awareness and for educating health professionals.
- **Surveillance:** It means close vigilance on occurrence and distribution of diseases and health-related problems, population dynamics, community behavior and environmental processes, resulting in increased risk of ill health in the community. It involves identification of missed and suspected cases and contacts, their confirmation by laboratory investigations, identifying source of infection and channel of transmission.
- **Monitoring** helps in keeping a continuous tract of health related states or events and accordingly plan replan and take correct measures. Epidemiologically, monitoring is specific and essential part of surveillance.

IMPORTANCE OF EPIDEMIOLOGY

Epidemiology process is bound to continue in future adding new challenges to the practice of public health. In these circumstances epidemiology is designed to play an increasingly important role in defining the magnitude of the problems, forecasting their long-term consequences and deriving appropriate strategies for their promotion and control. Presently the use of epidemiology is mainly confined to following areas:

- **Disease antecedents:** Epidemiology has always stressed the importance of exploring the natural history of disease in their entirely, with special stress on the identification of disease antecedents rather than disease consequents.
- **Disease correlates:** Epidemiology has revolutionized the concept of etiology and etiogenesis. Epidemiological studies identified a variety of disease correlates not all of which are casually associated diseases, and some of which are risk factors. The risk factors increase the probability of contracting a particular disease.
- **Disease behavior:** Epidemiological surveillance is applied to disease of international significance. Disease behavior is studied by a process of epidemiological surveillance whereby diseases are kept under constant observation firstly to identify their normal distribution patterns and normal temporal fluctuations, and secondly to detect any deviation in their expected behavior patterns.
- **Disease and causation:** Epidemiological studies not only establish cause effect association of many noncommunicable diseases, but also estimate the strength of associations in terms of relative and absolute risks. The most notable example is the cause effect associations established by epidemiological studies between smoking and lung cancer and smoking and coronary heart diseases.
- **Strategy formulation:** Epidemiology plays an important role in strategy formulation for disease control programs and improves program efficiency and effectiveness. Control and eradication of disease is much more complex than their prevention or treatment. A sound control strategy is one that epidemiologically relevant and operationally feasible.
- **Program evaluation:** Program performance is evaluated by measuring achievements in various operational areas of the program. Evaluation of public health program is both managerial and epidemiological process.

DISEASE CYCLE

This cycle includes phases of growth, consolidation, change of structure, multiplication/reproduction, spread, and infection of a new host. The combination of these phases is called the development of the pathogen. The transmission of pathogens from current to future host follows a repeating cycle. This cycle can be simple, with a direct transmission from current to future host, or complex, where transmission occurs through (multiple) intermediate hosts or vectors. This cycle is called the transmission cycle of disease, or transmission cycle. The transmission cycle has different elements:

- **Pathogen:** The organism causing the infection
- **Host:** The infected person or animal 'carrying' the pathogen
- **Exit:** The method of the pathogen uses to leave the body of the host
- **Transmission:** How the pathogen is transferred from host to susceptible person or animal, which can include

developmental stages in the environment, in intermediate hosts, or in vectors
- **Environment:** The environment in which transmission of the pathogen takes place
- **Entry:** The method the pathogen uses to enter the body of the susceptible person or animal. The susceptible person or animal. The potential future host who is receptive to the pathogen.

MODES OF DISEASE TRANSMISSION

Communicable disease may be transmitted from the reservoir or source of infection to a susceptible individual in many different ways, depending upon the infectious agent, portal entry and the local ecological conditions.

- **Direct contact:** Infection may be transmitted by direct contact from skin to skin, mucosa to mucosa or mucosa to skin of the same or another person. For example, during touching, kissing, sexual intercourse (STD, AIDS, leprosy, skin infections) and scratching through fingers.
- **Droplet infection:** Droplet infection occurs due to contact transmission by infections agents contained in most respiratory secretions. The microorganisms from nasopharyngeal secretions during coughing, sneezing, speaking and spitting into the surrounding atmosphere (e.g., respiratory infections, TB, meningitis, etc.).
- **Contact with soil:** Infectious agent (microorganisms) present in soil can cause disease, when the host comes into contact with soil (e.g., hookworm, tetanus, etc.)
- **Inoculation into skin or mucosa:** The disease agent may be inoculated directly into the skin or mucosa. Transmission of infection occurs by direct inoculation into skin with syringe, needles or animal bite, e.g., rabies virus infection after dog.
- **Transplacental (vertical):** Transmission of infectious agent can occur transplacentally.

SPECTRUM OF DISEASE

Natural history of disease refers to the progression of a disease process in an individual overtime, in the absence of treatment. For example, untreated infection with HIV causes a spectrum of clinical problems beginning at the time of seroconversion (primary HIV) and terminating with AIDS and usually death. It is now recognized that it may take 10 years or more for AIDS to develop after seroconversion. Many, if not most, diseases have a characteristic natural history, although the timeframe and specific manifestations of disease may vary from individual to individual and are influenced by preventive and therapeutic measures.

The onset of symptoms marks the transition from subclinical to clinical disease. Most diagnoses are made during the stage of clinical disease. In some people, however, the disease process may never progress to clinically apparent illness. In others, the disease process may result in illness that ranges from mild to severe or fatal. This range is called the spectrum of disease. Ultimately, the disease process ends either in recovery, disability or death **(Fig. 4.3)**.

DISEASE CAUSATION

A number of models of disease causation have been proposed. Among the simplest of these is the epidemiologic triad or triangle, the traditional model for infectious disease. The triad consists of an external agent, a susceptible host, and an environment that brings the host and agent together. In this model, disease results from the interaction between the agent and the susceptible host in an environment that supports transmission of the agent from a source to that host.

Cause of Disease

It is an event, condition, characteristic or a combination of these factors which plays an important role in producing the disease. The causes of disease can be classified into two:
1. **Primary causes:** These are the factors which are necessary for a disease to occur, in whose absence the disease will not occur. The term "etiologic agent" can be used instead of primary cause for Infectious causes of diseases. For example "*Mycobacterium tuberculosis*" is the primary cause (etiologic agent) of pulmonary tuberculosis.
2. **Risk factors (contributing, predisposing, or aggravating factors):** These are not the necessary causes of disease but they are important for a disease to occur. A factor associated with an increased occurrence of a disease is risk factor for the exposed group; and a factor associated with a decreased occurrence of a disease is a risk factor for the nonexposed group. Risk factors could be related to the agent, the host and the environment.

EPIDEMIOLOGICAL TRIAD (FIG. 4.4)

The etiology of a disease is the sum total of all the factors (primary causes and risk factors) which contribute to the occurrence of the disease. It is the interaction of the agent,

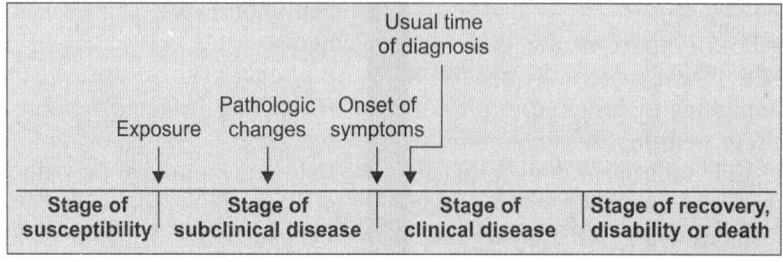

Fig. 4.3: Spectrum of disease.

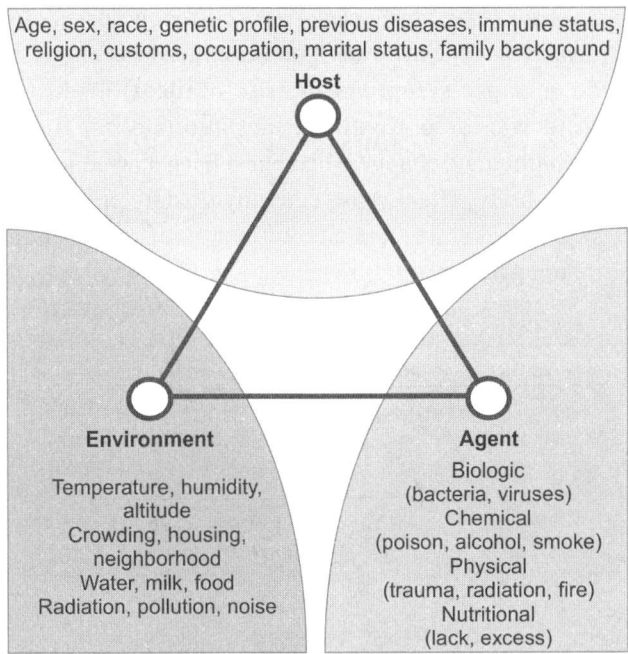

Fig. 4.4: Epidemiological traid.

the host, and the environment which determines whether or not a disease develops, and this can be illustrated using the epidemiologic triangle. The epidemiology demands a broader concept of disease causation that synthesized the basic factors of agent, host and environment. An individual's health is never static and is always in a dynamic equilibrium with his environment. The condition of health is seen as the resultant of various ecologic interactions which determines the health status of the human body.

- **Agent factors:** Disease causing agent are in the environment may be classified into the following categories. Inanimate group of agents are mainly responsible for non-communicable diseases such as physical agents, chemical agents, nutritional agents.
  - *Physical agents*—heat, light, radiation, etc.
  - *Chemical agents*—acids, alkalies, metals, etc.
  - *Nutritional agents*—lack or excess nutritional factors.
  - *Biological agents*— the disease caused are always transmissible from one individual to another individual. Therefore, they are called communicable diseases. Some of the communicable diseases are transferable only through another medium like insects, where the agents undergo certain changes in their life cycle.
- **Environmental factors:** Environment is the aggregate of all external conditions and influence factors affecting the life and development of an organism. It is classified as below:
  - *Physical environment*—all those inanimate objects like air, water, food, etc.
  - *Biological environment*—all those animate objects like animals, insects and other humans.
  - *Socioeconomic environment*—social and economic factors like housing, social group, education, etc.

- **Host factors:** Age, sex, habits and customs, general and specific defence mechanism, genetic makeup and psychobiological characteristics of the host are some of the important factors which determine the outcome of interaction between the agents and host in a suitable environment.

NATURAL HISTORY OF DISEASES

Every disease has a period before man is involved and this is called the 'period of prepathogenesis where the interrelations, of the various agents, host and environmental factors which bring the agent and host that follow, will take place. If the host is able to withstand the stimulus the disease process will not be allowed to progress. If the agent takes the upper hand the disease progresses within the tissue and physiological changes in the body.

- During the early part of this period (early pathogenesis) the disease will not be recognized (unless special examinations like the vaginal test, i.e. PAP test in the detection of cervical cancer are available), may be missed.
- Further progression of the disease produces signs and symptoms of the disease.
- This may progress further, if not recognized and treated early, into disability, defect or death, or to a complete recovery without any disability depending on the host factors and effectiveness of treatment taken.
- Disease results from a complex interaction between man, an agent (or cause of disease) and the environment. The term natural history of disease is a key concept in epidemiology.
- Each disease has its own unique natural history, which is not necessarily the same in all individuals, so much so any general formulation of the natural history of disease is necessarily arbitrary.

Prepathogenesis Phase (Fig. 4.5)

Prepathogenesis phase is a period preliminary to the onset of disease in man. The disease agent has not yet entered man, but the factors which favor its interaction with the human host already exist in the environment. The causative factors of disease may be classified as agent, host and environment. Prepathogenesis period is not sufficient to start disease in man. There is an interaction of these factors to initiate the disease process in man.

Pathogenesis Phase

Pathogenesis phase begins with the entry of the disease agent in the susceptible human host. The further events in the pathogenesis phase are clear cut in infectious disease. The disease agent multiplies and induces tissue and pathological changes. The disease progresses through a period of incubation and later through early and late pathogenesis. The final outcome of the disease may be recovery, disability or death.

Four Stages in the Natural History of a Disease

The "natural history of disease" refers to the progression of disease process in an individual over time, in the absence of intervention. There are four stages in the natural history of a disease. These are: 1. Stage of susceptibility 2. Stage of pre-symptomatic (sub-clinical) disease 3. Stage of clinical disease 4. Stage of disability or death (**Fig. 4.6**).

1. **Stage of susceptibility:** In this stage, disease has not yet developed, but the groundwork has been laid by the presence of factors that favor its occurrence. For example, unvaccinated child is susceptible to measles.
2. **Stage of pre-symptomatic (sub-clinical) disease:** In this stage, there are no manifestations of the disease but pathologic changes (damages) have started to occur in the body. The disease can only be detected through special tests since the signs and symptoms of the disease are not present.

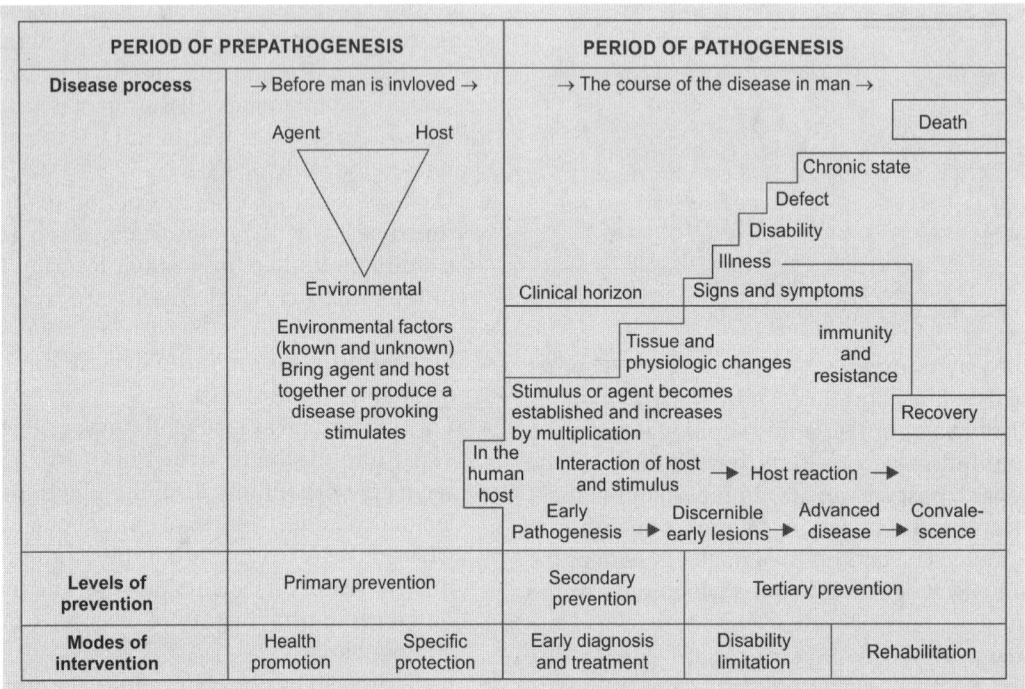

Fig. 4.5: Levels of health prevention.

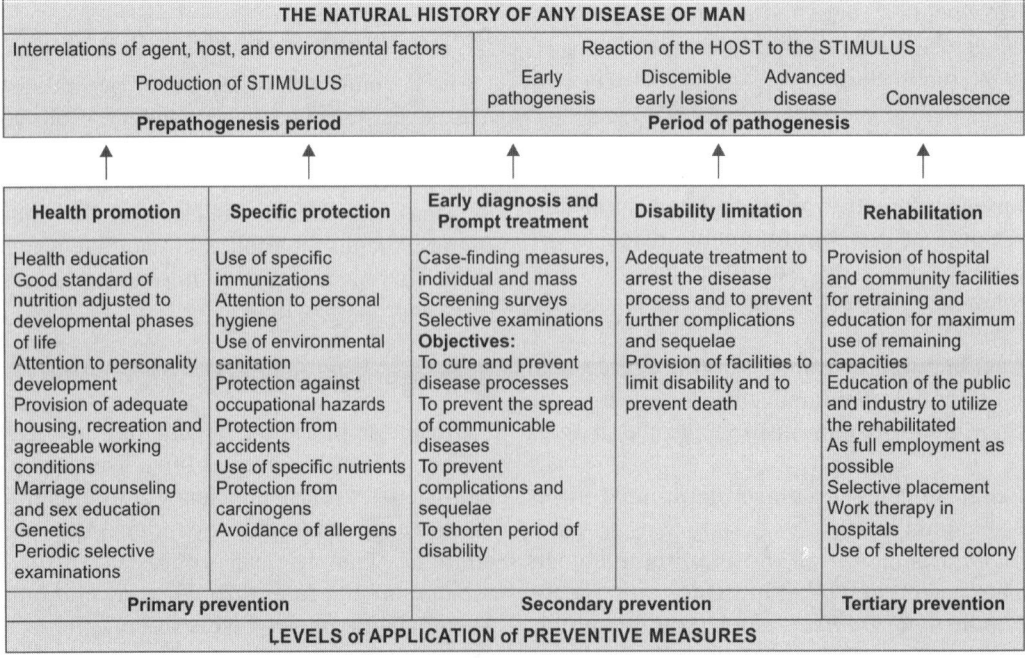

Fig. 4.6: History of natural causes of illness.

Examples:
- Detection of antibodies against HIV in an apparently healthy person.
- Ova of intestinal parasite in the stool of apparently healthy children.

The pre-symptomatic (sub-clinical) stage may lead to the clinical stage, or may sometimes end in recovery without development of any signs or symptoms.

3. **Clinical stage:** At this stage, the person has developed signs and symptoms of the disease. The clinical stage of different diseases differs in duration, severity and outcome. The outcomes of this stage may be recovery, disability or death.

   Examples:
   - Common cold has a short and mild clinical stage and almost everyone recovers quickly.
   - Polio has a severe clinical stage and many patients develop paralysis becoming disabled for the rest of their lives.
   - Rabies has a relatively short but severe clinical stage and almost always results in death.
   - Diabetes mellitus has a relatively longer clinical stage and eventually results in death if the patient is not properly treated.

4. **Stage of disability or death:** Some diseases run their course and then resolve completely either spontaneously or by treatment. In others the disease may result in a residual defect, leaving the person disabled for a short or longer duration. Still, other diseases will end in death. Disability is limitation of a person's activities including his role as a parent, wage earner, etc

   Examples:
   - Trachoma may cause blindness
   - Meningitis may result in blindness or deafness. Meningitis may also result in death.

LEVELS OF DISEASE PREVENTION

The disease process, in many instances is susceptible to interruption in order to limit its further progress or the speed of its progression. As disease involves interaction of host, agent and environment, prevention can be achieved by altering one or more of these three elements so that interaction does not take place or is interrupted in favor of the host. Effective preventive measure requires that the disease process be interrupted as early in its course as possible.

The interaction between the agent and the host can be avoided either by the elimination of the agent in the environment or by converting the human host immune to the attack of the agent.

Those attempts to bring about changes in the three elements before the disease stimulus is produced are grouped under one type of prevention, namely primary prevention. When the disease stimulus has already been practiced and the disease process has crossed over to the period of pathogenesis measures taken are grouped under two types of prevention, namely secondary and tertiary prevention **(Fig. 4.7)**.

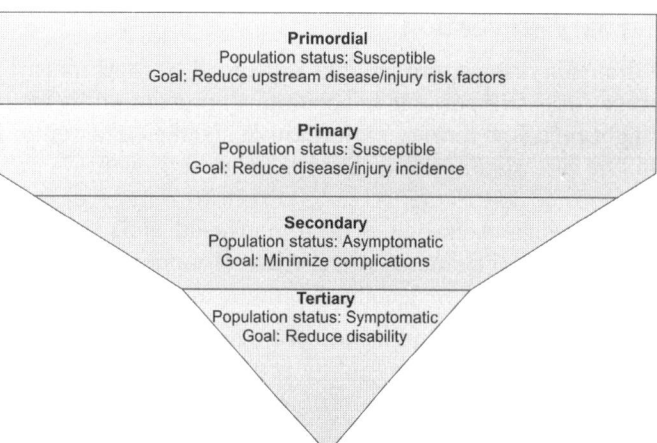

Fig. 4.7: Phase of illness prevention.

Primary Prevention

Primary prevention can be defined as an action taken prior to the onset of disease which removes the possibility that a disease will ever occur. It signifies intervention in the prepathogenesis phase of a disease or health problem or other departure from health. Primary prevention is applied at the prepathogenic period; it includes health promotion and specific protection.

- **Health promotion:** The first level of prevention is by promoting and maintaining the health of the host by nutrition, health education, good heredity and other health promotion activities.
- **Specific protection:** It may be directed towards the agent like disinfection of contaminated particles, materials water, food and other particles on the assumption that the agent has escaped into these vehicles or environment. Specific protection can also be achieved by immunizations to increase the resistance of the host so that the host will be able to withstand the onslaught of the agent. This is done by the active and passive immunizations.

Secondary Prevention

Secondary prevention can be defined as an action which halts the progress of a disease at its incipient stage and prevents complications. The specific interventions are early diagnosis, e.g., screening tests, case-finding programs) and adequate treatment. The secondary prevention is done by early diagnosis and treatment. Early diagnosis and prompt treatment comes under secondary prevention. If primary prevention fails or when suitable measures are not available (as in cancer) the disease stimulus is bound to be produced. Early detection of the disease is possible by periodic examinations of population groups who are at special risks like antenatal mothers, growing children, industrial worker, etc.

Monitoring of persons of middle age and above is one of the modern methods of early detection of cancer. In many instances, this detection of the diseases condition is possible only after the onset of the signs and symptoms. Early detection of the disease ensures prompt treatment so that the disease will not progress further.

Tertiary Prevention

When the disease process has advanced beyond its early stages, it is still possible to accomplish prevention by what might be called tertiary prevention. It signifies intervention in the late pathogenesis phase. Tertiary prevention can be defined as all measures available to reduce or limit impairment and disabilities, from good health and to promote the patient's adjustments to irremediable conditions. Tertiary prevention includes disability limitation and rehabilitation.

Disability limitation: It is necessary that the disability that is caused should be limited by active medical or surgical treatment so that there is no further deterioration of the health.

Rehabilitation: Those with permanent disability as in the case of leprosy, tuberculosis, polio, mental retardation, etc. will not be able to lead an independent life unless they are rehabilitated. This level will be needed only when it has failed in the application of previous levels of prevention.

CONTROL OF INFECTIOUS DISEASES

The control of communicable disease implies mainly the prevention of disease, primary prevention or secondary prevention or combination of both. Tertiary prevention is not so significant in the disease control. The term disease eradication indicates absolute termination of the disease. It implies the cessation of infection and disease. The term disease elimination comes in middle category between the control and eradication.

Objectives of Disease Control

- To decrease mortality and morbidity
- To reduce disease occurrence
- To reduce the risk of disease transmission
- To reduce the financial burden to the population
- To decrease the duration of illness
- To prevent from possible complications.

Techniques Used for Disease Control

- **Disinfection:** Killing or destroying most infectious agents outside the body by physical, chemical or any means. Disinfection classified into concurrent and terminal disinfection. Concurrent disinfection is disposal of contaminated material or equipment as early as possible. Terminal disinfection is disposal of contaminated articles after patient gets transfer or discharge or death.
- **Antiseptic:** A chemical substance that destroys microorganisms or inhibits their growth. Antiseptics destroy microorganisms or inhibit their growth. Antiseptics are less strong and are safe enough to be used on living tissues.
- **Sterilization:** It is a process of destroying all forms of microorganisms (including spores). It is the complete destruction of all pathogenic, nonpathogenic microorganisms and viruses or elimination of all viable organisms.

Host Defences by Immunization

A person is said immune when he possess specific protective antibodies or cellular immunity as a result of previous infection or immunization or is so conditioned by such previous experience as to respond adequately to prevent infection and/or clinical illness following exposure to a specific infectious agent.

Active Immunity

Active immunity depends upon the humoral and cellular responses of the host. The immunity produced is specific for a particular disease, i.e. the individual in most cases is immune to further infection with the same organism or antigenically related organism for varying periods depending upon the particular disease.

- **Humoral immunity:** It comes from the B–cells (bone marrow derived lymphocytes) which proliferate and manufacture specific antibodies after antigen presentation by macrophages. The antibodies are localized in the immunoglobulin fraction, subpopulations able to help B-lymphocytes.
- **Cellular immunity:** It plays a fundamental role in resistance to infection. It is mediated by the T-cells, which differentiate into subpopulations able to help B-lymphocytes.
- **Combination of the above:** In addition to the B and T lymphoid cells, which are responsible for recognizing self and non-self very often, the macrophages and human K (killer) cells and their joint functions constitute the complex events of immunity.

Passive Immunization

It is a process of conferring immunity by administrating readymade antibodies of human or animal origin. The immunity offers specific protection for a limited period, lasting for a few months.

- **Normal human Ig:** It is used to prevent measles in highly susceptible individuals and to provide temporary protection (up to 12 weeks) against hepatitis A infection for travelers to endemic areas and to control institutional and household outbreaks of hepatitis infection.
- **Specific human Ig:** These preparations are made from the plasma of patients who have recently recovered from an infection or are obtained from individuals who have been immunized against a specific infection. Specific human Igs are used for chickenpox prophylaxis and for post exposure prophylaxis of hepatitis B and rabies, and tetanus prophylaxis in the wounded.
- **Antisera or antitoxins:** These are prepared from non-human sources such as horses. Antitoxins are used against tetanus, diphtheria, botulism, gas gangrene and snake bite. Administration of antisera may occasionally give rise to serum sickness and anaphylactic shock due to abnormal sensitivity of the recipient.

DISINFECTION

Disinfecting uses chemicals (disinfectants) to kill germs on surfaces and objects. Some common disinfectants are bleach and alcohol solutions. You usually need to leave the disinfectant on the surfaces and objects for a certain period of time to kill the germs. Disinfecting does not necessarily clean dirty surfaces or remove germs.

Definition: Disinfection is defined as the treatment of surfaces/equipment using physical or chemical means such that the amount of microorganisms present is reduced to an acceptable level.

Methods of Disinfection

Chemical Disinfectants
- Alcohol
- Chlorine and chlorine compounds
- Formaldehyde
- Glutaraldehyde
- Hydrogen peroxide
- Iodophors
- Ortho-phthalaldehyde (OPA)
- Peracetic acid
- Peracetic acid and hydrogen peroxide
- Phenolics
- Quaternary ammonium compounds

Miscellaneous Inactivating Agents
- Other germicides
- Metals as microbicides
- Ultraviolet radiation
- Pasteurization
- Flushing- and washer-disinfectors

ROLE OF COMMUNITY HEALTH NURSE IN EPIDEMICS

Epidemiology and community health nursing are utmost essential in the field of health science. Epidemiology and nursing are closely related for the attainment of optimal health of the individuals, families and communities. Community health nurse take active role to identify and investigates the problem during outbreak of epidemics.

- Community health nurse has a greater concern with the occurrence of disease, health problems and risk factors prevalent in the community. The community health nurse works for the prevention and control of disease at various levels.
- Community health nurse participate as one of the team member especially when it is large scale investigation. For example, occurrence of any epidemic or community level general health survey or specific health survey, surveillance activities and screening, etc.
- Community health nurse take active participation in prevention and control of communicable diseases such as notification of certain specific disease like measles, diphtheria, tetanus, hepatitis rabies and STD to the health authority. And also identify sources of infection and methods of spread of infection.
- Community health nurse provide health education for the community regarding preventive and control measures for epidemics. Because of this she plays a key role in the health information system in the community.
- Community health nurse takes vital role during any unusual occurrence of any disease. She investigates regarding frequency and distribution and possible determinants. Community health nurse analyses the information collected, compares it with previous findings and with rates at the national level. They are also involved in planning and implementation of prevention and control program.

CONCLUSION

Epidemiology studies the three components, i.e., disease frequency, distribution of disease and determinants of disease. The first component indicates that epidemiology is measurement of frequency of disease, disability or death and summarizing this information in the form of rates and ratio, i.e., prevalence rate, incidence rate, death rate, etc. The second component concerned with describing the distribution of health status in terms of age, sex, race, geography, etc. and the third involves interpretation of the distribution in terms of the possible causal factors. Hence, it is a science developed from the study of the unusual to find out an explanation for unusual happenings.

BIBLIOGRAPHY

1. Beaglehole, Robert, Bonita, Ruth, Kjellström, Tord & World Health Organization. Basic epidemiology, Updated reprint. World Health Organization; 1993.
2. Benenson AS (Ed). Control of Communicable Diseases in Man, Fifteenth edition.
3. Cates WJ. Epidemiology: Applying principles to clinical practice. Contemp Ob/Gyn 1982; 20:147–61.
4. Centers for Disease Control. Case definitions for public health surveillance. MMWR 1990; 39 (No. RR-13):4–43.
5. Centers for Disease Control and Prevention. Framework for evaluating public health surveillance systems for early detection of outbreaks: recommendations from the CDC Working Group. MMWR May 7, 2004; 53(RR05);1–11.
6. Epidemiology: Man and Disease. New York: Macmillan Publishing Co., 1970:315–27.
7. Gordis, L. Epidemiology (Fifth edition.). Philadelphia, PA: Elsevier Saunders; 2014.
8. Hennekens CH, Buring JE. Epidemiology in Medicine, Lippincott Williams & Wilkins, 1987.
9. Marica Stannope, Veanetle Lancaster. Textbook of community and public health nursing, 6th edn. Mosby Publications, Missouri 2004.
10. National Center for Health Statistics. Health, United States, 1990. Hyattsville, MD: Public Health Service. 1991.
11. Orenstein WA, Bernier RH. Surveillance: Information for action. Pediatr Clin North Am 1990; 37:709–34.
12. Peterson DR. The practice of epidemiology. In: Fox JP, Hall CE, and Elveback LR.

REVIEW QUESTIONS

Long Essays

1. Discuss the history of epidemiology and population health.
2. Define epidemiology. Explain aims, objectives and functions of epidemiology.
3. Discuss the used of epidemiology in community health nursing.
4. Describe the epidemiological methods used in community health nursing.
5. Explain the natural history of diseases.
6. Enumerate the levels of disease prevention.
7. Role of community health nurse in epidemics.

Short Essays

1. Types of epidemiology.
2. Tools of measurement in epidemiology.
3. Components of epidemiology.
4. Principles of epidemiology.
5. Scope of epidemiology.
6. Dichotomies in epidemiological studies.
7. Epidemiological approaches.
8. Analytical method.
9. Importance of epidemiology.
10. Disease cycle.
11. Epidemiological triad.
12. Stages in the natural history of a disease.
13. Techniques used for disease control.
14. Methods of disinfection.

Short Answers

1. Carrier.
2. Contact.
3. Reservoir.
4. Pathogen.
5. Epidemic.
6. Eradication.
7. Experimental epidemiology.
8. Disease behavior.
9. Advantages of epidemiology.
10. Case control study.
11. Cohort study.
12. Spectrum of disease.
13. Disease causation.
14. Levels of health prevention.
15. Prepathogenesis phase.
16. Tertiary prevention.
17. Disability limitation.
18. Active immunity.
19. Objectives of disease control.

Multiple Choice Questions

1. Which of the following is not a part of continuum of natural history of the disease?
   a. Stage of susceptibility
   b. Stage of preclinical
   c. Stage of prevention
   d. Stage of recovery
2. Which of the following are also known as retrospective studies?
   a. Cohort studies
   b. Descriptive studies
   c. Experimental studies
   d. Case control studies
3. Total number of deaths reported during a given time interval from estimated mid-interval population is called:
   a. Death rate
   b. Crude death rate
   c. Mortality rate
   d. Proportional mortality
4. Use of statistics to analyze characteristics or changes to a population is termed as:
   a. Population pyramid
   b. Vital statistics
   c. Population statistics
   d. Population dynamics
5. Which of the following is not a basic measurement in epidemiology?
   a. Rate
   b. Nominator
   c. Ratio
   d. Proportion
6. Which of the following is usually expressed as percentage?
   a. Rate
   b. Nominator
   c. Ratio
   d. Proportion
7. Measurement of current status of disease is termed as:
   a. Prevalence
   b. Incidence
   c. Cumulative incidence
   d. Mid interval population
8. The modes of transmission of infectious diseases are as follows, *except*:
   a. Direct
   b. Indirect
   c. Physiological
   d. Biological
9. The number of new cases occurring in a defined population during a specified period of time is called:
   a. Prevalence
   b. Incidence
   c. a and b
   d. Cumulative incidence
10. Measure of the frequency of occurrence of death in a defined population during a specified interval is called:
    a. Crude death rate
    b. Mortality rate
    c. Death ratio
    d. Mortality
11. Public health surveillance does not consists on the following step:
    a. Systematic collection
    b. Analysis
    c. Planning
    d. Interpretation

ANSWERS

1. c	2. d	3. b	4. c	5. b	6. b	7. a	8. c	9. b	10. b	11. c

CHAPTER 5: Family Health Nursing Care

LEARNING OBJECTIVES

1. Family as a unit of health
2. Concept, goals, objectives
3. Family healthcare services
4. Family healthcare plan and nursing process
5. Family health services—Maternal, child care and family welfare services
6. Roles and function of a community health nurse in family health service
7. Family health records

TERMINOLOGY

Family: Family is a group of two or more persons joined by ties of marriage, blood or adoption who constitute a single household, who interact with each other in their respective familial status, positions and roles, to create and maintain a common subculture.

Family health: Family health is concerned for the most part with the care of well, families, with non-hospitalized sick persons and their families, with groups of people and with health peoples that affect the community as a whole.

Assimilation: Individuals or group from one culture identifying more strongly with the dominant culture in values, activities and daily living.

Community resources: A collection of healthcare providers or supportive care providers who share common interests or a sense of unity.

Family developmental task: The usual and expected family psychological, cognitive or psychomotor skills at certain persons in life, failure to master a developmental task can lead to unhappiness and difficulty with later tasks.

Family functions: Active or behavior of families that maintains the unity of the family and meets the family's needs.

Family structure: The characteristics of individuals (age, gender, number) who make up the family unit.

Family system theory: A theory that says the family is a collection of people who are integrated, interacting and dependent and that the actions of the other members.

Community-based nursing: Nursing care within the context of the clients family and community with a prevention focus that enhances the clients ability for self care, a collaborative effort to maintain continuity of care.

Home visit: Assessment, diagnosis, planning and evaluation of nursing care in the client's home.

INTRODUCTION

Family healthcare nursing is an art and a science that has evolved over the last 20 years as a way of thinking about and working with families. Family nursing comprises a philosophy and a way of interacting with clients that affects how nurses collect information, intervenes with patients, advocate for patients, and approach spiritual care with families. This philosophy and practice incorporates the assumption that health affects all members of families that health and illness are family events, and that families influence the process and outcome of health care.

DEFINITIONS

- **Family:** Two or more individuals coming from the same or different kinship groups who are involved in a continuous living arrangement, usually residing in the same household, experiencing common emotional bonds, and sharing certain obligations toward each other and toward others.
- **Family health:** A condition including the promotion and maintenance of physical, mental, spiritual, and social health for the family unit and for individual family members.
- **Family process:** The ongoing interaction between family members through which they accomplish their instrumental and expressive tasks. The nursing process considers the family, not the individual, as the unit of care.
- **Family centered nursing:** Nursing that considers health of the family as a unit in addition to the health of individual family members.

FAMILY

The word family is derived from the Roman word "Famulus" which means a "servant". In Roman law, the word denotes "the group of producers and slaves and other servant as well as other members" connected by common descent or marriage". A family is a group of individuals united by bonds of blood or marriage. The group lives together and consumes food from a common kitchen. The members of the group interact with one another in various capacities and discharge their roles in accordance with the family tradition and cultural norms of the society to which they belong. A family is a primary unit of a society in many aspects social, biological, economical epidemiological and operational.

Definitions of Family

- Family is a group of biologically related persons living together and sharing common kitchen and purse
- A primary group of people living in household in consistent proximity and intimate relationships
- A group of individual bounded together by the common interests of its members—by Hymovich
- The family involves people who are related in a traditional or non-traditional sense by marriage, blood adoption or friendship
- Family can be defined as a group of two or more individuals united by blood, marriage, adaptation or mutual consent who live together under the same roof, eat from the common kitchen, pool, and share al the resources for the benefit of all members, who interact and intercommunicate with each other in their respective familial role and who create and maintain a common subculture.

Concept of Family

- **Biological concepts:** This based on the biological functions of the family. A family is a biological unit because all its members are bonded together by blood or marriage and in consequence share common gene pool.
- **Psychological concept:** Murray and Zentnen say that family is the basic unit of growth experience and adaptation.
- **Economical concept:** A family is an economical unit because its members pool income from all sources and distribute it among all its members, earning as well as non-earning.
- **Sociological concept:** A family is a social unit because it is an instrument of preserving, protecting and propagating the habits, practices, customs and traditions of the society with which it is in continuous interaction.
- **Epidemiological concept:** A family is an epidemiological unit because its members share a common genetic, nutritional, environmental, social and cultural milieu that influences their health and disease status.
- **Operational concept:** A family is an operational unit because it confirms to the service requirements of family medicine and primary health care.
- **System's theory:** System's theory concept is more applicable for community health nursing because of the focus on internal and external relationship and dynamics.

Family Types

- **Nuclear family:** It consists of husband, wife, and their unmarried children. This form of family is universal, found in all societies at every age. A nuclear family is economically independent. Nuclear families are symbol of female emancipation and empowerment. In the absence of the moralizing influence of a joint family system, there is an erosion of religious and cultural values in nuclear families.
- **Joint family:** A joint family comprises two or more couples united by bonds of blood of patrilineal descent. Joint families usually originate as two generation families in situations where sons do not separate even after marriage. The merit of the joint family system is that it is based on the motto "union is strength". There is a sharing of responsibilities practically in all matters which gives the family a greater economic and social security.
- **Three generation family:** It occurs usually when young couples are unable to find separate housing accommodation, and continue to live with their parents and have their own children. Thus, representatives of three generations related to each other by direct descent live together.

Functions of Family

- **Home or comfort:** Family creates the home and provides a homely life. A family is sanctuary for comfort, relief, relaxation and satisfaction. A home is the most cherished possession of man, a personal property, identification and an address that denotes an appropriate placement of an individual in his society.
- **Economical security:** Family provides an ideal security for its members which appear to be based on a socialistic philosophy "from every member as per his capacity and to every member as per his needs". Family provides economic security to its productive as well as non-productive members.
- **Procreation and rearing of children:** Bearing of children is an important function of the family to perpetuate race. This function is achieved through affection and sex between husband and wife. Both parents participate in rearing of children.
- **Physical and emotional care:** Family is committed to meet physical an emotional need of its members by providing food, shelter, clothing, healthcare, love and emotional environment provides member's sense of security and confidence, helps them build their self-concept, self-esteem and emotional stability.
- **Education:** A family is the first school for toddlers who learn the most elementary lessons from their parents at home. An educated family provides an ideal setting for learning experiences of preschool children in an atmosphere of loving, care and personalized attention.

- **Socialization:** The process of socialization first starts in the family. The family transmits the knowledge of its cultural practices which includes customs, traditions, religious virtues and rituals, behavior pattern, dressing up, speech, language relationship with people, etc.
- **Division labor:** Every member in the family has defined status, roles, functions and responsibilities to carry on various functions and tasks of the family. There is increasing sharing responsibilities between the partners especially related to earning for living and support due to industrialization inflation increasing individual and family needs.
- **Social care and control:** The family function to regulate and control the social behavior of members within the acceptable norms and family and society. It regulates behavior of members with reference to their daily routine personal and social habits, martial activities, sex relations through incest and taboo, etc.

FAMILY AS A UNIT OF COMMUNITY HEALTH SERVICES

The family is the unit of services in all generalized community health nursing programs. The health of one member affects the welfare of every other member in the family. Interdependency implies a dynamic interaction between members where by physical, psychosocial, cultural and spiritual needs are met.

A family is a primary unit of society in many respects social biological, economical epidemiological and operational. The family is affected by every aspect of community life. The community provides work, education, medical care. Community healthcare services, recreation and government for the people. The facilities in a given community are provided by the people through democratic action.

An effective family health service provides for a study of the family as a whole and the factor that affects the health and welfare of each members. The family record or folder provides a guide for collecting basic facts such as identification of each member, economic status, housing and environmental sanitation nutritional status of each member and other pertinent facts.

Rationale for Family as a Unit

- The family is considered the "National and fundamental unit of society." The family members have strong emotional ties, social and legal obligations by virtue of their family members, family structure and familial roles.
- The family as a group generates prevents tolerates and corrects health problems within its membership. Family as a group works together in improving knowledge, competencies and other resources and helps itself in preventing many of the health problems which may emerge any time.
- The health problems of families are interlocking; the health status of any one member in the family is likely to affect it the health of other members of the family.
- The family provides crucial environment force for its members to develop health attitude, values and health practices.
- The family is the most frequent locus of health decisions and actions in personal care. It is very important to build up proper decision making and care giving abilities of the family as a whole rather than of the individual alone.
- The family is an effective and available channel for much of the community health nursing efforts. The community health nurse has the opportunity to work with families constantly and provide need based comprehensive health care services.

Characteristics of Family as a Unit

- Family is a product of time and place families in developed areas differ to families in developing areas in terms of size, structure values, general behavior for decision-making, its differs from one to another.
- The family develops its own lifestyle families develop their own power system/controlling authority for decision making, it differs from one another.
- The family operates as a group—some families discuss the problems with all the members in a group and each one participate in decisions-making and share the responsibilities.
- The family accommodates to the needs of individual members – the natural family balance is attained between family needs and individual needs.
- The family relates to the community the character of the family differs and each family may also differ over time with respect to character.

FAMILY HEALTH CARE

Family health is defined as art and science of preventing disease, prolonging life and promoting health and efficiency of family through organized family efforts for the safe family environment, prevention and control of communicable diseases, reproductive and child health education of members in personal hygiene, seeking medical and nursing services for early diagnosis and treatment, development of social system and coping abilities to ensure normal development and optimum health status of family members.

Determinants/Factors of Family Health

- **Human biology:** It is composed of family size, structure, composition and characteristics, genetic inheritance and self-concept.
- **Environment:** It is composed of physical, biological and social environment of the family.
- **Lifestyle:** It is composite of daily living activities, behavioral and cultural practices including customs and traditions practiced by the family.
- **Health and allied resources:** It includes health services, health related facilities, socioeconomic conditions, political system and health related services, etc.

Aims of Family Health Care

- Reduction of maternal, infant and child mortality and morbidity rates.
- Family planning to space out children and ensure Planned Parenthood.
- Improve nutritional status of all family members.
- Health education of the family in all preventive, promotive, curative and rehabilitative aspects of healthcare.

Objectives of Family Health Care

- Identify and appraises health problems of the family.
- Ensure family's understanding and acceptance of the problem.
- Provide prompted and proper services according to the health needs of the family.
- Helps to develop the competence in the members to take care of their family as and when required.
- Contributes desired materials to personal and social development of the family members.
- Helps to promote the utilizing of available resources to maintain all aspects of health of the rehabilitative measure.

Principles of Family Health Care

- Establish good professional relationship with the family.
- Provide proper health education and guidance to family to take care of themselves.
- Collect all relevant information about family and community to identify problems and set priorities.
- Provide support to the family based on their needs.
- Encourage and motivate family members to participate healthcare services to improve their health status.
- Healthcare services should be provided to the family irrespective of sex, age, income, religion, etc.
- Duplication of health services should be provided to the family irrespective of sex, age, income, religion, etc.
- Proper health message to be communicated to family in every contact.

FAMILY HEALTH NURSING

Definition and meaning of family health nursing: Family health nursing is a nursing aspect of organized family health care services which are directed or focused on family as the unit care with health as the goal. It is thus synthesis of nursing care and health care. It helps to develop self-care abilities of the family and promote, protect and maintain its health. Family health nursing is generalized, well balanced and integrated comprehensive and continuous are requiring comprehensive planning to accomplish its goal. The goals of the family health nursing include optimal functioning for the individual and for the family as a unit."

Objectives of Family Health Nursing

The broad objectives of family health nursing are as under:
- To identify health and nursing needs and problems of each family.
- To ensure family's understanding and acceptance of these needs and problems.
- To plan and provide health and nursing services with the active participation of family members.
- To help families develop abilities to deal with their health needs and health problems independently.
- To contribute to family's performance of developmental functions and tasks.
- To help family make intelligent use of promotive, preventive, therapeutic and rehabilitative health and allied facilities and services in the community.
- To educate, counsel and guide family members to cultivate good personal health habits, practice safe cultural practices and maintain wholesome physical, psychosocial, and spiritual environment.

Principles of Family Health Nursing

- Provide services without discrimination
- Periodic and continuous appraisal and evaluation of family health situation
- Proper maintenance of record and reports.
- Provide continuous services
- Health education, guidance and supervision as integral part of family health nursing.
- Maintain good IPR.
- Plan and provide family health nursing with active participation of family.
- Services should be realistic in terms of resources available.
- Encourage family to contribute towards community health.
- Active participation in making healthcare delivery system.

Advantages of Family Health Nursing

- Family health nursing of patients saves hospital beds that can be utilized for critical cases.
- Family health nursing is cheaper than hospital nursing.
- Patient under family health nursing enjoys privacy and emotional support.
- Patients on family health nursing can continue with their routine pursuits.
- If the patient resides in a sanitary house, family health nursing is better than hospital nursing since he can control inimical environmental influences better.

Disadvantages of Family Health Nursing

- Family health nursing requires the nurse to carry portable laboratory machinery to the patent's home.
- If the patient resides in a substandard house, family health nursing could delay his recovery.

FAMILY-CENTERED NURSING APPROACH

The four approaches included in the family health nursing care views are:
1. Family as the context
2. Family as the client
3. Family as a system
4. Family as a component of society

Family as the Context

- When the nurse views the family as context, the primary focus is on the health and development of an individual member existing within a specific environment (i.e., the client's family). Although the nurse focuses the nursing process on the individual's health status, the nurse also assesses the extent to which the family provides the individual's basic needs.
- These needs vary, depending on the individual's development level and situation. Because families provide more than just material essentials, their ability to help the client meet psychological needs must also be considered.
- Family members may need direct interventions themselves.

Family as the Client

- The family is the foreground and individuals are in the background. The family seems as the sum of individuals family members.
- The focus is concentrated on each and every individual as they affect the whole family. From this perspective, a nurse might ask a family member who has just become ill.

Family as a System

- The focus is on the family as a client and it is viewed as an international system in which the whole is more than the sum of its parts.
- This approach focuses on the individual and family members become the target for nursing interventions. For example, the direct interaction between the parent and the child. The system approach to the family always implies that when something happens to one affected.
- It is important to understand that although theoretical and practical distinctions can be made between the family as context and the family as client, they are not necessarily mutually exclusive, and both are often used simultaneously, such as with the perspective of the family as system.

Family as a Component of Society

- The family is seen as one of many institutions in society, along with health, educational, religious, or economic institution.
- The family is a basic or primary unit of society, as are all the other units and they are all a part of the larger system of society.
- The family as a whole interacts with other institutions to receive exchange or give communications and services.
- Community health nursing has drawn many of its clients from this perspective as it focuses on the interface between families and communities.
- Family health nursing practice like any nursing practice begins with the nursing process.
- By using this process, the nurse practicing with family perspectives is potentially able to effectively intervene at any of the levels.

- After an assessment of the individuals, family unit, and supra system, the nurse is ready to begin to identify areas of concern or need.

FAMILY HEALTH NURSING PROCESS

Definition of Family Health Nursing Process

- Family health nursing process is a orderly, systematic steps to assess the health needs, plan, implement and evaluate the services to achieve the health. It is the systematic steps to analyze health problems and their solutions. It helps in achieving desire goals of health promotion, prevention and control of health problems.
- **Family nursing process:** The family nursing process, suggested by these authors, consists of the following steps adapted specifically with family as the focus group.

Elements of Family Nursing Process

- Assessment of client's problem
- Diagnosis of client response needs
- Planning of client's care
- Implementation of care
- Evaluation and documentation.

Assessment of Client's Problem

- The home health nurse assesses not only the healthcare demand of the client and family but also the home and community environment.
- Assessment actually begins when the nurse contacts the client for the initial home visit and reviews documents received from the referral agency.
- The goal of the initial visit is to obtain a comprehensive clinical picture of the client's need.
- During the initial home visit, the home health nurse obtains a health history from the client, examines the client, observe the relationship of the client and caregiver, and assess the home and community environment.
- Parameters of assessment of the home environment include client and caregiver mobility, client ability to perform self care, the cleanliness of the environment, the availability of caregiver support, safety, food preparation, financial supports and the emotional status of the client and caregiver.

Diagnosis of Client Response Needs

- As in other care environments, the nurse identifies both actual and potential client problems.
- Examples of common nursing diagnoses for home care include Deficient Knowledge, Impaired Home Maintenance, and Risks for caregiver Role strain.
- Client education is considered a skill reimbursed by Medicare and other commercial insurance carriers, it is important for the nurse to include Deficient Knowledge in the plan of care.

- The deficit in knowledge may relate to client's lack of information about their disease process, medications, and self-care skills and so on.

Planning of Client's Care

During the planning phase the nurse needs to encourage and permit client's to make their own health management decisions. Alternatives may need to be suggested for some decisions if the nurse identifies potential harm from a chosen course of action. Strategies to meet the goals generally include teaching the client family techniques of care and identifying appropriate resources to assist the client and family maintaining self-sufficiency.

Implementation of Care

To implement the plan, the home health nurse performs nursing interventions, including teaching, coordinates and uses referrals and resources, provides and monitors all levels of technical care; collaborates with other disciplines and providers; identifies clinical problems and solutions from research and other health literature, supervises ancillary personnel, and advocates for the client's right to self-determination. Technical skills commonly performed by home health nurses include blood pressure measurement; body fluid collection (blood, urine, stool, and sputum), wound care, respiratory care, and all types of intravenous therapy, eternal nutrition, urinary catheterization and renal dialysis.

Evaluation and Documentation

- Evaluation is carried out by the nurse on subsequent home visits, observing the same parameters assessed on the initial home visit and relating findings to the expected outcomes or goals.
- The nurse can also teach caregivers parameters of evaluation so that they can obtain professional intervention if needed.
- Documentation of care given and the client's progress toward goal achievement at each visit is essential.
- Notes also may reflect plan for subsequent visits and when the client may be sufficiently prepared for self care and discharge from the agency.

FAMILY HEALTH ASSESSMENT

Establishing a Working Relationship

- The family and nurse maintain a working relationship. It is relationship which is maintained while working together by developing trust, confidentiality and empathy.
- These are essential components or elements to find out the facts from families and making correct decisions. A working relationship must have scope of two way communication.
- The family members must be given equal opportunity to give their views and ideas and express the feelings and vice versa.
- The nurse must have enough interactions with family members to guide and help them to solve the problem.

Assessment of health needs: Assessment is a continuous process which becomes more accurate as knowledge of people deepens.

Family structure, characteristics and dynamics: Include the composition and demographic data of the members of the family/household, their relationship to the head and place of residence; the type of, and family interaction/communication and decision-making patterns and dynamics.

Socioeconomic and cultural characteristics: Include occupation, place of work, and income of each working member; educational attainment of each family member; ethnic background and religious affiliation; significant others and the other role(s) they play in the family's life; and, the relationship of the family to the larger community.

Home and environment: Include information on housing and sanitation facilities; kind of neighborhood and availability of social, health, communication and transportation facilities in the community.

Health status of each member: Includes current and past significant illness; beliefs and practices conducive to health and illness; nutritional and developmental status; physical assessment findings and significant results of laboratory/diagnostic tests/screening procedures.

Values and practices on health promotion/maintenance and disease prevention: Include use of preventive services; adequacy of rest/sleep, exercise, relaxation activities, and stress management or other healthy lifestyle activities, and immunization status of at-risk family members.

METHODS OF DATA COLLECTION

- **Observation:** Method of data collection through the use of sensory capacities, sight, hearing, smell and touch. Data gathered through this method have the advantage of being subjected to validation and reliability testing by other observers.
- **Physical examination:** Done through inspection, palpation, percussion, auscultation, measurement of specific body parts and reviewing the body systems.
- **Interview:** Completing the health history of each family member. The health history determines current health status based on significant past health history. The second type of interview is collecting data by personally asking significant family members or relatives questions regarding health, family life experiences and home environment to generate data on what wellness condition and health problems exist in the family. Productivity of the interview process depends upon the use of effective communication techniques to elicit the needed responses.
- **Record review:** Reviewing existing records and reports pertinent to the client. Individual clinical records of the family members; laboratory and diagnostic reports; immunization records; reports about the home and environmental conditions.

- **Laboratory/Diagnostic tests:** Performing laboratory tests, diagnostic procedures or other tests of integrity and functions carried out by the nurse herself and/or other health workers.

ASSESSMENT OF HEALTH PROBLEMS

Health Deficits

Health deficits refer to instances of failure in health maintenance and development. Health deficits include:
- Diagnosed/ suspected illness states of family members
- Sudden or premature or untimely death illness or disability and failures to adapt reality of life emotional control and stability
- Deviations in growth and development
- Personality disorders

Health Threats

- Practices health threats refer to conditions which predispose to disease, accident, poor or retarded growth and development and personality disorder and a failure to realize one's health potentials.
- These situations are incomplete immunization among children, environmental hazards, poverty, family history of chronic illness, e.g., diabetes.

Foreseeable Crisis or Stresses

- Foreseeable crisis situations or stress points, refers to anticipated periods of unusual demands on the individual or the family in terms of adjustment or family resources.
- These demands may be pregnancy, retirement from work and adolescence.
- Though these conditions are expected but still lead to various types of crisis in family.

ASSESSMENT OF FAMILIES

- **Assessment of environmental condition:** The environment of the family home should be examined carefully, the type of house, hygienic conditions, facilities available and safety factors.
- **Health status assessment:** The physical and emotional health status assessment must be done for all family members by using the available assessment tools. Each family member should be evaluated even if she/he is not primary person whom you are seeing. For example, name, age, sex, height, weight, immunization, developmental stages; health history and current health history.
- **Family health practices:** Finding out their practices towards healthy living of nutritional status, sleeping pattern, exercises, rest and alcoholism, smoking, etc. use of health facilities. The type and ways in which a family uses health resources and providers give the information about health, will make community health nurse aware of their health practices about their strengths and weaknesses.
- **Family lifestyle:** Observe and describe family's interrelationship and communication pattern. Try to identify the role of each family member, patterns of decision making and family's attitude towards health care.

Assessment of Health Risk Families

Health risk families are those who experience a particular event or other events of any disease repeatedly, that make them more prone towards physical, psychological and environmental response.

Assessment through Family

- **Health records:** The family information can also be collected through family records. Family records are important sources of all family members' health information. The previous family records and reports are important means to gather information about family.
- **Clinics:** The family members coming to health centers to attend the clinics for medical care can also contribute to identify the health risk. Community health nurse can make observation and relate to the present health situation.
- **Observation:** In community health nursing, certain situations need direct observation. It is important to get acquainted with family environment along with patient, and many things can be learnt by observation, e.g., in a family how mother holds the infant.
- **Physical health assessment:** Community health nurse may require to do physical examination of each family member to find individual's physical state of health. This may help her early diagnosis and treatment and appropriate referral.

PLANNING FOR NURSING ACTION

Goal setting and selection of appropriate strategy: A good assessment will make the selection of appropriate goals and strategies easier. Families determine the degree of change required. Often people can easily identify their own goals. However community health nurse has to assist in making a clear goal statement by achievable means. Be sure that neither community health nurse nor families are too ambitious. Goal should be clear and concise statement. Clearly written goals give a sense of direction in how to proceed in the care of the family. This increases the self confidence and trust and confidence of the family in you and your ability to provide care.

Formulation of Nursing Diagnosis

- Once assessment is complete, review all the data, compile the risk factors and formulate nursing diagnosis. Since assessment is an ongoing process, it should be periodically reviewed, deleted and revised as per need.
- It is important to look at assessment data in totality and compile as overall functioning and health of the family.
- The final step of family assessment is formulation of nursing diagnosis. The nurse, who practices in the community just like those practicing in other health care settings, formulates nursing diagnosis based on assessment data with complete data available.

- She can formulate more accurate and scientific diagnosis. This forms the foundation for development of a health care plan.

Resources Available

- Availability of health related resources and financial resources used by family members. Sometimes families need help in identifying these resources; they may not define as broad as community health nurse can do.
- Discussing the family's financial status may be difficult initially, and family may be reluctant to disclose their finances, to a stranger.

IMPLEMENTING THE PROGRAM

Implementation of nursing process in family healthcare is foundation of nursing practice. Nurse uses family healthcare process to promote the health of families and differentiate from work with individual events. Implementing the healthcare requires home visits, working closely with families, community leaders, health workers, and other related agencies like social welfare and educational institution, etc. for comprehensive system to care. As the implementation process goes on, it may be necessary to change or omit certain strategies according to situation. Nurse can also facilitate the growth of the well-planned program. Family's satisfaction serves as the stimulus for adding further goal. Sometimes nurse observes the family's readiness and raises the possibility of care.

EVALUATION OF PROGRAM ACTION

Evaluation is not an end to family healthcare program, it is continuing process integrated in the other phases. The ultimate goal of community health nurse is for the family to be self-supporting and independent in identifying the presence or absence of preventive health behavior and skills in determining strategies and using appropriate resources. The evaluation is based on the set objectives for family. For success in evaluation, it is better to involve family in setting the objectives to bring the desired changes in attitude. The nurse should observe for change in attitude during and after the intervention of care. If she notices the failure brings to the desired change, then she needs to go back to reset the objective, replan and reimplement the programming.

NURSING CARE PLAN

Family care plan is the blueprint of the care that the nurse designs to systematically minimize or eliminate the identified health and family nursing problems through explicitly formulated outcomes of care (goals and objectives) and deliberately chosen of interventions, resources and evaluation criteria, standards, methods and tools.

Qualities of a Nursing Care Plan

- It should be based on clear, explicit definition of the problems. A good nursing plan is based on a comprehensive analysis of the problem situation.
- A good plan is realistic.
- The nursing care plan is prepared jointly with the family. The nurse involves the family in determining health needs and problems, in establishing priorities, in selecting appropriate courses of action, implementing them and evaluating outcomes. The nursing care plan is most useful in written form.

Importance of Planning Care

- They individualize care to clients.
- The nursing care plan helps in setting priorities by providing information about the client as well as the nature of his problems.
- The nursing care plan promotes systematic communication among those involved in the health care effort.
- Continuity of care is facilitated through the use of nursing care plans. Gaps and duplications in the services provided are minimized, if not totally eliminated.
- Nursing care plans, facilitate the coordination of care by making known to other members of the health team what the nurse is doing.

NURSING CARE

Steps in Developing a Family Nursing Care Plan

- The prioritized condition/s or problems based on:
  - Nature of condition or problem
  - Modifiability
  - Preventive potential
  - Salience
- The goals and objectives of nursing care.

Expected Outcomes

- Conditions to be observed to show problem is prevented, controlled, resolved or eliminated.
- Client response/s or behavior
- Specific, measurable, client-centered statements/competencies
- The plan of interventions.

Measures to help family eliminate:
- Barriers to performance of health tasks
- Underlying cause/s of non-performance of health tasks
- Family-centered alternatives to recognize/detect, monitor, control or manage health condition or problems
- Determine Methods of Nurse-Family Contact
- Specify resources needed
- The plan for evaluating
- Criteria/outcomes based on objectives of care
- Methods/Tools

CORE COMPETENCIES FAMILY HEALTH NURSE

These core competencies will be achieved through a process of developing the underpinning competencies, i.e., those which will enable Family Health Nurses effectively and efficiently to:

- Identify and assess the health status and health needs of individuals and families within the context of their cultures and communities;
- Make decisions based on ethical principles;
- Plan, initiate and provide care for families within their defined caseload;
- Promote health in individuals, families and communities
- Apply knowledge of a variety of teaching and learning strategies with individuals, families and communities;
- Use and evaluate different methods of communication;
- Participate in disease prevention;
- Coordinate and manage care, including that which they have delegated to other people and personnel;
- Systematically document their practice;
- Generate, manage and use clinical, research-based and statistical information (data) for planning care and prioritizing health- and illness-related activities;
- Support and empower individuals and families to influence and participate in decisions concerning their health
- Set standards and evaluate the effectiveness of family health nursing activities;
- Work independently and as members of a team;
- Participate in the prioritization of health- and illness-related activities;
- Manage change and act as agents for change;
- Maintain professional relationships and a supportive collegiate role with colleagues; and
- Display evidence of a commitment to lifelong learning and continuing professional development.

FAMILY HEALTH SERVICES—MATERNAL, CHILD CARE AND FAMILY WELFARE SERVICES

According to WHO (1976), Maternal and child health services can be defined as "promoting, preventing, therapeutic or rehabilitation facility or care for the mother and child". Thus, maternal and child health service is an important and essential service related to mother and child's overall development.

Aims and Objectives of MCH Program

- Reducing maternal and child mortality and morbidity rates.
- Child survival
- Promoting reproductive health or safe motherhood
- Ensure birth of healthy child
- Prevent malnutrition
- Prevent communicable diseases
- Early diagnosis and treatment of the health problems
- Health education and family planning services.

Activities of MCH Program

Maternal and child health services are an important part of primary health care. Traditional activity areas of this program:
1. Complete health check-up and care of the child and mothers from conception to birth.
2. Studying health problems of mothers and children.
3. Providing health education to parents for taking care of children.
4. Training to professional and assistant workers.

Need for MCH Program

There are four main reasons why mother and child health must be given top priority in health program:
1. Mother and child below the age of 15 years make up the majority of the population in almost countries.
2. Mother and children constitute a "special risk" or vulnerable group in the case of illness, deaths, in the terms of pregnancy, childbirth of mothers, and growth and development in the case of children.
3. By improving the health of mother and children we can improve the health of the family and community.
4. Ensuring child survival is a future investment for the family and community.

Recent Trends in MCH Service Program

- **Integration of care:** Earlier maternal and child health care services were divided into antenatal, child care and family planning. Naturally it is helpful in increasing the capability and effectiveness of service.
- **Risk approach:** This new thought was born from the lack of resources and their availability. As per this, the risk group among mother and infant is identified special care is given to them.
- **Manpower changes:** According to new concept, maternal and child health services should be left to traditional health workers(ANMs, health visitors) rather than specialist of field and child volunteers and workers of NGOs.
- **Primary health care:** It makes available information about protection and protection and resources for mother and child healthcare.
- **Reproductive and child health:** As per the decision taken in world women' conferences, Beijing (1995), maternal and child health services have been included in reproductive and child health services.

Principles

The guiding principle for the maternal and child health program are:
- **Consultation and participation:** Consultation with, and participation by, families is integral to the services. Services will be informed by, and seek to meet, the young needs of young children and their families.
- **Access and availability:** All families with young children should be able to readily access the information, services and resources that are appropriate for, and useful to, them.
- **Primacy of prevention:** Prevention of harm or damage is preferable to repairing it later. Early detection of risk factors is required, and intervention, where appropriate.
- **Capacity building:** Promotion of resilience and capacity is preferable to allowing problems to undermine health or autonomy.

- **Equity:** All children should be able to grow up actively learning, healthy, sociable and safe-irrespective of their family circumstances and background.
- **Family-centered:** The identification and management of child and family needs requires a family-centered approach that focuses on strength.
- **Inclusion:** Inclusive practices are essential for all children to get the best start, irrespective of their family circumstances, differing abilities and background.
- **Partnership:** Quality services are archived through integrated services delivery and partnership with other early childhood and specialist services, and with family.
- **Quality:** All families with young children must be confident of the quality of information, services and resources provided to them.

Maternal and Child Health Service Program Standards

- The maternal and child health services provide universal access to its services for children from birth to school age and their families.
- The maternal and child health services promote optimal health and development outcomes for children from birth to school age through a focus on the child, mother and family.
- The maternal and child health services builds partnership with families and communities and collaborates and integrates with other services and organizations.
- The maternal and child health services is delivered by a competent and professional workforce.
- The maternal and child health service, supported by local government or the governing authority, provides a responsive and accountable

RESPONSIBILITIES OF COMMUNITY HEALTH NURSE IN MCH SERVICES

Antenatal Care

i. **Contact:** Contacting every pregnant mother in the primary stage of pregnancy.
ii. History-taking of general health, previous child birth and present pregnancy.
iii. **Antenatal examination:**
   a. Calculate obstetric examination, etc.
   b. Calculating the expected date of delivery
   c. Identifying high risk of mothers
   d. Providing counseling and health education
   e. Helping mother and other family members in planning the delivery.

Intranatal Care

- Preparing the place for delivery
- Arranging necessary equipment
- Giving mental support to mothers
- Preparing mother for delivery
- Examine position of fetus, dilatation of cervix, and heart of fetus, observing the position of bladder and uterine contraction
- Noting general condition of the pregnant mother, process of pain and time of membrane rupture
- Ensuring safe delivery, examining umbilical cord and noting abnormalities
- If necessary, taking help of doctor or referring patient to a specialist
- Maintaining through asepsis during delivery
- Should be ready to handle complications like bleeding, malpresentation, cord prolapse, etc.
- Noting the correct time of birth.

Postnatal Care

The week immediately after the child birth is called postnatal period. The responsibilities of community health nurse are:
- Observing the blood pressure, temperature and pulse of mother immediately after the delivery and then during the following period
- Collecting information about the general condition of mother, food, sleep, pain and elimination, etc. and, accordingly the nursing care
- Observing fundus, perineum, lochia, bladder, etc.
- Observing breast and nipples
- Protecting the mother from complications like puerperal sepsis, breast inflammation, postpartum hemorrhage, urinary incontinence, urinary retention and Thrombophlebitis and providing required treatment.

Neonatal Care

- Observing the respiration of newborn, immediately after birth and if necessary providing resuscitation
- Taking care of the umbilical cord and cutting the Cord and tying it using proper techniques
- Taking notice of abnormalities or congenital defects and informing the relatives
- Assessing the physical condition of the newborn by his apgar score (9 or 10 is ideal score)
- Cleaning the newborn child (giving bath to the newborn has become less popular
- Taking care of the newborn skin and eyes.
- Keeping the newborn child on safe bed and providing breastfeeding to baby at the earliest
- Maintaining normal body temperature of the newborn
- Give kangaroo care.

Functions Related to Maternal Clinics

Home visits: During home visit, community health nurse should try to focus the attention of mother on the following points:
- Antenatal check up and its importance.
- Anatomy, physiology, and psychology of pregnancy
- Diet during pregnancy
- Plans of delivery
- Neonatal care
- Family planning.

Managerial Functions

- Organizing and managing the nursing homes.
- Playing the role of liaison officer under referral system, for sending the mother to hospital for safe delivery.
- Taking part in community activities.
- Explaining the importance of reproductive and child health in community.
- Supervising the work of midwives and female health workers and giving them appropriate suggestions.
- Organizing and managing maternal clinics.
- Coordinating between the doctor, family and patients.
- Storing and maintaining the records of maternal and child health services.
- Assisting the research work in the field of maternal and child health services.

Educational Functions

- Providing health education to mother and family either individually or in the group.
- Educating (using demonstration) pregnant mothers and relatives about maternal nursing.

Community health nurse should discuss following topics with pregnant mothers:

- Importance of regular antenatal check-up.
- Personal hygiene and proper diet.
- Clean environment (including mental environment)
- Importance of hospital delivery or delivered or delivery by trained worker.
- Taking care of infant.
- Thus, community health nurse has a multifaceted role in maternal services. It is only through proper discharge maternal and infant mortality can be reduced to targeted rate.

ROLES AND FUNCTION OF A COMMUNITY HEALTH NURSE IN FAMILY HEALTH SERVICE

The roles of healthcare nurses are evolving along with the specialty. Each healthcare setting affects roles that nurses assume with families, and many of these roles may occur in the same setting as well.

- **Health teacher:** The family nurse teaches about family wellness, illness, relations, and parenting, to name a few. The teacher educator function is ongoing in all settings in both formal and informal ways.
- **Coordinator, collaborator, and liaison:** The family nurse coordinates the care that families receive, collaborating with the family to plan care.
- **Deliverer and supervisor of care and technical expert:** The family nurse either delivers or supervises the care that families receive in various settings. To do this, the nurse must be a technical expert in terms of both knowledge and skill.
- **Family advocate:** The family nurse advocates for families with whom they work; the nurse empowers family members to speak with their own voice or the nurse speaks out for the family.
- **Consultant:** The family nurse serves as a consultant to families whenever asked or whenever necessary. In some instances, he or she consults with agencies to facilitate family centered care.
- **Counselor:** The family nurse plays a therapeutic role in helping individuals and families solve problems or change behavior.
- **Case finder and epidemiologist:** The family nurse gets involved in case finding and becomes a tracker of disease.
- **Environmental modifier:** The family nurse consults with families and other healthcare professionals to modify the environment.
- **Clarifier and interpreter:** The family nurse clarifies and interprets data to families in all settings.
- **Surrogate:** The family nurse serves as a surrogate by substituting for another person. For example, the nurse may stand in temporarily as a loving parent to an adolescent who is giving birth to a child by herself in the labor and delivery room.
- **Researcher:** The family nurse should identify practice problems and find the best solution for dealing with these problems through the process of scientific investigation.
- **Role model:** The family nurse is continually serving as a role model to other people through his or her activities. A school nurse who demonstrates the right kind of health in personal self-care serves as a role model to parents and children alike.
- **Case manager:** Although case manager is a contemporary name for this role, it involves coordination and collaboration between a family and the healthcare system. The case manager has been formally empowered to be in charge of a case.

FAMILY HEALTH RECORDS

A record is a permanent written communication that documents information relevant to a client's healthcare management, e.g., a client chart is a continuing account of client's healthcare status and need—Potter and Perry An effective health record shows the extent of the health problems' needs and other factors that affect individuals their ability to provide care and what the family believes. What has been done and what to be done now also can be shown in the records. It also indicates the plans for future visits in order to help the family member to meet the needs.

Purposes of Records

- Supply data that are essential for program planning and evaluation.
- To provide the practitioner with data required for the application of professional services for the improvement of family's health.
- Records are tools of communication between health workers, the family, and other development personnel.
- Effective health records shows the health problem in the family and other factors that affect health.
- A record indicates plans for future.

- It provides baseline data to estimate the long-term changes related to services.
- Legal documents: poisoning, assault, rape, LAMA, burn, etc.
- Research or statistics: rates
- Audit and nursing audit
- Quality of care
- Continuity of care
- Informative purposes: census
- Teaching purpose of students
- Diagnostic purposes: test reports

Importance of Records and Reports

- Assess health level of the community
- Helps in collecting data
- Assessment and evaluation of work
- Basis for formulating plans
- Tool or medium for health education
- Determine needs of resources
- Legal documentation
- Means of communication
- Provide information of good nursing
- Conduct training and research work
- Assess health problems

CONCLUSION

Family nursing is a part of the primary care provided to patients of all ages, ranging from infant to geriatric health. Nurses assess the health of the entire family to identify health problems and risk factors, help develop interventions to address health concerns, and implement the interventions to improve the health of the individual and family. Family nurses often work with patients through their whole life cycle. This helps foster a strong relationship between healthcare provider and patient. Family nursing is not as much patient-centered care as it is centered on the care of the family unit. It also takes a team approach to healthcare. A family nurse performs many duties commonly performed by a physician. They have the ability to write prescriptions, and need a broader base of knowledge and skills in order to care for their patients. Nurses may work in clinics, private offices, hospitals, hospice centers, schools and homes to care for their patients.

BIBLIOGRAPHY

1. BT Basavanthapa, "Community Health Nursing", 2nd edition, chapter-6, Family Health Nursing, Jaypee Brothers Medical Publishers (P) Ltd, 2008;108–36.
2. Krishna Kumari Gulani. "Community Health Nursing (Principles and Practices)", 1st Edition, Chapter-11, Maternal and Child Health, Kumar Publishing House, 2005;354–66.
3. Marcia Stanhope, Jeanette Lancaster. "Foundations of Nursing in the Community" (Community-Oriented Practice), 2nd edition, chapter-18, Family Development and Family Nursing Assessment, Mosby Elsevier, 321–39.
4. Park K. Essential of Community Health Nursing, 4th edition, Premnagar, Jabalpur, 2014;278–80.
5. Park K. Preventive and Social Medicine, 22nd edition 2013, Premnagar, Jabalpur, 2013;481–514.
6. Rao Sundar Kasthuri Mrs. Dr., An Introduction to Community Health Nursing, 4th edition (reprint) 2005, B.I. Publication (P) Ltd.
7. Shirely May Harmon Hanson. Family Health Care Nursing—Theory, Practice and Research 3rd edition. New Delhi: Jaypee Brothers Medical Publishers (P) Ltd; 2007.
8. Sunita Patney. "Textbook of Community Health Nursing", First edition, Chapter-8, Family Health Care, Modern Publishers, 2005;88–103.
9. Swarnkar Keshav. Community Health Nursing, 2nd edition, N.R. Brothers, Indore, 2007;83–87.

REVIEW QUESTIONS

Long Essays

1. Define family. Explain the types and functions of the family.
2. Enumerate family as a unit of community health services.
3. Define family health nursing. Explain the objectives, principles, advantages and disadvantages of family health nursing.
4. Define family health nursing process. Explain the steps in detail.
5. Describe in detail about the assessment of health problems.
6. Enumerate the core competencies family health nurse.
7. Explain family health services—maternal, child care and family welfare services.
8. Discuss the responsibilities of community health nurse in MCH services.

Short Essays

1. Characteristics of family as a unit.
2. Family health care.
3. Determinants/factors of family health.
4. Aims and objectives of family health care.
5. Principles of family health care.
6. Family-centered nursing approaches.
7. Family health assessment.
8. Methods of data collection.
9. Assessment of families.
10. Formulation of nursing diagnosis.
11. Steps in developing a family nursing care plan.
12. Recent trends in MCH service program.
13. Roles and function of a community health nurse in family health service.
14. Family health records.

Short Answers

1. Family health.
2. Family structure.
3. Family system theory.
4. Community-based nursing.
5. Socialization.
6. Family as a system.
7. Family as a component of society.
8. Nursing care plan.
9. Qualities of a nursing care plan.
10. Aims and objectives of MCH program.
11. Activities of MCH program.
12. Functions related to maternal clinics.

Chapter 5: Family Health Nursing Care

13. Purposes of records.
14. Importance of records and reports.

Multiple Choice Questions

1. Determinants/factors of family health is the following, *except*:
    a. Human biology
    b. Technology
    c. Environment
    d. Lifestyle
2. Principles of family health care is:
    a. Professional relationship
    b. Communication
    c. Priority based care
    d. All of the above
3. Elements of family nursing process includes all, *except*:
    a. Assessment and diagnosis of client's problem
    b. Planning and implementation of care
    c. Quality assurance
    d. Evaluation of the success of implemented care
4. Methods of data collection in family health care are:
    a. Observation
    b. Interview
    c. Record review
    d. All of the above
5. Aims and objectives of MCH program:
    a. Reducing maternal and child mortality and morbidity rates
    b. Promoting reproductive health or safe motherhood
    c. Ensure birth of healthy child
    d. All of the above

ANSWERS

| 1. b | 2. d | 3. c | 4. d | 5. d |

CHAPTER 6

Family Healthcare Settings

LEARNING OBJECTIVES

Home Visit
1. Purposes, principles
2. Planning and evaluation
3. Bag technique

Clinic
4. Purposes, type of clinics and their functions
5. Function of health personnel in clinics

TERMINOLOGY

Healthcare setting means a licensed home health organization, licensed hospice program, licensed hospital or nursing home, licensed assisted living facility, (licensed adult day care program), or licensed mental health or developmental services facility.

Healthcare services means services for the diagnosis, prevention, treatment, cure, or relief of a health condition, illness, injury, or disease.

Home healthcare services means medical and nonmedical services, provided to ill, disabled or infirm persons in their residences. Such services may include homemaker services, assistance with activities of daily living and respite care services.

Basic healthcare services means in and out-of-area emergency services, inpatient hospital.

Healthcare plan means any contract, policy or other arrangement for benefits or services for medical or dental care or treatment under:

Healthcare entity means any healthcare provider, health plan or healthcare clearinghouse.

Medicare select issuer means an issuer offering, or seeking to offer, a Medicare Select policy or certificate.

Foster care services means the provision of a full range of casework, treatment and community

Healthcare worker means a person other than a healthcare professional who provides medical, dental, or other health-related care or treatment under the direction of a healthcare professional with the authority to direct that individuals activities, including medical technicians, medical assistants, dental assistants, orderlies, aides, and individuals acting in similar capacities.

Home care services means skilled or personal care services provided to clients in their place of residence for a fee; Healthcare decision means any decision regarding the health care of the prospective donor.

Acute care hospital means any hospital that provides emergency medical services on a 24-hour basis.

Family health: A condition including the promotion and maintenance of physical, mental, spiritual, and social health for the family unit and for individual family members.

Family process: The ongoing interaction between family members through which they accomplish their instrumental and expressive tasks.

Primary healthcare center: A center that provides services which are usually the first point of contact with a health professional. They include services provided by general practitioners, dentists, community nurses, pharmacists and midwives, among others.

INTRODUCTION

Family health nursing process is a systematic approach to help family to develop and strengthen its capability to meet its health needs and solve health problem. Family health nursing process is closely related to community health nursing process. Nurses must address the needs of patients, but also caregivers, and this care must be integrated, dynamic and family-centered, which is composed of the affected person, caregiver, and the rest of the family. If we ensure that family members can perform their function at the lowest cost for their quality of life and satisfaction, this would have positive socioeconomic consequences in terms of health. In this way, the Nursing would develop better forms of approach that would allow him to return to his essence, to the meaning of his actions and to their experiences of the day to day that gives him the practice in the real scenario.

Chapter 6: Family Healthcare Settings

DEFINITIONS

1. Healthcare setting is defined as any setting devoted to both the diagnosis and care of persons, such as CHD clinics, hospital emergency departments, urgent care clinics, substance abuse treatment clinics, primary care settings, community clinics, mobile medical clinics and correctional healthcare facilities.
2. Family health services can be defined as having the skills and resources to carry out family development tasks. It is special care given to family members to promote their health, prevent health problems, and for the well-being of the family.
3. Home visit refers to meeting the health needs of people at their doorsteps. Health services given at home for patient, family and the community in general for nursing service and health counseling.
   Family-centered nursing: Nursing that considers health of the family as a unit in addition to the health of individual family members.

CONCEPT OF HEALTHCARE SETTING

Healthcare setting means any place where health care, including physical, dental, or behavioral health care is delivered and includes, but is not limited to any healthcare facility or agency licensed such as hospitals, ambulatory surgical centers, birthing centers, special inpatient care facilities, long-term acute care facilities, inpatient rehabilitation facilities, inpatient hospice facilities, nursing facilities, assisted living facilities, and residential facilities, behavioral health residential facilities, home health care, hospice, pharmacies, in-home care, vehicles or temporary sites where healthcare is delivered or is related to the provision of healthcare (for example, mobile clinics, ambulances, nonemergency medical transport vehicles (NEMT), secure transportation, and street based medicine), outpatient facilities, such as dialysis centers, healthcare provider offices, dental offices, behavioral healthcare offices, urgent care centers, counseling offices, school-based health centers, offices that provide complementary and alternative medicine such as acupuncture, homeopathy, naturopathy, chiropractic and osteopathic medicine, and other specialty centers.

Role of Nurse in Family Health

- Care provider
- Educator
- Coordinator and Collaborator
- Advocate
- Consultant
- Counselor
- Environmental modifier
- Researcher
- Case manager

Qualities of Family Health Nurse

Family centered approach, Holistic approach (wellness), Non-judgmental during approach, accepting different values and beliefs, self-awareness, able to work in adverse conditions, being flexible, sensitive towards time and efforts, skillful, independent and maintain positive attitude, able to cope and manage stress, able to handle situation and finally terminate relationship with family.

HEALTHCARE SETTINGS

There are several levels of health care including primary, secondary, and tertiary care. Each of these levels focuses on different aspects of health care and is typically provided in different settings.

Primary Care

- Primary care promotes wellness and prevents disease. This care includes health promotion, education, protection (such as immunizations), early disease screening, and environmental considerations.
- Settings providing this type of health care include physician offices, public health clinics, school nursing, and community health nursing.

Secondary Care

- Secondary care occurs when a person has contracted an illness or injury and requires medical care. Secondary care is often referred to as acute care.
- Secondary care can range from uncomplicated care to repair a small laceration or treat a strep throat infection to more complicated emergent care such as treating a head injury sustained in an automobile accident.
- Whatever the problem, the patient needs medical and nursing attention to return to a state of health and wellness.
- Secondary care is provided in settings such as physician offices, clinics, urgent care facilities, or hospitals.
- Specialized units include areas such as burn care, neurosurgery, cardiac surgery, and transplant services.

Tertiary Care

- Tertiary care addresses the long-term effects from chronic illnesses or conditions with the purpose to restore a patient's maximum physical and mental function.
- The goal of tertiary care is to achieve the highest level of functioning possible while managing the chronic illness. For example, a patient who falls and fractures their hip will need secondary care to set the broken bones, but may need tertiary care to regain their strength and ability to walk even after the bones have healed.
- Patients with incurable diseases, such as dementia, may need specialized tertiary care to provide support they need for daily functioning.
- Tertiary care settings include rehabilitation units, assisted living facilities, adult day care, skilled nursing units, home care, and hospice centers.

Healthcare Team

- No matter the setting, quality health care requires a team of healthcare professionals collaboratively working together to deliver holistic, individualized care.

- Nursing students must be aware of the roles and contributions of various healthcare team members.
- The healthcare team consists of healthcare providers, nurses (licensed practical nurses, registered nurses, and advanced registered nurses), unlicensed assistive personnel, and a variety of interprofessional team members.

Healthcare Providers

- The Wisconsin Nurse Practice Act defines a provider as, "A physician, podiatrist, dentist, optometrist, or advanced practice nurse."
- Providers are responsible for ordering diagnostic tests such as blood work and X-rays, diagnosing a patient's medical condition, developing a medical treatment plan, and prescribing medications.
- In a hospital setting, the medical treatment plan developed by a provider is communicated in the "History and Physical" component of the patient's medical record with associated prescriptions (otherwise known as "orders").
- Prescriptions or "orders" include diagnostic and laboratory tests, medications, and general parameters regarding the care that each patient is to receive.
- Nurses should respectfully clarify prescriptions they have questions or concerns about to ensure safe patient care. Providers typically visit hospitalized patients daily in what is referred to as "rounds."
- It is helpful for nurses and nursing students to attend provider rounds for their assigned patients to be aware of and provide input regarding the current medical treatment plan, seek clarification, or ask questions.
- This helps to ensure that the provider, nurse, and patient have a clear understanding of the goals of care and minimize the need for follow-up phone calls.

Nurses: There are three levels of nurses as defined by each state's Nurse Practice Act: Licensed Practical Nurse/Vocational Nurse (LPN/LVN), Registered Nurse (RN), and Advanced Practice Nurse (APRN).

SCOPE OF PRACTICE FOR REGISTERED NURSES

General nursing procedures: An RN shall utilize the nursing process in the execution of general nursing procedures in the maintenance of health, prevention of illness or care of the ill. The nursing process consists of the steps of assessment, planning, intervention, and evaluation. This standard is met through performance of each of the following steps of the nursing process:

- **Assessment:** Assessment is the systematic and continual collection and analysis of data about the health status of a patient culminating in the formulation of a nursing diagnosis.
- **Planning:** Planning is developing a nursing plan of care for a patient, which includes goals and priorities derived from the nursing diagnosis.
- **Intervention:** Intervention is the nursing action to implement the plan of care by directly administering care or by directing and supervising nursing acts delegated to LPNs or less skilled assistants.
- **Evaluation:** Evaluation is the determination of a patient's progress or lack of progress toward goal achievement, which may lead to modification of the nursing diagnosis.

Performance of Delegated Acts

In the performance of delegated acts, an RN shall do all of the following:

- Accept only those delegated acts for which there are protocols or written or verbal orders.
- Accept only those delegated acts for which the RN is competent to perform based on his or her nursing education, training or experience.
- Consult with a provider in cases where the RN knows or should know a delegated act may harm a patient.
- Perform delegated acts under the general supervision or direction of provider.

Supervision and Direction of Delegated Acts

In the supervision and direction of delegated acts, an RN shall do all of the following:

- Delegate tasks commensurate with educational preparation and demonstrated abilities of the person supervised.
- Provide direction and assistance to those supervised.
- Observe and monitor the activities of those supervised.
- Evaluate the effectiveness of acts performed under supervision.

TYPES OF HOME HEALTHCARE SERVICES

The range of home healthcare services a patient can receive at home is limitless. Depending on the individual patient's situation, care can range from nursing care to specialized medical services, such as laboratory workups. You and your doctor will determine your care plan and services you may need at home. At-home care services may include:

- **Doctor care:** A doctor may visit a patient at home to diagnose and treat the illness(es). He or she may also periodically review the home healthcare needs.
- **Nursing care:** The most common form of home healthcare is some type of nursing care depending on the person's needs. In consultation with the doctor, a registered nurse will set up a plan of care. Nursing care may include wound dressing, ostomy care, intravenous therapy, administering medication, monitoring the general health of the patient, pain control, and other health support.
- **Physical, occupational, and/or speech therapy:** Some patients may need help relearning how to perform daily duties or improve their speech after an illness or injury. A physical therapist can put together a plan of care to help a patient regain or strengthen use of muscles and joints. An occupational therapist can help a patient with physical, developmental, social, or emotional disabilities relearn how to perform such daily functions as eating, bathing, dressing, and more. A speech therapist can help a patient with impaired speech regain the ability to communicate clearly.

- **Medical social services:** Medical social workers provide various services to the patient, including counseling and locating community resources to help the patient in his or her recovery. Some social workers are also the patient's case manager—if the patient's medical condition is very complex and requires coordination of many services.
- **Care from home health aides:** Home health aides can help the patient with his or her basic personal needs such as getting out of bed, walking, bathing, and dressing. Some aides have received specialized training to assist with more specialized care under the supervision of a nurse.

HOME VISIT

The community health nurse work with families in different settings including clinics, schools, support groups, office and the family home. Home visits give a more accurate assessment of the family structure and behavior in the natural environment. Home visits also provide opportunities to observe the home environment and to identify barriers and support for reaching family health promotion goods. Health services in the home requires technical skills, knowledge of preventive and therapeutic measures, teaching ability, judgment and a full understanding of human relations.

Concepts of Home Visiting

- Home visiting provides opportunity to make direct observation on home environment, family structure, familial roles and relationships, lifestyle, cultural practices, group dynamics, etc., and make family health assessment.
- In home visiting the members are relaxed, have more time and privacy and feel free to raise questions, seek clarifications and sort out their problems.
- It provides opportunities to make direct observation of care given by family members in planning and implementing family healthcare services.
- It provides opportunities to contact and interact with most of the family members and establish report with the family as a whole.
- It also makes possible to have active participation of family members in planning and implementing family healthcare.
- It makes feasible to plan and provide comprehensive family health care with major emphasis on promotive and preventive care.

Purposes of Home Visiting

- It is a routine part of a planned visiting program by a community health personnel.
- It helps to investigate the source of infectious diseases.
- To do follow-up on some problems identified in the health center, school, industry or hospital.
- To assess the nutritional and immunization status, environmental hazards.
- To give health education to the individual, family and community.
- To supervise and guide other health workers.

Principles of Home Visiting

- **Need based**—Home visiting should be planned and conducted based on the identified needs of the people.
- **Priority based**—The home visit should give to the existing problem in the family. It may be maternal and child health services or antenatal check-up.
- **Regularity**—Plan for regular home visiting programme based on family needs. It should be conducted at regular intervals.
- **Flexibility**—The community health nurse should adopt a flexible approach based on prevailing circumstances at home.
- **Scientific based**—Be sure of the scientific soundness of the subjects used for discussion. Use of technical skills includes handwashing an inspection.
- **Analysis based**—Collect facts about the home, the patient and the environment and make on objective analysis of the facts as an initial step in visiting the home.
- **Developing relationship**—Work with the person and family plan jointly. Home visiting helps to establish good working relationship in the family.
- **Sensitivity**—The community health nurse should be sensitive to the persons feeling and needs at the time of the visit. Listen to the family and understand the other person's point of view.
- **Educative**—Evaluate your own work remember the quality of care is more important than the number of hoe visits. It is essential to evaluate home visits from time to time.

Steps in Home Visiting

Initial phase: The community health nurse should collect information from clinical and other records before planning for a visit. During home visit, she has to assess or observe and make a note in initial visit. The community health nurse should introduce and establish a friendly relationship by using simple language. Assess physical and environmental status, family's cultural background, occupation and income of family member, age, educational factors and psychological factors influences.

Action phase: The inter-personal relationship starts when nurses enter into the house. The nurse should use their effective communication skills to implement the nursing process. During home visit, nurse practice a variety of roles when interviewing in patient care. The community health nurse has to take a role as collaborator, consultant, co-coordinator, preventor of disease, promoter of health, health educator and an epidemiologist and takes steps to implement nursing process.

During action phase the community health nurse provides nursing care, e.g., taking temperature, physical examination and dressing, etc. Demonstrating and teaching, e.g., teaching insulin self-administration. She makes diagnosis and tentative nursing care plan based on establishing priorities.

Termination phase: Nurse patient goals are reached, health is restored and the patient can function without actions. The nurse records the important events in the family and reports the problems of the family. Evaluation of home visit is a continuous process, through at the end of every visit community health nurse evaluate and document.

Advantages of Home Visit

- The nurse can directly observe home and family atmosphere.
- The nurse can directly observe the care given to patient by the family members.
- It is possible to discover new health problems.
- The family members will be more relaxed in their own surroundings.
- The family gains confidence and feels to clear their doubts.
- This helps to apply the gained knowledge and skills in the homes assisting and solving individuals and families health problems.

BAG TECHNIQUES

The community health nurse requires some tools and instruments for doing procedures during home visits. The purpose of community bag is to carry out nursing procedures in home, which includes weighing the children, performing minor dressing and to conduct delivery in emergency situations.

Definitions

- The community health bag can be made of khaki material or any material with an aluminum or iron frame to fit inside. Leather bags can also be used if the agency can afford this. It is designed to carry equipment and material needed during a visit to the home, school or factory.
- The nursing bag is a vehicle for carrying the material and equipment needed during home made to attend family healthcare needs. The bag should have outside packets for keeping a note book, Waste paper bad, folder, newspaper, stationeries and tablet container.

Importance of Community Bag

- It is essential during each home visit school and industrial visit to do some nursing procedures.
- The community bag and material required are kept ready to use at any time.
- The community bag helps to demonstrate some procedure nursing procedure during home visit.
- The community bag acts as a vehicle for carrying the tools during a home visit.
- The community bag is an excitement demonstration of cleanliness.

Principles of Bag Technique

- The community bag must be kept scrupulously clean and ready for use at all times.
- The community bag should be kept in clean areas without danger of being contaminated by the children or domestic animals.
- Clean or boil the instruments after use and replace it safety.
- Avoid unnecessary exposure while doing procedure.
- Secure the bag by often cleaning and cover it properly.
- The community bag placed in a clean surface or piece of newspaper or a plastic sheet.
- Remove the soap, towel and nail brush and wash the hands well.
- Open the bag and remove only the needed articles and close the bag.
- Carry out the procedure placing soiled swabs inside a newspaper bag for disposal by burning or any other suitable method.
- Carry the bag. Fold used paper or plastic sheet with exposed side innermost and keep it in the outside pocket of the bag.
- Write brief note of the observation, procedure done or instructions given.
- Check the bag daily, washing hands before opening it and make necessary replacements.

Articles Used in Community Bag

- **Outside packet:** Newspaper, stationeries, family folders, flash cards and waste paper bag.
- **Side flap:** Tablets containers should have paracetamol, septran multivitamin or B-complex, Anthelmintics, flagyl anti-inflammatory, etc., solutions—antiseptic, savlon, Betadine, Benedict's solution, acetic acid, methylated spirit and eye drops or ointment.
- **Lower compartment:** Urine analysis kit, specimen bottle, kidney tray test tubes, test tube holder, spirit lamp and match box.
  The handwashing items—soap, towel, nail brush, small mackintosh or plastic sheet and plastic aprons.
  Physical assessment instruments—fetoscope, inch tape, shakir tape and spring balance to check weight.
- **Sterile compartment:** Instruments—artery forceps, thumb forceps, small towel and scissors. A pair of disposable glove or paper gloves.
- **Miscellaneous articles:** Mucus suckers, tallquist paper for checking hemoglobin and small catheter.

Steps of Procedure with Community Bag

- Select a work area according to the convenient of the family.
- Place the bag in a mat in a veranda on newspaper.
- Unbutton the bag of lower compartment.
- Remove handwashing equipment and wash hands properly.

- Remove apron from the bag and put it on.
- Remove the need items from the outside compartment.
- Give nursing care based on the plan.
- When procedure is over, wash hands with soap an water.
- Place the articles to the bag after cleaning.
- Fold used newspaper with used side inside.
- Close the bag.
- Record your procedures and observation and instructions given.

HOME HEALTH NURSING PROCEDURES

The community health nurse primary responsibility to meet health needs of the family, it is necessary to provide nursing care on a selective basis and to demonstrate the care to some responsible member of the family. It is recognized that nurses working in the community health field have been trained in many different hospitals and schools, they were taught procedures have changed community.

Principles

- **Resources usage:** Standard procedures should be followed as far as possible utilizing materials and equipment found in the home.
- **Demonstration:** Demonstration of nursing care in the home is most effective method of teaching.
- **Standing orders:** Medical instructions in the form of standing instructions or individual instructions must be available before administering medicine or treatment.
- **Prevent spread of disease:** The health worker must know to check the disease at its sources. The practice of medical asepsis and the habit of thorough cleanliness at all time sis basic to all procedures.
- **Respect the families** practice as far as possible custom and habits is sacred to the family. Habit changes are slow and come wit knowledge ad action which the nurse may initiate and or participate in through individual and group teaching.
- **Comfort and relationship:** Consider comfort and relationship when selecting the patients unit. The nurse must select the place where the patient will get rest, privacy and clean air. The sick person may be housed comfortably and at the same time, prevent the spread of infectious material.
- **Economical use** supplies and equipment economically, always consider the high cost of fuel, the hardship in getting water and the family economics.
- **Teaching:** The community health nurse should teach the patient and responsible member of the family, teach with proper demonstration and also encourage to do return demonstration.
- **Record keeping:** Adequate records and reports are an integral part of every good nursing services. Records should be maintained up to date.
- **Prevention of accidents:** Write name of the drug ad instructions for taking using the language of the people. Inform the family to keep all drugs locked in their cupboards and out of reach of children.
- **Health promotion:** Safe water, latrines, drainage, cooking arrangements, bathing, absence or presence of animals within the compound or in the house is of major important in the promotions of health.
- **Nutritional observation:** Observation and action relative to the nutritional status of the family is a primary responsibility of the nurse.

HANDWASHING

Handwashing is most important and basic technique used in preventing and controlling, transmission of pathogens. It is vigorous brief rubbing together of all surfaces of hands lathered in soap and followed by rinsing under a stream of water.

Purposes

- To remove soil and transient microorganism.
- To reduce total microbial counts overtime.
- To prevent cross infection
- To protect herself from infection and prevents the spread of infection to others.

Articles Needed

- Soap in a soap dish
- Tab water or water in a container
- Nail brush
- Bucket to receive water
- A mug or chamber for pouring water
- Towel to wipe wet hands.

Procedure

- Place the community bag on newspaper.
- Remove watch, bangles, rings in a safe place or place it in the packet.
- Open unsterile compartment and remove hand washing set.
- Place newspaper and keep handwashing things near the washing area.
- Turn on the tap or ask family member to pour water.
- Scrub for 2-3 minutes with nail brush, wash soap and hands with water.
- Hold hands up to prevent water from coming back down.
- Dry hands with hand towel.

CLEANING, DISINFECTING AND STERILIZATION

Definitions

Cleaning: Cleaning is the removal of dirt including some organism from the hands skin and articles by using friction with soap, soap nut or clean ash and thoroughly rinsing with water.

Disinfection: Disinfection is the process of destroying microorganisms (except spores) by physical and chemical agents all microorganisms including spores.

Sterilization: It refers to eliminates, eliminates, or renders inactive all life forms, notably microorganisms like fungi, bacteria, spores, and unicellular eukaryotic organisms, as well as other biological agents like prions, that are present in or on a given surface, object, or fluid.

Principles

- Allow enough time for articles to be thoroughly disinfected or sterilized.
- The articles contaminated with blood, feces, pus, sputum or other substances to prevent coagulation and adherence of solids, rinse with cold water.
- Use the right disinfectant the right strength and the right time.
- Select the right procedure to render the article safe for use and to prevent spread of infection.

Cleaning

- Soap and water are the most universally used cleaning agents. Soap and water have limited bacterial power. To be most effective, use warm water, lather, rub vigorously and rinse thoroughly.
- **Detergent:** A good detergent increases cleaning power of water and leaves no film or scum.
- **Dusting and sweeping:** Some disease producing organisms travel from person to person through dust particles. Demonstrate and encourage use of long handle brooms for sweeping.

Sterilization and Disinfection

Physical Agents

- **Stream under pressure:** It is the most effective method for destroying spores and other disease producing organisms. Medical Research Council recommends safety margin of 20 Ibs pressure and temperature of $260°$ F for 30 minutes for destroying spores.
- **Boiling:** Boiling water is the most universally used method of disinfection. For sterilization the articles must be completely submerged in boiling water for 5 minutes. This will kill all nonspore formers.
- **Dry heat:** Ironing destroys most pathogenic organisms. Dampen the cloth that is to be used for dressing organisms. Dampen the cloth that is to be used for dressing a wound or for perineal pad and press with hot iron until dry.
- **Scorching:** Hold the cloth or dressing over live coals and apply directly to the wound. This procedure is often used to disinfect the cloth used for cord dressing.
- **Exposure to sunlight:** The efficiency of sunlight is believed to be due to a combination of ultra violet rays, visible rays and infrared heat wears.
- **Chemical disinfection:** Chemical disinfection is safe only when "tested" chemicals are used in the correct strength and when proper time is allowed. Commonly used chemicals are ethyl alcohol 70%, Dettol 2% in soft water, chloride of lime or bleaching powders.

THERMOMETER TECHNIQUES

A clinical thermometer is a special instrument designed to measure the temperature of the body. Two thermometers one oral and one rectal are essential equipment which the nurse always carries in her bag. Elevation in temperature is an indication that the body is reacting to an infection.

Principles

- Meticulous cleaning of thermometer before and after use is essential to prevent the spread of infection.
- Temperature is usually taken by mouth. Rectal temperatures are most accurate while auxiliary temperatures are least accurate.
- Shake the mercury to $95°$ F before taking the temperature.
- Keep all thermometers in the shade and in the coolest part of the building.
- Accuracy in temperature helps in effective treatment and medical decision.

Equipment

- Ten small cotton swabs
- Kidney basin to hold moist cotton swabs
- Thermometer
- Lubricant for rectal temperature
- Paper bag

Procedure

- Use bag technique as per standard precautions
- Remove the thermometer swab up to bulb and read
- Place the thermometer at proper site.
- Rinse the thermometer thoroughly under cool running water after reading.
- Replace it in the community bag and wash hands
- Record it in the TPR sheet.

MEASUREMENT OF WEIGHT AND HEIGHT

Weight and height measurements are an index of a person continuing growth and developments and may index to the maintenance of health. A person's height and weight is influenced by varying factors such as inheritance, nutrition, incidence of sickness, the endocrine system, etc.

Measurement of weight and height is the responsibility of the community health nurse and health visitors to explain the significance of weight and height to the person's being weighed. Weight and measurement of the child at planned specific periods is important to determine the rate of growth to detect deviation in his own growth curve.

Principles

- The weighing scales must be accurate
- The baby scales platform must be safe and secure to prevent the child from falling.
- The mother or nurse must stay with the child when he is being weighed to prevent falling.
- Record of the weight as soon as the scale is read. Adjust the scales each time.
- Emphasize importance of weighing during the growth period.
- Keep the scale locked when not in use, return bar to o after each weight has been read.

- To prevent cross infection, the nurse should stand behind or to the side of the person being weighted to prevent contact with the person's face and mouth.

Equipment
- Scales—with height rod
- Scales—bathroom or weight balance
- Tape measure
- Records or packet dairy

Procedure
- Place the scales and measuring in a well lighted and ventilated area
- Place a clean paper or clean plastic on the scale
- Look at the record and note the last recorded weight
- Place the child flat on weighing scale
- Record the present weight and remove the baby gently
- Record immediately on the chart
- Height can be measured by place the tape measure or measuring rod on a table or firm surface and place the infant alongside the measure. Hold the head and heel firmly and read the measure.

RECORDS AND REPORTS PERTAINING TO FAMILY HEALTH CARE

Reports are written when the information is to be used by several people or is more or less of permanent value. A written report should show an awareness of time and thinking. It should concentrate on the past present and future state of patient or family or the event. Description and conclusion of action that influence further planning and decision-making are necessary.

The family health records and report should be clear, unbiased observation of persons, relationship and events is needed to write a meaningful report. When reports are needed for information that will be used by a number of people or as a source of reference requirements for further consideration as for research and legal purpose for further consideration as for research and legal purpose.

Presenting good report is an art. It is a skill that is developed by definite effort. In a community health service, the community health nurse or health worker is responsible for keeping both administrative and service records about community. The nursing service may require reports on the work of staff nurses, nurse aids and other professional workers.

NURSING CLINIC

A broad definition of a nurse-led clinic defines these clinics based on what nursing activities are performed at the site. Nurses within a nurse-led clinic assume their own patient case-loads, provide an educative role to patients to promote health, provide psychological support, monitor the patient's condition and perform nursing interventions. Advanced practice registered nurses, usually nurse practitioners, may have expanded roles within these clinics, depending on the scope of practice defined by their state, provincial or territorial government.

Definition

A nurse-led clinic is any outpatient clinic that is run or managed by registered nurses, usually nurse practitioners or Clinical Nurse Specialists in the UK. Nurse-led clinics have assumed distinct roles over the years, and examples exist within hospital outpatient department's public health clinics and independent practice environments.

Community Clinic Services

Clinic setting is a place where family members come to seek medical and healthcare services as desired by them from the members of healthcare team including physician stationed there. Clinics are arranged at the following locations: Sub-center, Primary health center, Community health center, Hospital, Slums, MCH and family welfare centers, Schools, Fair places, etc.

Reasons for Clinics
- To offer care for people's felt need.
- To provide care for actual needs of people.

Types of Clinics
- General clinics
- Separate clinics
- Specialty clinics

General Clinics

Any person can be attended with any of the health problem. These are more convenient because:
- All clients can be dealt with at the same time. For example, pregnant mother, malnourished child, father having fever, grandmother having indigestion; they all together can attend the same clinic.
- An individual person can use the same visit to have all the problems seen on one single occasion. For example, a mother needing antenatal check up, having sore eyes, cut injury and requesting information about child care.

Separate Clinics

There are a number of separate clinics run on different days of the week. This system of clinics is used where access is very easy and client's number is very large. The important clinics under this category include:
- Antenatal clinics
- Postnatal clinics
- Under five clinics
- Family welfare clinics
- Reproductive and child health clinics

- It must be seen that community health nurse must not spend all the days in the clinic. It is useful to spend time for community healthcare activities. Clinic must be a part of community programme so that the clinic can provide service to the needy people.

Specialty Clinic

These provide medical and counseling services for specific disorders. These clinics are run by specialist Doctors and Nurses. Some of the important clinics under this category include:
- TB clinic
- Diabetes clinic
- STDs clinic
- Nutrition clinic
- Cardiac clinic
- Chest clinic

Location of the Clinic

- Clinic should be set up within the community or as near to the community as possible. No one should need to travel more than 1 hour of easy journey.
- The location should be acceptable to all.
- The clinic and waiting area must be safe for children.

Criteria for a Good Clinic

- Clinic is located close to the community. The location should be acceptable and accessible.
- The clinic should be well organized with effective flow pattern from one station to another.
- Provision for follow-up care and referral.
- There should be effective system of recording and reporting.
- There should be effective system of health education for people coming to the clinics.

Functions of Community Health Nurse

- Setting up of clinic and arranging equipment and supplies.
- Placement of health worker at a particular service area and assigning responsibilities accordingly.
- Assessment of health status of patients.
- Proving need based nursing care services.
- Giving necessary instructions to patient and family members.
- Conducting health education sessions as needed.
- Assisting the Doctor/Specialist.
- Supervision and guidance of health workers.
- Monitoring of health records and registers.
- Maintaining and preserving the health records, registers and reports of the clinic services provided.
- Helping in promoting good working environment at the clinic.

Functions of MPHW (F)

- Helps in setting up of clinic.
- Does registration of cases attending the clinic.
- Takes and records their weight if required.
- Does assessment of health status as per guidelines.
- Provides treatment and care based on needs as per standing order.
- Gives necessary instructions to patient and family members.
- Participates in health education sessions.

Nurses Role in Clinics

The primary role of a nurse is to advocate and care for individuals and support them through health and illness. However, there are various other responsibilities of a nurse that form a part of the role of a nurse, including to:
- Record medical history and symptoms
- Collaborate with teams to plan for patient care
- Advocate for the health and wellbeing of patients
- Monitor patient health and record signs
- Administer medications and treatments
- Operate medical equipment
- Perform diagnostic tests
- Educate patients about management of illnesses
- Provide support and advice to patients

Patient Care

- A nurse is a caregiver for patients and helps to manage physical needs, prevent illness, and treat health conditions. To do this, they need to observe and monitor the patient, recording any relevant information to aid in treatment decision-making.
- Throughout the treatment process, the nurse follows the progress of the patient and acts accordingly with the patient's best interests in mind. The care provided by a nurse extends beyond the administration of medications and other therapies.
- They are responsible for the holistic care of patients, which encompasses the psychosocial, developmental, cultural, and spiritual needs of the individual.

Patient Advocacy

- The patient is the first priority of the nurse. The role of the nurse is to advocate for the best interests of the patient and to maintain the patient's dignity throughout treatment and care.
- This may include making suggestions in the treatment plan of patients, in collaboration with other health professionals.
- This is particularly important because patients who are unwell are often unable to comprehend medical situations and act as they usually would.
- It is the role of the nurse to support the patient and represent the patient's best interests at all times, especially when treatment decisions are being made.

Planning of Care

- A nurse is directly involved in the decision-making process for the treatment of patients.

Chapter 6: Family Healthcare Settings

- It is important that they are able to think critically when assessing patient signs and identifying potential problems so that they can make the appropriate recommendations and actions.
- As other health professionals, such as doctors or specialists, are usually in charge of making the final treatment decisions, nurses should be able to communicate information regarding patient health effectively.
- Nurses are the most familiar with the individual patient situation as they monitor their signs and symptoms on an ongoing basis and should collaborate with other members of the medical team to promote the best patient health outcomes.

Patient Education and Support

- Nurses are also responsible for ensuring that patients are able to understand their health, illnesses, medications, and treatments to the best of their ability.
- This is of the essence when patients are discharged from hospital and need to take control of their own treatments.
- A nurse should take the time to explain to the patient and their family or caregiver what to do and what to expect when they leave the hospital or medical clinic. They should also make sure that the patient feels supported and knows where to seek additional information.

Nursing in India

- As India struggles with doctor shortage, government gives a push to nurse-led clinics. If changes come through, a nurse practitioner may be allowed to prescribe medicines, conduct invasive procedures under supervision of senior doctors. Nursing professionals may soon be allowed to run autonomous clinics in India.
- At the behest of the government, the Indian Nursing Council, the regulatory body for nurses and their education, is preparing a draft bill to amend a 1947 Act which will bring nurse practicing rights in the country up to global standards.
- The program may allow nurse practitioners (registered nurses educated to a master's degree level) to prescribe medicines for primary care and conduct invasive procedures in the presence of senior doctors. It is also expected to institute a new examination process to issue nursing licenses.
- Once the draft bill is ready, it will be sent to the ministry of health and family welfare for approval and introduction in Parliament. The council is likely to send the draft in the next three months.
- "Nurse practitioner programs and licentiate examination for nurses are among the key initiatives under the National Health Policy 2017 of the government of India. The ministry of health and family welfare has entrusted the Indian Nursing Council with their implementation in a time-bound manner."

BIBLIOGRAPHY

1. Child Trends. World Family Map: Mapping Family Change and Child Well-Being Outcomes. Child Trends: Springer; 2013.
2. Universal declaration of human rights, Article 16.3. United Nations General Assembly, Paris: Springer; 1948.
3. Wright LM, Leahey M. Nurses and families: A guide to family assessment and intervention. Philadelphia, USA: FA Davis Company; 2009.

REVIEW QUESTIONS

Long Essays
1. Define healthcare settings. Describe primary, secondary and tertiary health care.
2. Describe the scope of practice for registered nurses.
3. Define home visiting. Give an account of purposes and principles of home visiting.
4. Define bag techniques. Explain the importance and principles of bag technique.

Short Essays
1. Healthcare team.
2. Healthcare providers.
3. Types of home healthcare services.
4. Steps in home visiting.
5. Articles used in community bag.
6. Steps of procedure with community bag.
7. Home health nursing procedures.
8. Principles of home health nursing procedures.
9. Sterilization and disinfection.
10. Measurement of weight and height.
11. Records and reports pertaining to family health care.
12. Functions of community health nurse.

Short Answers
1. Healthcare setting.
2. Healthcare services.
3. Home healthcare services.
4. Healthcare worker.
5. Family health.
6. Primary healthcare center.
7. Role of nurse in family health.
8. Qualities of family health nurse.
9. Advantages of home visit.
10. Handwashing.
11. Cleaning.
12. Disinfection.
13. Community clinic services.
14. Criteria for a good clinic.
15. Patient advocacy.
16. Functions of MPHW (F).
17. Nurses role in clinics.

Multiple Choice Questions
1. Healthcare setting is any setting devoted to both the diagnosis and care of persons in:
    a. Clinics, hospital emergency departments
    b. Primary care settings, community clinics

c. Mobile medical clinics and correctional healthcare facilities
  d. All of the above
2. Role of nurse in family health, *except*:
  a. Problem solver
  b. Care provider
  c. Educator
  d. Counselor
3. The purposes of home visiting are:
  a. It is a routine part of a planned visiting program by a community health personnel
  b. To do follow-up on some problems identified in the health center, school, industry or hospital
  c. To assess the nutritional and immunization status, environmental hazards
  d. All of the above
4. The PHN bag is an important tool in providing nursing care during a home visit. The most important principle of bag technique states that it:
  a. Should save time and effort
  b. Should minimize if not totally prevent the spread of infection
  c. Should not overshadow concern for the patient and his family
  d. May be done in a variety of ways depending on the home situation, etc.
5. To maintain the cleanliness of the bag and its contents, which of the following must the nurse do?
  a. Wash his/her hands before and after providing nursing care to the family members
  b. In the care of family members, as much as possible, use only articles taken from the bag
  c. Put on an apron to protect her uniform and fold it with the right side out before putting it back into the bag
  d. At the end of the visit, fold the lining on which the bag was placed, ensuring that the contaminated side is on the outside

ANSWERS

| 1. d | 2. a | 3. d | 4. b | 5. a | | | | | | | |

Referral System

LEARNING OBJECTIVES

1. Levels of health care and healthcare settings
2. Referral services available—steps in referral
3. Role of a nurse in referral

TERMINOLOGY

Referral: A process in which a health worker at one level of the health system, having insufficient resources (e.g., drugs, equipment, skills), manages a clinical condition, seeks the assistance of a better or differently resourced facility at the same or higher level to assist in or take over the management of a client's case.

Initiating/referring facility): The facility (e.g., organization, clinic) that starts the referral process. This is the point in the referral process where an outward referral is prepared to communicate the client's condition and status.

Receiving facility: The facility (e.g., organization, clinic) that accepts the referred client's case and provides needed services.

Initiating/referring service: The type of service from which the referral was initiated (e.g., family planning, antenatal care or general primary care).

Receiving service: The type of service to which the client is referred (e.g., family planning, antenatal care or HIV testing and counseling).

Facilitated referral: Every beneficiary is referred through a specific protocol, which includes triad of proper information transfer (referral slip, counseling); feedback and tracking (completion of referral loop) and evidence of efforts overcoming barriers (geographical, financial, etc.).

Counter-referral: The process in which clients are directly reaching the facility, then the facility staff after providing the necessary treatment sends clients to their respective UPHCS. The UPHC staff then completes the loop at the community level.

Back referral: The process by which the receiving facility sends the client back to the initiating facility with information about services provided there and any needed follow-up. This completes the referral loop between the two facilities.

Referral network: The interconnected group of service providers among which referrals are made. Referral systems are used to integrate networks of service providers.

Referral protocols/healthcare pathways: For any particular clinical condition or service, each beneficiary has to go through multiple stages of management. Each stage needs him/her to pass through a series of health facilities and health providers.

Initiating facility: The facility that starts the referral process is called the initiating facility, and they prepare an outward referral to communicate the client condition and status.

Receiving facility: The facility that accepts the referred case is called the receiving facility and at the end of their involvement, they prepare a back referral on the lower part of the forms to let the initiating facility know what has been done. This completes the referral loop between the two facilities.

Referral register: It is a means of maintaining a list of all outward and inward referrals for one facility or service provider. Information registered includes client referred, to where, when and why, whether the case is closed or continuing, and whether it was an appropriate referral or if there were any issues.

Directory of services: Some areas maintain a directory of services that lists all organizations providing specialist care. Such a directory can facilitate the search for the most appropriate service provider for a particular referral. Where such a directory is used, it is important that the contact information is kept up-to-date.

INTRODUCTION

A referral system is a mechanism that enables a patient's health needs to be comprehensively managed using resources beyond those available at the location they access care from, be it in a community unit, dispensary, health center or a

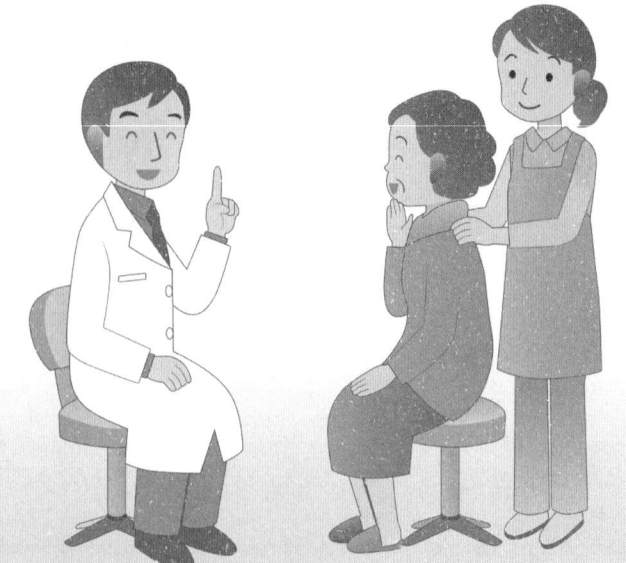

Fig. 7.1: Referral services.

higher level health facility. The main objective of a referral system is to improve and streamline communication among the various people involved in the healthcare process—from primary healthcare physicians to super-specialists **(Fig. 7.1)**.

DEFINITIONS

- Referral system is defined as a system of transferring cases which are beyond the technical competence of one infrastructure to a higher level infrastructure/institution having technical competency and all other resources to provide desired health services.
- Referral system is defined as a system of transferring cases which are beyond the technical competence of one infrastructure to higher level infrastructure/institution having technical competency and all other resources to provide desired health services.
- In another word "a referral can be defined as a process in which a health worker at a one level of the health system, having insufficient resources (drugs, skills, equipment) to manage a clinical condition, seeks the assistance of a better or differently resourced facility at the same or higher level to assist in, or take over the management of, the client's case.

REFERRAL IN HEALTH SYSTEMS

A referral can be defined as a process in which a health worker at one level of the health system, having insufficient resources (drugs, equipment, skills), manages a clinical condition, and seeks the assistance of a better or differently resourced facility at the same or higher level to assist in or take over the management of, the client's case.

Key reasons for deciding to refer either an emergency or routine case is shown in **Box 7.1**.

The health system in India is hierarchical, like most others in the world, starting with primary care to secondary care facilities and ending at the highest level of care. This consists of tertiary level facilities that provide highly specialized services.

However, in most developing countries, health referral systems across the various levels of care are weak at present, affecting the overall performance of the health system. An active referral system ensures a handy relationship between every level of health care delivery system, i.e., primary, secondary and tertiary health care. It also ensures optimal utilization of health services as it connects the populations with service locations which they may chose on preference or proximity or both. To create a good referral system **(Box 7.2)**, it is important to consider the following points:

- Patients should be given optimal care at the right level, right time and right cost
- Optimal and cost-efficient utilization of healthcare systems
- Optimal and appropriate utilization of specialist services for patients in need
- Optimal utilization of primary healthcare services.

PURPOSES OF HEALTH SYSTEMS

Referral is a process of directing someone to another source of assistance. Referral is the act or instance of sending or directing someone for treatment, aid, information or a decision

- To provide need based comprehensive care within the technical competencies and resources at each level of primary healthcare infrastructure efficiently and effectively.
- To help people avail specialized services available at higher level institution which are beyond their reach.
- To streamline the appropriate use of PHC infrastructure and specialized services in order to prevent overloading of specialized institution by direct uses.

LEVELS OF HEALTH CARE AND HEALTHCARE SETTINGS

There are several levels of health care including primary, secondary, and tertiary care. Each of these levels focuses on different aspects of health care and is typically provided in different settings.

Box 7.1: Key reasons for referral.

Key reasons for deciding to refer either an emergency or routine case include:
- To seek expert opinion regarding the client
- To seek additional or different services for the client
- To seek admission and management of the client
- To seek use of diagnostic and therapeutic tools.

Box 7.2: Good referral system ensures.

A good referral system can help to ensure:
- Clients receive optimal care at the appropriate level and not unnecessarily costly.
- Hospital facilities are used optimally and cost-effectively.
- Clients who most need specialist services can accessing them in a timely way.
- Primary health services are well utilized and their reputation is enhanced.

Chapter 7: Referral System

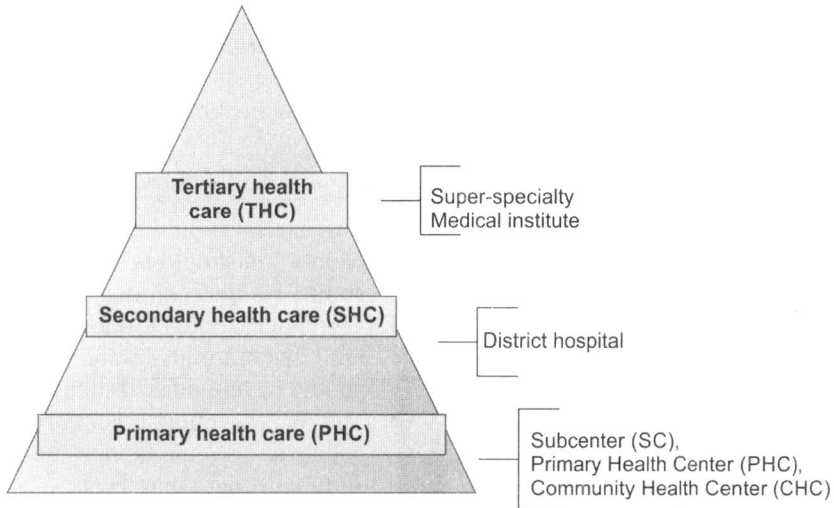

Fig. 7.2: Pyramid of level of health care.

Definition: There are three different levels of healthcare systems which are primary, secondary, and tertiary (**Fig. 7.2**). In this chapter, you'll get to know more about these healthcare systems. These referral systems are interlinked or interconnected to one another.

Primary Health Care

- Primary health care denotes the first level of contact between individuals and families with the health system. According to Alma Ata Declaration of 1978.
- Primary health care was to serve the community it served; it included care for mother and child which included family planning, immunization, prevention of locally endemic diseases, treatment of common diseases or injuries, provision of essential facilities, health education, provision of food and nutrition and adequate supply of safe drinking water.
- In India, primary health care is provided through a network of Subcenters and Primary Health Centers in rural areas, whereas in urban areas, it is provided through Health posts and Family Welfare Centers.
- The Subcenter consists of one Auxiliary Nurse Midwife and Multipurpose Health worker and serves a population of 5000 in plains and 3000 persons in hilly and tribal areas.
- The Primary Health Center (PHC), staffed by Medical Officer and other paramedical staff serves every 30000 population in the plains and 20,000 persons in hilly, tribal and backward areas. Each PHC is to supervise 6 subcenters.

Secondary Health Care

Secondary health care refers to a second tier of health system, in which patients from primary health care are referred to specialists in higher hospitals for treatment. In India, the health centres for secondary health care include District hospitals and Community health center at block level.

- Secondary health care includes specialists such as cardiologists, dermatologists, urologists and other specialists.
- Individuals reach out to the secondary medical care providers through the referral of the primary healthcare professionals.
- In few countries, the individuals cannot consult the specialists without the referral of the medical practitioner at the primary care level.
- The secondary healthcare providers act as a liaison between the patient and the advanced medical care.

Tertiary Health Care

- Tertiary health care refers to a third level of health system, in which specialized consultative care is provided usually on referral from primary and secondary medical care.
- Specialized Intensive Care Units, advanced diagnostic support services and specialized medical personnel on the key features of tertiary healthcare.
- In India, under public health system, tertiary care service is provided by medical colleges and advanced medical research institutes.

Examples of tertiary care services include specialist cancer management, neurosurgery, cardiac surgery, transplant services, plastic surgery, treatment for severe burns, advanced neonatology services, palliative, and other complex medical and surgical interventions.

- This is the care that comes into the picture as a referral to patients by the primary and healthcare providers.
- The individuals may require advanced medical procedures such as major surgeries, transplants, replacements and long-term medical care management for diseases such as cancer, neurological disorders.
- Specialized consultive medical care is the highest form of healthcare practice and performs all the major medical procedures.
- Advanced diagnostic centres, specialized intensive care units and modern medical facilities are the key features in Tertiary Medical Care.
- The practices that provide tertiary medical care could be part of the government or a combination of both public and private sectors.

Quaternary Health Care

Quaternary health care has been defined as an extension of tertiary care in reference to advanced levels of medicine which are highly specialised and not widely accessed, and usually only offered in a very limited number of national or international centers. Experimental medicine and some types of uncommon diagnostic or surgical procedures are considered quaternary care.

CONCEPT OF REFERRAL SYSTEM

A referral system is a powerful tool that helps healthcare providers keep track of the referrals made by their patients. The main objective of a referral system is to improve and streamline communication among the various people involved in the healthcare process—from primary healthcare physicians to super-specialists.

- The referral system is vertical in nature. The cases can be referred from village health post to SC/PHC, from SC to PHC/CHC and from PHC to CHC/secondary or tertiary level hospital and from CHC to secondary or tertiary level hospital.
- Provision is made for bypassing 1 or 2 level depending upon the nature and seriousness of cases so that required medical and nursing care can be given on time to the case and mortality and morbidity can be prevented and controlled.

COMPONENTS OF A REFERRAL SYSTEM (FIG. 7.3)

A referral system at all levels of the health care can facilitate the flow of patient referrals among government and private healthcare providers. When implemented efficiently, referral systems contribute to high standards of care and optimal use of medical services and resources. It is a critical component of quality healthcare as a functioning referral system both decreases costs and improves patients' health. An optimal referral process should be in place for the effectiveness, safety and efficiency of high standard medical care. A referral process is an inherently complex activity that has two aspects—Referral Decision and Referral Communication. A referral decision is a clinical decision made by doctors or other healthcare providers on whether a referral is needed, and at what level the referral must be made. Referral Communication deals with interactions between referring and referred-to providers once a referral decision is made. To have an efficient referral mechanism, it is important to prioritize both components and the implementation of effective healthcare provision with a government health set up.

PRINCIPLES OF A REFERRAL SYSTEM (FIG. 7.4)

- The referral should meet the needs and objectives of the clients and should be necessary and appropriate—there should be merit in referral.
- The client should be able to use the referral in an efficient, effective manner—it should be practical. The referral should be individualized to the client.
- The referral should meet the needs and objectives of the clients and should be necessary and appropriate—there should be merit in referral.
- The client should be able to use the referral in an efficient, effective manner—it should be practical. The referral should be individualized to the client.

RATIONALE, BENEFITS AND OBJECTIVES

While the most vulnerable and poor communities of urban populations are the target population for improvements made to the urban public healthcare system, the rationale for implementing an effective referral mechanism, is far wider. A referral mechanism can support quality health service delivery to entire urban populations in India (**Fig. 7.4**) in the following ways:

- Coordination and standardization of referral services.
- Continuity of care across the different levels of care.
- Cost-effectiveness of health services provided to the community.
- Promotion of universal coverage and equity in provision of health services.
- Healthcare planning based on performance monitoring of the referral system.

A well-functioning referral system will have the following benefits:

- Maximize efficiency of the health system by ensuring appropriate use of health services.

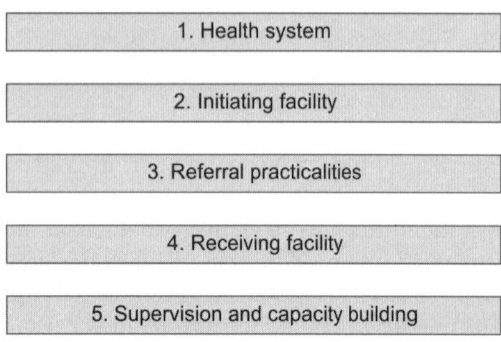

Fig. 7.3: Components of a referral system.

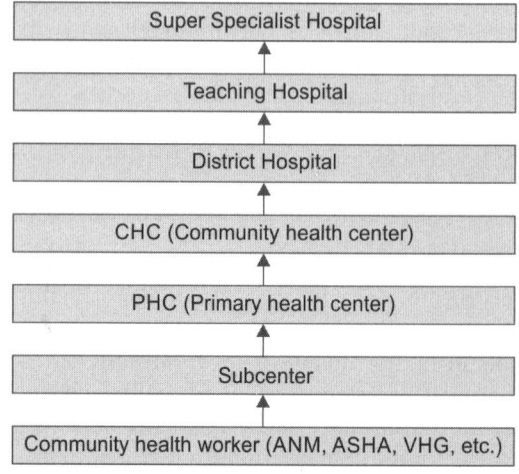

Fig. 7.4: Referral services in India.

- Strengthen lower-level facilities and improve capacity for decision-making by health workers at all levels.
- Create opportunities for balanced distribution of funds, services, and human resources.
- Promote linkages across the different levels of care and between public and private entities.
- Ensure that care is provided at the lowest possible cost. A referral mechanism has the following objectives:
- Increase the use of services at lower levels of the healthcare system
- Reduce self-referral to the higher levels of care
- Develop service providers' capacity to offer services and appropriately refer at each level of the healthcare system
- Improve the health system's ability to transfer patients, patient parameters, specimens and expertise between the different levels of the healthcare system.
- Improve supportive supervision, thereby ensuring up-to-date management practices are used across the country.
- Improve referral performance monitoring and coordination and referral feedback information systems including procedures for counter-referral.
- Strengthen outreach systems for provision of referral health services to marginalized and vulnerable populations.

NEED OF REFERRAL SYSTEM

Super Specialist Hospital

A single super specialty hospital is defined as a hospital that is primarily and exclusively engaged in the care and treatment of the patients suffering from a specific illness.

Purposes

- To provide need based comprehensive care within the technical competencies and resources at each level of primary healthcare infrastructure efficiently and effectively.
- To help people avail specialized services available at higher level institution which are beyond their reach.
- To streamline the appropriate use of PHC infrastructure and specialized services in order to prevent overloading of specialized institution by direct uses.

Referral units of PHC system need to:
- Well trained required number of professionals, medical equipment and supplies, organization structure, etc.
- Continuing training, guidance and supervision of community health workers.
- Guidance on sanitary measures and to disseminate information on disease control methods.
- Conduct health education sessions.
- Provide logistic supports in terms of equipment and supplies required at PHC.
- Establish liaison and functional relation with other sectors involved in social and economic development.
- Organize transportation facilities for cases to be referred.

The referral hospital at secondary and tertiary level need to:
- Provide specialized clinical outpatient and inpatient care continuously.
- Back up primary healthcare system by providing PH care messages/teaching.
- Discourage people attending OPD's directly, i.e., to attend OPD when they have referral card/letter or a genuine emergency.
- Act as teaching center for health professionals including community health workers.

Selection of Referral Cases

- The very serious patient requiring immediate medical care and treatment.
- Patients presenting serious signs and symptoms. He/she may not be sick but requires immediate referral.
- When special diagnostic procedures are required for diagnosis.

IMPORTANCE OF REFERRAL

- Providing diagnostic services to patient and community.
- Providing specialist's services to the patient.
- Propagating the purposes of referral system among health workers.
- Teaching the nursing personnel for reviewing of patients sent for referral.
- Preventing further complications and for appropriate treatment.
- Sending the patients comfortably to the referral institute.

ADVANTAGES OF REFERRAL CASES

- Beneficial to patients because they receive effective care at the primary level which is near to their home.
- Beneficial to health workers because they are able to take care of patients which are within their level of competence and are not frightened to handle difficult cases because they can refer them to higher level centers and referral units.
- Beneficial to management because it is economical as highly trained and highly paid doctors, nurses and other professionals take care of patients with serious and complex problems at higher level referral unit and patients with simple and minor problems are taken care at much low cost by health workers at lower level.

LEVELS OF HEALTH CARE: REFERRAL SYSTEM (FIG. 7.5)

Level-1

- **Primary healthcare clinic:** A Primary Healthcare Clinic is the first step in the provision of healthcare and offers services such as immunization, family planning, antenatal care, and treatment of common diseases, treatment and management of Tuberculosis, HIV/AIDS counseling, amongst other services.

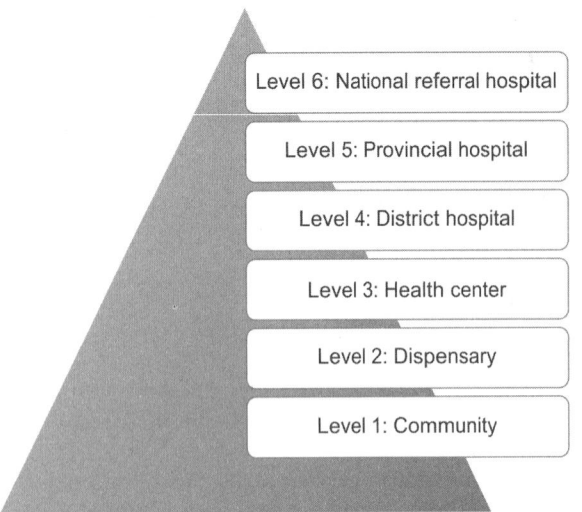

Fig. 7.5: Levels of referral services.

If the clinic cannot assist, they will refer the patient to a Community Health Center.
- **Community healthcare centre:** A Community Healthcare Centre is the second step in the provision of healthcare but can also be used for first contact care. A Community Healthcare Center offers similar services to a Primary Healthcare Clinic with the addition of a 24 hours maternity service, emergency care and casualty and a short stay ward. The Community Healthcare Center will refer a patient to a District Hospital when necessary.
- **District hospital:** This is the third step in the provision of healthcare. These hospitals will normally receive referral from and provide generalist support to community health centers and clinics such as diagnostic, treatment, care, counseling and rehabilitation services. Clinical services include Surgery, Obstetrics and Gynecology, Outpatients Department, Medicine, Pediatrics, Mental Health, Geriatrics, Casualty and Clinical Forensic Medical Services amongst other services. These hospitals receive referrals from the Community Health Centers and Clinics. Most care will be delivered by doctors and primary healthcare nurses. If the District Hospital cannot help a patient they will be referred to the local Regional Hospital for treatment.

Level-2

Regional hospital: This is the second level of healthcare. These hospitals will normally receive referral form and provide specialist support to a number of district hospitals. If the Regional Hospital cannot help they will refer to the Provincial Tertiary Hospital.

Level-3

Provincial tertiary hospital: These hospitals will receive referral from and provide sub-specialist support to a number of regional hospitals and is the third level of health care. These hospitals are staffed by specialists and generalists and offer services such as neurosurgery, neurology, Plastic and reconstructive surgery, Cardiology, Urology, Pediatric surgery, maxillofacial surgery, Psychiatry, Occupational health and Orthopedics amongst other services. If a Provincial Tertiary Hospital cannot help they will refer to a National Central Hospital.

Level-4

- **Central hospitals:** The fourth and highest level of healthcare. These hospitals will consist of very highly specialized referral units which together provide an environment for multi-specialty clinical services, innovation and research. People are referred to these hospitals by Provincial Tertiary Hospitals.
- **Specialized hospital:** These hospitals will provide care only for certain specialized groups of patients. They will include chronic psychiatric and TB hospitals, as well as specialized spinal injury and acute infectious disease hospitals.

IMMEDIATE REFERRAL

Cases requiring immediate care the cases that may require immediate referral are as under:
- Cases presenting any problem which cannot be handled during pregnancy, labor and postnatal period.
- Severe diarrhea with dehydration or not responding to treatment.
- Pain in abdomen and vomiting with or without presence of bowel sounds.
- Heart burn, dyspepsia, dysphagia, hematemesis and malena, etc.
- Continuous cough with or without sputum, hemoptysis.
- Fever with stiff neck.
- Fever not responding to treatment.
- Fever with severe joints pain, rashes, bleeding under the skin.
- Breathing difficulty while walking, sleeping, doing physical work.
- Chest pain with/without pain in the left arm, restlessness and vomiting.
- Jaundice, loss of appetite.
- Convulsions with fever.
- Coma, paralysis, fracture, severe injury, hemorrhage, poison, etc.

REFERRAL FORM

A referral form has the following information:
- Patient details (name, location, age and sex)
- Detail of referral doctor or hospital
- Reasons for referral
- Degree of urgency for appointment
- Clinical problem
- Important previous history
- Findings and physical examination
- Findings on investigation
- Detail of given mediation, treatment and any drug sensitivities.
- Expected outcome and desirable follow-up.

BENEFITS OF REFERRAL SYSTEM

- **Prevents revenue leakage:** The benefits of a referral management system are far-reaching. It not only makes your organization more efficient, and better equipped to serve patients, but also stops revenue leakage and makes the organization prosperous.
- **Decreased lead times:** Many times, primary healthcare providers refer patients to a specialist. However, studies have shown that up to 65% of these referrals are not required. This unnecessarily puts pressure on the specialists and leads to longer waiting times for patients, who really need to see them.
  With an efficient referral system, these unwanted appointments can be avoided.
  This would result in shorter waiting time for genuine patients, higher patient satisfaction, and more patients being attended ultimately.
- **Completing the loop:** When a physician refers a patient to a specialist, he has no way to track whether the patient has met the specialist or not. But with a referral management system, you can track the status of each referral. This creates greater transparency, improved healthcare, and completes the loop of healthcare.
- **Improved utilization:** Being able to track a patient's progress through a referral system, helps both the provider and staff. With online scheduling, doctors can see more patients, and also the waiting time for patients is reduced. This way it helps both, the patients and the healthcare providers.
- **Enhanced healthcare system:** Most referral management systems are built on value-based care models, which require an integrated communication system to maintain a standard healthcare quality.
- **Improved patient access:** One more benefit of the referral management system is improved patient access. The system gives the power to patients to schedule appointments as per their availability, and the availability of the specialist. In case they cannot visit the doctor, or it is no critical, a patient may even use an e-consult facility to communicate with the specialists. This strengthens patient retention and prevents referral leakage.
- **Quality patient time:** Finally, a referral management system frees a specialist from routine administrative tasks. This gives the specialists additional time to spend with their patients. This quality time spent with the patients goes a long way in improving patient experience, which helps your healthcare practice grow resulting in more referrals and increased revenue.

BARRIER TO REFERRAL PROCESS

- **Resource barriers:** Attitude of healthcare professionals physical accessibility of resources cost of resources client barriers priorities motivation previous experience with resources lack of knowledge about available resources lack of understanding regarding need for referral client self- image (-ve) cultural factors finance accessibility.
- **Establishing criteria for referral:** The community health nurse uses outcome-based clinical evidence to establish guidelines for initiating the referrals. Screening test results that fall outside of normal parameters and require follow-up evaluation indicate the need for referral.

NURSE'S ROLE IN REFERRAL SYSTEM

- Observe and collect information about the illness, trauma, related situation, factors, etc.
- Identifies the nature of illness/emergency and its seriousness.
- Provides immediate treatment care within her competence, standing orders and resources available.
- Assures the casualty/family members/any other person accompanying.
- Explains about the seriousness of the problem situation and need for reference to the casualty.
- Fills up the referral form as desired and hands over the same with related documents to be given to health professionals in referred health center.
- Arranges for transport of the patient according to feasibility as soon as possible.
- May do the telephonic consultation or provide information to referred health center.
- May accompany the casualty/patient if required and feasible.
- Maintains the records and reports.
- Provides follow-up care as per treatment and instructions prescribed by the referral unit.

Responsibilities of Nurse in Referral System

- Offering Advice and Support to Lower-Level Health Facilities.
- Providing Quality Assurance and improvement.
- Education and Training.
- Management and Administration.
- Research and Innovation.
- All nursing personnel working in subcenter PHCs/CHCs or in district hospital should have the knowledge of Referral system.
- Patients should be carefully selected for Referral system.
- Nurses should be aware of their limitations and responsibilities in their referral system.

CONCLUSION

There is a need to establish a strong referral mechanism in urban India to ensure high quality of healthcare and optimum utilization of each health facility, improve coordination and governance, regulate private formal and informal sectors, strengthen public health capacities, and reduce pocket expenditure. At each level of healthcare infrastructure, there is need for support from higher level of health structure and also from secondary and tertiary level hospitals for better care and promote credibility of primary healthcare system.

An effective referral system ensures a close relationship between all levels of the health system and helps to ensure people receive the best possible care closest to home. It also assists in making cost-effective use of hospitals and primary healthcare services. Support to the centers and outreach services by experienced staff from hospitals or district health office helps build capacity and enhance access to better quality care.

BIBLIOGRAPHY

1. Freeman and Heinrich. Community Health Nursing Practice 2nd edition; 1998.
2. Gulani KK. Community Health Nursing: Principles and Practices. 1st edition Delhi: Kumar Publishing House; 2008.
3. Judith AA, Barbara WS. Community Health Nursing Concept and Practice 5th edition; 2001.
4. Lucita M. Public Health and Community Health Nursing in the New Millennium. 1st edn. Chennai: B.I. Publications (P)Ltd. 2006.
5. Stanhope M, Lancaste J. Community Health Nursing: Promoting Health of Aggregates, Families and Individuals. 4th edition; St. Louis: Mosby; 1996.

REVIEW QUESTIONS

Long Essays
1. Describe the levels of health care and healthcare settings.
2. Enumerate the benefits of referral system.
3. Describe the barrier to referral process.
4. Explain the nurse's role in referral system.

Short Essays
1. Define referral system. Explain the purposes of referral system.
2. Components of a referral system.
3. Principles of a referral system.
4. Describe the need of referral system.
5. Importance of referral.
6. Levels of health care: referral system.
7. Immediate referral.
8. Responsibilities of nurse in referral system.

Short Answers
1. Referral.
2. Facilitated referral.
3. Referral protocols.
4. Referral register.
5. Quaternary health care.
6. Advantages of referral cases.
7. Primary healthcare clinic.
8. Community healthcare centre.
9. District hospital.
10. Regional hospital.
11. Provincial tertiary hospital.

Multiple Choice Questions
1. Referral is a process in which a health worker at one level of the health system, having insufficient resources, *except*:
   a. Drugs
   b. Water and electricity
   c. Equipment
   d. Personals
2. To create a good referral system, it is important to consider:
   a. Patients should be given optimal care at the right level, right time and right cost
   b. Optimal and cost-efficient utilization of healthcare systems
   c. Optimal and appropriate utilization of specialist services for patients in need
   d. All of the above
3. First Referral Unit in India is _____ which is a clinical facility equipped to provide emergency care.
   a. CHC
   b. PHC
   c. DHC
   d. All of the above
4. A good referral system can help to ensure:
   a. Clients receive optimal care at the appropriate level and not unnecessarily costly
   b. Hospital facilities are used optimally and cost-effectively
   c. Primary health services are well utilized and their reputation is enhanced
   d. All of the above

ANSWERS

| 1. b | 2. d | 3. a | 4. d |

CHAPTER 8: Records and Reports in Community Health Nursing

LEARNING OBJECTIVES

1. Types and uses
2. Essential requirements of records and reports
3. Preparation and maintenance

TERMINOLOGY

- **Standing order:** Standing orders are the directions and orders of specific nature. On the basis, in the non-availability of doctor, the nurse and health workers and provide treatment to patients, at home, hospital or health institution and community.
- **Family folder:** Family folder provides essential and complete information about the family to complete information about the family to the community health nurse to plan, organize and to implement nursing care to the family.
- **Record:** It is a written communication relevant to a client's health care and management. It is a continuing account of the client's healthcare needs.
- **Informed consent:** It is a person's agreement to allow something to happen based on full disclosure of facts needed to make an intelligent decision. The consent must be given voluntarily by a mentally competent adult.
- **Incident report:** An incident report is field when something arises that could or did cause injury and which was not dealt with good care, so the detail incidental report should be given by the particular staff or person.
- **Contract:** A contract is a written or oral agreement between two people in which there is a mention of goods or services exchanged.
- **Documentation:** In the medical record, it provides the only credible proof in court to prove the appropriate care was given and the standards of care was met with.
- **Patient care standards:** They are guides for collaborative practice responding the predicted care requirement for patients. They are based on an analytical and problem solving of assessment, planning, intervention and evaluation.
- **Field review:** It is a method; appraisal of worker is done by the personal officer by collecting oral rating about them from the supervisor at the place of work. The personal offer later writes his notes and invites the supervisor to make additions or corrections.
- **Protocol:** A protocol is a written plan specifying the procedures to be followed during care of a client with a selected clinical condition or situation.

INTRODUCTION

Nursing documentation is a vital component of safe, ethical and effective nursing practice, regardless of the context of practice or whether the documentation is paper-based or electronic. This document is intended to provide registered nurses (RNs) with guidelines for professional accountability in documentation and to describe the expectant for nursing documentation in all practice settings, regardless of the method or storage of that documentation. The main aim of the document is to assist the registered nurse to meet their standards of practice related to documentation.

CONCEPT OF RECORD AND REPORT

An effective health record shows the extent of the health problems' needs and other factors that affect individuals their ability to provide care and what the family believes. What has been done and what to be done now also can be shown in the records. It also indicates the plans for future visits in order to help the family member to meet the needs.

Relation of Record and Report

- Record and report are mutually interdependent. Report can be prepared on the basis of records.
- Similarly, report can be presented as record.
- Record is always in the written form while report can be oral as well.
- Report especially oral report, can be forgotten while record can be preserved for a long time.
- Despite being literally different, records and reports are interrelated; also they are essential and important component of community health, management and nursing.

Record the memory of the internal and external transactions of an organization. Records contain a written evidence of the activities of an organization in the form of letters, circulars, reports, contracts, invoices, vouchers, minutes of meeting, books of account, etc. It is a written communication that permanently documents information relevant to a client's healthcare management. It is a continuing account of the client's healthcare needs.

DEFINITIONS OF RECORDS AND REPORTS

Records

- Records are written formal and legal individual family and community. It may provide information about personal socioeconomic, psychological environmental and health.
- Records are facts and figures, arranged in a logical order, that a new worker may be able to maintain continuity if service to individuals families and communities.
- A record or documentation is defined as anything written or printed that is relied on as a record of proof for authorized persons.
- A record or documentation is defined as anything written or printed that is relied on as a record of proof for authorized persons.
- It is a written communication that permanently documents information relevant to a client's healthcare management. It is a continuing account of the client's healthcare needs.

Reports

- Reports offer a summary of activities or observations seen, performed or heard is exchanged among healthcare team members, clients and family members.
- A Report summarizes the services of the nurses or the agency. Reports may be in the form of an analysis of some aspect of a service. Reports are usually written daily, weekly, monthly and yearly.
- Report is an oral or written account by one member to another in the health team which includes the end of shift handing over report.

MEANING OF RECORDS AND REPORTS

- Records and reports are a practical and indispensable aid to the doctor, nurse and paramedical personnel in giving the best possible service to individual, family and to the community.
- Documentation is important in healthcare today. Documentation is defined as anything written or presented that is relied on as a record of proof for authorized persons.
- A medical records should be comprehensive declaration of the individual family and community health status and needs, as well as the service provided for the client care.
- Recorded facts have a value and scientific accuracy for more than mere impression of memory and these are guidelines for better administration of family health services.
- Records are the means of communication between the health workers and the family, for example, any health or socioeconomic problem observed by the health workers during home visit is recorded, which may require the attention of the doctor or other members of the health team.
- Family records serve as a guide to nursing care as they are major practice tools today in the community health practice.
- Consumerism, accountability and quality assurance plays a vital role on legal written documents. It is necessary to have adequate records to record the care provided and other information which will help to assess and improve the quality of care given.
- Records and reports express or presenting the facts, records, means record is the "written presentation of information."
- Patient's clinical record is a brief account of the personal and medical history of the patient, results of diagnostic tests, findings of medical examination, treatment, nursing care, daily progress notes are recorded.
- A record is a permanent written communication that documents information relevant to a client's healthcare management. Health records give information about members, activities carried out, and achievements.

CHARACTERISTICS OF GOOD RECORDING AND REPORTING

- **Accuracy:** Information should be correct to prevent serious mistakes. Use of correct spelling and the institutions accepted abbreviation and symbols ensure accurate interpretation of information. It should be always complete with accurate signature. Do not use nick names.
- **Conciseness:** Use a few words as possible to give the necessary information.
- **Thoroughness:** Even a concise record or report must contain complete information.
- **Up-to-date:** Recording should be done on time. A definite time and routine for the reporting make more time and routine for the reporting makes more efficient management. Delay in recording can result in serious omissions and delay the work.
- **Organization:** Communicate all the information in a logical format or order.
- **Confidentiality:** The information should be confidential.
- **Objectivity:** Presentation of facts not personal feelings, to give true picture.

IMPORTANCE OF REPORTS AND RECORDS

Records

- It provides facts of health services.
- It provides a basis for analyzing needs and direct towards goal achievement.

Chapter 8: Records and Reports in Community Health Nursing

- Provides a basis for short and long-term planning.
- It prevents duplication of services and helps follow-up services effectively.
- It helps the nurse to evaluate the care and teaching which she has given.
- It enables the nurse to judge the quality and quantity of work done.
- It serves as a guide to professional growth.
- Records help to become aware of and recognize their health needs of the individual and the family.
- Records can be used as a teaching tool to the individual and family.
- The record serves as a guide for diagnosis, treatment and evaluation for the doctors.
- The record helps identify families needing service and those prepared to accept help.
- The record helps the supervisor evaluate the services rendered, teaching done and person's actions and reactions.

Reports

- Complete report establishes the nurse's accountability in being sure that client care is uninterrupted.
- It provides a baseline for comparison during the next shift.
- It shares significant information about family members as it relates to client's problems.
- It relays to staff significant changes in the way therapies are given.
- It evaluates results of nursing and medical care measures.
- It describes instructions given in teaching plan and clients' families and community response.

PURPOSES OF RECORDING AND REPORTING

Recording

- **Communication:** The record is a means by which healthcare team members communicable and contributes to health of an individual family and community.
- **Financial billing:** The client care record is a document that shows the extent to which healthcare agencies should be reimbursed for services. It is client's bill.
- **Educational:** The record contains variety of information, including medical and nursing diagnosis, signs and symptoms of disease, successful and unsuccessful therapies, diagnostic findings and clients behaviors. Students of nursing medicine and other health related disciplines use these records as educational resources.
- **Assessment:** The record provides data that nurses uses to identify and support nursing diagnosis and plan proper investigations of care. Information from the record adds to the nurse's observations and assessment.
- **Research:** Statistical data relating to the frequency of clinical disorders, complications, use of specific medical and nursing therapies, deaths and recovery from illness can be gathered from clients records.

- **Auditing and monitoring:** A regular review of information in client records gives a basis for evaluation of the quality and appropriateness of care provided in an institution.
- **Legal administration:** A medical record must be accurate because it is a legal document. Accurate documentation is one of the best defenses for legal claims associate with nursing care.

Reporting (Written Reports)

- To show the kind and amount of services rendered over a specified period.
- It helps to illustrate progress in reaching goals.
- It acts as an aid in studying health conditions.
- It aids in planning.
- It helps to interpret the services to the public and to the other interested agencies.

VALUES AND USES OF RECORDS

- Record provides basic facts for services. Records show the health condition as it is and as the patient and family accepts it.
- Provides a basis for analyzing needs in terms of what has been done, what is being done, what is to be done and the goals towards which means are to be directed.
- Provides a basis for short and long-term planning.
- It prevents duplication of services and helps follow-up services effectively.
- Helps the nurse to evaluate the care and the teaching which she has given.
- It helps the nurse organize her work in an orderly way and to make an effective use of time.
- It serves as a guide to professional growth.
- It enables the nurse to judge the quality and quantity of work done.
- Records help them to become aware of and to recognize their health needs. A record can be used as a teaching tool too.
- Record serves as a guide for diagnosis, treatment and evaluation of services.
- It indicates progress
- It may be used in research
- The record helps identify families needing service and those prepared to accept help.
- It enables him to draw the nurse's attention towards any pertinent observation he has made.
- The record helps the supervisor evaluate the services rendered, teaching done and a person's actions and reactions.
- It helps in the guidance of staff and students—when planned records are utilized as an evaluation tool during conferences.
- It helps the administrator assess the health assets and needs of the village or area.
- It helps in making studies for research, for legislative action and for planning budget.
- It is legal evidence of the services rendered by each worker.
- It provides a justification for expenditure of funds.

PRINCIPLES OF RECORDING AND REPORTING

Principles of Recording

- Records should be written clearly, accurately, appropriate and legibly.
- Nurses should develop their own method of expression and form in record writing.
- Records are confidential documents, so it should be handled carefully.
- Care to be taken not to make any errors on the records if anything is crossed out, it should be dated and initialed.
- All records should be written with black ink or typed for better legibility.
- Record should be written in chronological order as to date and time. When recording medications and treatments, note exact time and date on which they are carried out.
- Records should be written immediately after an interview.
- Record system is essential for efficiency and uniformity of services.
- Record should provide for periodic summary to determine progress and to make future plans.
- Select relevant facts and the recording should be brief and accurate.

Principles of Reporting

- Report should be truthful, accurate appropriate clear, confidential, brief, complete and legible.
- Good reports will indicate the efficiency of the health team in carrying out their assignments.
- Good reports will avoid duplication of work.
- Good reports will help the relieving personnel to plan the future care of the patient's without wasting time unnecessarily.
- Patient receives better care when the reports are through and give all pertinent data.
- Good report tells us about the problems relating to supplies and equipment.
- Use only standard abbreviations.
- All entries should be signed by the individual who writes them.

Principles of Maintaining Records

- Specific purpose which should be clearly understood
- Items on forms and in registers should be conveniently grouped so as to make their completion as easy as possible.
- The wording should be easily understood, and where doubt is likely to arise, instructions to facilitate interpretation should be included.
- Records should permit some freedom of expression.
- Records which are required by the teaching staff should be easily accessible to them.
- Person responsible for maintaining records should be aware of their particular responsibility and every effort should be made to keep records up-to-date and accurate.
- Provision for periodic review of all records to ensure that they keep pace with the changing needs of the program.
- Adequate supply of stationery to permit records to be maintained on the proper forms and in the proper registers at all times.
- Sufficient number of filing cabinets and appropriate equipment to operate a filing system which is simple and safe and requires the minimum possible time.
- Adequate, safe, fireproof storage arrangements

CARE OF THE RECORDS

- The records are kept under the safe custody of the nurse in each ward.
- No individual sheet is separated from the complete record.
- Records are kept in a place, not accessible to the patients and visitors.
- Records are never sent out of the hospital without the doctor's permission.
- All the records should be handled carefully. Careless handling can destroy the records.
- Records are not handled over to the legal
- All the hospital personnel are legally and ethically obligated to keep in confidence all the information provided in the records.

TYPES OF RECORDS, REPORTS AND REGISTERS IN COMMUNITY HEALTH NURSING

Types of Records

- **Cumulative or continuing records:** The system utilizing one record for home and clinic services in which home visits are recorded in red and clinic visit in blue ink helps coordinate the service and save the time of all the personnel concerned. Continuing record save time and much filling space by avoiding repetition.
- **Family records:** All the records which relate to members of one family should be placed in the single family folder. In this way the doctor and health workers can see the total situation and give effective economical service to the family as a whole. The family folder which contains all the individual records of one family.
- **Anecdotal records:** It is a brief description of an observed behavior that appears significant for evaluation purposes, done by the community health nurse during home visit. It provides information about particular one incident.
- **Clinical records:** It is used in the hospital; investigations special treatments and procedures are written and signed.
- **Doctor ordersheet:** Doctor orders regarding medications, investigations, special treatments and procedures are written and signed.
- **Nurses sheet:** Nurses notes are a record of treatments and nursing measures carried out by the nurses, their effects, the observations made on the patient.
- **Other records:** TPR chart, lab report sheet, diet sheets, concern form, intake output chart, anesthesia chart, physiotherapy sheet, special treatment sheets, etc.

Types of Reports

- **Oral reports:** Oral report is sometimes used in an emergency and followed by a written report later. An oral report is made by the nurse who is assigned to patient care to another nurse who is supposed to relieve her.
- **Written reports:** It should concentrate on the past, present and future state of the patient or event. Description and conclusions of action the influence further planning and decision-making are necessary.
- **24 hours reports:** Nursing supervisor and nursing administration personnel need to be kept informed of what is happening in all patient care areas.
- **Census report:** The daily census or the number of patients are admitted in the hospital. This report helps in planning of healthcare services and knows about the morbidity and mortality statistics.
- **Accidental reports:** Writing a detailed report on mistakes or accidents that has taken place in the care of patients. It should be promptly informed to the higher authorities by writing accidental report.
- **Change of shift report:** At the end of each shift nurses report information about their assigned clients to the nurses working on the next shift.
- **Transfer report:** It involves communication of information about clients from the nurse on the sending to the nurse on the receiving unit.
- **Other reports:** It includes reports among the members of the nursing team, reports between the head nurse and her assistant, reports between the head nurse and her assistant, reports between the head nurse and the nursing superintendent, reports to the physician, evaluation reports, etc.

Types of Registers

The register usually provides only an indication of the total volume of service and of the types of cases seen. It gives no idea of quality of services or the results achieved. It is necessary to keep each register up-to-date and accurate. A good record system provides all the information available from the usual clinic register.

Register maintains the statistics. In all community health centers, hospital system and education institutions maintain registers. Every hospital maintains registers such as birth and deaths, register for operations and delivered, census register, register for the admission and discharges, OPD attendants, etc. In community healthcare daily clinic attendance register, immunization register, clinic attendance registers, family planning registers, birth registers and death registers, etc.

LEGAL IMPLICATIONS OF RECORDS AND REPORTS

Legal Records

- **Incidental reports:** The nurse has a moral and legal responsibility to report to the health agency any accidents, losses or unusual occurrences. The primary purpose is to ensure that there is a record of the details of the incident and subsequent action taken, in the event that legal proceedings are instituted.
- **Informed consent:** One of the most fundamental rights of patients is the right to consent to treatment. It is indeed a well established principle of law that an adult of sound mind has the right to decide what shall or shall not be done to his body. In emergency when treatment is matter of life and death and the patient unable to give permission consent may be implied.

Legal Implication in Record Maintenance

- Informed consent is essential before surgery or investigation for the patients.
- Confidential record and report should be shown to authorized persons only.
- Registration of births, deaths and stillbirths are the important vital events.
- Medicines should be administered as per the order of physician and also under supervision.
- Checking of labels appearance of drug and also should be charted accurately before administration.
- Recording and reporting accidents, errors and incompetent behaviors.
- Identification of babies in labor ward by disks.
- Identification of dead bodies in mortuary.

Legal Approaches in the Community

- **Individual approach:** Birth death report individual health record, immunization chart, maternal description, etc, all records and reports have legal importance.
- **Community approach:** Records and reports present the legal basis through which changes can be levied against medical administration and political system coming in the implementation of health programs, mistakes in the evaluation and medical and administrative inactivity.
- **Nursing approach:** Preserving the individual and family health records of the patients, maintaining the confidentiality and privacy of the records. Records related to medicolegal cases, dying declaration and will, etc., should be handled carefully for giving witness whenever needed.

ROLE OF COMMUNITY HEALTH NURSE IN RECORDING AND REPORTING

Records and reports are the essential components of implementation and evaluation of community health activities. It is necessary for the community health nurse to have thorough knowledge of their maintenance.

Securing Record Information

- Records are started in the center or in the home at a time when the individual is seeking some service or when the health worker recognizes the need for service. The nurse and the individual should be comfortably seated in a

private quiet area so that confidential information can be given and kept at a professional level.
- The record should show chronologically to what extent progress is being made towards the goal of better health for the individual and the family. This is particularly important in regard to better nutrition and sanitation.
- The individual and family cooperation in making out the record is important. Explain the reason for making the record, how the record will be used and the confidential nature of the record.

Record filling: Correct filing of records is essential. Hours of time and effort are served when records are set up and maintained in a systematic planned and organized manner. Some agencies file records alphabetically and others use a numerical system.

Precautions in the maintenance: The community health nurse should take following precautions in the maintenance of records and reports:
- The records should be kept carefully at a clean place.
- The records should be protected against mice, termites and insects, etc.
- Good filling system should be developed for the records and reports.
- Records should be easily available on time.
- Confidential record and report should be shown to authorize persons only.

School health records: It is essential to maintain complete, accurate and continuous health records of school children. It also helps to evaluate the school health services and assist in further development and improvement of health services rendered to school children. It should include information about identification and personal aspect, personal and family health history, findings of physical and medical examination, findings of routine investigations and screening and services rendered and the prognosis.

NURSES RESPONSIBILITY FOR RECORD KEEPING AND REPORTING

Records and reports must be functional, accurate, complete, current organized and confidential.
- **Fact:** Information about clients and their care must be functional. A record should contain descriptive, objective information about what a nurse sees, hears, feels and smells.
- **Accuracy:** A client record must be reliable. Information must be accurate so that health team members have confidence in it.
- **Completeness:** The information within a recorded entry or a report should be complete, containing concise and thorough information about a client care or any event or happening taking place in the jurisdiction of manager.
- **Promptness:** Delays in recording or reporting can result in serious omissions and untimely delays for medical care or action legally, a late entry in a chart may be interpreted on negligence.
- **Organization:** The nurse or nurse manager communicates information in a logical format or order. Health team members understand information better when it is given in the order in which it is occurred.
- **Confidentiality:** Nurses are legally and ethically obligated to keen information about client's illnesses and treatments confidential.

COMMUNITY HEALTH NURSING REGISTERS

It provides indication or the total volume of service and type of cases seen. Clerical assistance may be needed for this. Registers can be of various types such as:
- Immunization register
- Clinic attendance register
- Family planning register
- Birth register
- Death register

Nurses responsibility for record keeping and reporting:
- Keep under safe custody of nurses
- No individual sheet should be separated
- Not accessible to patients and visitors
- Strangers are not permitted to read records
- Records are not handed over the legal advisors without written permission of the administration
- Handed carefully, not destroyed
- Identified with bio-data of the patients such as the name, age, admission number, diagnosis, etc. (Legal issues)
- Never send outside of the hospital without the written administrative permission.

Patient Verification

- Two identifiers: Patient's name and birth date
- Compare of ID Band, consents, diagnostic images, and all other patient documentation related to the procedure.

System of Medical Record

- In the modern age, medical record has the utility and the usefulness and is a very broad based indicator of patients care.
- The policy is to keep indoor patient records for 10 years.
- The OPD registers for 5 years.
- The record which is register for legal purposes is maintained for 10 years for till final decision at the court of the law.

Functions of Medical Record Department

- Daily receipt of case sheets pertaining to discharge and expired patients from various wards, there checking and assembly.
- Daily compilation of hospital census report.
- Maintains and retrieval of records for patient care and research study.
- Completion and processing of hospital statistics and preparation on different periodical reports on morbidity and mortality.

- Online registration of vital event of birth and death.
- Issuing birth and death certificated up to one year.
- Dealing with medicolegal records and attending the courts on summary.
- Arrangement and supervision of inquiry and admission office.

CONCLUSION

Records are an account of something, written to perpetuate knowledge of events. Records and reports and indispensable aids to all who are responsible for giving best possible service to individuals, families and community. Good reports are time savers. They prevent duplication of work, decrease errors and show efficiency level of the staff. Records and reports hold an important place in the process of educational administration. The teacher should prepare records and reports after implementation of a plan over project and the educational administrator himself is expected to prepare a report about the organization and its function periodically.

BIBLIOGRAPHY

1. Barriet J. Ward Management and Teaching. 2nd edition. Delhi: EBS Publishers; 1967.
2. District hospitals—Guidelines for Development. WHO. Geneva: HTBS Publishers; 1994.
3. Gopalakrishnan, Sunderasan. Material Management, Prentice Hall of India (P) Ltd. New Delhi; 1979.
4. Gupta S, Kanth S. Hospital Stores Management, an Integrated Approach. 1st edition New Delhi: Jaypee Brothers Medical Publishers; 2004.
5. Jha SM. Hospital Management. 1st edition Mumbai: Himalaya Publishers; 2007.
6. Koontz H, Weihrich H. Essentials of Management an International Perspective. 1st edition New Delhi: Tata McGraw Hill Publishers; 2007.
7. Koontz H, Weihrich H. Management a Global Perspective. 1st edition New Delhi: Tata McGraw Hill Publishers; 2001.
8. Kulkarni GR. Managerial Accounting for Hospitals. Mumbai: Ridhiraj Enterprise; 2003.
9. Kumar R, Goel SL. Hospital Administration and Management. Vol 1, 1st edition. New Delhi: Deep & Deep Publications.
10. Wise PS. Leading and Managing in Nursing. 1st edition Philadelphia: Mosby Publications; 1995.

REVIEW QUESTIONS

Long Essays

1. Define of records and reports. Describe the characteristics of good recording and reporting.
2. Enumerate the principles of recording and reporting.
3. Discuss the types of records, reports and registers in community health nursing.
4. Describe the role of community health nurse in recording and reporting.

Short Essays

1. Importance of reports and records.
2. Purposes of recording and reporting.
3. Values and uses of Records.
4. Principles of maintaining records.
5. Cumulative or continuing records.
6. Legal implications of records and reports.
7. Legal implication in record maintenance.
8. Legal approaches in the community.
9. Nurses responsibility for record keeping and reporting.
10. Community health nursing registers.

Short Answers

1. Standing order.
2. Family folder.
3. Informed consent.
4. Incident report.
5. Documentation.
6. Patient care standards.
7. Protocol.
8. Care of the records.
9. Anecdotal records.
10. Family records.
11. Clinical records.
12. Change of shift report.
13. Transfer report.
14. Record filling.
15. Functions of medical record department.

Multiple Choice Questions

1. The main aim of the document is to assist the registered nurse to meet their _____ of practice related to documentation.
    a. Standards
    b. Policy
    c. Procedure
    d. All of the above
2. Characteristics of good recording and reporting:
    a. Accuracy
    b. Conciseness
    c. Up-to-date
    d. All of the above
3. Community health nursing registers includes all, *except*:
    a. Immunization register
    b. Family planning register
    c. Birth and death register
    d. Cumulative record
4. Records should be clear, intelligible and _____.
    a. Accessible
    b. Available
    c. Annotated
    d. Accurate
5. When writing in patients' notes what must always be there?
    a. Date, time, signature, printed name, position held, mentor's signature
    b. Date, time, ward, signature
    c. Date, time, signature, printed name, position held
    d. Date, time, signature, printed name

Chapter 8: Records and Reports in Community Health Nursing

6. Which one of the following is a legal requirement to be complied with in relation to records?
   a. Data Protection Act
   b. Caldicot principles
   c. NMC record keeping
   d. Code of professional conduct
7. If you make a mistake in a record how should it be corrected?
   a. With correction fluid
   b. Scribble it out
   c. Put a single line through the record
   d. Tell your mentor
8. The NMC (2015) code states that nurses must 'collect, treat and store all data and research findings _____.
   a. In the ward office
   b. Appropriately
   c. Confidentially
   d. As soon as possible
9. The NMC (2015) code states that nurses must identify any _____ or problems that have arisen and take steps to deal with them.
   a. Issues
   b. Incidents
   c. Accidents
   d. Risks
10. The NMC (2015) code states that nurses must 'complete all records accurately and without any _____.
    a. Falsification
    b. Interference
    c. Patients present
    d. Mistakes.

ANSWERS

| 1. a | 2. d | 3. d | 4. d | 5. c | 6. ?? | 7. a | 8. b | 9. d | 10. a | | |

9. Minor Ailments

LEARNING OBJECTIVES
1. Principles of management
2. Management as per standing instructions/orders

TERMINOLOGY

- **Standing orders:** They are the direction and orders of specific nature, on the basis of these, in the non-availability of doctors, the nurses and health workers can provide treatment to patients at home, hospital or health institution and community.
- **Institutional standing orders:** This category includes standing orders prepared with a view of the available resources, staff position and objectives of medical institution or hospitals.
- **Specific standing orders:** These types of standing orders are prepared for the trained medical personnel, mainly for nurses. Technical knowledge and special skills are required to implement these orders.
- **General standing orders:** Due to large population and geographical area and shortage of health resources some standing orders are used to propagate the health messages to the masses. Common man is expected to follow these.
- **Minor ailments:** It indicates mild illness; it also includes emergencies of smaller nature. Some illness may be acute, which needs immediate care.
- **General minor ailments:** It includes common accidents and emergencies which need immediate first aid, e.g., fracture, high fever and dog bite.
- **Systemic minor ailments:** It includes the mild ailments which affects the various system of the body, e.g., earache, sore throat and toothache.
- **Criteria:** It refers to the signs or indications of expected level of performance against which actual performance of nurse or client or both is compared to determine the extent of achievements of goals and objectives.
- **Emergency:** Psychological, medical or traumatic condition that requires immediate care or care within one hour to prevent further deterioration.
- **Disease:** Any deviation from or interruption of the normal structure or function of any part, organ or system of the body, manifesting with a characteristic set of signs and symptoms.

INTRODUCTION

A minor ailment is a less serious medical condition that does not require lab or blood tests. Examples include cold sores, mild eczema, oral thrush, heartburn, hay fever, skin rash, fungal skin infections and yeast infections. Minor ailments are described as health conditions that can be managed with minimal treatment and/or self-care strategies. Additional criteria include: Usually a short-term condition, Lab results are not usually required, Low risk of treatment masking underlying conditions, Medications and medical histories can reliably differentiate more serious conditions, Only minimal or short-term follow-up is required.

DEFINITIONS

- Minor ailments are generally defined as medical conditions that will resolve on their own and can be reasonably self-diagnosed and self-managed with over-the-counter medications. Examples of minor ailments include headache, back pain, insect bites, heartburn, nasal congestion, etc.
- Standing orders are the directions and orders of specific nature on the basis of these in the non availability of doctor, the nurse and health workers can provide treatment to patients at home, hospital or health institution and community.

BASIC PRINCIPLES OF CARE DURING MINOR AILMENTS AND ACCIDENTS AILMENTS

Community health nurse have to spend most of your time in prevention of illness and promotion of health. An illness may be acute or chronic. Acute illness is the one that is of short duration and usually ends in full recovery. In some cases, it ends in death or it may become chronic. Chronic illness takes time to develop and lasts longer with only partial recovery. In general, the basic principles of care are same as listed below.
- Refer the patient if you are in any doubt in diagnosis or progress in restoration to health.

- Treat the sick person promptly in order to prevent complications.
- Make sure that treatments are carried out as ordered by doctor.
- Make observations of the patient's condition including vital signs and record accurately and report to the doctor.
- Attend to the physical needs, comfort and personal care of the patient.
- Understand and care for the patients intellectual and spiritual needs.
- Consider each patient as an individual and plan care based on patient's particular problems and needs.
- Ensure a safe and healthful environment for patient. If disease is infectious, take precautions to prevent the spread.
- Remember that people are more ready to listen to advice when there is an accident or illness.
- Be prepared to give health teaching when and where this is appropriate.
- Follow-up patients returning to their homes in your community.
- Make sure they understand and carry out treatments and rehabilitation measures necessary to restore their good health.
- Educate the patient and his relatives on continuing self-care and healthful living.

MANAGEMENT OF MINOR AILMENTS

- **History-taking** should include asking questions like, What is your complaint? Do you have any pain? Does it hurt you all the time? How and when did the trouble Start? Did anyone else have these problems? These answers will give you details of illness and epidemiology of the diseases. This will also help in identifying sources of disease.
- **Examine patient** carefully in good light for general appearance, skin, and color of eyes pallor or any signs of shock. Look at eyes and observe for signs of any difference in size of pupil. Check for condition of ears, mouth, tongue, throat and tonsils. Observe for any gland enlargement and note any stiffness of neck or jaw. Observe for any kind of discomfort in abdomen, observe any wound, swelling, scars, patches, sores, rashes or loss of sensation and behavior. If it is a child, observe road to health card if available and immunization status.
- **Give treatment** depending upon the nursing diagnosis after examination. This treatment is mostly on standing orders as prescribed by the agency. Nursing measures which may relieve symptoms may be carried out and further explained to the relatives if they are in a position to do so like giving cold compress, hot water bottle, eye care, etc.
- **Recognize** any sign/symptom which cannot be managed and refer the case.

MINOR AILMENTS IN RESPIRATORY TRACT

- **Allergic rhinitis:** The patient complains of water discharge from the nose with sneezing and itching. Patient may be allergic to dust, feathers pollens or some food item. Give antihistaminics like Tab Avil (25 mg) and try to find out causes of allergic reaction and if there is no improvement; refer for treatment.
- **Sinusitis:** This is a common complication of cold. Patient usually complains of pain and tenderness above or below eyes and headache. There may be fever, stuffy nose, thick mucus or pus in the nose. If the trouble becomes chronic the discharge starts smelling, treatment includes giving steam inhalation, hot wet compress over the tender congested area.

Decongestant (otrivin) nasal drops usually help to relieve symptoms and pain. If pain is not relieved give aspirin and paracetamol (50–100 mg/kg). If there is still no improvement in 3 to 4 days refer patient.

Sore throat: Sore throat is a very common problem. Sore throat can be along with tonsilitis or other infection of throat. You need to familiarize about handling Acute Respiratory Infection (ARI) of children from your doctor. Treat these patients with hot saline gargles, steam inhalation and medicine as per standing orders. The patient should take rest and smoking should not be allowed. If it continues after 3 days refer to a doctor.

Cough: Cough is also a very common symptom of respiratory disease. You should find out when the cough how frequent it is, if there is any irritation due to sputum, type; of sputum, breathing problem or, wheezing sounds. If cough is associated with fever, it could be tonsilitis, pneumonia, tuberculosis, whooping cough or chronic heart failure. Treatment for dry and simple cough is steam inhalation, taking hot fluids, as this loosens mucus. Expectorant or cough sedatives relieve symptoms of cough.

MINOR AILMENTS IN EYES AND EARS

Eyes and ears are important organs and need to be protected to preserve hearing and sight. Common conditions of eye are:

- **Eye accidents:** Injuries may be caused by fall, fireworks, foreign bodies and chemicals. In case of injury, immediate first aid may be given to protect eyes from danger. First aid care includes washing eye with clean water. If any foreign body is visible try to remove with minimum discomfort to the patient. Bleeding can be controlled by eye or ear bandage and dressing. Refer the client to doctor as early as possible.
- **Eye infections:** Besides accidents, infections are also very common. On examination, the eye looks red and there is discharge from the eyes and eyelids are swollen. Often there is an epidemic of sore eyes. The patient complains of pain in the eyes. Treatment of infected eyes will start by

taking history of when and how it started, and observation of signs and symptoms. If problem is acute clean the eyes carefully and treat with eye drops (locula) or ointment (terramycin).
- **Ear problems** are mostly present as earache and this is most common among children. Problem may be with the external ear, the middle ear or the inner ear. Middle or inner ear infection is serious and is likely to be associated with other conditions like fever, throat infection, presence of foreign body, etc. Treatment depends upon what is the cause. If infection is local apply ear drops and keep the ear clean and dry. If associated with fever give sulpha preparation as per standing orders. For pain analgesics are given.

MINOR AILMENTS IN CARDIOVASCULAR SYSTEM

The conditions which we may need to handle are hemorrhage, high blood pressure, chest pain, edema due to heart problem or anemia.
- **High blood pressure**: High blood pressure may be associated with other diseases like kidney problem, toxemia of pregnancy, anxiety, etc.
    - Patient complains of frequent headache, shortness of breath, fatigue and palpitation.
    - Diagnosed case under treatment should be advised to take medicine regularly.
    - New case should be referred to the hospital for treatment. Health teaching plays an important part in treatment. Health teaching should include: avoid overweight salt restriction avoid smoking and alcohol learn to relax and take moderate exercise.
- **Chest pain:** Chest pain usually indicates the disease of heart. Coronary heart disease is either angina pectoris or myocardial infarction.
    - Coronary arteries supplying the blood to the heart muscle become diseased.
    - Pain may be relieved with rest but still it should not be neglected.
    - In myocardial infarction blood clots in diseased coronary arteries shut off blood supply to the part of myocardium. When pain gets worse even with rest, urgent medical attention is required. Refer to the district hospital.
- **Rheumatic heart disease:** This disease is more common among young people. The heart valves are damaged due to bacterial infection.
    - The patient may have a history of repeated sore throat. To prevent this disease, any child with pain and swelling in joints should be referred without delay.
- **Anemia:** Anemia is a very common problem but it is more common among women and children. The patient complains of feeling tired, weak, giddy or fainting and short of breath. There may be swelling of feet.

MINOR AILMENTS IN DIGESTIVE SYSTEM

Most of the conditions related to digestive system are due to poor food personal or environmental hygiene.

Common problems which you may have to face or need to take care are toothache, soreness of mouth, diarrhea, abdominal pain, distension, intestinal obstruction or hemorrhoids.
- **Toothache:** A person coming with toothache will complain of pain, swelling of face and sometimes fever also.
  Examine the patient carefully for any swelling or abscess locally. If gum is swollen patient may have fever. Treatment is to give antiseptic mouthwash, analgesics and if local abscess or infection is observed, antibiotics or sulpha drugs can be given, depending upon the condition.
  To prevent further problems, advise about oral hygiene and how to care for teeth, gums and mouth.
- **Soreness of mouth:** Cracks at the corner of the mouth are often signs of malnutrition, especially riboflavin deficiency. It is most common in children who should be given food rich in vitamins such as whole grain, green vegetables, nuts, milk and eggs.
  Soreness in the mouth often comes when a person has fever or severe cold. It lasts for a few days.
  Advise oral hygiene, saline mouth washes and apply hydrogen peroxide.
- **Diarrhea:** This is a most common complaint among children and we may need to handle these problems through the rural or urban health centers.
  Timely action taken can prevent complications. You need to discuss more with your doctor the latest directives on the management of diarrheal diseases.
- **Abdominal pain and distention:** Abdominal pain could be due to any problems of organs situated in the abdomen. To identify the exact problem examine the patient carefully and locate the pain region which will help you to know likely cause of it.
- **Hemorrhoids:** Hemorrhoids mean varicose veins in the anus. It often causes pain and bleeding. During constipation it is worse. Treatment includes sitz bath, suppositories and diet containing more roughage to avoid constipation.

MINOR AILMENTS IN URINARY SYSTEM

- Urinary system may be affected due to infection, renal stones or tumors. A common symptom which we may need to handle as a minor ailment is burning micturition. You should enquire for discharge from urethra or vagina, fever, change in color of urine or any venereal disease.
- Advise for plenty of fluid intake, personal hygiene and refer the patient to hospital for specific treatment.
- Renal stones may form and remain in kidney without any symptoms till a stone enters the ureter. There is sudden onset of renal colic (severe shooting pain). There may be vomiting, sweating, and difficulty with urination and blood in urine.
- Treatment is mostly surgical for stones but to relieve pain tablets of Baralgan can be given; advise patient to have lot of fluids.

MINOR AILMENTS IN NEUROMUSCULAR SYSTEM

Headache

- Headache is a very common complaint. The headache may be occasional, persistent, dull or severe.
- Headache due to worry, nervous tension, lack of sleep or food, eye strain, indigestion, constipation or menstruation is called as simple headache and can be mostly relieved by analgesics and rest.
- Advise to improve personal health habits and counseling wherever needed.

Pressure Headache

- Pressure headache due to emotional disturbances and tight band around head can be relieved by gentle massage or counseling.
- Headache with other disorders like common cold, fever, discharging ears, sinusitis, and stiffness of neck may be relieved by rest, cold compress or treating the condition with which headache is related.
- Patient should be referred for specific treatment.

Back Pain

- Back pain is also a symptom of various disorders. Careful history to find out site of pain, type of pain, association of pain with heavy work, injury, exposure to cold, menstruation, pregnancy, old age or worries.
- Examine patient carefully at the site of pain for any tenderness of spine or abdomen, poor posture, fever, or any muscle strain, low backache is usually associated with menstruation, pregnancy or retroverted uterus.

MINOR AILMENTS IN REPRODUCTIVE SYSTEM

Menstruation Problems

- Amenorrhea means absence of menstruation. Observe for any signs of pregnancy, other possible causes could be lactation, menopause, emotional trauma, etc.
- If amenorrhea continues without pregnancy in child bearing age, she should be referred to hospital for investigations.

Dysmenorrhea

- It means painful menstruation. Advise to take moderate exercise if pain is dull, and the backaches. Avoid constipation, empty the bladder frequently. If necessary, she can take Aspirin tablet or Baralgan tablet.
- If dysmenorrhea continues, refer to doctor. Heavy bleeding during between menstrual periods can be treated with calcium gluconate tablet and Vit. C tablet. If there is no improvement, refer to hospital.

Sores or Discharges

- Sores and discharge from genital organs are very common problems A sore on genital organ is a hard swelling which may be painful or painless, and is likely to be due to syphilis which is a sexually transmitted disease: urethral discharge in males is commonly caused by gonorrhea.
- There is difficulty in passing urine and if not treated there is danger of sterility. Both these diseases are sexually transmitted.
- The patient should have blood tests and should not have sexual intercourse with anyone, as far as possible, or else use mechanical contraceptive device, till treatment is completed. Find the source of infection and get it treated.

Vaginal Discharge

- There is some normal vaginal discharge which has no smell; but any discharge greater in quantity and of bad smell is a sign of disease. It may be infection due to thrush, Trichomonas, Gonorrhea, after IUD insertion or childbirth.
- Treatment mainly requires personal hygiene and washing with antiseptic lotions; and if there is no improvement, refer to doctor.

STANDING ORDERS

Standing orders are specific instructions regarding treatment for conditions that nurses and other health workers may meet in homes, schools and in industries where a doctor is not readily available. The standing orders are intended to provide treatment only in emergencies and temporarily in the absence of a doctor, they should be limited.

Purposes of Standing Orders

- To meet the emergency situation in the rural areas
- To deliver care at home, schools and communities
- To provide temporary treatment in the absence of a doctor.
- To promote health services in the community.

Objectives

- To maintain the continuity of treatment of the patient
- To protect the life of the patient/to resuscitate him
- To create the feeling of responsibility in the members of health team.

Uses

- Providing treatment during emergency
- Enhancing the quality and activity of the health services
- Strengthening of primary health services in the community
- Decentralization of health responsibilities
- Developing the feeling of confidence and responsibility in nursing and other health worker
- Protecting the general public from quacks.

General Instructions

- The standing order instructions should be issued jointly by an authorized medical officer and a nurse or a committee with a nurse representative.
- The community health nurse working in rural areas may be the only qualified professional person more readily available to the family, so standing instructions must be used with caution and discretion.
- The medical officer is legally responsible for issuing standing orders, he has faith in the sound judgment of his staff and express them to use.
- To promote health services in the community.
- To reduce danger in acute conditions.
- To create the feeling of responsibility in the members of health team.
- Every health service should issue standing instructions to meet the needs of the health problems in the area.

Types of Standing Orders

- **Institutional standing orders:** They are prepared with a view of the available resources, staff position and objectives of medical institution or hospitals, e.g., standing orders of primary health centers can be different than those of district hospitals.
- **Specific standing orders:** These types of standing orders are prepared for the trained medical personnel, mainly for nurses. Technical knowledge and special skills are required to implement these orders, for example, giving injection oxygen therapy and home care, etc.
- **General standing orders:** Due to large population and geographical area and shortage of health resources some standing orders are used to propagate the health message to the massage, e.g., ORS therapy in cases of dehydration.

Role of Nurse in Standing Orders

- The community health nurse should be skillful in history collection and physical examination skills to detect abnormalities.
- The community health nurse should prompt enough to deliver appropriate action for particular situations to manage.
- The nurse should maintain a record of vital signs and other details to the patient.
- The nurse has thorough knowledge to identify the actual problem of the patient and to plan appropriate nursing interventions.
- The nurse should intervene the services according to the given community standing orders.
- The nurse should develop a good therapeutic relationship with the individual and family.
- The nurse should use the referral system if it is possible.
- The nurse should inform to the health officer immediately about the communicable disease.
- Place the medications safe and ready to follow standing orders.
- Ensure a safe and healthful environment for patient.
- Recording and reporting is essential part in community health services.

Advantages

- Community standing orders providing treatment during emergency.
- It enhances the quality and activity of health services.
- It provides feeling of confidence and responsibility in the nursing and other health workers.
- It helps to decentralize the health responsibilities.
- It helps to strengthen the primary health services in the community.

CARE OF PATIENT WITH FEVER

Fever or pyrexia is defined as a rise in the body temperature above 99°F.

Causes of Fever

The causes of fever are infectious diseases of the nervous system, certain malignant neoplasm, blood diseases such as leukemia, embolism and thromboses, heat stroke from exposure to hot environment, dehydration, surgical trauma and crushing injuries, skin abnormalities that interfere with heat loss, allergic reactions to foreign proteins and pyrogens, etc.

Clinical Manifestations

In fever, all the systems of the body are affected. It may vary with the nature of the disease. The primary signs and symptoms are shallow and rapid breathing, increased pulse rate, dry mouth, coated tongue, loss of appetite, nausea, vomiting, diminished urine output, burning maturation, headache, restlessness, irritability, insomnia, fatigue, body pain and heavy sweating.

Types of Fever

- **Chronic fever:** Chronic fever persists for weeks or months and is present in chronic condition like tuberculosis. Untreated acute illness like malaria can also cause acute fever.
- **Intermittent fever:** Intermittent fever rises and falls to normal level frequently. It may come daily or after longer periods. Urinary tract infections, Malaria sore throat and filariasis are common examples.
- **Continuous fever:** Continuous fever remains throughout the illness without fluctuating more than one degree. Typhoid, pneumonia, meningitis and cerebral malaria are the examples.
- **Remittent fever:** It also fluctuates by more than one degree F, but it never touches normal temperature level throughout the day.

Standing Orders

- Check the vital signs (**Fig. 9.1**): TPR and blood pressure.
- Collect data about other signs and symptoms accompanied
- Provide rest and liquid diet
- Obtain blood smear (thick and thin) for Malaria
- Provide antipyretic- Paracetamol tablet/syrup
- Advise plenty of oral fluid to the patient
- If temperature is more than 39°C , give cold sponging.

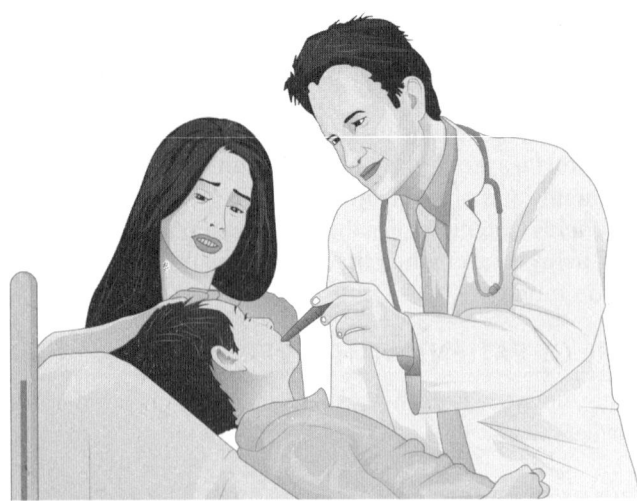

Fig. 9.1: Measurement of oral temperature.

- Observe the pattern of fever and wait for 2 days.
- Refer the patient immediately to the doctor in case of delirium, convulsions and unconscious accompanied with hyperpyrexia.

CARE OF PATIENT WITH SORE THROAT

Sore throat is a very common illness in children and adults. Infection due to virus/bacteria is the most common cause of some throat, but this is not the only cause.

Causes

Sore throat caused by infection due to virus/bacteria, allergic factors, irritant substances (dust and gases) and even over use. Some organisms stay in the upper respiratory tract and may invade the system, when body resistance is low.

Clinical Manifestations

A feeling of "rawness" in the throat is an early symptom. A sensation of "pricking" in the throat and difficulty in swallowing solids is also common. Gradually, there is pain in the throat and person find it difficult to speak. There may be redness and swelling of the mucous membrane seen in the throat. Differences between bacterial and viral infections are shown in **Figure 9.2**.

Standing Orders

- **Check the vital signs:** Temperature, pulse and respiration and record.
- **Physical examination**—inspect the throat for the evidence of redness and white patches.
- **Send throat swab to laboratory**—if facilities are available.
- **Advice saline gargle**—if it pharyngitis
- Provide tab 'Aspirin'.
- If there is history of recurrent tonsillitis refer to hospital for treatment.

CARE OF PATIENT WITH SORE EYE

Sore eye (conjunctivitis) is inflammation of the conjunctiva due to germs, irritants or allergens. It is difficult to

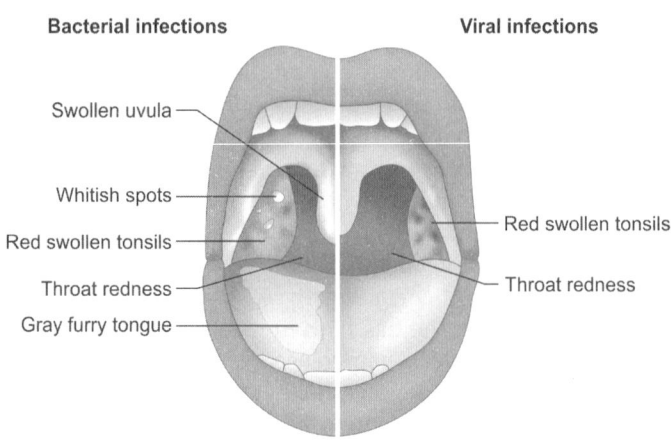

Fig. 9.2: Differences between bacterial and viral infections.

identify the cause. It usually affects both the eyes clinical presentation of.

Causes

Sore eye caused by bacteria and certain viruses cause infective illness. It also spreads by articles such as handkerchiefs used by the patient or through water in a swimming tank. Infective conjunctivitis commonly occurs in epidemics. Infection spreads quickly among families and other contacts.

Clinical Manifestations

Common features are a sensation of "grit" in the eye, redness, watering, pain, swelling of the conjunctiva, photophobia (difficulty in facing light), and sticky flow that often makes it difficult to open the eye. **(Figs. 9.3A and B)**.

Infective conjunctivitis causes pus. Allergic illness causes a watery flow rather than pus.

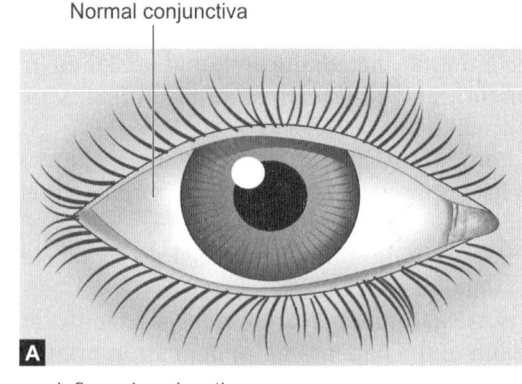

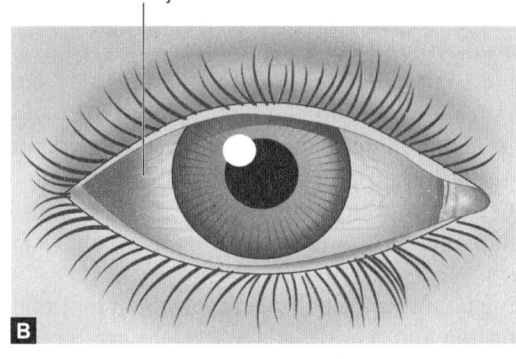

Figs. 9.3A and B: Normal and inflamed conjunctiva.

Standing Orders Management

- Irrigate the eye with clean water and wipe with clean cotton swab.
- Apply sulphacetamide (29%) eye drops or chloromycin eye ointment.
- Demonstrate cleaning and application of eye ointment.
- Cover the eye with sterile eye pad and bandage.
- Refer the patient to hospital, if there is any wound, cuts or ruptures the eyeball.
- Inform to local health officer regarding any epidemics of infective conjunctivitis.

CARE OF PATIENT WITH CONVULSIONS

Convulsion or epilepsy episodes can vary from a nerve local muscle involvement to general convulsions followed by sleep or unconsciousness. Grandmal epilepsy consists of sudden generalized convulsions followed by unconsciousness.

Causes

The exact cause of convulsion is not known. Injury to the brain at the time of birth is a possible cause. There could be other causes for convulsions like cause. There could be other causes for convulsions like a brain tumor, diabetes or low calcium level in the blood.

In children under 5 years, the causes could be high fever, infection of brain or brain coverings, tetanus, consumption of certain poisons, calcium deficiency and injury to brain due to accidents.

Standing Orders/Management (Fig. 9.4)

- Place the patient in side lying or turn the head to one side
- Prevent tongue bit by placing a bit of wood covered with a clean cloth.
- Do not try to restrain during a fit.
- Protect him from any danger like fire, sharp instruments or objects, etc.
- Provide ventilation by clearing the people around him.
- Loosen the clothes so that he gets enough fresh air.
- After he recovers from the fit, give him hot tea with plenty of sugar.
- Refer the patient to hospital.

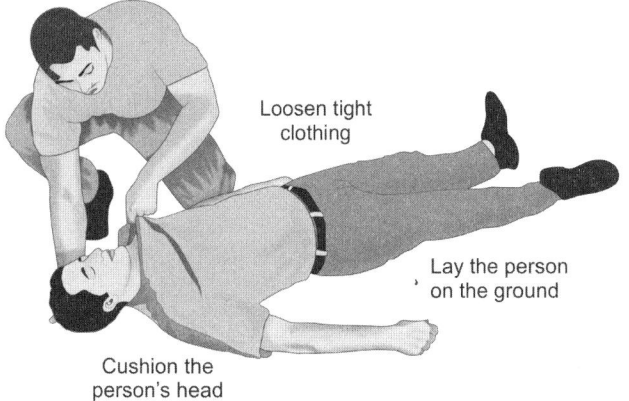

Fig. 9.4: First-aid: Convulsions.

CARE OF PATIENT WITH DIARRHEA

Diarrhea or loose motions are the commonest of abdominal complaints in all age groups. Diarrhea is defined as more than three motions in 24 hours.

Causes (Fig. 9.5)

- Both bacteria and viruses can cause watery diarrhea. About half of "watery" motion episodes in children are due to viral infections.
- Ameba and giardia cause greenish semi liquid or semi-solid stools in the acute phase, but chronic amebiasis tends to cause soft or semisolid stools once or twice a day.
- Diarrhea caused by worm is either semi liquid or semisolid.
- Blood or mucus without feces are a sure sign of bacillary infection.

Clinical Manifestations

- Vomiting is common in illness like cholera, viral diarrhea and food poisoning. This group can be called gastroenteritis.
- Abdominal pain is usually absent in viral diarrhea. Abdominal pain is likely with large bowel diseases, worms in the intestines and food poisoning.
- Foul smell is typical of worms, amebiasis and giardiasis,.
- Greenish stools ameba or giardia. Frothing usually accompanies giardial infection. Giardiasis causes "hurry".

Factors Affect Diarrhea

- Poor personal hygiene.
- Poor environmental sanitation.
- Improper preparation and storage of food.

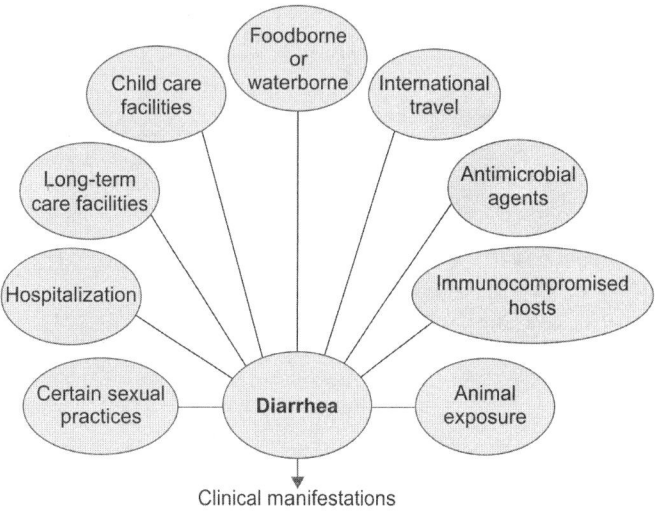

Fig. 9.5: Causes and features of diarrhea.

Home Level

This is the level where a number of primary decisions and actions take place, without which the rest of the programme will not benefit children. These actions include: correct feeding of the child who has diarrhea, i.e., continuing breastfeeding and maintaining adequate fluid intake, using safe and appropriate solutions; recognition of dehydration and ability to take appropriate action when it occurs, e.g., seeking care, obtaining ORS packets and using them correctly; knowledge and practice of personal hygiene with regard to the handling of food and water, and proper use of latrines and the disposal of excreta; informing health authorities of suspected outbreaks of diarrheal disease as soon as possible **(Fig. 9.6)**.

Community Level

The community has a number of ways of giving support to the home level as well as to the health program itself, through its various groupings. In addition, there are a number of tasks related to diarrheal disease control that can, or should, take place as communal actions, initiated by the Community Development Committees or similar bodies and involving community groups as well as volunteering or selected community members. Some examples are: performance of tasks related to the provision of safe water and basic sanitary facilities; informing health authorities of suspected outbreaks of diarrheal diseases as soon as possible; implementation of appropriate measures to control outbreaks, e.g., decontamination of water, proper waste disposal.

Health Service (Including First Health Facility and First Referral Level)

The health personnel carry out very important activities in support of those performed at the home and communal levels. These include: determining the cause of diarrheal disease (as far as possible) and providing treatment that is appropriate to the cause and to the degree of dehydration; packaging and supplying oral dehydration ingredients, i.e., ORS investigating the cause of outbreaks of diarrheal diseases and determining appropriate methods for their control; establishing and managing temporary treatment, centers during serious outbreaks of diarrheal diseases; training and supervising all categories of health workers, including non-medical personnel, required in support of the necessary treatment and control measures; educating family members and the community about the importance of the tasks related to the provision of safe water and basic sanitary facilities.

Standing Orders/Management

- Observe the signs and symptoms of dehydration.
- Provide ORS preparation (take 1 liter of boiled and cooled water add 4 tip of sugar, jaggery or honey, half tea spoon of salt and 1 pinch of sodium bi carbonate).
- In case of severe dehydration—refer the patient immediately to community health center or Hospital.
- Encourage to take plenty of fluids like rice water, coconut water, lemon juice, light tea.
- If any epidemic of vomiting and diarrhea sample should be sent for stool test.

1. Wash your hands thoroughly with soap and water

2. Pour all the ORS powder from a packet into a clean container

3. Measure one litre of clean drinking water and pour it into the container in which you poured ORS. (If you have ORS packets for 1/2 litre of water then take 1/2 litre water)

4. Stir until all the powder in the container has been mixed with water and none remain at the bottom of the container

5. Taste ORS solution before giving it to the child. It should taste like tears – neither too sweet nor too salty. If it tastes too sweet or too salty then throw away the solution and prepare ORS solution again

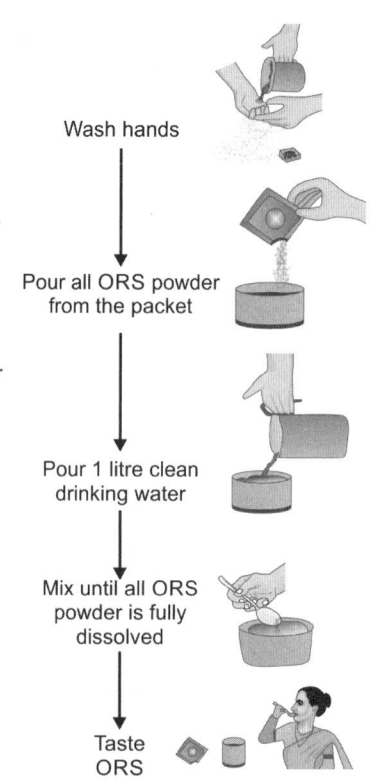

Fig. 9.6: Steps of preparing oral rehydration solution.

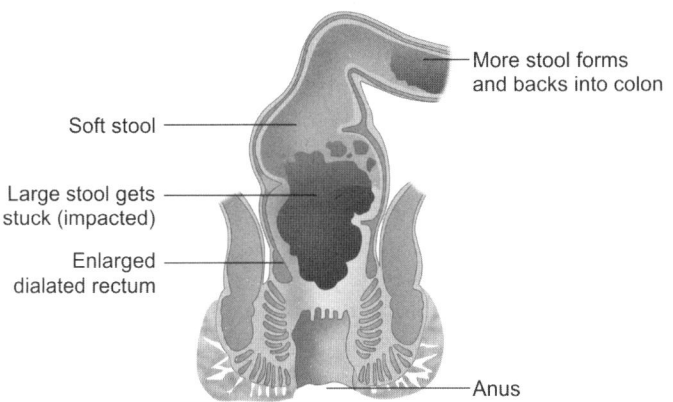

Fig. 9.7: Chronic constipation.

- Educated the patient about proper disposal of stools, hygiene, and sanitary measures.
- Advise the importance of drinking boiled and cooled water and fly control measures.
- Inform the occurrence of the condition to higher health officials, when an epidemic is suspected.

CARE OF PATIENTS WITH CONSTIPATION

Constipation is defined has not passed stools for two days. Occasional constipation is more common than habitual constipation **(Fig. 9.7)**.

Causes

Constipation occurs due to changes in diet and sleep. Habitual constipation is quite common but should not be ignored because it could be a sign of serious illness like large bowel cancer. Chronic amebic infection and warms are also common causes of constipation. Lack of fiber in the diet is a common cause of constipation.

Clinical Manifestations

- Loss of appetite
- Inadequate intake of milk in children.

Community Standing Orders

- Assess the habitual pattern of bowel movement.
- Advise fluids, fruits, green leafy vegetables and food with natural fibers like tapioca.
- Encourage to have regular daily walk and exercises.
- Provide mild laxatives to patients suffering from constipation.
- Refer to the community health center or hospital for further investigation or diagnostic purposes.

CARE OF PATIENTS WITH ANIMAL BITE—DOG BITE

Animal bites may result in puncture wounds, lacerations and avulsions, especially if the client pulled away from the animal while its teeth were clenched. There is a potential for infection from bacterial normally residing in the animals mouth **(Fig. 9.8)**.

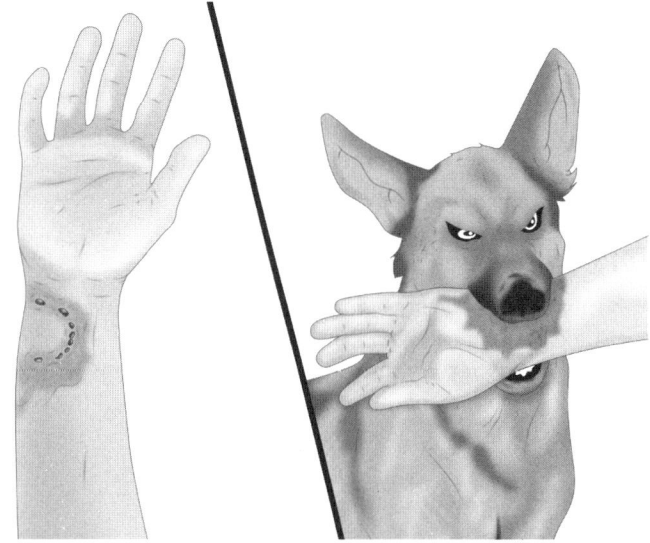

Fig. 9.8: Dog bite.

Rabies is an infectious virus that affects the central nervous system, especially brain. The incidence of rabies in domestic animals especially by dog bite.

Immediate Care of Dog Bite

Dogs often tear the skin, creating a laceration with ragged edges. So as a community health nurse you will do the immediate care followed:
- Wash the wound with betadine. Soak in warm water with salt
- Watch for pain, bleeding and wound, swelling
- Wound dressing is needed after applying antiseptic
- Watch the dog if possible to know the condition of the dog or any symptoms of rabies
- To rush nearby health center or hospital for antirabies vaccine if needed.

Community Standing Orders/Management

- Obtain the history of bite
- Assess the general condition of the patient
- Wash the wound thoroughly with soap and water
- Administer injection tetanus toxoid
- Clean and dress the wound with betadine or tincture iodine.
- If the animal is without symptoms, watch the animal for 10 days.

If the dog shows signs and symptoms of rabies:
- Clean the area with soap and water or hydrogen peroxide before referring to hospital
- Do not cover the wound
- Administer injection tetanus toxoid 5 mL and antirabies vaccine for 14 days.
- Refer the person to a primary health center or hospital
- Inform to the health officer/sanitary inspector for killing the animal and other control measures at community level.

CARE OF PATIENT WITH SNAKE BITE (FIG. 9.9)

- Snakes bites are more common in summer and during the rain because snakes emerge from their holes either due to the heat or the rain
- About 2 lakh events of snake bite occur in India every year and about 15 thousand of these are fatal.

Important Snakes

- Only about 20% bites are due to poisonous snakes.
- Snakes mostly strike in the early morning or when it is dark when they venture out for food.
- Snake bites mostly on the leg and arms, 70% of the bites occur on the lower part of leg.

Aims of First-aid

- Attempt to retard systemic absorption of venom.
- Preserve life and prevent complications before the patient can receive medical care
- Control distressing or dangerous early symptoms of envenoming.
- Arrange the transport of the patient to a place where they can receive medical care.

Immediate Care of Snake Bite

- Keep the bitten part down.
- Construct a band above the bitten part (if it is kept for long time then it is harmful) remove all jewellery or tight fitting clothing.
- Watch for spreading pain, oozing blood and swelling, bluish discoloration. If possible suction device is important.
- Cold pack method can be applied.
- Bite is simply cleansed and rapidly apply antiseptic cleanser to the entire area and a cold compress is positioned directly over the wound.
- Check constriction bands periodically as swelling may occur and loose as appropriate.
- Keep victim warm and immobilize.
- Monitor few symptoms of shock and be prepared to administer appropriate treatment.
- Standby with relatives.
- Providing useful information of incident facts
- To rush to nearby health center or hospital because antivenom is needed.

Community Standing Order/Management

- Check history of snake bite and look for obvious evidence of a bite (fang puncture marks, bleeding, swelling of the bitten part, etc.). However, in krait bite no local marks may be seen. It can be noted by magnifying lens as a pin head bleeding spot with surrounding rash.
- Reassure the patient as around 70% of all snake bites are from non-venomous species.
- Immobilize the limb in the same way as a fractured limb. Use bandages or cloth to hold the splints (wooden stick), but do NOT block the blood supply or apply pressure. Ideally the patient should lie in the recovery position (prone, on the left side) with his/her airway protected to minimize the risk of aspiration of vomitus
- Nil by mouth till victim reaches a medical health facility.
- Traditional remedies have no proven benefit in treating snake bite.
- Shift the victim to the nearest health facility (PHC or hospital) immediately.
- Arrange transport of the patient to medical care as quickly, safely and passively as possible by vehicle ambulance (toll free no. 102/108/etc.), boat, bicycle, motorbike, stretcher etc.
- Victim must not run or drive himself to reach a Health facility. Motorbike Ambulance may be a feasible alternative for rural India.
- If possible PHC medical officer can accompany with patient to know the progress and management and facilitate resuscitation on the way.
- Inform the doctor of any symptoms such as progress of swelling, ptosis or new symptoms that manifest on the way to hospital.
- Remove shoes, rings, watches, jewellery and tight clothing from the bitten area as they can act as a tourniquet when swelling occurs.
- Leave the blisters undisturbed.

CARE OF PATIENT WITH FRACTURE

Fracture defined as disruption of normal bone continuity that occurs when more stress is placed on a bone than it is able to absorb. First-aid for fracture is shown in **Figure 9.10**.

Types of Fracture

- **Simple fracture:** It is one without any external or open injury. It is also known as closed fracture.

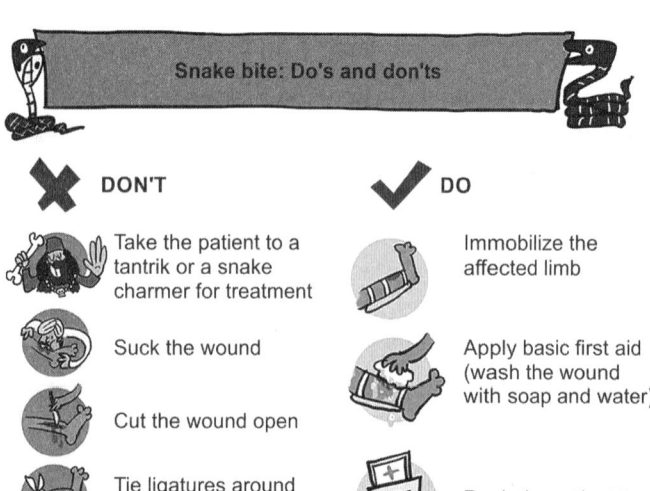

Fig. 9.9: Care of patient with snake bite.

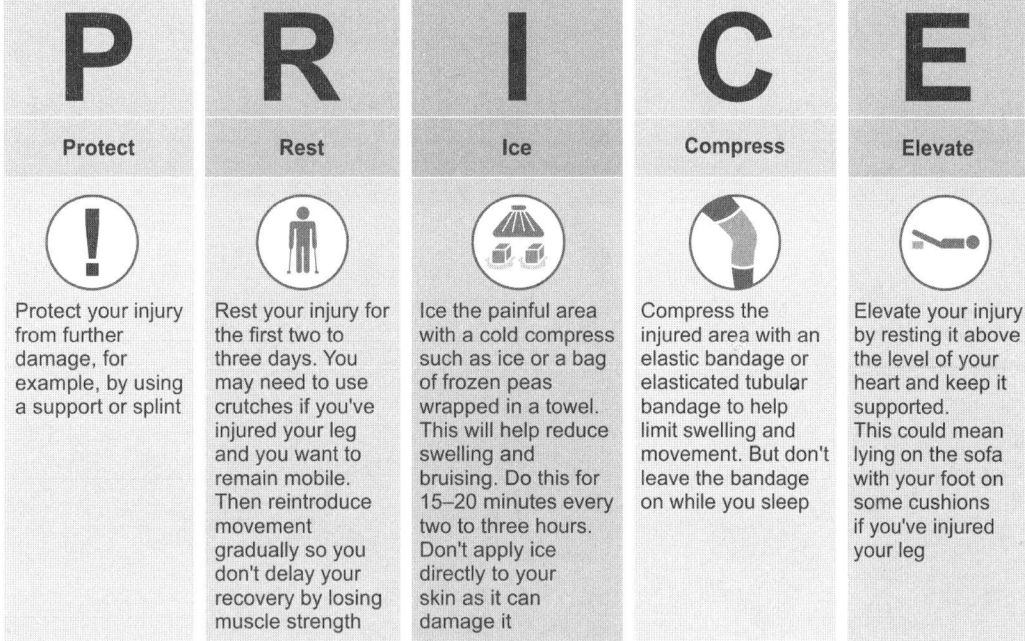

Fig. 9.10: First-aid for fracture.

- **Compound fracture:** It involves both the bone and the soft tissues, especially the skin.
- **Green stick fracture:** It occurs in childhood and could affect the long bones, since in this age group the long bones are slightly elastic, much like a green stick. The fractured ends may remain stuck together, even after fracture.
- **Communicated fracture:** in which the bone breaks into small pieces. This is more difficult to heal since more pieces lose their blood supply and may suffer tissue death.

Clinical Manifestations

- Pain—due to fracture is often unbearable and may cause fainting. The pain helps to locate the site of fracture.
- Tenderness—may be present at the site of the fracture.
- Limitation of movement is a very important clue to the fracture.
- Swelling and deformity are usually clear indications as to the nature of damage.
- Crepitus—is the crackling sound as the broken pieces of the bone rub against each other. This is a sure sign of fracture.

Community Standing Order/Management

- Assess the general condition of the patient.
- Superficial wounds can be cleaned with sterile water.
- Cover the area with sterile cloth.
- Immobilize the part with wooden scale, foot boards
- Support the injured part by means of bandages and slings.
- Administer injection tetanus toxoid 0.5 mL by intramuscularly.
- Administer analgesic to minimize the pain
- Monitor the general condition of the patient
- Refer the patient to primary health center.

CARE OF PATIENT WITH ANEMIA (FIG. 9.11)

Anemia is a reduction in red blood cells (erythrocytes), which in turn decreases the oxygen-carrying capacity of the blood. Anemia is not a diseases, it reflects the abnormality in red blood cell number, structure and function.

Causes of Anemia

- Deficiency in RBC production—disease conditions, inadequate intake of protein, iron and B-12, worm infestation, blood donation and accidents.
- Blood loss—due to menstruation, menorrhagia, thalassemia and valvular diseases.
- Hemolytic—occurs due to malaria and destruction of RBCs.

Clinical Manifestations

- Giddiness, self-care deficit, indigestion, and paleness can be assisted in conjunctiva and tongue, puffiness in face, ankle of the feet, in progressive anemia shortness of breath occurs also at rest.
- Pale yellowish face, pale pigmented tongue, dilation of blood vessels, jugular vein pulsation and enlargement of spleen.

Community Standing Order/Management

- Assess the patient and find out the correct cause by obtaining detail history.
- Sent stool to laboratory for stool analysis.
- Check the blood hemoglobin level.
- Administer mebendazole or albendazole 100 mg bd for 3 days or 400 mg bd single dose.
- Advise the patient walks with chapels and explains the importance.

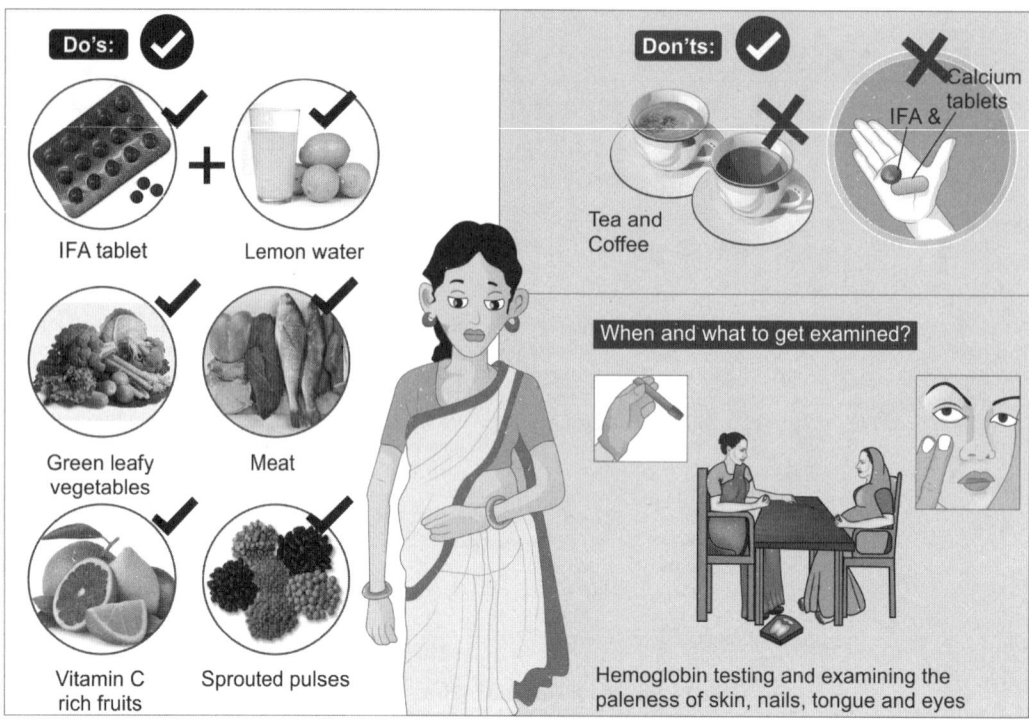

Fig. 9.11: Care of patient with anemia.

- Encourage the person to eat ragi, green leafy vegetables, peas, jaggery, egg and liver.
- If Hb is very low (less than 40%) refer to a primary health center or hospital.
- Condition likes bleeding piles, menstrual disorders with excessive bleeding and other bleeding conditions have to be referred to primary health center hospital immediately.

CARE OF PATIENT WITH EPITASIS (NOSE BLEEDING) (FIG. 9.12)

Epitasis (nose bleeding) may result from irritation, trauma, infection or tumors. In addition, epitasis may also be the result of systemic disease (such as atherosclerosis, hypertension, and blood dyscrasia).

Community Standing Order/Management

- Make patient sit up with head erect and bent forward.
- Loosen all clothes at neck.
- Ask patient to apply pressure by pinching the anterior portion of the nose for a minimum of 5 to 10 minutes.
- Inform the patient not to blow the nose.
- Apply a cold compress.
- If the bleeding is not controlled refer the patient to hospital or primary health center.

CARE OF PATIENT WITH HEAT STROKE (FIG. 9.13)

Heat stroke is a condition that the body fails to cope up the environment heat. Heat stroke is an intense injury due to excessive heat in the atmosphere.

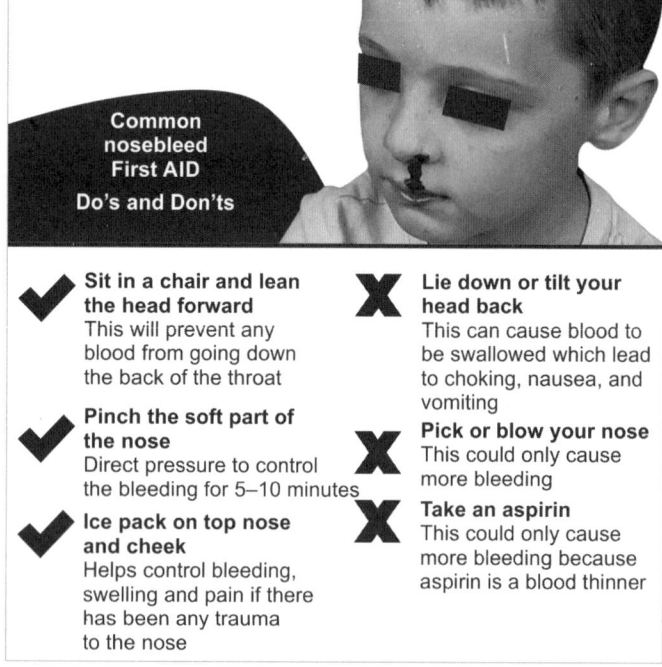

Fig. 9.12: First-aid in nose bleeding.

Clinical Manifestations

- Mild affects causes heat exhaustion, heat fatigue, heat syncope (fainting) and sunburn.
- vomiting, face flushed and full and bounding pulse.
- Unconsciousness and death occurs soon if temperature is not lowered.

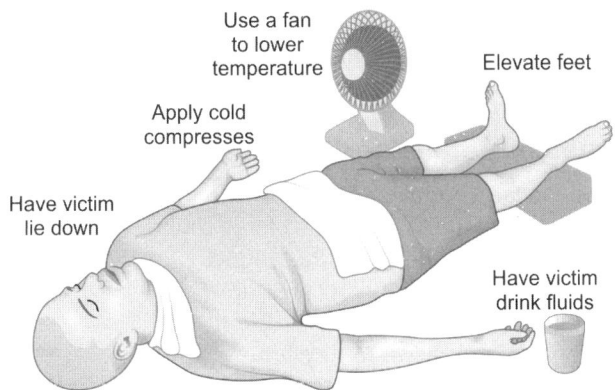

Fig. 9.13: First-aid in heat stroke.

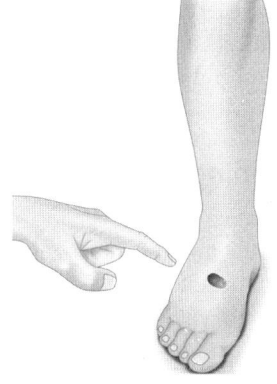

Fig. 9.14: Edema/swelling assessment.

Community Standing Order/Management

- Check the general condition of the patient
- Monitor and record the temperature, pulse, respiration and blood pressure.
- Bring and place the patient under the shade and a well-ventilated place.
- Remove all clothes of the person and wrap him in a wet sheet.
- Keep him wrapped in the wet sheet till the temperature falls at 38 degree centigrade.
- If the patient is conscious, give him cold water mixed salt and other cold drinks.
- Keep continuous observation over temperature.
- Refer the patient to a hospital.

CARE OF PATIENT WITH EDEMA

Edema is a condition occurs due to increased fluid retention in the intravascular and interstitial spaces.

Causes of Edema

Edema occurs due to heart failure, renal disorders, cirrhosis of the liver, increased ingestion food containing high amounts of sodium such as packaged foods and excessive amount of intravenous fluids containing sodium.

Clinical Manifestations

- Edema is the presence of excess interstitial fluid. An area of edema appears swollen, shiny and taut and tends blanch the skin color or if accompanied by inflammation, may redden the skin **(Fig. 9.14)**.
- Generalized edema is most often an indication of impaired venous circulation and in some cases reflects cardiac dysfunction or vein abnormalities.

Community Standing Order/Management

- Assess the general condition of the patient.
- Check the temperature, pulse, respiration and blood pressure.
- Check the daily weight
- Record and maintain intake and output daily
- Examine the urine for albumin
- Advise low salt diet
- Refer the patient top primary health center or hospital.

CARE OF PATIENT WITH SCABIES

Scabies is a contagious disease caused by a mite, sarcoptes scabiei, the disease is spread through contact with individuals or rarely through contact with infected clothes, bed linen or towels.

Causes of Scabies

- Unhygienic living condition
- Lack of personal hygiene
- Sharing of cloths and bedding
- Neglected health.

Clinical Manifestations

- The main complaint is itching. It starts in the evenings and is generally during the day. Often scabies starts in the hands, later the insects spread to the wrist, trunk, elbows, armpits, waist, genitals, and buttocks and under the breasts in women **(Fig. 9.15)**.

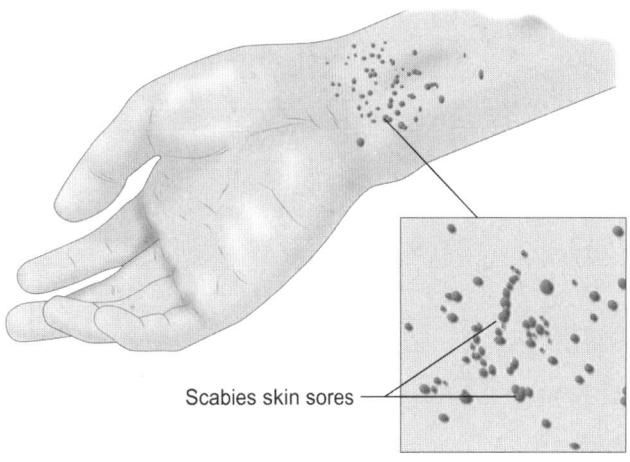

Fig. 9.15: Features of scabies.

- Scabies lesions are dry, if infected by bacteria, the lesion look messy since there is pus. Infection also causes fever. Natural itching also leads to ulcer to scratching by fingers.

Community Standing Order/Management

- Assess the general condition
- Examine the family members for scabies
- Secondary infections should be treated with antibiotics
- Provide bath, scrub well with scrap and water and dry
- Apply Benzyl benzoate—25 percent emulsion external use all over the body at night except face—continuously 3 days.
- Advise to wash all the linens in hot water used by the patient and dry under the sunlight.
- Sulphur ointment can also be used in a similar manner for 3 days.
- Inform the patient that treatment is incomplete unless one more cause of treatment for 3 days is done after a period of two weeks.
- Examination and treatment should be given for schoolmates, playmates and family members.
- Health education should be given to the family members.

CARE OF PATIENT WITH WOUNDS

Wounds are defined as disruption of the normal continuity of the body structure internally or externally.

Types of Wounds

- Incised wounds are caused by sharp instruments like knife, razor, etc. The blood vessels are 'clean out' and so these wounds bleed very much.
- Contused wounds are caused by blow by blunt instruments or by crushing. The tissues are bruised.
- Lacerated wounds are caused by machinery, falls on rough surfaces, pieces of shells, claw of animals, etc. These wounds have turn and irregular edges and they bleed less.
- Punctured wounds are caused by stabs by any sharp instruments like a knife or a dagger. They have small openings, but may be very deep.

Community Standing Order/Management

- Assess the general condition of the patient
- Check the extent and nature of the wound
- Check the bleeding from the wounds
- Stop bleeding by applying pressure
- Clean the wound by sterile water
- Cover the area with sterile cloth
- Administer injection Tetanus toxoid 0.5 mL
- Do not apply any ointment and antiseptic over the wound
- Refer the patient to primary health center or Hospital.

CARE OF PATIENT WITH TOOTHACHE

Toothache is a very common illness in all ages.

Causes of Toothache (Fig. 9.16)

- Loss of enamel cover, exposing the inner dentine, causing toothache on exposure to sour, hot or cold substances.
- Throbbing pain is due to pus in the tooth or in the bone below the roots, with or without swelling of cheek.
- Chewing and intake of hot and cold foodstuff increase the pain of fractured tooth.

Community Standing Order/Management

- Assess the general condition (**Fig. 9.17**).
- Examine the dental hygiene and condition.
- If toothache without fever, ask to do mouth wash with potassium permanganate.
- Provide health education on oral care.
- Advise for periodical dental check-up.
- Refer the patient to primary health center or hospital.

CARE OF PATIENT WITH SHOCK

Shock defined as a life-threatening state in which there is a serious reduction of cardiac output with inadequate

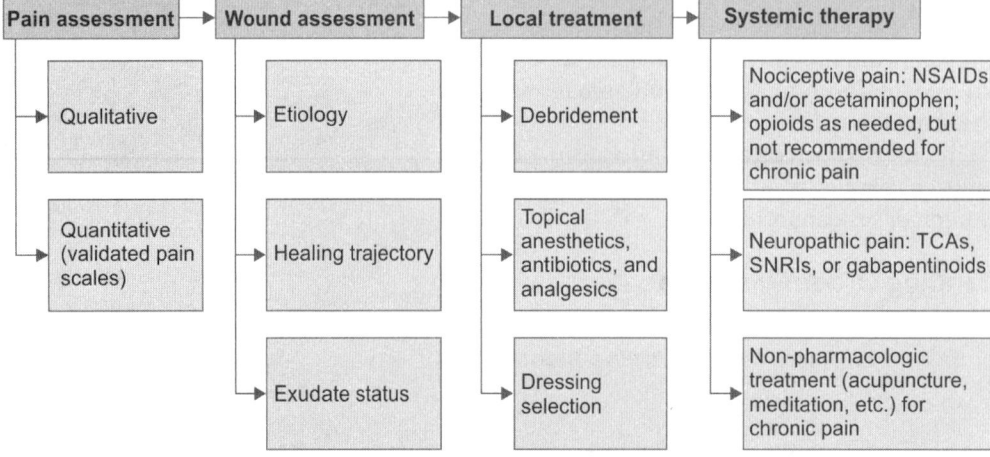

Fig. 9.16: Causes of common type of dental pain (Toothache).

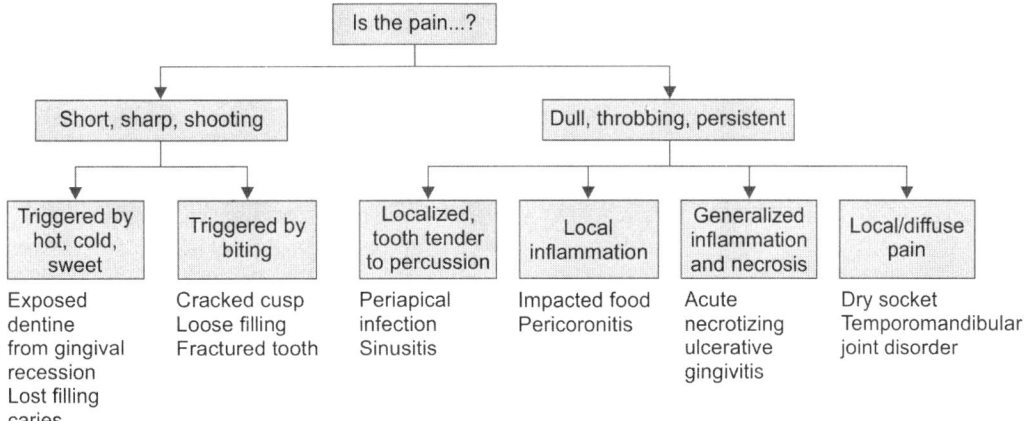

Fig. 9.17: Assessment of pain.

perfusion of organs such as kidneys, brain and liver. Pathology physiology of shock is shown in **Figure 9.18**.

Types of Shock

- **Hypovolemic shock:** Failure of venous return, to the heart due to decreased circulatory blood volume.
- **Cardiogenic shock:** Acute deficiency in cardiac filling and emptying.
- **Neurogenic shock:** It occurs due to interruption of neural mechanisms that maintain vascular tone, cardiac output and venous return.
- **Anaphylactic shock:** Due to antigen and antibody reaction. Laryngeal edema and bronchospasm are the leading causes of death resulting in respiratory insufficiency.
- **Septic shock:** It is otherwise called endotoxin or gram negative shock. Severe toxemia paralyzing vasomotor system and causing pooling of blood in small vessels. Most common organisms are gram negative bacteria such as *E. coli* and *Pseudomonas*.

Community Standing Order/Management

- Assess the general condition of the patient
- Check temperature, pulse, respiration and blood pressure

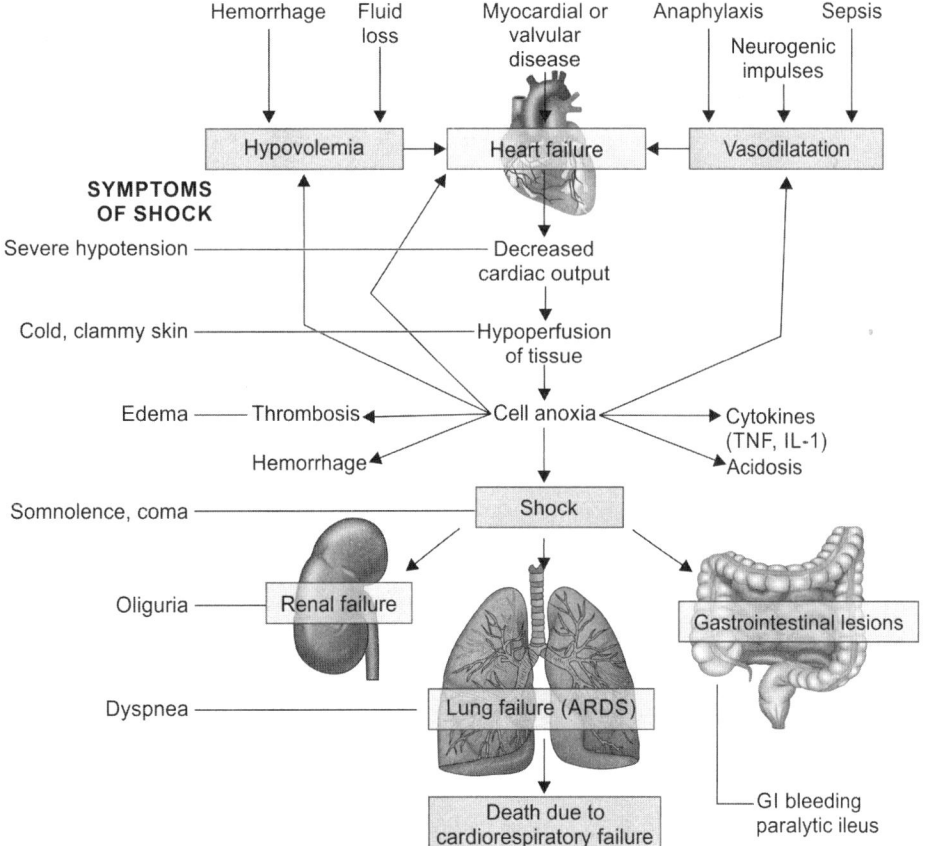

Fig. 9.18: Pathophysiology of shock.

- Keep the airway pattern clear
- Make the patient to lie flat
- Keep him warm and reassure
- If the patient is conscious, provide psychological support and strong hot tea with plenty of sugar.
- If the patient is altered level of conscious—refer immediately to hospital.

CARE OF PATIENT WITH UNCONSCIOUS

Unconscious is a lack of awareness of one's environment and the inability to respond to external stimuli. Clinical features of unconsciousness is depicted in **Figure 9.19**.

Causes of Unconscious

- Head injuries
- Epilepsy
- Infections like meningitis or encephalitis
- Renal failure
- Poisoning or anesthesia
- Hypoglycemia or hyperglycemia
- Emergency condition—shock due to hemorrhage.

Community Standing Order/Management (Fig. 9.20)

- Assess the general condition of the patient
- Check the level of consciousness

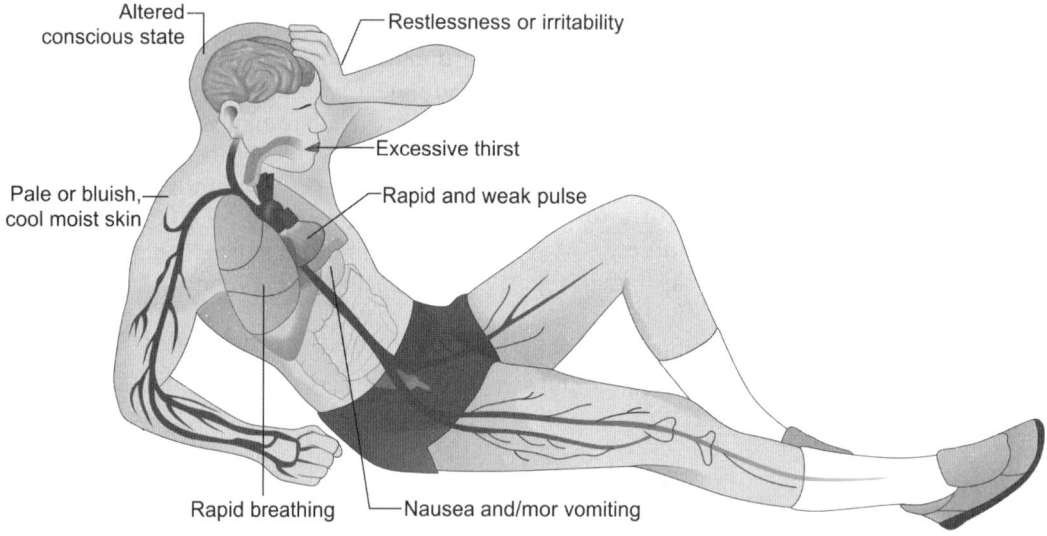

Fig. 9.19: Clinical features of unconsciousness.

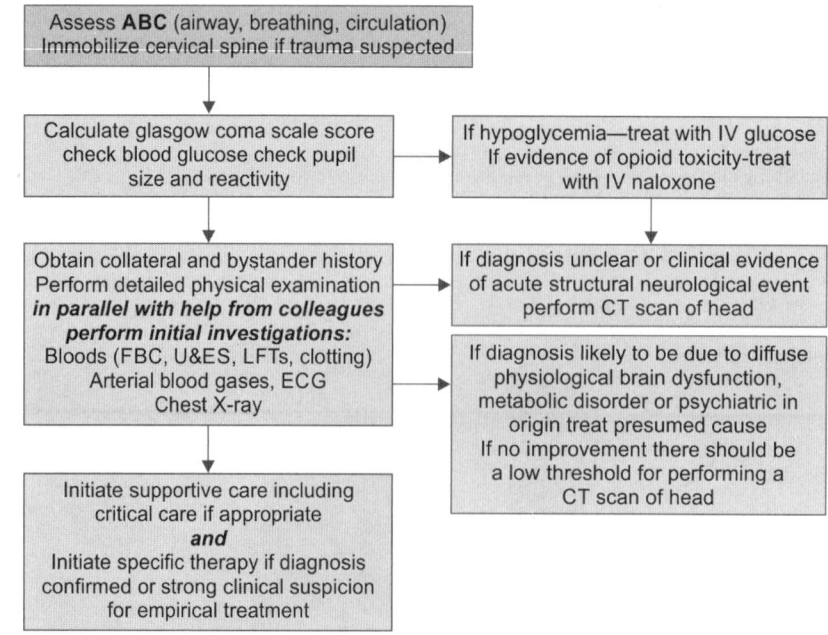

Fig. 9.20: First-aid for unconscious patient.

- Check the temperature, pulse, respiration and blood pressure.
- Make the patient lie on sides.
- Maintain the airway pattern clear.
- Provide adequate ventilation.
- Loosen the tight clothes at neck, chest and wrist.
- Maintain airway, breathing and circulation
- Provide airway or tongue depressor or mouth gauge to prevent tongue falling back.
- Refer the patient to hospital.

CONCLUSION

One of the elements of primary healthcare approach to health problems is treatment of minor ailments and accidents at various levels of care. A community health nurse needs to develop skill in caring for the sick so that restoration to health is achieved in the best and quickest way for the individual, the family and the community. She also has the responsibility to deal appropriately with various accidents occurring in her area of work. She also must know what could be done at what level for the sick and injured so that prompt referral could be done by her through the community participation in terms of primary health care.

BIBLIOGRAPHY

1. International Pharmaceutical Federation. Statement of principle self-care including self-medication: The professional role of the pharmacist.1996; 1–5.
2. World Health Organization. Good pharmacy practice (GPP) in community and hospital pharmacy settings. Geneva. 1996; 1–10.

REVIEW QUESTIONS

Long Essays

1. Explain the basic principles of care during minor ailments and accidents ailments.
2. Define standing orders. Explain the purposes, objectives and uses of standing orders.
3. Describe care of patients with animal bite (dog bite).
4. Discuss the standing order for patient with unconscious.

Short Essays

1. Management of minor ailments.
2. Minor ailments in eyes and ears.
3. Minor ailments in cardiovascular system.
4. Minor ailments in digestive system.
5. Minor ailments in urinary system.
6. Minor ailments in neuromuscular system.
7. Types of standing orders.
8. Role of nurse in standing orders.
9. Care of patient with fever.
10. Care of patient with sore throat.
11. Care of patient with convulsions.
12. Care of patient with diarrhea.
13. Care of patients with constipation.
14. Care of patient with anemia.
15. Care of patient with epitasis.
16. Care of patient with scabies.
17. Care of patient with wounds.
18. Care of patient with shock.

Short Answers

1. Standing orders.
2. Minor ailments.
3. Systemic minor ailments.
4. History-taking.
5. Eye infections.
6. Menstruation problems.
7. Dysmenorrhea.
8. Intermittent fever.
9. Care of patient with sore eye.
10. Care of patient with snake bite.
11. Care of patient with fracture.
12. Care of patient with heat stroke.
13. Care of patient with edema.
14. Types of wounds.
15. Care of patient with toothache.
16. Hypovolemic shock.
17. Causes of unconscious.

Multiple Choice Questions

1. The examples of minor ailment treatments in community health include all, *except*:
    a. Cold sores, mild eczema
    b. Oral thrush, heartburn
    c. Hay fever, skin rash
    d. Shock
2. Standing orders are the directions and orders of specific nature on the basis of these in the nonavailability of doctor at:
    a. Home and hospital
    b. Health institution
    c. Community
    d. All of the above
3. A minor ailment in cardiovascular system includes all, *except*:
    a. High blood pressure
    b. Thoracenthesis
    c. Chest pain
    d. Anemia
4. Minor ailments in reproductive system:
    a. Menstruation problems
    b. Dysmenorrhea
    c. Vaginal discharge
    d. All of the above
5. The objectives of standing orders are:
    a. To maintain the continuity of treatment of the patient
    b. To protect the life of the patient/to resuscitate him
    c. To create the feeling of responsibility in the members of health team
    d. All of the above
6. Fever or pyrexia is defined as a rise in the body temperature above:
    a. 97°F   b. 98°F
    c. 99°F   d. 100°F

7. Grandmal epilepsy consists of sudden generalized convulsions followed by _____.
   a. Unconsciousness
   b. Drowsy
   c. Consciousness
   d. All of the above
8. Most common organisms are gram negative bacteria causes septic shock is:
   a. Streptococci
   b. Pseudomonas
   c. Staphylococci
   d. All of the above
9. Causes of unconscious include all, *except*:
   a. Head injuries
   b. Epilepsy
   c. Infections like meningitis or encephalitis
   d. Diabetes mellitus
10. Edema is a condition occurs due to increased fluid retention in the:
    a. Interstitial spaces
    b. Extravascular
    c. Both a and b
    d. None of the above

ANSWERS

| 1. d | 2. d | 3. b | 4. d | 5. d | 6. c | 7. a | 8. b | 9. d | 10. a | | |

Health System in India

LEARNING OBJECTIVES

Organization and administration of health system in India at:
1. **Central level**
   - Union Ministry
   - Directorate General of Health Services
   - Central Council of Health
2. **State level**
   - State Health Administration
   - State Ministry of Health
   - State Health Directorate
3. **District level**
   - Subdivisions
   - Tehsils/ Talukas
   - Villages
   - Municipalities and Corporation
   - Panchayats

TERMINOLOGY

- **Panchayati Raj:** It is a system of rural, local self-government in India, which represents the local inhabitants, posing a range or degree of autonomy. It was integrally connected with community development.
- **Primary health care:** Primary health care is an essential healthcare based on practical, scientifically sound and socially acceptable methods and technology. It is made universally accessible to individuals and families in the community through their full participation and at that cost that the community and country can afford to maintain at every stage of their development in the spirit of self-reliance and self-determination.
- **Health for all:** Health for all is defined as attainment of a level of health that will enable every individual to lead a socially and emotionally productive life.
- **Health administration:** It is about public health administration, which deals with matters relating to the promotion of health, preventive services, medical care, rehabilitation, and delivery of health services, development of manpower, medical education and training.
- **Public health administration:** It is the science and art of organizing and coordinating government agencies, whose purpose is to improve the physical, mental and social well-being of people. It aims at prevention of disease.
- **Primary health center:** It is a center which provides essential healthcare, made universally accessible to individuals and families in the community by means acceptable to them, through their full participation and at a cost that the community and country can afford.
- **Community development:** It is defined as the process in which people unite with the government authorities in order to improve the economic, social and cultural conditions of the communities, thus contributing fully to national progress.
- **Comprehensive health care:** The term was first used by Bhore Committee in 1946; it means provision of integrated preventive, curative and promotional health services from womb to tomb to every individual residing in a defined geographic area.
- **Basic health service:** A basic health service is understood to be a network of coordinates, peripheral and intermediate health units capable of performing effectively. A selected group will function according to the need of health care of an area and assuring the availability of competent, professional and auxiliary personnel to perform these functions.
- **Administration:** Administration is the organization and direction of human and material resources to achieve desired goals.

INTRODUCTION

The healthcare system in India is primarily administered by the states. India's Constitution tasks each state with providing health care for its people. In order to address lack of medical coverage in rural areas, the national government launched the National Rural Health Mission in 2005. Health administration is a branch of public administration, which deals with matters relating to the promotion of health, preventive services, medical care, rehabilitation and delivery of health services, development of health, manpower, medical education and training. Public health administration is the science and art of organizing and coordinating government agencies, whose purpose is to improve the physical, mental and social well-being of people. It aims at prevention of disease, preservation and promotion of health.

DEFINITIONS

- **Health:** Health is defined as, "a dynamic state of complete physical, mental and social well-being and not merely an absence of disease or infirmity." (WHO)
- **Health care:** Health care is defined as, "multitude of services rendered to individuals, families or communities by the agents of the health services or professions for the purpose of promoting, preventing, maintaining, monitoring or restoring health."
- **System:** A set of interrelated and independent parts designed to achieve a set of goals.

HEALTH SYSTEM

- Health system covers a whole extent of health activities, health programs, institutions providing medical care such as hospitals, clinics and primary healthcare centres and the policies enunciated by governments to provide optimal health care for its citizens. Levels of healthcare system is depicted in **Figure 10.1**.
- In general health system defines as "Complex of facilities, organizations, and trained personnel engaged in providing health care within a geographical area."
- Health system as described by WHO is the "sum total of all the organizations, institutions and resources whose primary purpose is to improve health."
- Health systems should be accessible, efficient, affordable and of a good quality.

- Health systems usually include the following:
  - Development of health policies, plan for their implementation and development of a system of regulation of health services.
  - Define and develop the institutional framework to deliver the health services within the purview of this system.
  - Allocate and mobilize financial and human resources for its functioning.
  - Plan, manage and deliver the health services.

AIMS AND GOALS OF HEALTH SYSTEM

Aims of Health System

Ultimately aim of health systems is to improve, maintain and restore the health status of the community at a cost that an individual and the community can afford to spend without substantial change in their financial status.

Goals of Health System

A health system has to provide for much more than routine delivery of services. It has to protect the health of its community, treat them with dignity and ensure that it responds fairly to the expectations of the population. The WHO has thus identified three overall goals for the health systems to be:
1. Effective in contributing to better health throughout the entire population.
2. Responsive to people's expectations, including safeguarding patient's dignity, confidentiality and autonomy and being sensitive to the specific needs and vulnerabilities of all population groups.
3. Fair in how individuals contribute to funding the system so that everyone has access to the services available and is protected against potentially impoverishing levels of spending.

DETERMINANTS OF HEALTH SYSTEM

Economic
- Affordability
- Availability

Political
- Priorities
- Appropriateness
- Accessibility
- Equity

Cultural
- Acceptability
- Utilization
- Participation

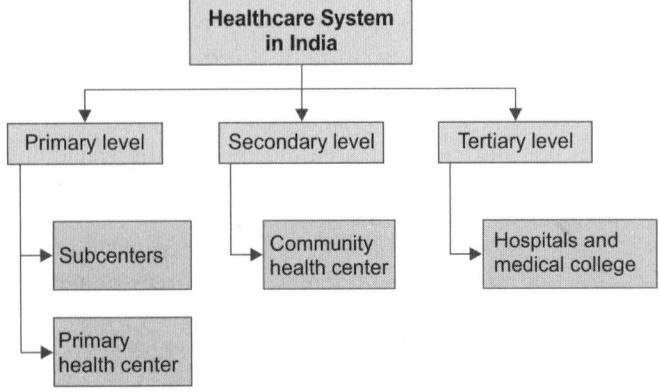

Fig. 10.1: Levels of healthcare system.

FORCES INFLUENCE THE HEALTH SYSTEM

- New emerging diseases
- Changing disease profile
- Technical and diagnostic advances
- Longevity of life
- Expectations of people
- Subsidies and cross-subsidies
- Increasing non-plan expenditure
- Competing priorities
- Improving awareness among people
- Rising Cost of healthcare delivery

HEALTH ADMINISTRATION

- Centralized direction and decentralized activity.
- When a special function is to be undertaken, it should be undertaken by or in co-operation with the official body.
- There should not be duplication and overlapping in rendering treatment and prevention of disease.
- Treatment and prevention of disease should be administratively combined.
- Administration must be based on a sound economic consideration and practical financial budgeting.
- A clear picture of the complete plan must be made before starting a program.
- A program of continuing staff education is essential.
- Program should be planned on a scientific priority basis.
- Periodic appraisal of service rendered, effectiveness of programs and evaluation of results is major responsibility of the health administration.
- Provision must be made for desirable working conditions for all members of the staff.

Objectives of Health Administration

- To increase the average length of human life.
- To decrease mortality and morbidity rates.
- To increase the physical, mental and social well-being of the individual.
- To provide total health care to enrich quality life.
- To increase the pace of adjustment of individual to his environment.
- To make provision of primary healthcare services to everyone.
- To develop health and manpower to provide proper services to the community.
- To formulate health policies and their periodic revision from time to time.

History of Health Administration in India

Health administration is a part of public administration of the country and is one of the aspects of the social welfare activities of the government. Modern public health organization and administration is designed to prevent disease, prolong life and to promote physical and mental efficiency through organized community efforts. Public health organization is an integral part of the government, responsible to central authority and interrelated in its activities with the general conduct of governmental affairs. Cooperation and co-ordination of service with schools, community, projects, welfare boards and with voluntary agencies (**Fig. 10.2**).

During pre-independence period, the medical and public health services at the central were administered by two separate departments headed by Director General of Indian Medical Services and commissioner of public health service respectively but after independence, these two offices were amalgamated into Directorate General of health services which was headed by Director of Health Services (**Fig. 10.3**).

- Post-independence era—Public health in post-independence year in 1947, after independence, a democratic regime was set up in India with a new concept aimed towards the establishment of a welfare state. The Bhore Committee report and recommendations became the basis for most of the planning and measures adopted by the National Government.
- 1947—Ministries of Health were established at the center and states. The post of Director General Indian medical service and of public health commissioner with government of India was integrated into the post of Director General of Health Science (DHS).
- 1948—India became a member of World Health Organization. The WHO is a specialized non-political health agency constituted on 7th April 1948 with an objective of attainment of the highest level of halt for all people. The Employee State Insurance Act (ESI) was passed in the parliament. The report of the environmental hygiene committee was published.
- 1949—The post of Registrar General, India was created in the Ministry of Home Affairs. The South East Asia regional office of the WHO was established in New Delhi. The Indian Council of Medical Research (ICMR) was formed.
- Planning commission—The Government of India set up a planning commission in 1950 to make an assessment of maternal capital and human resources of the country and to draft developmental plans for the most effective utilization of these resources. Over the years, the planning commission has been formulating successive five year plans.
- Five Year Plan—The five year plans were conceived to rebuild rural India, to lay foundations of industrial progress and to secure the balanced development of all parts of the country. The broad objectives of five year plans are control or eradication of major communicable diseases, strengthening the basic health services through the development of health, manpower and resources.
- National Health Policy—The Ministry of Health and Family Welfare, Government of India evolved a National Health Policy in 1983, keeping in view the national commitment to attain the goal of 'health for all by the year 2000'. The main objective of this policy was to achieve an acceptable standard of good health amongst the general population of the country.

Chapter 10: Health System in India

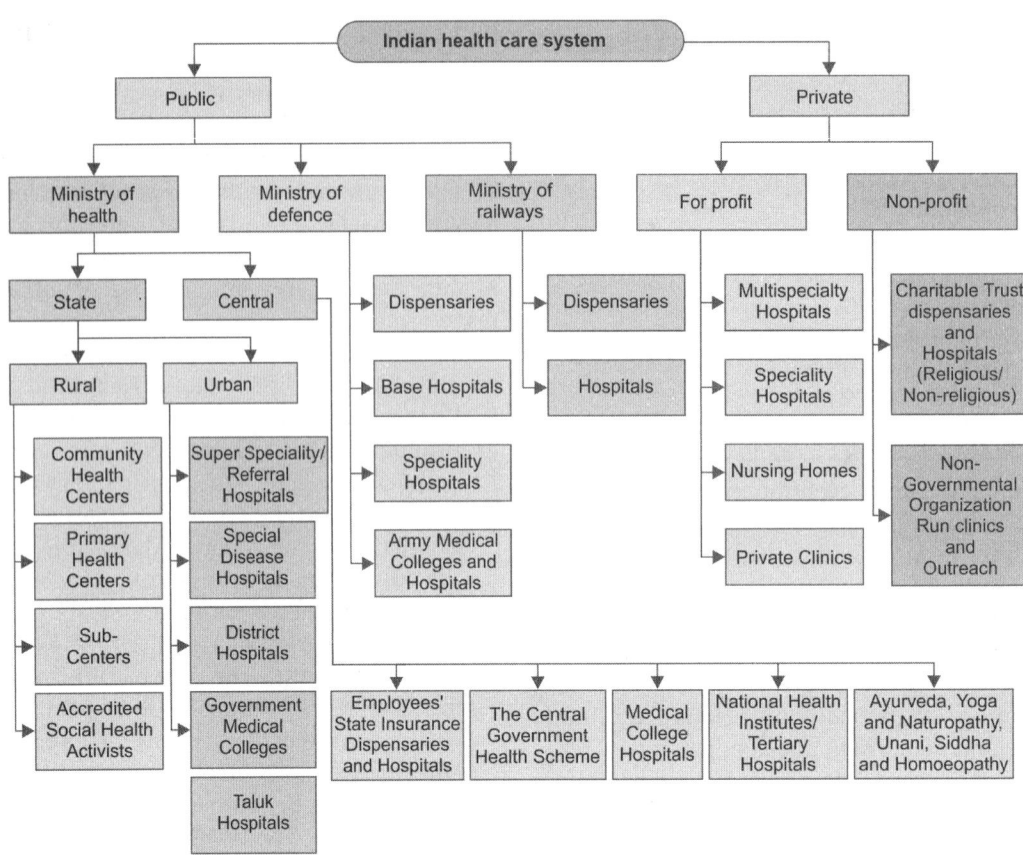

Fig. 10.2: Public and private healthcare system in India.

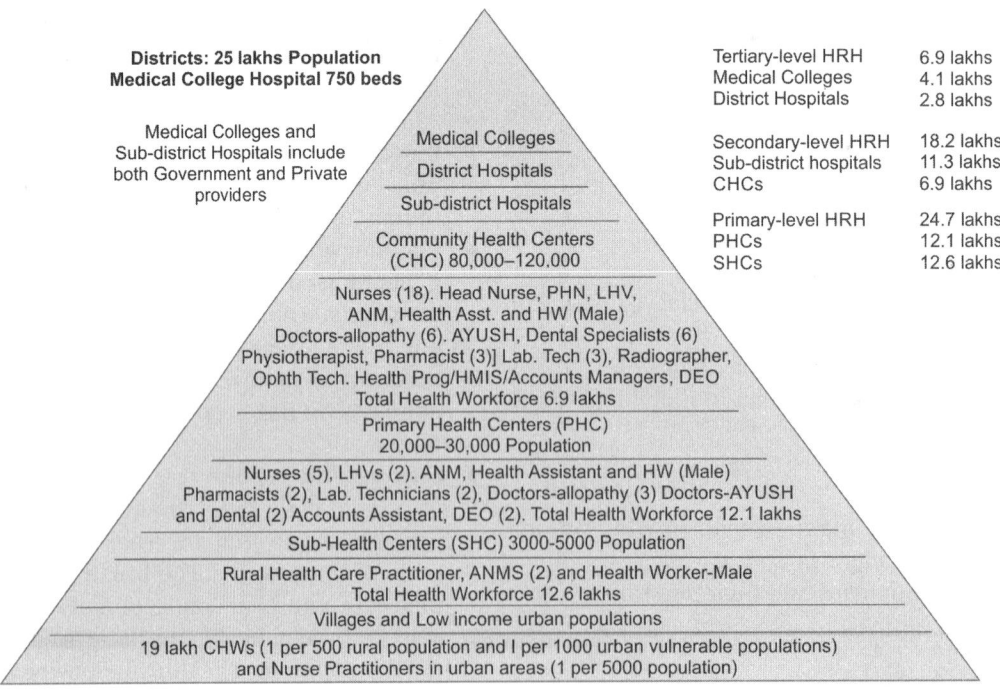

Fig. 10.3: Population coverage in healthcare system.

MODEL OF HEALTHCARE DELIVERY SYSTEM (FIG. 10.4)

The challenge that exists today in many countries is to reach the whole population with adequate healthcare services and to ensure their utilization. For that the numerous models have been developed for the delivery of healthcare services. One of the simplest models is:

- The "inputs" are the health status or health problems of the community; they represent the health needs and health demands of the community. Since sources are always limited to meet the many health needs, priorities have to be set.

Chapter 10: Health System in India

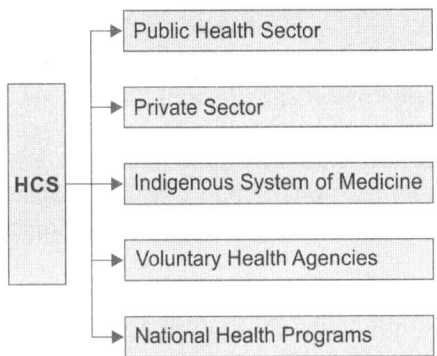

Fig. 10.4: Healthcare delivery model.

- The "healthcare services" are designed to meet the health needs of the community through the use of available knowledge and resources. The services provided should be comprehensive and community-based.
- The "healthcare system" is intended to deliver the healthcare services; it constitutes the management sector and involves organizational matters.
- The final outcome or output is the changed health status or improved health status of the community which is expressed in terms of lives saved, deaths averted, diseases prevented, etc.

ORGANIZATION AND ADMINISTRATION OF HEALTH SYSTEM IN INDIA

Health administration is the science of the organizing and coordinating government agencies whose purpose is to improve the physical, mental and social well-being of the people of the country. It is a part of the public administration.

India is a Union of 28 States and 7 Union territories. Under the Constitution of India, the States are largely independent in matters relating to the delivery of healthcare to the people. Each State has developed own system of healthcare delivery, independent of the Central Government.

The Central responsibility of an organization of policy making, planning, guiding, assisting, evaluating, and coordinating the work of the State Health Ministries, so that health services cover every part of the country, In order to achieve the goal to "Health for All – 2020". Health administration governed in India at four levels:
1. National level (Central level)
2. State level
3. District level
4. Community level

CENTRAL LEVEL HEALTHCARE ADMINISTRATION (FIG. 10.5)

The healthcare system or health organization in India has three main links, i.e., central, state and local or peripheral. Under the constitution of India, the states are largely independent in matters relating to the delivery of healthcare to the people. The central responsibility consists mainly of policy making, planning, guiding, assisting, evaluating and coordinating the work of the State Health Ministries. The official "organs" of the health system at the national level consist of:

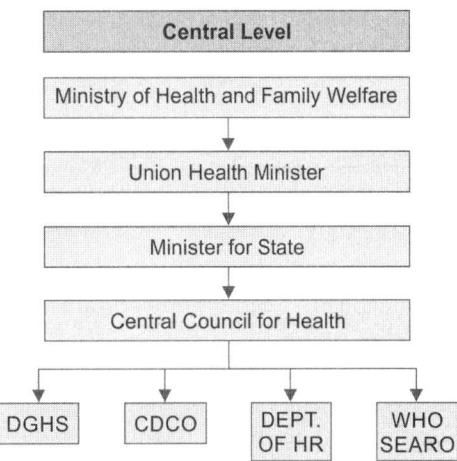

Fig. 10.5: Central level healthcare administration.

- The Ministry of Health and Family Welfare;
- The Directorate General of Health Services; and
- The Central Council of Health and Family Welfare.

Union Ministry of Health and Family Welfare

The Union Ministry of Health and Family Welfare is headed by a cabinet minister, a minister of state and a deputy health minister, these are political appointments. The Union Ministry of Health and Family Welfare at the Center plays a vital role in the governmental efforts to enable the citizen to live a healthier and useful life. Currently, the union ministry has the following departments:

Organization: The Union Ministry of Health and Family Welfare is headed by a Cabinet Minister, a Minister of State and a Deputy Health Minister. The Union Ministry has three departments:
1. Departments of health
2. Departments of family welfare
3. Departments of Indian Systems of Medicine and Homoeopathy (ISM and H)

The department of family welfare was created in 1966 within the ministry of health and family welfare, for the administrative purpose of the union health and family welfare, minister seeks the help of health secretariat headed by Secretary. The secretary is assisted by a number of additional, joint, deputy and assistant secretaries and various administrative staff. Department of health deals with planning, coordination, programming and evaluation of medical and public health matters including drug control and prevention of food adulteration. The department of health functions through the Directorate General of Health Service.

Department of family welfare is headed by Secretary to the Government of India, ministry of health and family welfare, who is supported and assisted by a team of two joint secretaries, two chief directors, number of deputy secretaries, deputy commissioners, directors and other technical and administrative officers in hierarchy.

Functions of the union health ministry: The functions of the Union Health Ministry are set out in the seventh schedule of Article 246 of the Constitution of India under:
- Union list
- Concurrent list.

Union List

The functions given in the Union list are:
- International health relations and administration of port quarantine
- Administration of central institutes such as the All India Institute of Hygiene and Public Health, Kolkata; National Institute for the Control of Communicable Diseases, Delhi, etc.
- Promotion of research through research centers and other bodies
- Regulation and development of medical, pharmaceutical, dental and nursing professions
- Establishment and maintenance of drug standards
- Census, and collection and publication of other statistical data
- Immigration and emigration
- Regulation of labor in the working of mines and oil fields
- Coordination with States and with other ministries for promotion of health.

Concurrent List

The functions listed under the concurrent list are the responsibility of both the Union and State governments. The concurrent list includes:
- Prevention of communicable diseases
- Prevention of adulteration of foodstuffs
- Control of drugs and poisons
- Vital statistics
- Labour welfare
- Ports other than major
- Economic and social planning
- Population control and family planning.

Functions of Department of Medical and Public Health

The functions of the Department of Medical and Public Health are:
- Health policy preparation
- National Health Programes conduction
- Drug Control
- PFA enforcement
- Diseases control
- Communicable/Non-communicable
- Supplies and Disposal maintenance
- CME and training
- Medical education and research
- Vital statistics and health intelligence
- International support

Functions of Department of Family Welfare

The functions of the Department of Family Welfare are:
- Policy preparation and planning
- Information collection and evaluation
- Contraceptive-Research/Supply
- Seeking international support for family welfare
- EPI/UIP/CSSM/RCH/ARI/ORT-Trainings and area development
- Maternal and Child Health Services.
- IEC—Information, Education and Communication.
- Rural Health Services
- Paraprofessional training
- NGO support
- Development of subcenter.

Functions of Department of IMS and H

The functions of the Department of IMS and H are:
- Upgrade the educational standards in the Indian Systems of Medicines and Homoeopathy colleges in the country.
- Strengthen existing research institutions and ensure a time-bound research program on identified diseases for which these systems have an effective treatment.
- Draw up schemes for promotion, cultivation and regeneration of medicinal plants used in these systems.
- Evolve Pharmacopoeial standards for Indian Systems of Medicine and Homoeopathy drugs.

DIRECTORATE GENERAL OF HEALTH SERVICES

Organization: Directorate General of Health Services (DGHS) is the principal adviser for the Union Government in both medical and public health matters. He is assisted by additional director, a team of deputies and a large administrative staff. It comprises of three units—medical care and hospital, public health and general health.

Functions: The general functions are surveys, planning, coordination, programming and appraisal of all health matters in the country. The specific functions are:
- **International health relations and quarantine:** All the major ports in the country and international air ports are directly controlled by the Directorate General of Health Services. All matters relating to the obtaining of assistance from International agencies and the coordination of their activities in the country are undertaken by the Directorate General of Health Services.
- **Control of drug standards:** The DGHS is headed by the Drugs Controller. Its primary function is to lay down and enforce standards and control the manufacture and distribution of drugs through both Central and State Government Officers.
- **Medical store depots:** The Union Government runs medical store depots. These depots supply the civil medical requirements of the Central Government and of the various State Governments. These depots also handle supplies from foreign agencies. The Medical Stores Organization endeavors to ensure the highest quality, cheaper bargain and prompt supplies.

- **Postgraduate training:** The DGHS is responsible for the administration of national institutes, which also provide postgraduate training to different categories of health personnel.
- **Medical education:** The Central Directorate is directly in charge of the following medical colleges in India: the Lady Harding, the Maulana Azad and the medical colleges at Pondicherry, and Goa. Besides these, there are many medical colleges in the country which are guided and supported by the Center.
- **Medical Research:** Medical Research in the country is organized largely through the Indian Council of Medical Research, founded in 1911 in New Delhi. The funds of the Council are wholly derived from the budget of the Union Ministry of Health.

Central Government Health Scheme

- **National Health Programes:** Health programs of this kind can hardly succeed without the help of the Central Government. The Central Directorate plays a very important part in planning, guiding and coordinating all the national health programs in the country.
- **Central Health Education Bureau:** An outstanding activity of this Bureau is the preparation of education material for creating health awareness among the people. The Bureau offers training courses in health education to different categories of health workers.
- **Health intelligence:** The Central Bureau of Health Intelligence was established in 1961 to centralize collection, compilation, analysis, evaluation and dissemination of all information on health statistics for the nation as a whole. It disseminates epidemic intelligence to States and international bodies. The Bureau has an Epidemiological Unit, a Health Economics Unit, a National Morbidity Survey Unit and a Manpower Cell.
- **National Medical Library:** The Central Medical Library of the Directorate General Health Services was declared the National Medical Library in 1966. The aim is to help in the advancement of medical, health and related sciences by collection, dissemination and exchange of information.

CENTRAL COUNCIL OF HEALTH

The Central Council of Health was set up by a Presidential Order on 9 August, 1952 under Article 263 of the Constitution of India for continuous consultation, mutual understanding and cooperation between the Center and the States in the implementation of all the programs and measures pertaining to the health of the nation.

Organization: The Union Health Minister is the Chairman and the State Health Ministers are the members.

Functions: The functions of the Central Council of Health are:
- To consider and recommend broad outlines of policy in regard to matters concerning health in all its aspects such as the provision of remedial and preventive care, environmental hygiene, nutrition, health education and the promotion of facilities for training and research.
- To make proposals for legislation in fields of activity relating to medical and public health matters and to lay down the pattern of development for the country as a whole.
- To make recommendations to the Central Government regarding distribution of available grants-in-aid for health purposes to the States and to review periodically the work accomplished in different areas through the utilization of these grants-in-aid.
- To establish any organization or organizations invested with appropriate functions for promoting and maintaining cooperation between the Central and State Health administrations.

STATE LEVEL HEALTHCARE ADMINISTRATION (FIG. 10.6)

- Organizational structure at the state level is on the similar pattern as that as that as the central level. Health being a state subject, the state govt. has autonomy in dealing with health matters.
- At present there are 28 States in India, with each state having its own health administration.

State Ministry of Health and Family Welfare

- The State Ministry of Health is headed by a Minister of Health and Family Welfare and a Deputy Minister of Health and Family Welfare. These are political appointments and they are elected members of legislative assembly.
- They have political responsibilities, responsibilities towards their constituencies as per their political agenda, and responsibilities for administration and management of Health and Family Welfare services in their state.

Health Secretariat

- The State Health and Family Welfare Minister is assisted for all administrative aspects of healthcare by the Health Secretariat, that is the official organ of his Ministry.
- The Health Secretariat is headed by the secretary who is assisted by Additional, Deputy and Assistant Secretaries and other hierarchy of administrative staff.

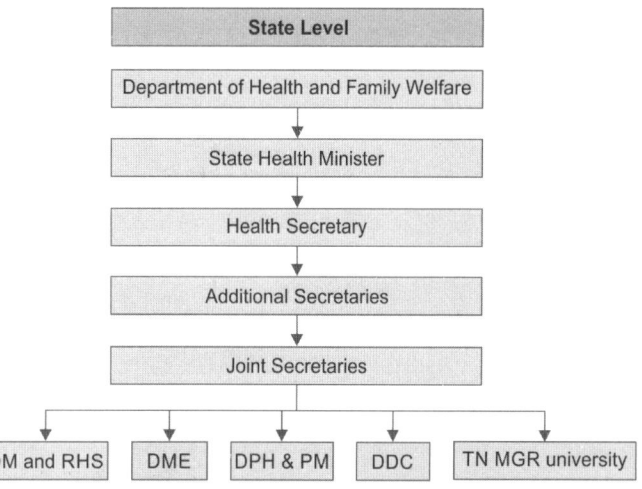

Fig. 10.6: State level health administration.

Functions: The major functions which are performed by the secretariat include helping minister in:
- Formulation, review and modification of broad policy outlines.
- Execution of policies programs, etc.
- Coordination with Government of India and other state Governments.
- Control for smooth and efficient functioning of administrative machinery.

State Health Directorate

- The State Health Directorate is the technical wing of state Ministry of Health and Family Welfare.
- Before independence, the Medical and Public Health Services at the State level like at the Centre were also administered by two separate departments headed by surgeon General and Inspector General of civil hospitals and Director of Public Health Services respectively.
- After independence these two departments' medical health and public health were integrated into State Directorate of Health Services as recommended by Dr. Bhore committee report in 1946.
- State Health Directorate is headed by Director of health services. In some States he is designated as Director of Health and Family Welfare.
- He is the chief technical advisor to the stale Government on all matters of Medical, Public Health and Family welfare.
- He is assisted by a number of Deputy and Assistant Directors to plan and provide healthcare services to meet healthcare needs of the State as per Govt. health policy.
- The Deputy and Assistant Directors of Health may be of two types—regional and functional. The Regional Directors inspect all the branches of public health within their jurisdiction, irrespective of their specialty. The Functional Directors are usually specialists in a particular branch of public health such as mother and child health, family planning, nutrition, tuberculosis, leprosy, health education, etc.

Functions

- It studies in department of the health problem and need of the state and planning for health services in the state.
- Implementation of national health programs and evaluating their achievements.
- Promoting providing and supervising all types of health services in the state such as primary health services; school health services; family planning services; MCH occupational health services, etc.
- Collection of vital statistics.
- Encouraging reproductive and child health (family welfare, maternal health, etc.)
- Improvement of nutrition program and Controlling food adulteration and also sanitation in milk and edibles.
- Medical and nursing education, training of nurses, female health workers and other health workers.
- Controlling rural and urban health services through district medical officer.
- Providing feedback to the state health ministry regarding health.

DISTRICT LEVEL HEALTHCARE ADMINISTRATION

District: An Administrative unit Defined Geographical boundary and Population. Within each district again, there are 6 types of administrative areas: Sub-divisions, Tehsils (Talukas), Community Development Blocks, Municipalities and Corporations (urban area), Panchayats (Villages) **(Fig. 10.7)**.

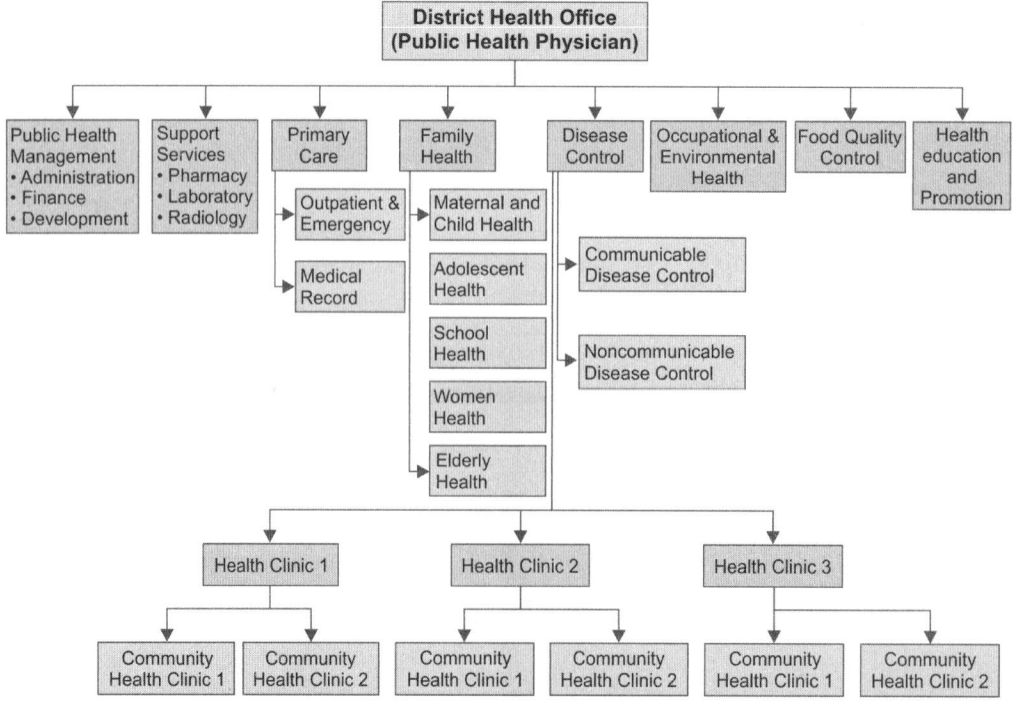

Fig. 10.7: District level healthcare administration.

- District is Peripheral most Planning unit
- It is a self-contained segment of National Health System
- Middle level management organization
- The principal unit of administration in India is the district under a Collector.
- It is a link between the State/regional structure on one side and the peripheral level structures such as PHC/Subcenter on the other side.

Organization

Chief Medical and Health Officer (CM and HO)

Chief Medical and Health Officer—CM and HO is a Director of health and family welfare service at the district in rural area and are overall in-charge of the health and family welfare programmes in the rural area. CM and HO is assisted by Dy. CMO, RCH officer and program officers. Dy. CMO and RCH officer are assisted by Block CMOs.

Principal Medical Officer (PMO)

Principal Medical Officer—PMO is a Director of health and family welfare service at the district in urban area and is overall in-charge of the health and family welfare programs in urban area.

Functions of District Health System

- Liaison between field units and headquarter
  - Field reports
  - Inspections
  - Meetings
- Implementation of policy and programs
- District level planning and action plans
- Rationale use of finance and resources
- Communication management: Plans/Schedules/Progress/Problems
- Control and monitoring.

COMMUNITY LEVEL HEALTHCARE ADMINISTRATION

Community health centre (CHC) has been established for every 80,000 to 120,000 population and this centre provides the basic specialty services in general medicine, Pediatric, surgery, obstetrics and gynecology.

Functions of CHC

- Care of Routine and emergency cases in medicine
- Care of Routine and emergency cases in surgery.
- Our delivery services, including normal and assisted deliveries.
- Essential and emergency obstetric care
- FP services including laparoscopic services
- Newborn care
- Routine and emergency care of sick children
- Other management including nasal packing, tracheotomy, foreign body removal, etc.
- All the National Health Programmes (NHP) should be delivered through the CHC.
- Other:
  - Blood storage facility
  - Essential laboratory services
  - Referral services.

Staffing Pattern at CHC

Existing clinical manpower

- General surgeon — 1
- Physician — 1
- Obstetrician/Gynecologist — 1
- Pediatrician — 1

Existing Support Manpower

- Nurse- Mid wife — 7+2
- Dresser — 1
- Pharmacist/Compounder — 1
- Lab technician — 1
- Radiographer — 1
- Ophthalmic assistant — 1
- Ward boy/Nursing orderly — 2
- Sweepers — 2
- Chowkidar — 1
- OPD attendant — 1
- Data Entry Operator — 5
- OT attendant — 1
- Registration Clerk — 1

Organization

Center	Population Norms	
	Plain Area	Hilly/Tribal/Difficult Area
CHC	1,20,000	80,000
PHC	30,000	20,000
Subcenter	5000	3000

Primary Health Center Level

At present there is one primary health center covering about 30,000 (20,000 in hilly, desert and difficult terrains) or more population. Many rural dispensaries have been upgraded to create these PHCs. The bed strength of Primary health center is 6 (but can be raised up to 10). Basic pillars of primary health care is depicted in **Figure 10.8**.

Functions of PHC

- Medical Care
- MCH including Family Planning
- Safe water supply and basic sanitation
- Prevention and control of locally endemic diseases.
- Collection and reporting of vital statistics.
- Education about health
- National health programs as relevant
- Referral services
- Training of health guides, health workers local dais and health assistants.
- Basic laboratory services.

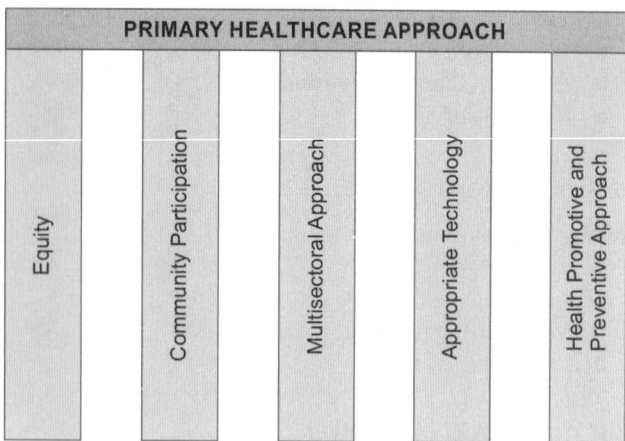

Fig. 10.8: The 5 basic pillars of primary health care.

Staffing Pattern of PHC

- Medical Officer — 1
- Pharmacist — 1
- Nurse Midwife — 1
- Health Worker (female)/ANM — 1
- Block Extension Educator — 1
- Health Assistant (Male) — 1
- Health Assistant (Female) — 1
- U.D.C (Upper Division clerk) — 1
- L.D.C (Lower Division Clerk) — 1
- Lab. Technician — 1
- Driver — 1
- Class IV — 4
- Total — 15

Subcenter Level

The subcenter is the peripheral outpost of exiting healthcare delivery system in rural areas. it provides interface with community at the grass root level, providing all the primary health services. one subcenter for every 5000 population in general and one for every 3000 population in hilly, tribal and backward areas. Each subcenter is manned by one male and one female multipurpose health worker.

Functions of Subcenter

- Mother and child healthcare
- Family planning and immunization
- It is proposed to extend the facilities at all subcenters for IUD insertion, and simple laboratory investigation like routine examination of urine for albumin and sugar
- The work at subcenters is supervised by male and female health assistants
- According to the revised norm, one female HA will supervise the work of 6 female Health Workers

Staffing Pattern of Subcenter

- Health Worker (Female)/ANM — 1
- Health Worker (Male) — 1
- Voluntary Worker — 1
- Total — 3

HEALTH ORGANIZATION AT DISTRICT LEVEL

Bhore committee 1946 recommended integrated services at all levels and the setting up of a unified health authority in each district. The principal unit of administration in India is the district under a collector. There are 593 (year 2001) districts in India. The districts vary widely in area and population. Healthcare workers in different levels of health care depicted in **Figure 10.9**.

- Each district has 6 types of administrative areas—subdivisions, Tehsils (Talukas), community development blocks, municipalities and corporations, villages and panchayats.
- Most of the districts in India are divided into (two or more subdivisions, each in charge of an assistant collector or subcollector. Each division is again divided into tehsils (taluks) in charge of a tehsildar. A tehsildar usually comprises between 200 to 600 villages.
- The district officer is in charge of all health administration and all National health programs are implemented in the district except family welfare program.
- The district family welfare and maternal and child health officer is in-charge of family welfare programme. Both of them have control over primary health center.
- The district health organization is headed by chief medical officer of health (CMOH) who is the director of health service at the district. He is assisted by a number of officers in charge of different programs.
- They are District Family Welfare Officer (DFWO) District Malaria Officer (DMO), District Leprosy officer (DLO), District Health officer (DHO), Civil Surgeon in charge district hospital. The health organization at the district level includes:
    - The chief medical officer of the district and his assistant staff
    - The district hospital and the district stores
    - The network of primary health centers and dispensaries

Functions of District Health Organization

- Primary health care
- Secondary and referral health care

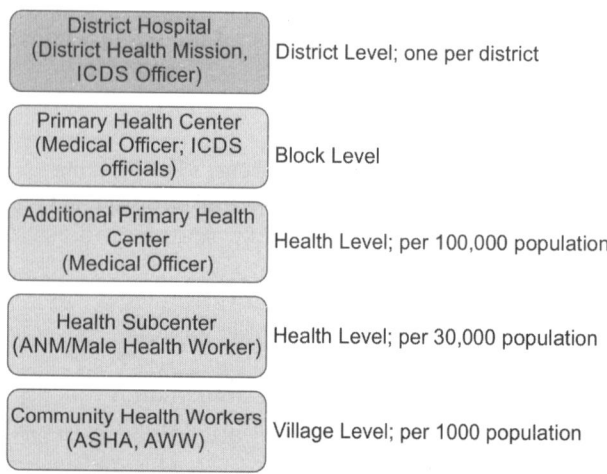

Fig. 10.9: Healthcare workers in different levels of health care.

- Family welfare
- National Health Programes

HEALTH ORGANIZATION AT BLOCK LEVEL

Health organization at block level comprises community health center, primary health centre, dispensaries and sub centers. Since the launching of the community development programme in India in 1952, the rural areas of the district have been organized into blocks, known as or may not coincide with a tehsil.

The block is a unit of rural planning and development and comprises approximately 100 villages and about 80,000 to 1,20,000 population in charge of a block development officer. The main functions of the block health organization are—Primary health care, referral care, National health programes, family welfare, community participation and intersectoral coordination and school health and ICDS scheme.

HEALTH ORGANIZATION AT SUBCENTER

Each primary center has 5 to 6 subcenters. This is the first unit of health system for the villagers. The subcenter covers population of 30,000 in general and 3000 in hilly/tribal and backward areas.

Staffing Pattern of Subcenter

- Multipurpose female health worker -1
- Multipurpose male health worker -1
- Voluntary/part time worker -1

Services Provided by Subcenters

- Maternal and child health services
- Family planning and welfare services
- Immunization services
- Health education
- Training and supervision of indigenous dais.

Maintenance of subcenters: Financial aid or support for most of the centers is made by union ministry of health and family welfare. Rest of the centers are financially assisted by the State government under minimum need program (MNP) or Basic minimum services (BMS).

HEALTH ORGANIZATION AT URBAN

The urban areas of the district are organized into local self-government such as town municipal council, city municipal council and corporations.

- **Town area committee**—The town area committee are set up in areas having population in the range of 5000 – 10,000. These are like panchayats and provide sanitary services in the area.
- **Municipal Boards**—Municipal boards are set up in areas having population between 10,000–200,000. The municipal board is headed by Chairman/president elected usually by its members. The term of the member ranges from 3–5 years. The function of municipal board are—construction and maintenance of roads, sanitation and drainage, street lighting, water supply, maintenance of hospitals and dispensaries, education, registration of births and deaths.
- **Corporations**—Corporations are set up in areas having population more than 200,000. The corporation is headed by a major. Its members are the councilors who are elected from various wards of the city. The corporation is headed by a major. Its members are the councilors who are elected form various wards of the city. The corporation has the executive agency headed by the commissioner.
- **The executive agency includes** the commissioner, the secretary, the engineer and the health officer. The activities are similar to those of the municipalities but on a larger and wider scale. The mayor is honored as the first citizen of the city. Every corporation has an honorary sheriff appointed by the state government by rotation on communal basis.
- **The corporation** has separate standing committee to look after each work such as education, finance health and works. The commissioner is the executive head of the corporation; usually he is an officer of IAS.

PANCHAYAT RAJ

Parallel to this official structure of administration, there are institutions of local self government in rural areas. This is refers to panchayat Raj system. This system is introduced since 1957 strengthen the administration at the gross root level.

Panchayat Raj is a 3 tire structure of the rural local self government. It is a complex system, which represents the local inhabitants, possessing a range or degree of autonomy. The panchayati Raj institutions are accepted as agencies public welfare. All development programmes are channeled through these bodies.

Panchayat Raj institutions strengthen democracy at its root and ensure more effective and better participation of the people in the government. It is a three tire structure.

Panchayati Raj at Village Level

- The primary unit or local government is the 'village' and the primary institution of local government is the 'village panchayat'. Panchayats has been in existence in India from Vedic age. They continued to exist till 1800 AD, when they were ruined and remained so until revived in 1948 (Fig. 10.10).
- Villages throughout the country are to be served by the panchayats for panchayats have a defined role in planning and implementing the programs in village.
- **Gram Sabha:** It is the assembly of all adult men and women of the village. The body meets at least twice in a year and discusses important issues and considers proposals for taxation; discuss the annual program and elects members of gram panchayat.
- **Gram panchayat:** It is executive organ of the gram sabha and an agency for planning and development at the village level. It consists of 15–30 elected members; it covers a population of 2000 to 5000. Every panchayat has an elected president (Sarpanch/mukhiya/sabhapati), a

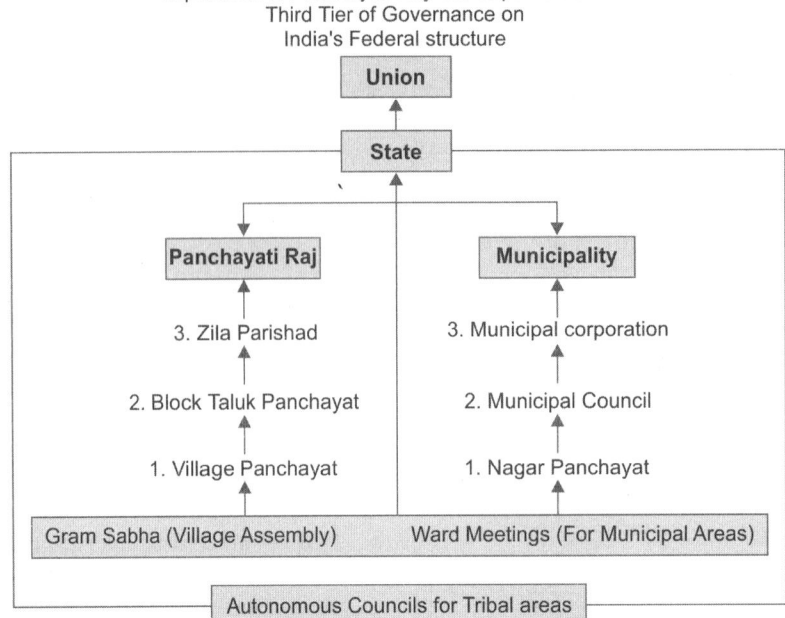

Fig. 10.10: Three tire system.

vice president and panchayat secretary. The panchayat secretary has been given powers to function for wide areas, such as maintenance of sanitation and public health, socioeconomic development of the villages, etc.

- **Nyaya panchayt:** It is composed of 5 members from the panchayat. It tries to solve the dispute between the panchayat. It tries to solve the dispute between the two parties/individuals over certain matters on mutual consent.

Functions

- **Developmental functions**—All developmental functions, e.g., agriculture, animal husbandry, cottage industries, medical relief and public health are to be implemented.
- **Judicial functions**—"Nyaya panchayat" which is to be established for a group of "Village panchayats" and its members are elected by Gram sabha.
- **Low and order functions**—The panchayat also helps in maintaining law and order in the village.
- **Administrative and civic functions**—The panchayat is expected to perform all the elementary civic functions such as arrangements of sanitation, conservancy, construction and repair of roads, water supply, street lights, etc.

Panchayati Raj at Block Level

The panchayati Raj institution at the block level is known as "Panchayat samiti". The body mainly works to arose and encourage the people to utilize their resourcefully for the development activities under the community development programme. The funds for the development activities are processed through panchayat samiti.

Each panchayat samiti office is headed by block development officer who is the secretary of the Panchayat samiti and is in charge of the entire administrative staff of the block for carrying out the functions maintains liaison with the medical officer PHC and CHC and provides help when requested **(Fig. 10.11)**.

Principles of Panchayat Samiti

- Scrutiny and approval for gram panchayat budget within a prescribed limit.
- Implementation of various development works concerning more than one panchayat.
- Coordination of the plan of the gram panchayat and necessary supervision and guidance in the execution of works.
- Settlement of disputes between the two or more panchayats.
- Provision of relief in case of natural calamities.
- Promotion of small scale industries, cottage industries and education.

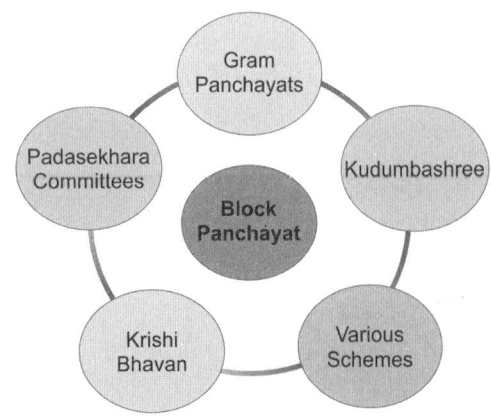

Fig. 10.11: Block panchayat.

Panchayati Raj at District Level

The Zila parishad/Zila panchayat is the agency of rural local self-governmental at the district level. The Zila parishad in general supervise and coordinate development programs being carried by the gram samitis in the block s of a district. The collector is designed as Advisor to the Zila Parishad.

Members of Zila Parishad

- District head of all departments who are ex-officials. This includes the district health officer.
- All the members of parliament in the districts.
- All chairman's of Block samitis.
- All members of state Legislature in the District
- Representatives of scheduled castes, scheduled tribes, and women.

Zila Parishad Functions

- It is the primarily a coordinating and supervisory agency.
- It plans such schemes or the district as a whole.
- Any special program may be assigned to Zila parishad by the State government from time to time.
- It scrutinizes and approves the budgets of the Block samitis.

Resources of Parishad

- Grants received from the State Government for specific development works to be carried out in the district.
- 15% of land revenue given to them by the government to meet the contingent expenditure of non-official members.

CONCLUSION

Health administration is a branch of public administration, which deals with matters relating to the promotion of health, preventive services, medical care, rehabilitation, and delivery of health services, development of health, manpower, medical education and training. Public health administration is the science and art of organizing and coordinating government agencies, whose purpose is to improve the physical, mental and social well-being of people. It aims at prevention of disease, preservation and promotion of health.

BIBLIOGRAPHY

1. Freeman & Heinrich. Community Health Nursing Practice 2nd edition; 1998.
2. Gulani KK. Community Health Nursing: Principles and Practices. 1st edition Delhi: Kumar Publishing House; 2008.
3. Judith AA, Barbara WS. Community Health Nursing: Concept and Practice 5th edition; 2001.
4. Lucita M. Public Health and Community Health Nursing in the New Millennium. 1st edition Chennai: B.I. Publications (P) Ltd; 2006.
5. Stanhope M, Lancaste J. Community Health Nursing: Promoting Health of Aggregates, Families and Individuals. 4th edition St. Louis: Mosby; 1996.

REVIEW QUESTIONS

Long Essays

1. Define health system. Explain the goals and determinants of health system.
2. Define health administration. Give an account of history of health administration in India.
3. Enumerate the organization and administration of health system in India.
4. Describe state level healthcare administration.
5. Define panchayati raj. Explain panchayati raj at village level.

Short Essays

1. Factors influence the health system.
2. Objectives of health administration.
3. Model of healthcare delivery system.
4. Central level healthcare administration.
5. Union ministry of health and family welfare.
6. Functions of department of medical and public health.
7. Directorate general of health services.
8. Central government health scheme.
9. Central council of health.
10. District level healthcare administration.
11. Community level healthcare administration.
12. Functions of subcenter.
13. Health organization at district level.
14. Health organization at block level.
15. Health organization at subcenter.
16. Health organization at urban.
17. Panchayati raj at block level.

Short Answers

1. Panchayati raj.
2. Primary health care.
3. Health administration.
4. Public health administration.
5. Primary health center.
6. Community development.
7. Comprehensive health care.
8. Basic health service.
9. Functions of Department of Family Welfare.
10. National Health Programs.
11. Central Health Education Bureau.
12. Health Secretariat.
13. State Health Directorate.
14. Functions of District Health System.
15. Functions of PHC.
16. Staffing pattern of PHC.
17. Functions of District Health Organization.
18. Staffing pattern of subcenter.
19. Services provided by subcenters.
20. Gram sabha.
21. Gram panchayat.
22. Nyaya panchyt.
23. Principles of panchayat samiti.
24. Members of zila parishad.
25. Zila parishad functions.
26. Resources of parishad.

Chapter 10: Health System in India

Multiple Choice Questions

1. What did the Central Council of Health recommend in 1966?
   a. To strengthen primary health centers and district hospitals
   b. To appoint separate assistants to undertake family planning duties
   c. To initiate the program of training community health workers
   d. To focus on integrated health services
2. What was the big milestone in the field of health?
   a. Appointment of social workers to support health social work part
   b. Rural Health Scheme
   c. Health for all by 2000 AD
   d. Appointment of Psychiatric Social Workers
3. What is the Central Council of Health?
   a. A council set up by the government to provide coordinated and concerted action between the center and the state in the implementation of all the programs and measures pertaining to the health of the nation
   b. A department of the Ministry of Health and Family Welfare created in 1964
   c. An apex body in health systems at the state level
   d. A directorate that works as the principal advisor to the Union Ministry in both medical and public health matters
4. Ministries of health were established at the center and states in the year:
   a. 1947
   b. 1948
   c. 1949
   d. 1950
5. The Indian Council of Medical Research (ICMR) was formed in the year:
   a. 1947
   b. 1948
   c. 1949
   d. 1950
6. Community health center (CHC) has been established for every _____ population and this center provides the basic specialty services in general medicine, pediatric, surgery, obstetrics and gynecology.
   a. 70,000 to 100,000 populations
   b. 80,000 to 110,000 populations
   c. 80,000 to 120,000 populations
   d. 80,000 to 130,000 populations
7. Functions of PHC includes all, *except:*
   a. Medical care
   b. MCH including family planning
   c. Referral services
   d. Rehabilitation care
8. Functions of District Health Organization is:
   a. Primary health care
   b. Secondary and referral health care.
   c. Family welfare
   d. All of the above
9. Panchayat raj system is introduced since _____ strengthen the administration at the gross root level.
   a. 1956
   b. 1957
   c. 1958
   d. 1959
10. Health administration is a branch of public administration, which deals with matters relating to:
    a. Promotion of health
    b. Preventive services
    c. Medical care and rehabilitation
    d. All of the above
11. _____ is an essential component of health care system.
    a. Referral system
    b. Graiage system
    c. Health care system
    d. None of the above
12. How much population is coming under one subcenter?
    a. 5000
    b. 10000
    c. 2000
    d. 2500

ANSWERS

| 1. a | 2. c | 3. a | 4. a | 5. c | 6. c | 7. d | 8. d | 9. b | 10. d | 11. a | 12. a |

Healthcare Delivery System

LEARNING OBJECTIVES

1. Health care concept and trends
2. Healthcare services—Public sector, Rural, Urban and Private sector
3. Public private partnership
4. Other agencies: Indigenous systems of medicine—Ayurveda, yoga, unani, siddha and homeopathy (AYUSH)
5. Voluntary health services
6. Nurse role in healthcare services

INTRODUCTION

Healthcare services in general are rendered by the government through a network of health centers from the grassroots areas to the block level in the rural areas and through hospitals, dispensaries, maternal, child health and family welfare centers in the urban areas. The hospitals in the subdivisional, Talukas level, district level, etc. provide referral services to the infrastructure in the rural area. There are also voluntary and private agencies which are functioning to deal with the health problems of people.

TYPES OF HEALTHCARE DELIVERY (FIG. 11.1)

Public or Government Sector

- Public sector is government sponsored system. It is funded by the public funds which are generated through general taxes.
- The services are rendered to the people at large in rural and urban areas by three tier system developed at the block level, district and state level.

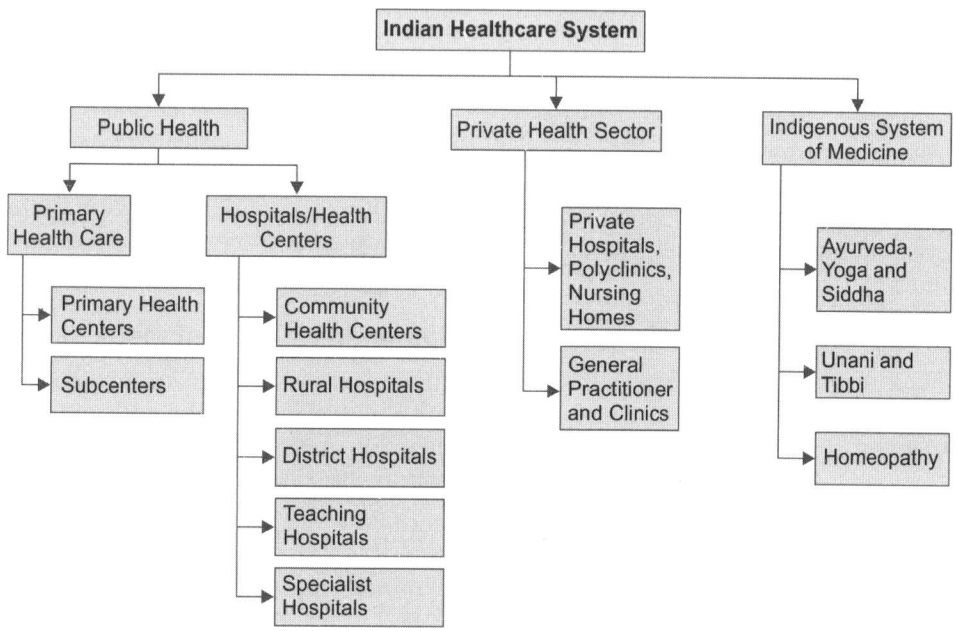

Fig. 11.1: Healthcare delivery system in India.

Rural Health Service

- The health services in the rural areas are rendered through a network of infrastructure developed from within the village and in continuum up to block level.
- The major emphasis is on promotive and preventive healthcare services and comprises primary health care.
- At the village level, elementary services are rendered by trained village health guides, birth attendants (local Dias) and anganwari workers. They belong to the village they serve and are non-governmental functionaries. They are included in the healthcare delivery system to promote and encourage community participation and to have a link between the community and the health functionaries.
- The village health guide provides simple treatment for common minor ailments, first aid during accidents and emergency, care to mother and children including family planning, health education, etc.
- The trained birth attendants work under the supervision and guidance of female health worker and provide personal and skillful care during prenatal period, give health education on child care, immunization, nutrition, and family planning.
- Anganwari workers work in Anganwaries and carry on the responsibility of health check-ups, supplementary nutrition, immunization, nonformal education of children enrolled in Anganwardi. They coordinate with the ANMs in their areas for some of the functions, e.g., immunization and health check-up of children. Each one serves a population of 1,000 in the village.
- The continuum of health centers which provide primary healthcare services include subcenters, primary health centers and community health centers. The subcenter serves a population of 5,000 in plain area and 3,000 in hilly, tribal and backward areas.
- The limited primary healthcare services which are provided from subcenters include maternal and child health, family planning, prevention and control of communicable diseases, treatment of minor ailments, record of vital events, emergency care, maintenance of record and reports, supervision and training of dais and village health guides.
- The services are rendered by, ANMs, i.e., health workers (F) and health worker (M) under the supervision and guidance of health supervisor (F and M) respectively.

Urban Health Services

- The services in the urban areas are rendered through district hospitals and medical college hospitals.
- There are also hospitals and institutes of higher education and research which are under Central Government and provide general as well as referral services.
- In addition to these hospital services, there are maternal and child health, family welfare centers, family planning clinics, dispensaries, maternity homes, community hospitals run by local Government to provide specific primary level services to defined population.

Health Insurance System

In India, health insurance system is restricted to factory/industrial workers and their families and central government employees and their families. They are covered by two different very well-organized health insurance schemes. These are:

1. **Employees state insurance:** The ESI scheme was started under the parliament Act in 1948 to provide medical benefits in kind and cash during sickness, employment injury, maternity, etc. the scheme is based on the contributions from the employer, employees and the government.
2. **Central Government Health scheme:**
   - This scheme is for the Central Government Employers. To start with it was introduced in Delhi in 1954 to provide comprehensive healthcare to central government employees.
   - Gradually, it was extended to other cities not only to central government employees and their family members but also other autonomous organizations employees, members of parliament, retired central government servants and widow receiving family pensions, Governors and retired judges.
   - The scheme is on the cooperative efforts and contribution basis from the employees and employer for their mutual benefits.
   - The services are given through a network of dispensaries, governmental hospitals, and identified private specialized hospitals in various systems of medicine.
   - The CGHS provides outdoor, domiciliary, indoor, specialists consultations, emergency, maternal and child welfare and family welfare services. It also supplies optical and dental aids at reasonable rates.

Other Agencies—Railway Hospitals and Military Hospitals

The services to these people and their families are rendered by specially organized armed forces medical services and railways health services respectively. Comprehensive preventive, promotive, curative and rehabilitative services are rendered through specially organized health units, clinics, hospitals, etc.

Indigenous System of Medicine

The indigenous systems of medicine form an important part of public system of healthcare delivery in both rural and urban areas. Services are rendered through out-patient departments, dispensaries and hospitals.

National Health Programe

- In addition to various levels are depicted in **Figure 11.2** of healthcare services through public system, the government of India has put in lot of efforts to deal with various health problems at the national level.
- These problems are related to communicable and non-communicable diseases, environmental sanitation problem, nutritional problems, population problems, etc.

Chapter 11: Healthcare Delivery System

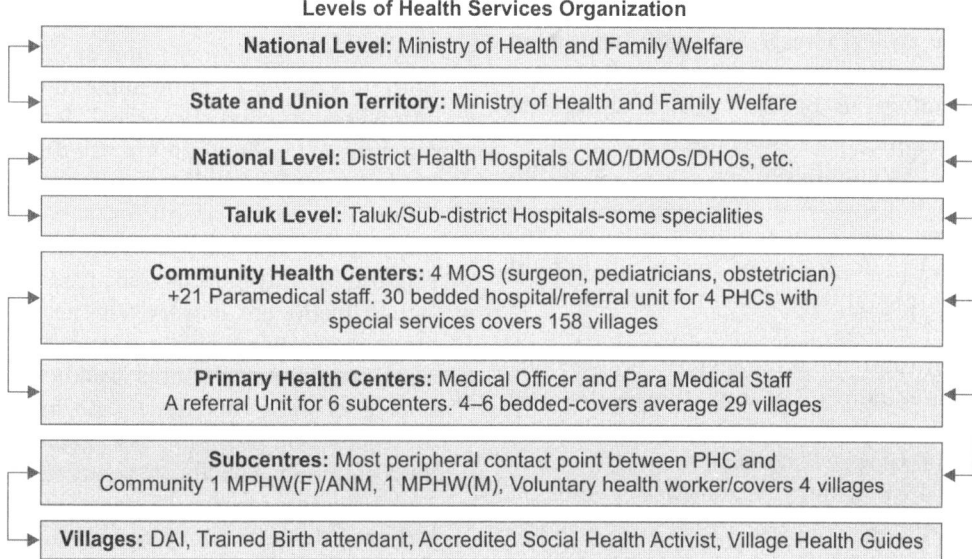

Fig. 11.2: Levels of healthcare organization in India.

- The government of India through its ministry of health and family welfare have launched ongoing various national health programs in successive five year plans since independence.
- The technical and material assistance have also been obtained by various international and bilateral agencies in planning and implementation of these programs. These organizations include WHO, UNICEF, Word Bank, UNFPA, DANIDA, etc.

Voluntary Health Agencies

- There are varieties of non-governmental organizations which are voluntary in nature and contribute tremendously in furthering the public health by providing health services, or health education, by advancing research, etc.
- The NGOs complement and supplement role of government agencies. There are also "not for profit" voluntary hospitals which generate funds to sustain and provide charitable services, e.g., Holy Family Hospital.

Private Sector

- Like voluntary health sector, the private health sector also occupies an important place in healthcare delivery system in the country. There has been extensive growth in the private owned facilities since independence but more so during the last decade, there has been significant increase in the number of medical practitioners.
- They range from herbal and witch doctors to modern unqualified or quasiqualified "quacks" to qualified practitioners of different system of medicine, many of whom also indulge in quackery.
- The different system of medicine includes Allopathy or Modern Medicine, Homeopathy, Ayurveda, Unani and Siddha. Apart from these, there are other like Yoga, Naturopathy and Chiropractic.
- There are large numbers of practitioners who have not qualified in any of the recognized systems. It is this diversity and complexity which is in part responsible for lack of regulation and quality control in private practice.
- Further, those who are qualified in modern medicine tend to locate themselves in urban areas and all others are equally locate themselves in urban areas and all others are equally located in urban and rural areas. There are three times more allopathic in urban than in rural areas.
- There has been increase in the number of private hospitals including those owed by the voluntary agencies.
- The private consultants are attached to these hospitals. They participate in the services organized by the hospital as well as they have their own private OPD/clinics and cases in hospital.
- The system is beyond the reach of even an average middle class family. It is not an organized system of providing healthcare services. Efforts are being put in to maintain the standards through legislation related to nursing homes and hospitals and consumer protection Act.
- The various diagnostic facilities are on the increase to assist in making diagnosis but these are very expensive and often exploited liberally. The government is putting in efforts to involve Medical Council of India and Indian Medical Association to regulate the system, etc.

Medical Tourism and Telemedicine

- Medical tourism is one of the major external drivers of growth of the Indian healthcare sector. This is a developing concept whereby people from world over visit India for their medical and relaxation needs.
- Most common treatments are heart surgery, joint replacement, orthopedic surgery, gastroenterology, ophthalmology, transplants, urology, cosmetic surgery and dental care. Hospital groups like The Global Hospitals Group, MIOT Hospitals, Fortis Healthcare, Apollo hospitals, Max Hospitals, Dharamshila Cancer Hospital and Research Centre have increased their presence in international market for medical tourism.

- In the current rapidly changing healthcare scenario the magnitude of the problem associated with healthcare delivery is enormous and extremely dynamic. However, present day technology has the solution for this problem. User-friendly equipment with compatibility to integrate technologies like telemedicine makes the solution simpler.
- Telemedicine system is growing rapidly in India, nearing 700 million rural populations of India will benefit enormously from digital data transmission related to healthcare.
- Both public and private entities are aggressively pursuing the use of telemedicine to hasten diagnostics and treatment of a variety of diseases. Private hospitals such as Apollo Hospital Group, Escorts Heart Institute and Fortis Healthcare are providing these services in India.

Challenges in Health System

- Manpower—number and norms
- Rural/Urban differential
- Geographical divide across States
- S-E groups—accessibility/reach
- Gaps between policy and action
- Health sector expenditure
- Newer infections

Role of Nurse in Healthcare Delivery System

- Care-provide
- Planner
- Sensitive observer
- Educator manager
- Organizer
- Evaluator
- Controller
- Administrator

INFRASTRUCTURE AND HEALTH SECTORS

Health infrastructure is an important indicator for understanding the healthcare policy and welfare mechanism in a country. It signifies the investment priority with regard to the creation of healthcare facilities. Infrastructure has been described as the basic support for the delivery of public health activities.

- India has systematically improved health conditions. Life expectancy has doubled from 32 years in 1947 to 66.8 years at present; infant mortality rate (IMR) has fallen to 50 per thousand live births. Further, it is estimated that public funding accounts for only 22% of the expenses on healthcare in India.
- Most of the remaining 78% of private expenditure is out-of-pocket expense. The share of the richest 20% of the population in total public sector subsidies is nearly 31%, almost three times the share of the poorest 20% of the population.

Healthcare System and Structure

- Healthcare has become one of India's largest sectors both in terms of revenue and employment. Healthcare comprises hospitals, medical devices, clinical trials, outsourcing, telemedicine, medical tourism, health insurance and medical equipment.
- The Indian healthcare sector is growing at a brisk pace due to its strengthening coverage, services and increasing expenditure by public as well private players.
- Indian healthcare delivery system is categorized into two major components public and private.
- The Government, i.e., public healthcare system comprises limited secondary and tertiary care institutions in key cities and focuses on providing basic healthcare facilities in the form of Primary Healthcare centers (PHCs) in rural areas.
- The private sector provides majority of secondary, tertiary and quaternary care institutions with a major concentration in metros, tier I and tier II cities.
- India's competitive advantage lies in its large pool of well trained medical professionals. India is also cost competitive compared to its peers in Asia and Western countries. The cost of surgery in India is about one-tenth of that in the US or Western Europe.
- Medical education infrastructure in India has shown rapid growth during the last 20 years. The country has 476 medical colleges, 313 colleges for BDS courses and 249 colleges which conduct MDS courses. There has been a total admission of 52,646 Medical Colleges and 27060 in BDS and 6233 in MDS during 2017–18.
- There are 3215 Institutions for General Nurse Midwives with admission capacity of 129,926 and 777 colleges for Pharmacy (Diploma) with an intake capacity of 46,795 as on 31st October, 2017.
- There are 23,582 government hospitals having 710,761 beds in the country. 19,810 hospitals are in rural area with 279,588 beds and 3,772 hospitals are in urban area with 431,173 beds. Seventy percent of population of India lives in rural areas and to cater to their need there are 156,231 Subcenters (SCs), 25,650 Primary Health Centers (PHC) and 5,624 Community Health Centers (CHC) in India as on 31st March 2017.

Towards Universal Access to Health Care

- Universal access to health care is a well-articulated goal for both global institutions and national government.
- India's national Health Policy, 2017 envisions the goal of attaining highest possible level of health and well-being for all at all ages through a preventive and promotive healthcare orientation in all developmental policies, and universal access to good quality healthcare services without financial hardship to the citizens.
- Under health related Sustainable Development Goal (SDG) no. 3 (Good Health and Well-Being), a commitment towards global effort to eradicate disease, strengthen treatment and healthcare, and address new and emerging health issues has been pronounced.

Chapter 11: Healthcare Delivery System

- The gains of India in many health related indicators helped the country to make progress in achieving MDGs.
- Ayushman Bharat Mission, world's largest health scheme announced in the Union Budget 2018–19, is the latest initiative for expanding the health insurance net and targets 10 crore poor and deprived rural families.
- There has been a concerted effort to improve the healthcare infrastructure as well as delivery mechanism in the last couple of years.
- Several schemes, programs and initiatives have been undertaken to bridge the gap to make the quantity as well as quality of the health services available to the last mile.

Major Government Initiatives

- Government of India has taken some major initiatives to promote Indian healthcare industry. On September 23, 2018, Government of India launched Pradhan Mantri Jan Arogya Yojana (PMJAY), to provide health insurance worth ₹500,000 (US$ 7,124.54) to over 100 million families every year.
- In August 2018, the Government of India has approved Ayushman Bharat National Health Protection Mission as a centrally Sponsored Scheme contributed by both Center and State governments at a ratio of 60:40 for all States and 90:10 for hilly North Eastern States and 60:40 for Union Territories with legislature. The Center will contribute 100% for Union Territories without legislature.

Pradhan Mantri Swasthya Suraksha Yojana (PMSSY): The Pradhan Mantri Swasthya Suraksha Yojana (PMSSY) has the objectives of correcting regional imbalances in the availability of affordable/ reliable tertiary healthcare services and also to augment facilities for quality medical education in the country.

PMSSY has two components:
1. Setting up of AIIMS like institutions
2. Upgradation of Government Medical College Institutions.

Six AIIMS-like institutions, one each in the States of Bihar (Patna), Chhattisgarh (Raipur), Madhya Pradesh (Bhopal), Orissa (Bhubaneswar), Rajasthan (Jodhpur) and Uttaranchal (Rishikesh) has been set-up under the PMSSY scheme. Approved cost of each new AIIMS in first phase was ₹820 crores, ₹620 crores towards cost of construction and ₹200 crores for procurement of Medical Equipment and modular operation theaters.

PMSSY also envisaged upgradation of several existing medical institutions in different states in the country. Initially the estimated outlay for upgradation was revised to ₹150 crores per institution (From initial estimate of ₹120 crore), with ₹125 crore as the share of Central Government.

Ayushman Bharat, Pradhan Mantri Jan Arogya Yojana (PMJAY)

- One of the most ambitious health insurance programs in the world today, the Pradhan Mantri Jan Arogya Yojana (PMJAY). Ayushman Bharat, gives India the chance to transform its healthcare infrastructure.
- Launched in September 2018, PMJAY aims to address the healthcare needs of India's poorest 100 million households. The path to success, however, is strewn with several challenges. If these hurdles are overcome and if PMJAY succeeds. India's largest health insurance scheme would also become its most effective healthcare initiative.
- PMJAY has the potential to institute reforms to the country's health care and health insurance systems at a lower cost to the exchequer. If streamlined, health information and monitoring systems can arrest the possibility of over-provisioning and cost-inflation.
- The idea to shift away from a decaying system of government-funded hospitals and people, towards a mix of private and government healthcare, governed by common principles and financed by low-cost health insurance–is a step in the right direction.

Kayakalp

- The Swachh Bharat Abhiyan launched by the Prime Minister on 2nd October 2014 focuses on promoting cleanliness in public spaces.
- Public healthcare facilities are a major mechanism of social protection to meet the healthcare needs of large segments of the population.
- Cleanliness and hygiene in hospitals are critical to preventing infections and also provide patients and visitors with a positive experience and encourages molding behavior related to clean environment.
- As the first principle of healthcare is "to do no harm" it is essential to have our healthcare facilities clean and to ensure adherence to infection control practices.
- Swachhta Guidelines for Public Health Facilities have been issued separately. To complement this effort, the Ministry of Health and Family Welfare, Government of India has launched a National Initiative to give Awards to those public health facilities that demonstrate high level of cleanliness, hygiene and infection control.
- "Kayakalp" is an initiative to promote sanitation and hygiene in public healthcare institutions. Facilities which outshine and exceed the set measures are awarded and incentivized under Kayakalp.
- Till date, "Kayakalp' initiative has been able to encourage public health facilities in the country to work towards attainment of excellence in cleanliness and hygiene.
- "Kayakalp" is becoming instrumental in building confidence of the users in public health facilities.

Mission Indradhanush: The Government of India has launched Mission Indradhanush with the aim of improving coverage of immunization in the country. It aims to achieve at least 90% immunization coverage by December 2018 which will cover unvaccinated and partially vaccinated children in rural and urban areas of India.

Private Sector in Health Care

- The Supreme Court in a recent judgment directed government hospitals in Delhi to refer poor patients to private hospitals. This decision has been described as a

pro-poor decision which aims at bringing the poor rural patients at par with the urban rich patients who till now had been the sole beneficiaries of such private institutions.
- The court directed that the private institutions would provide medical care free of cost the poor, pending preparation of a scheme which would involve private players in treating the poor.
- The appeal was filed against an earlier decision of the Delhi High Court whereby, the High court had directed certain private hospitals to ensure free treatment to 10% in-patients and 25% outpatients, this mandatory ruling was given on the ground that the land' for construction was given on an undertaking which bound the private players to provide free healthcare to people who belong to economically weaker sections of the society.
- The apex court directed that the Delhi Government and Private Health institutions should come together and draw up a plan for serving the poor. This decision would go a long way in strengthening the public health system.
- The issues of access to quality healthcare may be addressed by collaboration between State Governments and private players.

Market Size

- The healthcare market can increase three fold to ₹ 8.6 trillion (US$ 133.44 billion) by 2022.
- India is experiencing 22–25% growth in medical tourism and the industry is expected to double its size for present (April 2017) US$ 3 million to US$ 6 billion by 2018.
- There is a significant scope for enhancing healthcare services considering that healthcare spending as a percentage of Gross Domestic Product (GDP) is rising.
- The government's expenditure on the health sector has grown to 1.4% in FY18E from 1.2% in FY14. The Government of Indian is planning to increase public health spending to 2.5% of the country's GDP by 2025.

Investment: The hospital and diagnostic centers attracted Foreign Direct Investment (FDI) worth US$ 5.25 billion between April 2000 and June 2018, according to data released by the Department of Industrial Policy and Promotion (DIPP).

Achievements

- In 2017, the Government of India approved National Nutrition Mission (NNM), a joint effort of Ministry of Health and Family Welfare (MoHFW) and the Ministry of Women and Child Development (WCD) towards a lifecycle approach for interrupting the intergenerational cycle of under nutrition.
- As of September 23, 2018, the world's largest government funded healthcare scheme, Ayushman Bharat was launched.
- As of November 15, 2017, 4.45 million patients were benefitted from Affordable Medicines and Reasonable Implants for Treatment (AMRIT) Pharmacies.
- As of December 15, 2017, the Government of India approved the National Medical Commission Bill 2017. It aims to promote medical education reform.

Road Ahead: Healthcare Infrastructure and Services

- India's healthcare industry is one of the fastest growing sectors and it is expected to reach $280 billion by 2020.
- The country has also become one of the leading destinations for high-end diagnostic services with tremendous capital investment for advanced diagnostic facilities, thus catering to a greater proportion of population. Besides, Indian medical service consumers have become more conscious towards their healthcare upkeep.
- Indian healthcare sector is much diversified and is full of opportunities in every segment which includes providers, payers and medical technology.
- With the increase in the competition, businesses are looking to explore for the latest dynamics and trends which will have positive impact on their business.
- The hospital industry in India is forecasted to increase to ₹8.6 trillion (US$ 132.84 billion) by FY22 from ₹4 trillion (US$13 61.79 billion) in FY17 at a CAGR of 16–17%.
- India's competitive advantage also lies in the increased success rate of Indian companies in getting Abbreviated New Drug Application (ANDA) approvals.
- India also offers vast opportunities in R and D as well as medical tourism. To sum up, there are vast opportunities for investment in healthcare infrastructure in both urban and rural India.
- Garg (2018) suggests that public healthcare service should ensure three "Es-Expand-Equity-Excellence". Access to adequate healthcare would need expansion of tertiary care facilities.
- Tertiary care should be equitably distributed to different segments of population.
- The setting tip of new facilities will have to address imbalances at three levels—regional, specialties, and ratio of medical doctors to nurses and other healthcare professionals.
- India is well poised to a better public healthcare infrastructure, facilities and services and hopefully with all the well intentioned initiatives we shall see health taking a top priority agenda in the coming years and delivering on the promises that the new and bold initiatives in the health sector.

DELIVERY OF HEALTH SERVICES AT SUBCENTER (SC)

- The subcentre is the most peripheral and first contact point between the primary healthcare system and the community.
- Subcenters are assigned tasks relating to interpersonal communication in order to bring about behavioral change and provide services in relation to maternal and child health, family welfare, nutrition, immunization, diarrhea control and control of communicable diseases programs.
- Each subcenter is required to be manned by at least one auxiliary nurse midwife (ANM)/female health worker and one male health worker.

- Under National Rural Health Mission (NRHM), there is a provision for one additional second ANM on contract basis.
- One lady health visitor (LHV) is entrusted with the task of supervision of six subcenters.
- Government of India bears the salary of ANM and LHV while the salary of the Male Health Worker is borne by the State governments.

Subcenter

The peripheral outpost of the health delivery system in
- Rural areas
- One s/c for 5,000 populations
- One for every 3,000 population in hilly, tribal and backward areas.

Services: All Primary Healthcare Services

- Immunization
- Antenatal, natal and postnatal care
- Prevention of malnutrition
- Family planning and counseling
- Medicines for minor ailments
  - ARI
  - Diarrhea
  - Fever
  - Worm infestation, etc.
  - Implementation of several national health and FW programs.

Staff at a Subcenter

- One ANM (Auxiliary Nurse Midwife) who is the Female Health Worker
- One Multipurpose Worker (Male) who is the Male Health Worker
- One voluntary health worker as a helper to ANM
  - Employed as and when needed
  - Two Health Assistants located at the PHC supervise six subcenters under the PHC.

They are supervised by:
- One Lady Health Visitor (LHV) who is the Health Assistant (female)
- One Health Assistant (male)

GOI provides the funds for:
- Salary of ANM
- Salary of LHV
- Rent of subcenter (if located in a rented building)
- Drugs, equipment and kits
- Contingency money for ANM which includes the stipend for the helper if employed
- State government pays for the: salary of the Male Health Worker.

DELIVERY OF HEALTH SERVICES AT PHC

- PHC is the first contact point between village community and the medical officer.
- The PHCs were envisaged to provide an integrated curative and preventive health care to the rural population with emphasis on preventive and promotive aspects of health care.
- The PHCs are established and maintained by the State governments under the Minimum Needs Program (MNP)/Basic Minimum Services (BMS) Program.
- As per minimum requirement, a PHC is to be manned by a medical officer supported by 14 paramedical and other staff.
- Under NRHM, there is a provision for two additional staff nurses at PHCs on contract basis. It acts as a referral unit for 6 subcenters and has 4-6 beds for patients.
- The activities of PHC involve curative, preventive, promotive and family welfare services.

Primary Health Center (PHC)

- One for every 30,000 population
- One for every 20,000 population in hilly, tribal and backward areas—25,020 PHC's established (as in March, 2014).

Functions of PHC

1. Medical care
2. MCH including FP
3. Safe water supply and basic sanitation
4. Prevention and control of locally endemic diseases
5. Collection and reporting of vital statistics
6. Health education
7. National Health Programs as relevant Referral services
8. Training of health guides, health workers, local dais and HAs
9. Basic laboratory services

Selected Surgical Procedures Facilities at PHC

- Vasectomy
- Tubectomy
- MTP
- Minor surgical procedures

ROME Program: (Reorientation of Medical Education)

- Three primary health centers have been attached to each medical colleges
- Purpose is to reorient the ME towards the needs of the country and community care

Staff at PHC

- Total 15
  - One medical officer
  - One pharmacist
  - One staff Nurse k/a Nurse—Midwife
  - One Health worker (F)
  - One Health Educator
  - Two Health Assistants—one male and one female
  - Two clerks
  - One laboratory technician

- One driver
- Four class-IV workers
- Recommended to increase under IPHS

Six beds per PHC are recommended: Secondary and Tertiary Healthcare in Public Health Sector.

DELIVERY OF HEALTH SERVICES AT CHC

- CHCs are being established and maintained by the State government under MNP/BMS program.
- As per minimum norms, a CHC is required to be manned by four medical specialists, i.e., surgeon, physician, gynecologist and pediatrician supported by 21 paramedical and other staff. It has 30 in-door beds with one OT, X-ray, labor room and laboratory facilities.
- It serves as a referral center for 4 PHCs and also provides facilities for obstetric care and specialist consultations.

Community Health Center (CHC)

- Established by upgrading PHCs
- One CHC covers a population of 80,000 to 1.20 lakhs
  - 30 beds
  - X-ray facility
  - Laboratory facilities

Medical Services at CHC

1. Surgery
2. Medicine
3. Obstetrics and gynecology
4. Pediatrics
    - One Community Health Officer
    - Selected from supervisory category of staff at PHC and district level
    - Should have minimum of 7 years of experience in rural health programs
    - Some states have not accepted CHO – and opted for a second medical officer instead

The specialists at CHC can refer patient to:
- Sub-divisional hospital
- District hospital
- OR if necessary, then directly to
- State level hospital
- Nearest Medical College Hospital

Staff at CHC

- Clinical manpower
- General Surgeon 1
- Physician 1
- Obstetrician/Gynecologist 1
- Pediatrician 1
- Support manpower
- Nurse—Midwife 7 + 2 (one ANM and one PHN under NRHM)
- Dresser (certified by Red Cross/St. Johns ambulance) 1
- Pharmacist 1
- Lab technician 1
- Radiographer 1
- Ophthalmic assistant 0–1 (can be employed on contractual basis)
- Ward boy/Nursing orderly 2
- Sweepers 3
- Chowkidar
- OPD attendant
- Statistical assistant/Data entry operator 5
- OT attendant
- Registration clerk
- Total essential 21 – 22 + 2

First referral units (FRUs): An existing facility (District Hospital, Subdivisional Hospital, Community Health Center, etc.) can be declared a fully operational First Referral Unit (FRU) only if it is equipped to provide round-the-clock services for emergency obstetric and New Born Care, in addition to all emergencies that any hospital is required to provide. It should be noted that there are three critical determinants of a facility being declared as a FRU:

- Emergency Obstetric Care including surgical interventions like cesarean sections;
- Newborn care; and
- Blood storage facility on a 24-hour basis.

Health and wellness centers: The National Health Policy, 2017 recommended strengthening the delivery system of Primary Healthcare, through establishment of "Health and Wellness Centers (HWCs)" as the platform to deliver Comprehensive Primary Healthcare.

- Government of India is committed towards creation of 150,000 Health and Wellness Centers (HWCs) by transforming existing subcenters (SCs) and Primary Health Centers (PHCs) as basic pillar of Ayushman Bharat to deliver Comprehensive Primary Health Care (CPHC).
- These centers delivers CPHC bringing health care closer to the homes of people covering both maternal and child health services and noncommunicable diseases, including free essential drugs and diagnostic services.
- Health and wellness centers are envisaged to deliver and expanded range of services to address the primary healthcare needs of the entire population in their area, expanding access, universality and equity close to the community.
- The emphasis of health promotion and prevention is designed to bring focus on keeping people healthy by engaging and empowering individuals and communities to choose healthy behaviors and make changes that reduce the risk of developing chronic diseases and morbidities.

ADMINISTRATION OF NURSING PERSONNEL

Nursing Administration at Center (Fig. 11.3)

- The nursing advisor is directly responsible to the deputy director general (medical). The nursing advisor is assisted by nursing officer and support staff for all her/his work.

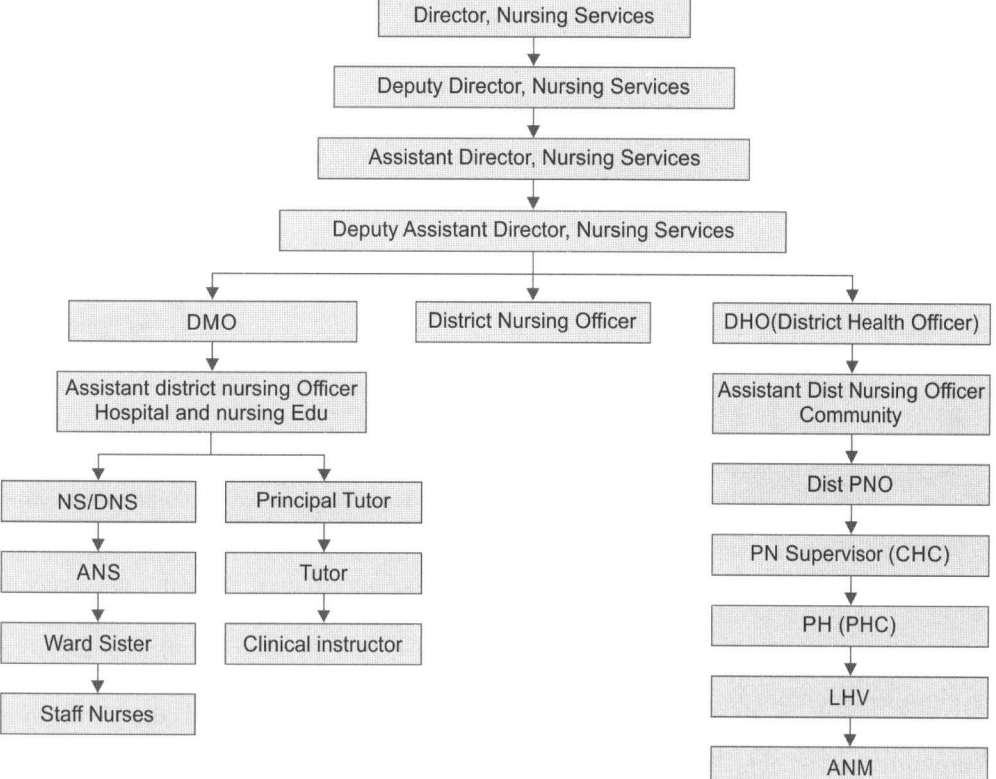

Fig. 11.3: Nursing administration at center level.

- Nursing advisor is the chief to coordinate all nursing programs in the country. There is an Indian Nursing council to assist and advice on matters of nursing education and service where in community health nursing is an integral part of the overall program.
- Deputy nursing advisor is working in rural health division to coordinate the activities of public health program.
- The recommended organization setup will need full administrative and financial support of the government.
- It will take after the overall nursing components, development of nursing standards, norms, policies, ethics, recruitments selection and placement rules for both hospital and community health nursing etc, developments in specialty nursing, higher education and research in nursing will promote professional standards, autonomy and accountability.

Nursing Administration at State Level

- State nursing is directed by a nurse designate as additional director of health services (nursing). In west Bengal, there are two nursing personnel of such position, one for education and another for general nursing administration.
- The nursing division is responsible for hospital as well as community nursing services, nursing manpower planning, in service and continuing education and all administrative work related for the nursing profession.
- The nursing person in charge at the State level is responsible for administration, planning, recruiting of staff both for hospitals and public health work and for planning and recruiting of students for nursing and auxiliary nursing courses.
- In Karnataka, there are three assistant directors of nursing Services, one for public health, one for Education training and one for nursing services.

Nursing Administration at District Level

- Bhore committee recommended posting on PHNs at the primary health centers, but unfortunately public health nurses are generally not placed in community centers and primary health centers.
- West Bengal as health being the state subject. The only position of professional public health nurse is at the district level in the district family welfare bureau, which is being created under the multipurpose health worker scheme, and funded through the family welfare budget.
- The major areas of responsibility are administration and management of nursing and midwifery services in district, supervision and guidance of health supervisor, In-service training program for nurse, participation in teaching programs of the school of nursing, helping organizing community health nursing field experience for nursing students and helping in collection and compiling reports form CHC/PHC in the district.

Nursing Administration at Community Development

- At district level, the public health nurse will keep herself informed of all the key persons involved in community

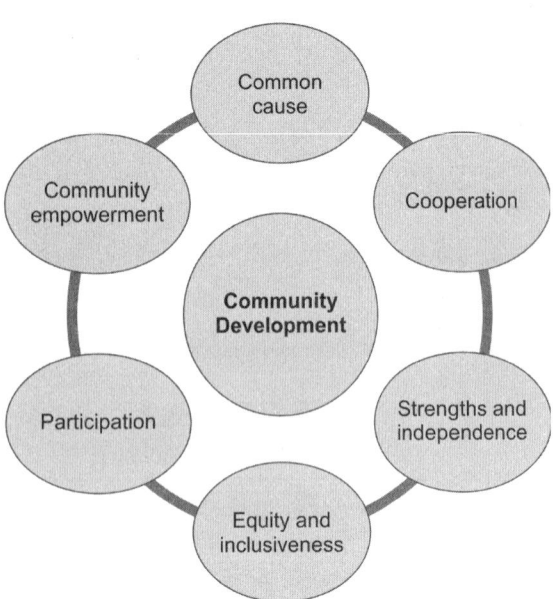

Fig. 11.4: Principles of community development.

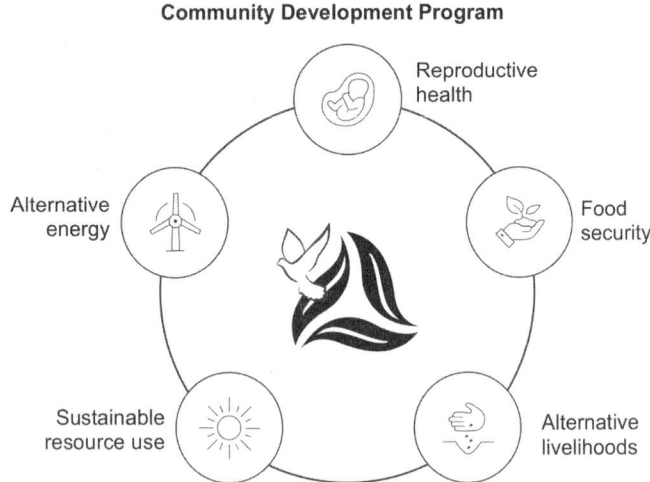

Fig. 11.5: Types of community development program.

development program, such as the President involved in community development members.
- She will take part in all relevant discussions of district coordination committee concerning the nursing services of the district through the district health officer who is the member of the committee.
- At the Block headquarters, the nurse and the female health worker (ANM) will keep in touch with the block development worker and with the village leaders for the villages which fall within the area of her work.
- At the subcenter, every female health worker must be acquainted wit the village officer and the sarpanch of the villages which fall within the area as the gram sevak, gram sevika, the president of mahila mandal, the yuvak mandal and the social education officer.
- The nurse must also get to know the important members of the village cooperatives, since they usually take care of village's financial matters. The nurse also assists in community development program and can completely change the look of the village, by building a healthy village community. Principles of community development are explained in **Figure 11.4**.

COMMUNITY DEVELOPMENT PROGRAM

- The community development program was launched 2nd October 1952 for the all round development of the rural areas. Provision of medical relief and preventive health services were part of the program. The program was hailed as program "of the people, for the people, by the people" to exterminate the three ill of poverty, disease and illiteracy depicted in **Figure 11.5**.
- The community development program was to involve the rural population in the process of planning their own welfare measures, under this program the rural areas of community have been organized into the community development blocks, each block comprising of approximately 100 villages and population of one lakh.
- Community development was defined as "a process designed to create conditions of economic and social progress for the whole community with its active participation and the fullest possible reliance up on the community's initiative.
- United Nations defined community development as "the process by which the efforts of the people themselves are united with those of governmental authorities to improve the economic, social and cultural conditions of communities to integrate those communities with the life of the nation and to enable them to contribute fully to national progress.

Organization Set Up

The community development program was envisaged as a multipurpose program. The rural areas of the country have been organized into a community blocks—each block comprising approximately 100 villages and a population of one lakh. There are about 6,000 community development block in the country. Each block is headed by a block developmental officer.

Functions of Community Development Blocks

The community development block activities are improvement of agriculture, improvement of communications, education health and sanitation, improvement of housing through self-help, social welfare and training in rural arts crafts and industries to local people.

Community Development Block Operation

- Each block passed through two stages of development stage 1 of year's intensive development by stage II of another 5 years. The Central government supported the program substantially by providing funds to the tune of ₹12 lakhs during first stage and ₹5 lakhs during second stage of development.
- At the end of 10 years, the blocks entered past stage II phase and their financial arrangements become the responsibility of the State Governments. The block

continues to be the permanent infrastructure for rural planning and development.

INTEGRATED RURAL DEVELOPMENT

- Integrated rural development program launched in April 1978 to eliminate rural poverty and improve the quality of life of the rural poor. The familiar targets of the program are agricultural laborers, small cultivators, village artisans and craftsman **(Fig. 11.6)**.
- They are provided with resources and skills, bank loans and subsidies by the government. The IRDP is being implemented through District Rural Development Agency. IRDP and initially taken up 100 development blocks and was expended to all 5,011 blocks on October 2, 1980.

IRDP Implementation

During ninth five year plan, it was implemented through an integrated approach under which the existing schemes.
- TRYSEM—(training of rural youth for self-employment and management)—this program aims at providing technical and management skills to rural youth in the age group of 18-35 from families living below the poverty line, helping them to take gainful self-employment.
- SITRA—Supply of improvement toolkits to rural artisans.
- DWCRA—Development of women and children in rural areas.
- GKY—Ganga Kalyan Yojana.

SUSTAINABLE DEVELOPMENT GOALS (SDGs)

In September 2015, the global community agreed the Sustainable Development Goals, setting out new development priorities for all countries, post-2015. The 17 new goals have been designed to integrate global ambitions on tackling poverty, reducing inequality, combating climate change, and protecting ecosystems including oceans, forests and biodiversity. It is an ambitious and universal agenda.

End Poverty in all its Forms Everywhere

Targets

- By 2030, eradicate extreme poverty for all people everywhere, currently measured as people living on less than $1.25 a day.
- By 2030, reduce at least by half the proportion of men, women and children of all ages living in poverty in all its dimensions according to national definitions.
- Implement nationally appropriate social protection systems and measures for all, including floors, and by 2030 achieve substantial coverage of the poor and the vulnerable.
- By 2030, ensure that all men and women, in particular the poor and the vulnerable, have equal rights to economic resources, as well as access to basic services, ownership and control over land and other forms of property, inheritance, natural resources, appropriate new technology and financial services, including microfinance.
- By 2030, build the resilience of the poor and those in vulnerable situations and reduce their exposure and vulnerability to climate-related extreme events and other economic, social and environmental shocks and disasters
  - Ensure significant mobilization of resources from a variety of sources, including through enhanced development cooperation, in order to provide adequate and predictable means for developing

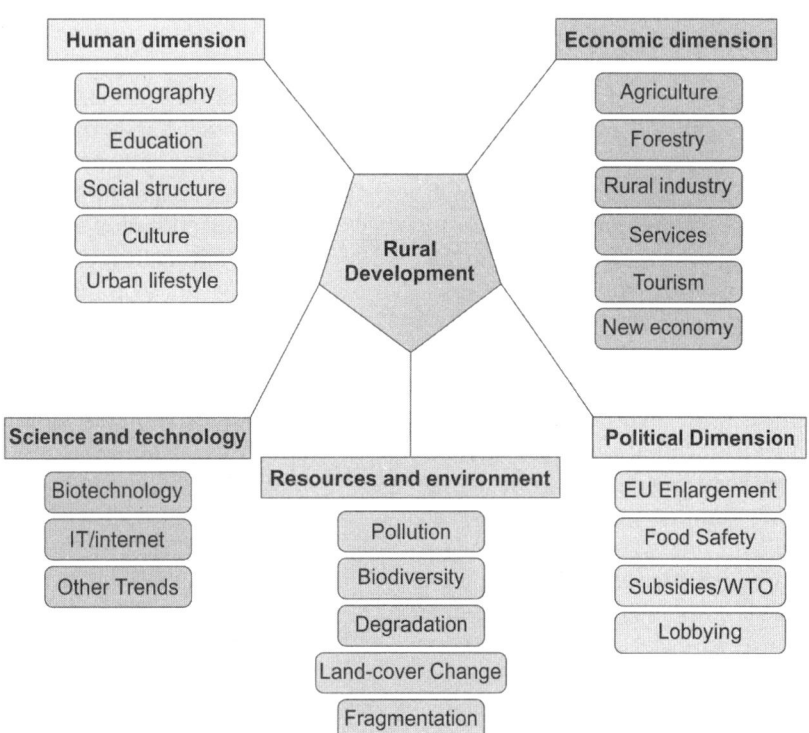

Fig. 11.6: Rural development programs.

countries, in particular least developed countries, to implement programs and policies to end poverty in all its dimensions.
- Create sound policy frameworks at the national, regional and international levels, based on pro-poor and gender-sensitive development strategies, to support accelerated investment in poverty eradication actions.

End Hunger, Achieve Food Security and Improve Nutrition and Promote Sustainable Agriculture

Targets

- By 2030, end hunger and ensure access by all people, in particular the poor and people in vulnerable situations, including infants, to safe, nutritious and sufficient food all year round.
- By 2030, end all forms of malnutrition, including achieving, by 2025, the internationally agreed targets on stunting and wasting in children under 5 years of age, and address the nutritional needs of adolescent girls, pregnant and lactating women and older persons.
- By 2030, double the agricultural productivity and incomes of small-scale food producers, in particular women, indigenous peoples, family farmers, pastoralists and fishers, including through secure and equal access to land, other productive resources and inputs, knowledge, financial services, markets and opportunities for value addition and non-farm employment.
- By 2030, ensure sustainable food production systems and implement resilient agricultural practices that increase productivity and production, that help maintain ecosystems, that strengthen capacity for adaptation to climate change, extreme weather, drought, flooding and other disasters and that progressively improve land and soil quality.
- By 2020, maintain the genetic diversity of seeds, cultivated plants and farmed and domesticated animals and their related wild species, including through soundly managed and diversified seed and plant banks at the national, regional and international levels, and promote access to and fair and equitable sharing of benefits arising from the utilization of genetic resources and associated traditional knowledge, as internationally agreed.
  - Increase investment, including through enhanced international cooperation, in rural infrastructure, agricultural research and extension services, technology development and plant and livestock gene banks in order to enhance agricultural productive capacity in developing countries, in particular least developed countries.
  - Correct and prevent trade restrictions and distortions in world agricultural markets, including through the parallel elimination of all forms of agricultural export subsidies and all export measures with equivalent effect, in accordance with the mandate of the Doha Development Round.
  - Adopt measures to ensure the proper functioning of food commodity markets and their derivatives and facilitate timely access to market information, including on food reserves, in order to help limit extreme food price volatility.

Ensure Healthy Lives and Promote Well-being for All at All Ages

Targets

- By 2030, reduce the global maternal mortality ratio to less than 70 per 100,000 live births.
- By 2030, end preventable deaths of newborns and children under 5 years of age, with all countries aiming to reduce neonatal mortality to at least as low as 12 per 1,000 live births and under-5 mortality to at least as low as 25 per 1,000 live births.
- By 2030, end the epidemics of AIDS, tuberculosis, malaria and neglected tropical diseases and combat hepatitis, water-borne diseases and other communicable diseases.
- By 2030, reduce by one third premature mortality from noncommunicable diseases through prevention and treatment and promote mental health and well-being.
- Strengthen the prevention and treatment of substance abuse, including narcotic drug abuse and harmful use of alcohol.
- By 2020, halve the number of global deaths and injuries from road traffic accidents.
- By 2030, ensure universal access to sexual and reproductive healthcare services, including for family planning, information and education, and the integration of reproductive health into national strategies and programs.
- Achieve universal health coverage, including financial risk protection, access to quality essential healthcare services and access to safe, effective, quality and affordable essential medicines and vaccines for all.
- By 2030, substantially reduce the number of deaths and illnesses from hazardous chemicals and air, water and soil pollution and contamination.
  - Strengthen the implementation of the World Health Organization Framework Convention on Tobacco Control in all countries, as appropriate.
  - Support the research and development of vaccines and medicines for the communicable and non-communicable diseases that primarily affect developing countries, provide access to affordable essential medicines and vaccines, in accordance with the Doha Declaration on the TRIPS Agreement and Public Health, which affirms the right of developing countries to use to the full the provisions in the Agreement on Trade-Related Aspects of Intellectual Property Rights regarding flexibilities to protect public health, and, in particular, provide access to medicines for all.
  - Substantially increase health financing and the recruitment, development, training and retention

of the health workforce in developing countries, especially in least developed countries and small island developing States.

Ensure Inclusive and Equitable Quality Education and Promote Life Long Learning Opportunities for All

Targets

- By 2030, ensure that all girls and boys complete free, equitable and quality primary and secondary education leading to relevant and effective learning outcomes.
- By 2030, ensure that all girls and boys have access to quality early childhood development, care and pre-primary education so that they are ready for primary education.
- By 2030, ensure equal access for all women and men to affordable and quality technical, vocational and tertiary education, including university.
- By 2030, substantially increase the number of youth and adults who have relevant skills, including technical and vocational skills, for employment, decent jobs and entrepreneurship.
- By 2030, eliminate gender disparities in education and ensure equal access to all levels of education and vocational training for the vulnerable, including persons with disabilities, indigenous peoples and children in vulnerable situations.
- By 2030, ensure that all youth and a substantial proportion of adults, both men and women, achieve literacy and numeracy.
- By 2030, ensure that all learners acquire the knowledge and skills needed to promote sustainable development, including, among others, through education for sustainable development and sustainable lifestyles, human rights, gender equality, promotion of a culture of peace and nonviolence, global citizenship and appreciation of cultural diversity and of culture's contribution to sustainable development.
  - Build and upgrade education facilities that are child, disability and gender sensitive and provide safe, non-violent, inclusive and effective learning environments for all.
  - By 2020, substantially expand globally the number of scholarships available to developing countries, in particular least developed countries, small island developing States and African countries, for enrolment in higher education, including vocational training and information and communications technology, technical, engineering and scientific programs, in developed countries and other developing countries.
  - By 2030, substantially increase the supply of qualified teachers, including through international cooperation for teacher training in developing countries, especially least developed countries and small island developing States.

Achieve Gender Equality and Empower All Women and Girls

Targets

- End all forms of discrimination against all women and girls everywhere.
- Eliminate all forms of violence against all women and girls in the public and private spheres, including trafficking and sexual and other types of exploitation.
- Eliminate all harmful practices, such as child, early and forced marriage and female genital mutilation.
- Recognize and value unpaid care and domestic work through the provision of public services, infrastructure and social protection policies and the promotion of shared responsibility within the household and the family as nationally appropriate.
- Ensure women's full and effective participation and equal opportunities for leadership at all levels of decision-making in political, economic and public life.
- Ensure universal access to sexual and reproductive health and reproductive rights as agreed in accordance with the Program of Action of the International Conference on Population and Development and the Beijing Platform for Action and the outcome documents of their review conferences.
  - Undertake reforms to give women equal rights to economic resources, as well as access to ownership and control over land and other forms of property, financial services, inheritance and natural resources, in accordance with national laws.
  - Enhance the use of enabling technology, in particular information and communications technology, to promote the empowerment of women.
  - Adopt and strengthen sound policies and enforceable legislation for the promotion of gender equality and the empowerment of all women and girls at all levels.

Ensure Availability and Sustainable Management of Water and Sanitation for All

Targets

- By 2030, achieve universal and equitable access to safe and affordable drinking water for all.
- By 2030, achieve access to adequate and equitable sanitation and hygiene for all and end open defecation, paying special attention to the needs of women and girls and those in vulnerable situations.
- By 2030, improve water quality by reducing pollution, eliminating dumping and minimizing release of hazardous chemicals and materials, halving the proportion of untreated wastewater and substantially increasing recycling and safe reuse globally.
- By 2030, substantially increase water-use efficiency across all sectors and ensure sustainable withdrawals and supply of freshwater to address water scarcity and substantially reduce the number of people suffering from water scarcity.

- By 2030, implement integrated water resources management at all levels, including through transboundary cooperation as appropriate.
- By 2020, protect and restore water-related ecosystems, including mountains, forests, wetlands, rivers, aquifers and lakes
  - By 2030, expand international cooperation and capacity-building support to developing countries in water- and sanitation-related activities and programs, including water harvesting, desalination, water efficiency, wastewater treatment, recycling and reuse technologies.
  - Support and strengthen the participation of local communities in improving water and sanitation management.

Ensure Access to Affordable, Reliable, Sustainable Modern Energy for All

Targets

- By 2030, ensure universal access to affordable, reliable and modern energy services.
- By 2030, increase substantially the share of renewable energy in the global energy mix.
- By 2030, double the global rate of improvement in energy efficiency.
  - By 2030, enhance international cooperation to facilitate access to clean energy research and technology, including renewable energy, energy efficiency and advanced and cleaner fossil-fuel technology, and promote investment in energy infrastructure and clean energy technology.
  - By 2030, expand infrastructure and upgrade technology for supplying modern and sustainable energy services for all in developing countries, in particular least developed countries, small island developing States, and land-locked developing countries, in accordance with their respective programs of support.

Promote Sustained, Inclusive Sustainable Economic Growth, Full and Productive Employment and Decent Work for All

Targets

- Sustain per capita economic growth in accordance with national circumstances and, in particular, at least 7% gross domestic product growth per annum in the least developed countries.
- Achieve higher levels of economic productivity through diversification, technological upgrading and innovation, including through a focus on high-value added and labor-intensive sectors.
- Promote development-oriented policies that support productive activities, decent job creation, entrepreneurship, creativity and innovation, and encourage the formalization and growth of micro-, small- and medium-sized enterprises, including through access to financial services.
- Improve progressively, through 2030, global resource efficiency in consumption and production and endeavour to decouple economic growth from environmental degradation, in accordance with the 10-year framework of programs on sustainable consumption and production, with developed countries taking the lead.
- By 2030, achieve full and productive employment and decent work for all women and men, including for young people and persons with disabilities, and equal pay for work of equal value.
- By 2020, substantially reduce the proportion of youth not in employment, education or training.
- Take immediate and effective measures to eradicate forced labor, end modern slavery and human trafficking and secure the prohibition and elimination of the worst forms of child labor, including recruitment and use of child soldiers, and by 2025 end child labor in all its forms.
- Protect labour rights and promote safe and secure working environments for all workers, including migrant workers, in particular women migrants, and those in precarious employment.
- By 2030, devise and implement policies to promote sustainable tourism that creates jobs and promotes local culture and products.
- Strengthen the capacity of domestic financial institutions to encourage and expand access to banking, insurance and financial services for all.
  - Increase Aid for Trade support for developing countries, in particular least developed countries, including through the Enhanced Integrated Framework for Trade-Related Technical Assistance to Least Developed Countries.
  - By 2020, develop and operationalize a global strategy for youth employment and implement the Global Jobs Pact of the International Labor Organization.

Build Resilient Infrastructure Promote Inclusive and Sustainable Industrialization and Foster Innovations

Targets

- Develop quality, reliable, sustainable and resilient infrastructure, including regional and transborder infrastructure, to support economic development and human well-being, with a focus on affordable and equitable access for all.
- Promote inclusive and sustainable industrialization and, by 2030, significantly raise industry's share of employment and gross domestic product, in line with national circumstances, and double its share in least developed countries.
- Increase the access of small-scale industrial and other enterprises, in particular in developing countries, to financial services, including affordable credit, and their integration into value chains and markets.
- By 2030, upgrade infrastructure and retrofit industries to make them sustainable, with increased resource-

use efficiency and greater adoption of clean and environmentally sound technologies and industrial processes, with all countries taking action in accordance with their respective capabilities.
- Enhance scientific research, upgrade the technological capabilities of industrial sectors in all countries, in particular developing countries, including, by 2030, encouraging innovation and substantially increasing the number of research and development workers per 1 million people and public and private research and development spending.
  - Facilitate sustainable and resilient infrastructure development in developing countries through enhanced financial, technological and technical support to African countries, least developed countries, landlocked developing countries and small island developing States.
  - Support domestic technology development, research and innovation in developing countries, including by ensuring a conducive policy environment for, inter alia, industrial diversification and value addition to commodities.
  - Significantly increase access to information and communications technology and strive to provide universal and affordable access to the Internet in least developed countries by 2020.

REDUCE INEQUALITY WITHIN AND AMONG COUNTRIES

Targets

- By 2030, progressively achieve and sustain income growth of the bottom 40% of the population at a rate higher than the national average.
- By 2030, empower and promote the social, economic and political inclusion of all, irrespective of age, sex, disability, race, ethnicity, origin, religion or economic or other status.
- Ensure equal opportunity and reduce inequalities of outcome, including by eliminating discriminatory laws, policies and practices and promoting appropriate legislation, policies and action in this regard.
- Adopt policies, especially fiscal, wage and social protection policies, and progressively achieve greater equality.
- Improve the regulation and monitoring of global financial markets and institutions and strengthen the implementation of such regulations.
- Ensure enhanced representation and voice for developing countries in decision-making in global international economic and financial institutions in order to deliver more effective, credible, accountable and legitimate institutions.
- Facilitate orderly, safe, regular and responsible migration and mobility of people, including through the implementation of planned and well-managed migration policies.
  - Implement the principle of special and differential treatment for developing countries, in particular least developed countries, in accordance with World Trade Organization agreements.
  - Encourage official development assistance and financial flows, including foreign direct investment, to States where the need is greatest, in particular least developed countries, African countries, small island developing States and landlocked developing countries, in accordance with their national plans and programs.
  - By 2030, reduce to less than 3% the transaction costs of migrant remittances and eliminate remittance corridors with costs higher than 5%.

MAKE CITIES AND HUMAN SETTLEMENT INCLUSIVE SAFE, RESILIENT AND SUSTAINABLE

Targets

- By 2030, ensure access for all to adequate, safe and affordable housing and basic services and upgrade slums.
- By 2030, provide access to safe, affordable, accessible and sustainable transport systems for all, improving road safety, notably by expanding public transport, with special attention to the needs of those in vulnerable situations, women, children, persons with disabilities and older persons.
- By 2030, enhance inclusive and sustainable urbanization and capacity for participatory, integrated and sustainable human settlement planning and management in all countries.
- Strengthen efforts to protect and safeguard the world's cultural and natural heritage.
- By 2030, significantly reduce the number of deaths and the number of people affected and substantially decrease the direct economic losses relative to global gross domestic product caused by disasters, including water-related disasters, with a focus on protecting the poor and people in vulnerable situations.
- By 2030, reduce the adverse per capita environmental impact of cities, including by paying special attention to air quality and municipal and other waste management.
- By 2030, provide universal access to safe, inclusive and accessible, green and public spaces, in particular for women and children, older persons and persons with disabilities.
  - Support positive economic, social and environmental links between urban, peri-urban and rural areas by strengthening national and regional development planning.
  - By 2020, substantially increase the number of cities and human settlements adopting and implementing integrated policies and plans towards inclusion, resource efficiency, mitigation and adaptation to climate change, resilience to disasters, and develop and implement, in line with the Sendai Framework for Disaster Risk Reduction 2015–2030, holistic disaster risk management at all levels.
  - Support least developed countries, including through financial and technical assistance, in building

sustainable and resilient buildings utilizing local materials.

ENSURE SUSTAINABLE CONSUMPTION AND PRODUCTION PATTERNS

Targets

- Implement the 10-year framework of programs on sustainable consumption and production, all countries taking action, with developed countries taking the lead, taking into account the development and capabilities of developing countries.
- By 2030, achieve the sustainable management and efficient use of natural resources.
- By 2030, halve per capita global food waste at the retail and consumer levels and reduce food losses along production and supply chains, including postharvest losses.
- By 2020, achieve the environmentally sound management of chemicals and all wastes throughout their life cycle, in accordance with agreed international frameworks, and significantly reduce their release to air, water and soil in order to minimize their adverse impacts on human health and the environment.
- By 2030, substantially reduce waste generation through prevention, reduction, recycling and reuse.
- Encourage companies, especially large and transnational companies, to adopt sustainable practices and to integrate sustainability information into their reporting cycle.
- Promote public procurement practices that are sustainable, in accordance with national policies and priorities.
- By 2030, ensure that people everywhere have the relevant information and awareness for sustainable development and lifestyles in harmony with nature.
  - Support developing countries to strengthen their scientific and technological capacity to move towards more sustainable patterns of consumption and production.
  - Develop and implement tools to monitor sustainable development impacts for sustainable tourism that creates jobs and promotes local culture and products.
  - Rationalize inefficient fossil-fuel subsidies that encourage wasteful consumption by removing market distortions, in accordance with national circumstances, including by restructuring taxation and phasing out those harmful subsidies, where they exist, to reflect their environmental impacts, taking fully into account the specific needs and conditions of developing countries and minimizing the possible adverse impacts on their development in a manner that protects the poor and the affected communities.

TAKE URGENT ACTION TO COMBAT CLIMATE CHANGE AND ITS IMPACTS

Targets

- Strengthen resilience and adaptive capacity to climate-related hazards and natural disasters in all countries.
- Integrate climate change measures into national policies, strategies and planning.
- Improve education, awareness-raising and human and institutional capacity on climate change mitigation, adaptation, impact reduction and early warning.
  - Implement the commitment undertaken by developed-country parties to the United Nations Framework Convention on Climate Change to a goal of mobilizing jointly $100 billion annually by 2020 from all sources to address the needs of developing countries in the context of meaningful mitigation actions and transparency on implementation and fully operationalize the Green Climate Fund through its capitalization as soon as possible.
  - Promote mechanisms for raising capacity for effective climate change-related planning and management in least developed countries and small island developing States, including focusing on women, youth and local and marginalized communities.

CONSERVE AND SUSTAINABLY USE THE OCEANS, SEAS AND MARINE RESOURCES FOR SUSTAINABLE DEVELOPMENT

Targets

- By 2025, prevent and significantly reduce marine pollution of all kinds, in particular from land-based activities, including marine debris and nutrient pollution.
- By 2020, sustainably manage and protect marine and coastal ecosystems to avoid significant adverse impacts, including by strengthening their resilience, and take action for their restoration in order to achieve healthy and productive oceans.
- Minimize and address the impacts of ocean acidification, including through enhanced scientific cooperation at all levels.
- By 2020, effectively regulate harvesting and end overfishing, illegal, unreported and unregulated fishing and destructive fishing practices and implement science-based management plans, in order to restore fish stocks in the shortest time feasible, at least to levels that can produce maximum sustainable yield as determined by their biological characteristics.
- By 2020, conserve at least 10% of coastal and marine areas, consistent with national and international law and based on the best available scientific information.
- By 2020, prohibit certain forms of fisheries subsidies which contribute to overcapacity and overfishing, eliminate subsidies that contribute to illegal, unreported and unregulated fishing and refrain from introducing new such subsidies, recognizing that appropriate and effective special and differential treatment for developing and least developed countries should be an integral part of the World Trade Organization fisheries subsidies negotiation.
- By 2030, increase the economic benefits to Small Island developing States and least developed countries from the sustainable use of marine resources, including through

sustainable management of fisheries, aquaculture and tourism.
- Increase scientific knowledge, develop research capacity and transfer marine technology, taking into account the Intergovernmental Oceanographic Commission Criteria and Guidelines on the Transfer of Marine Technology, in order to improve ocean health and to enhance the contribution of marine biodiversity to the development of developing countries, in particular small island developing States and least developed countries.
- Provide access for small-scale artisanal fishers to marine resources and markets.
- Enhance the conservation and sustainable use of oceans and their resources by implementing international law.

PROTECT, RESTORE AND PROMOTE SUSTAINABLE USE OF TERRESTRIAL ECOSYSTEM, SUSTAINABLY MANAGE FOREST, COMBAT DESERTIFICATION AND HALT AND REVERSE LAND DEGRADATION AND HALT BIODIVERSITY LOSS

Targets
- By 2020, ensure the conservation, restoration and sustainable use of terrestrial and inland fresh water ecosystems and their services, in particular forests, wetlands, mountains and dry lands, in line with obligations under international agreements.
- By 2020, promote the implementation of sustainable management of all types of forests, halt deforestation, restore degraded forests and substantially increase a forestation and reforestation globally.
- By 2030, combat desertification, restore degraded land and soil, including land affected by desertification, drought and floods, and strive to achieve a land degradation-neutral world.
- By 2030, ensure the conservation of mountain ecosystems, including their biodiversity, in order to enhance their capacity to provide benefits that are essential for sustainable development.
- Take urgent and significant action to reduce the degradation of natural habitats, halt the loss of biodiversity and, by 2020, protect and prevent the extinction of threatened species.
- Promote fair and equitable sharing of the benefits arising from the utilization of genetic resources and promote appropriate access to such resources, as internationally agreed.
- Take urgent action to end poaching and trafficking of protected species of flora and fauna and address both demand and supply of illegal wildlife products.
- By 2020, introduce measures to prevent the introduction and significantly reduce the impact of invasive alien species on land and water ecosystems and control or eradicate the priority species.
- By 2020, integrate ecosystem and biodiversity values into national and local planning, development processes, poverty reduction strategies and accounts.
  - Mobilize and significantly increase financial resources from all sources to conserve and sustainably use biodiversity and ecosystems.
  - Mobilize significant resources from all sources and at all levels to finance sustainable forest management and provide adequate incentives to developing countries to advance such management, including for conservation and reforestation.
  - Enhance global support for efforts to combat poaching and trafficking of protected species, including by increasing the capacity of local communities to pursue sustainable livelihood opportunities.

PROMOTE PEACEFUL AND INCLUSIVE SOCIETIES FOR SUSTAINABLE DEVELOPMENT; PROVIDE ACCESS TO JUSTICE FOR ALL AND BUILD EFFECTIVE, ACCOUNTABLE AND INCLUSIVE INSTITUTIONS AT ALL LEVELS

Targets
- Significantly reduce all forms of violence and related death rates everywhere.
- End abuse, exploitation, trafficking and all forms of violence against and torture of children.
- Promote the rule of law at the national and international levels and ensure equal access to justice for all.
- By 2030, significantly reduce illicit financial and arms flows, strengthen the recovery and return of stolen assets and combat all forms of organized crime.
- Substantially reduce corruption and bribery in all their forms.
- Develop effective, accountable and transparent institutions at all levels.
- Ensure responsive, inclusive, participatory and representative decision-making at all levels.
- Broaden and strengthen the participation of developing countries in the institutions of global governance.
- By 2030, provide legal identity for all, including birth registration.
- Ensure public access to information and protect fundamental freedoms, in accordance with national legislation and international agreements.
  - Strengthen relevant national institutions, including through international cooperation, for building capacity at all levels, in particular in developing countries, to prevent violence and combat terrorism and crime.
  - Promote and enforce non-discriminatory laws and policies for sustainable development.

STRENGTHEN THE MEANS OF IMPLEMENTATION AND REVITALITY THE GLOBAL PARTNERSHIP FOR SUSTAINABLE DEVELOPMENT

Targets

Finance

- Strengthen domestic resource mobilization, including through international support to developing countries, to improve domestic capacity for tax and other revenue collection.
- Developed countries to implement fully their official development assistance commitments, including the commitment by many developed countries to achieve the target of 0.7% of ODA/GNI to developing countries and 0.15 to 0.20% of ODA/GNI to least developed countries; ODA providers are encouraged to consider setting a target to provide at least 0.20% of ODA/GNI to least developed countries.
- Mobilize additional financial resources for developing countries from multiple sources.
- Assist developing countries in attaining long-term debt sustainability through coordinated policies aimed at fostering debt financing, debt relief and debt restructuring, as appropriate, and address the external debt of highly indebted poor countries to reduce debt distress.
- Adopt and implement investment promotion regimes for least developed countries.

Technology

- Enhance North-South, South-South and triangular regional and international cooperation on and access to science, technology and innovation and enhance knowledge sharing on mutually agreed terms, including through improved coordination among existing mechanisms, in particular at the United Nations level, and through a global technology facilitation mechanism.
- Promote the development, transfer, dissemination and diffusion of environmentally sound technologies to developing countries on favorable terms, including on concessional and preferential terms, as mutually agreed.
- Fully operationalize the technology bank and science, technology and innovation capacity-building mechanism for least developed countries by 2017 and enhance the use of enabling technology, in particular information and communications technology.

Capacity-building

Enhance international support for implementing effective and targeted capacity-building in developing countries to support national plans to implement all the sustainable development goals, including through North-South, South-South and triangular cooperation.

Trade

- Promote a universal, rules-based, open, non-discriminatory and equitable multilateral trading system under the World Trade Organization, including through the conclusion of negotiations under its Doha Development Agenda.
- Significantly increase the exports of developing countries, in particular with a view to doubling the least developed countries' share of global exports by 2020.
- Realize timely implementation of duty-free and quota-free market access on a lasting basis for all least developed countries, consistent with World Trade Organization decisions, including by ensuring that preferential rules of origin applicable to imports from least developed countries are transparent and simple, and contribute to facilitating market access.

Systemic Issues

Policy and Institutional coherence
- Enhance global macroeconomic stability, including through policy coordination and policy coherence.
- Enhance policy coherence for sustainable development.
- Respect each country's policy space and leadership to establish and implement policies for poverty eradication and sustainable development.

Multi-stakeholder Partnerships

- Enhance the global partnership for sustainable development, complemented by multi-stakeholder partnerships that mobilize and share knowledge, expertise, technology and financial resources, to support the achievement of the sustainable development goals in all countries, in particular developing countries.
- Encourage and promote effective public, public-private and civil society partnerships, building on the experience and resourcing strategies of partnerships.

Data, Monitoring and Accountability

- By 2020, enhance capacity-building support to developing countries, including for least developed countries and small island developing states, to increase significantly the availability of high-quality, timely and reliable data disaggregated by income, gender, age, race, ethnicity migratory status, disability, geographic location and other characteristics relevant in national contexts.
- By 2030, build on existing initiatives to develop measurements of progress on sustainable development that complement gross domestic product, and support statistical capacity-building in developing countries.

BIBLIOGRAPHY

1. Baride JP, Kulkarni AP. Textbook of community medicine. 3rd edition Mumbai: Vora Medical Publications; 2006.
2. BT Basavanthappa. Community Health Nursing. 2nd edition Bangalore (India): Jaypee Brothers Medical Publications; 2008.
3. Diwakar G. Healthcare delivery system in India. The Heinz school review; 2006;3(2):34–36.
4. George S. Healthcare delivery system; social science research network; 2005(5):19–21.

Chapter 11: Healthcare Delivery System

5. Kamalam S. Essentials in community health nursing practices. 1st edn. New Delhi: Jaypee Brothers Medical Publications, 2005.
6. Kishore J. National health programs of India; 7 Ed; 2007:58-61.
7. Madura G. India launches national rural health mission. British Medical Journal. 2005; 4 (3):33-35.
8. Navarro, Vicente: 'Introduction' in V. Navarro (Ed) Imperialism, Health and Medicine, Baywood, New York, 1981.
9. NCAER: Household Survey of Medical Care, National Council for Applied Economic Research, New Delhi, 1991.
10. Shrivastav Committee: Report of the Group on Medical Education and Support Manpower, MoHFW, New Delhi, 1975.
11. Simon Committee: National Water Supply and Sanitation Committee, GOI, New Delhi, 1960.

REVIEW QUESTIONS

Long Essays

1. Describe the levels of healthcare organization in India. Explain the rural health services.
2. Explain healthcare system and structure.
3. Enumerate delivery of health services at subcenter (SC).
4. Discuss nursing administration at community development.
5. Describe community development program. Explain the organization set-up and functions of community development blocks.
6. Explain sustainable development goals (SDGs).

Short Essays

1. Types of healthcare delivery.
2. Urban health services.
3. Health insurance system.
4. National Health Programme.
5. Voluntary health agencies.
6. Medical tourism and telemedicine.
7. Pradhan Mantri Swasthya Suraksha Yojana (PMSSY).
8. Ayushman Bharat, Pradhan Mantri Jan Arogya Yojana (PMJAY).
9. Private sector in health care.
10. Delivery of health services at PHC.
11. ROME Program (Reorientation of Medical Education).
12. Delivery of health services at CHC.
13. Nursing administration at center.
14. Integrated rural development.

Short Answers

1. Healthcare services.
2. Public or government sector.
3. Employee's state insurance.
4. Central Government Health Scheme.
5. Railway Hospitals and Military Hospitals.
6. Indigenous system of medicine.
7. Challenges in health system.
8. Role of Nurse in healthcare delivery system.
9. Kayakalp.
10. Mission Indradhanush.
11. Staff at a subcenter.
12. Functions of PHC.
13. Community health center (CHC).
14. Medical services at CHC.
15. First referral units (FRUs).
16. Health and wellness centers.

Multiple Choice Questions

1. Three tier system of health care delivery in rural area based on the recommendations of:
    a. Bhore committee
    b. Mudaliar committee
    c. Srivastav committee
    d. Kartar Singh committee
2. First and foremost, element of PHC is:
    a. Immunization
    b. FP/MCH
    c. Health education
    d. Provision of safe drinking water
3. Panchayat Raj means:
    a. Local health care centre
    b. Community health care centre
    c. Primary health care
    d. Local self rule government
4. The community development programme is means:
    a. To bring about a special and economic change in village life through the effort of the villagers themselves
    b. To arrange welfare programmes for women and children
    c. To improve agriculture product through better manure and seeds
    d. To plan development program in a village high population of 60 and 80 thousand
5. Community health centre:
    a. Has 100 beds
    b. Covers a population of approx one lakh
    c. Has X-Ray and laboratory facilities
    d. Acts as a referral hospital for the community development block
6. Elements of primary health care:
    a. Promotion of food supply and proper nutrition
    b. Adequate supply of safe water and sanitation
    c. Maternal and child health care
    d. All the above
7. In community health nursing focus in on:
    a. Sick people
    b. Vulnerable groups
    c. Whole community with entire people
    d. Mothers and children
8. Objective of community health nursing is:
    a. Maintenance of health
    b. Monitoring of health
    c. Restoration of health
    d. All of the above
9. Elements of primary health care include all of the following, except:
    a. Providing essential drugs
    b. Adequate supply of safe water and basic sanitation
    c. Sound referral system
    d. Health education
10. Primary health care:
    a. First level health care
    b. Second level health care
    c. Tertiary health care
    d. All of the above

ANSWERS

| 1. c | 2. d | 3. b | 4. a | 5. b | 6. d | 7. c | 8. d | 9. c | 10. a | | |

CHAPTER 12: Health Planning in India

LEARNING OBJECTIVES
1. National Health Planning
2. Five Year Plans
3. Health Committees and Reports
4. National Health Policy

TERMINOLOGY

- **Planning:** An organized, conscious and continuous attempt to select the best available alternatives to achieve specific goals.
- **Health planning:** The orderly process defining national Health problems, identifying the unmeet needs, surveying the resources to meet them, and establishing the priority goals to accomplish the purpose of proposed program.
- **Policy:** Policy is a system, which provides the logical framework and rationality of decision-making for the achievement of intended objectives.

INTRODUCTION

Health planning in India is an integral part of national socio-economic planning. The guidelines for national health planning were provided by a number of committees. Health planning is a complex process with at least three distinctive features (health being a labor-intensive sector, complex relationships between different actors, and the balance between clinical and public health perspectives). Planning is the product of values, techniques, and power relationships between different groups. Health planning is a continuous process and the production of a plan should not be seen as the end product of this process.

DEFINITIONS

- **National health planning:** National health planning has been defined as the orderly process of defining national health problems, identifying unmet needs and surveying the resources to meet them, establishing priority goals that are realistic and feasible and projecting administrative action to accomplish the purpose of the proposed Program.
- **National development planning:** National development planning has been defined as "continuous, systematic, coordinated planning for the investment of the resources of a country in programs."

HEALTH PLANNING

- **Health planning** has been defined as the orderly process of defining community health problems, identifying the unmet needs and surveying the resource to meet them, establishing priority goals that are realistic and feasible and projecting administrative action to accomplish the purpose of the proposed program **(Fig. 12.1)**.
- **National development planning** has been defined as continuous, systematic, planning for the investment of the resources of a country (men, money and materials) in programs aimed at achieving the most rapid and social development possible.

Purposes of Planning
- To match the limited resources with existing problems.
- To eliminate wasteful expenditure or duplication of expenses.
- To develop the best course of action for accomplishing a defined objective.

Steps of Planning
- Plan formation
- Execution
- Evaluation

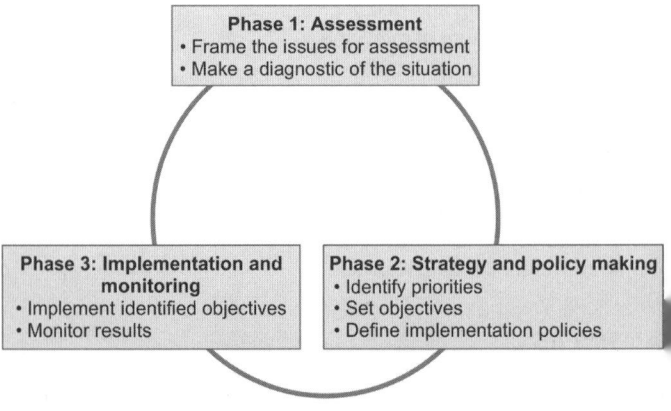

Fig. 12.1: Health planning phases.

Purposes of Health Planning

- The purpose is to meet the health needs and demands of the people. Health needs have been defined as deficiency in health that calls for preventive, curative, control or eradication measures. Health needs include need of medical care, safe water supply, adequate nutrition, immunization, family planning, etc.
- Health needs may be perceived by people in a different way from that seen by experts. Sometimes some health needs may both perceive at all by the people, while others are vaguely perceived. Also the needs are conditioned by the aspirations of the people.

Objectives, Targets and Goals

- An objective is precise, it is either achieved or not objective is a planned end point of all activities.
- A target—often refers to a discrete activity such as the number of blood films collected or vasectomies done, it permits the concept of degree of achievement.
- Goal—is defined as the ultimate desired state towards which objectives and resources are directed.
- Plan—planning results in the formation of plan. A plan is a blue print for taking action.

Elements of Plan

- **Objectives:** This is the statement of desired changes in behavior or state of excellence, expected as a result of particular program or activity.
- **Policies:** Written statement of the terms of a contract of insurance. It is a plan of action, statement of ideals, etc. proposed or adopted by a Government or political or activity.
- **Programs:** An organized order of performances of events.
- **Schedules:** It is a program of work to be done or of planned events.
- **Budget:** It is a concrete precise picture of the total operation of an enterprise in monetary terms.

SPECIFIC QUANTITATIVE GOALS AND OBJECTIVES

Health Status and Program Impact

Life Expectancy and Healthy Life

- Increase Life Expectancy at birth from 67.5 to 70 by 2025.
- Establish regular tracking of Disability Adjusted Life Years (DALY) Index as a measure of burden of disease and its trends by major categories by 2022.
- Reduction of TFR to 2.1 at national and subnational level by 2025.

Mortality by Age and/or Cause

- Reduce under Five Mortality to 23 by 2025 and MMR from current levels to 100 by 2020.
- Reduce infant mortality rate to 28 by 2019.
- Reduce neonatal mortality to 16 and stillbirth rate to "single digit" by 2025.

Reduction of Disease Prevalence/Incidence

- Achieve global target of 2020 which is also termed as target of 90:90:90, for HIV/AIDS i.e., 90% of all people living with HIV know their HIV status, 90% of all people diagnosed with HIV infection receive sustained antiretroviral therapy and 90% of all people receiving antiretroviral therapy will have viral suppression.
- Achieve and maintain elimination status of Leprosy by 2018, Kala-Azar by 2017 and Lymphatic Filariasis in endemic pockets by 2017.
- To achieve and maintain a cure rate of >85% in new sputum positive patients for TB and reduce incidence of new cases, to reach elimination status by 2025.
- To reduce the prevalence of blindness to 0.25/ 1000 by 2025 and disease burden by one third from current levels.
- To reduce premature mortality from cardiovascular diseases, cancer, diabetes or chronic respiratory diseases by 25% by 2025.

HEALTH SYSTEMS PERFORMANCE

Coverage of Health Services

- Increase utilization of public health facilities by 50% from current levels by 2025.
- Antenatal care coverage to be sustained above 90% and skilled attendance at birth above 90% by 2025.
- More than 90% of the newborn are fully immunized by one year of age by 2025.
- Meet need of family planning above 90% at national and subnational level by 2025.
- 80% of known hypertensive and diabetic individuals at household level maintain "controlled disease status" by 2025.

Cross-sectoral Goals Related to Health

- Relative reduction in prevalence of current tobacco use by 15% by 2020 and 30% by 2025.
- Reduction of 40% in prevalence of stunting of under-five children by 2025.
- Access to safe water and sanitation to all by 2020.
- Reduction of occupational injury by half from current levels of 334 per lakh agricultural workers by 2020.
- National/State level tracking of selected health behavior.

HEALTH SYSTEMS STRENGTHENING

Health Finance

- Increase health expenditure by Government as a percentage of GDP from the existing 1.15 % to 2.5 % by 2025.
- Increase State sector health spending to > 8% of their budget by 2020.
- Decrease in proportion of households facing catastrophic health expenditure from the current levels by 25%, by 2025.

Health Infrastructure and Human Resource

- Ensure availability of paramedics and doctors as per Indian Public Health Standard (IPHS) norm in high priority districts by 2020.
- Increase community health volunteers to population ratio as per IPHS norm, in high priority districts by 2025.
- Establish primary and secondary care facility as per norm in high priority districts (population as well as time to reach norms) by 2025.

Health Management Information

- Ensure district level electronic database of information on health system components by 2020.
- Strengthen the health surveillance system and establish registries for diseases of public health importance by 2020.
- Establish federated integrated health information architecture, Health Information Exchanges and National Health Information Network by 2025.

HEALTH PLANNING STEPS (FIG. 12.2)

- Analysis of the health situation
- Establishment of objectives and goals
- Assessment of resources
- Fixing priorities
- Write-up of formulated plan
- Programming and implementation
- Monitoring
- Evaluation

Analysis of the Situation

- The first step in health planning is the analysis of the current situation.
- The different aspects to be studied are:
  - Population—age and sex structure, religion, SES, etc.
  - Morbidity and mortality rates
  - Morbidity and mortality rates due to the disease under consideration
  - Epidemiology and geographic distribution of the disease under consideration
  - Existing healthcare facilities
  - Technical manpower available
  - Facilities for training healthcare staff
  - Awareness and attitude of the community regarding the disease, etc.

Establishment of Objectives and Goals

- This step is to identify the desirable future state for the issue under consideration. The program has to work for achieving this.
- Hence, goals and objectives, establish the standards against which current disease will be compared for assessing the performance of program.
- If there are no clear objectives and goals, a plan cannot be implemented efficiently and haphazard wasteful activity will result.
- At the central level, the objectives would be more general and with each successive level, the objectives will become more specific.
- Management techniques are usually used to determine objectives, for example, cost-benefit analysis.
- These analysis will assess the feasibility of attaining the desired results in optimum cost and time.
- The objective can be defined like: "To reduce the prevalence to the level of 0.5%".

Assessment of Resources

- The available manpower, money, material, skills, knowledge and Techniques should be accessed.
- A balance is to be struck between the available resources and the attainment of the objectives.

Fix Priorities

- The resources are usually not enough to attain all the objectives.
- So priority goals should be listed out and resources should be allocated to these.
- Various considerations in fixing priorities can be:
  - In order of magnitude
  - Lower costs needed to achieve the objectives
  - Saving the lives of younger people
  - Political commitments and pressure, etc.
- Once the priority objectives have been decided.
- Alternative ways of achieving them should be assessed.
- Management techniques for comparing the efficiency of alternative plans may be useful for deciding priority.

Write-up Formulated Plan

- Once priorities are laid out, a systematic plan should be made to attain them.
- All the major steps should be included with the:
  - Resources (input) required for each step

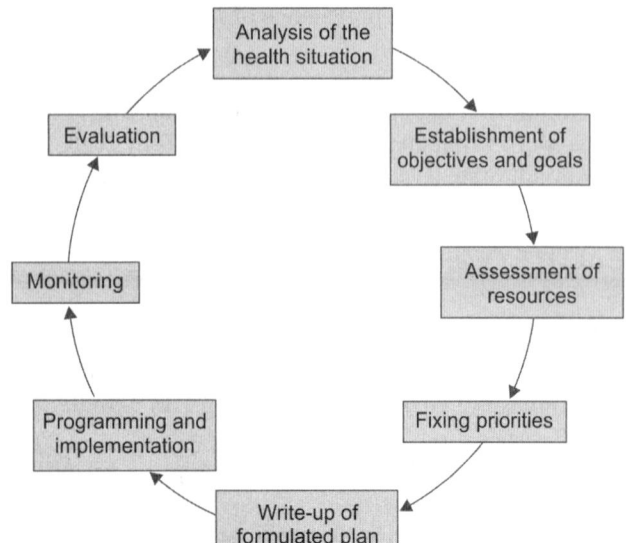

Fig. 12.2: Steps in health planning.

- The expected outcome (output) and
- Time period specified for each step
- Also include are:
  - Precise guidelines for procedures
  - Fixation of responsibility (identify individual responsible for the execution of each step).

Programming and Implementation

- Once the plan has been approved it has to be implemented.
- Implementation requires an effective organization to run the routine procedures and referrals.
- The real shortcomings or impracticalities of the program may be revealed at this stage.
- Main considerations at this stage are:
  - Definition of roles and tasks
  - Selection and training of personnel
  - Organization and communication so that all workers are aware of their responsibility and remain motivated
  - The involved institutions should work efficiently.

Monitoring

- Monitoring refers to the day to day follow-up of functioning of program.
- It is to be ensured that the activities are: proceeding as planned and are on schedule.
- Immediate corrective action is to be taken in case of deviations.
- Monitoring is thus defined as "the continuous process of observing, recording and reporting on the activities of the organization or project.

Evaluation

- Evaluation refers to the assessing the final outcome of the plan.
- Evaluation is in terms of:
  - Degree to which objectives are achieved.
  - How efficiently have the resources been utilized (output-input, cost-benefit analysis, etc.) in achieving these.
  - What were the factors responsible for shortfalls?
  - Factors responsible for better performance if any.
  - Difficulties faced during the implementation of and possible solutions for them.
- Based on the results of the evaluation, one of the following decisions may be taken:
  - To continue running the program as the results are satisfactory.
  - To make a few changes to overcome inefficiencies and let the program continue.
  - To change the objectives as the disease profile has changed due to the effect of the program.
  - To abandon the approach and analyze alternative approaches:
    - The program failed to achieve the objectives or
    - A new and much more effective technology has been developed for controlling the disease and needs to be incorporated in the program or
    - A new and more dangerous health problem has emerged and the priority needs a change.

PLANNING CYCLE

Planning may be defined as a process of analyzing a system or defining a problem, assessing the extent to which the problem exists as a need, formulating goals and objectives to alleviate or ameliorate those unidentified needs, examining and choosing from the alternative intervention strategies, initiating the necessary action for its implementation, monitoring the system to ensure proper implementation of the plan and finally evaluating the results of intervention in terms of the stated objectives.

Steps of Planning Cycle

- **Analysis of the health situation:** It involves the collection assessment and interpretation of information in such a way to give a clear picture of the health situation.
- **Establishment of objectives and goals:** Objective may be short-term or long-term, in setting these objectives time and resources are important factors. Objectives are guides to action and also a yard-stick to measure work after it is done.
- **Assessment of resources:** Resources implies the manpower, money, materials, skills, knowledge and techniques needed or available for the implementation of the health programs. These resources are assessed and a balance is struck between what is required and what is available.
- **Fixing priorities:** In fixing priorities, attention is paid to financial constraints, mortality and morbidity data, diseases which can be prevented at low cost.
- **Write-up of formulated plan:** The plan must be complete in all respect for the execution of a project. The plan must contain working guidance to all those responsible for execution. It must also contain a "built-in system evaluation.
- **Programming and implementation:** The organizational structure must incorporate well defined procedures to be followed and sufficient delegation of authority to and fixation of responsibility of different workers for achieving the predetermined objectives during the period prescribed.
- **Monitoring:** Monitoring is a continuous process of observing, recording and reporting on the activities of the organization or project. Thus consists of keeping track of the course of activities and identify deviations and taking corrective action if excessive deviation occurs.

- **Evaluation:** Evaluation measures the degree to which objectives and targets are fulfilled and the quality of the result obtained. It measures the productivity of available resources in achieving clearly – defined objectives.

Constrains of Health Planning

- Lack of adequate health information system for planning, monitoring and for evaluation.
- Natural resistance to change
- The relatively low priority often accorded to health by the political decision makers and the public.
- The frequency of governmental political and administrative changes with concurrent changes in commitment to support the plan.
- The imperfect state of the art planning, i.e. the absence of trained health administrators and planners are particularly the lack of precise tool to measure need, demand cost and benefit.
- The long time gap between planning and implementation particularly refers the supply of additional health man power and enactment of necessary legislation.
- The division of health professional into compartments and resultant lack of adequate interprofessional communication.
- The inflexibility of the educational system.
- Inefficient administrative practices that limit the flexibility of the budgets promote fragmented programs, and result in inappropriate personnel system.
- Inadequate coordination of planning between the various ministries and departments concerned with socio-economic development.

HEALTH PLANNING IN INDIA

Good health planning in India will enable the country to establish a healthcare system which will be socially acceptable, medically sound, and cost-effective enough for every Indian. Establishing health planning in India is a key to improving the health of the Indian Population. The Ministry of Health and Family Welfare has been facilitating Health needs in India by establishing various schemes and organizations. The Government is conscious of the need for dynamic Indian health planning and management. Innovative healthcare and development programs are the need of the hour. For this, major organizations like the National AIDS Control organization have been established by the Health Ministry. The areas to focus on in Health Planning have been laid down by the Ministry's National Health Policy. Some of them are mentioned below:

- **Increasing healthcare programs:** To be implemented in various socio-economic settings of different States of India.
- **Increasing public health infrastructure:** More hospitals, Outdoor medical facilities, Medical equipment.
- **Efficient doctors and nurses:** To ensure minimum standards of patient care.
- **Family medicine:** Establishing more personnel for family healthcare.
- **Low cost drugs and vaccines:** Keeping in view of the possible globalization induced high costs.
- **Mental health:** Need for increase in hospitals and professionals.
- **Health research:** Medical innovation and specialization is needed.
- **Disease control:** More database needs to be collected in this regard in order treat and prevent diseases.
- **Women's health:** Adequate access to public healthcare facilities is a necessity which in turn will improve family health as well.

List of National Health Programes organized by the health ministry are National Vector-Borne Disease Control Program (NVBDCP), National Iodine Deficiency Disorders Control Programme, National Leprosy Eradication Programme, National Programme for Control of Blindness, National Filaria Control Programme, National Programme for Prevention and Control of Deafness, National Cancer Control Programme, National Aids Control Programme, Universal Immunization Programme (RTI ACT, 2005), Revised National TB Control Programme, and National Mental Health Program.

Some more endeavors for health planning in India are Medical Health Division, Hospital Services Consultancy Corporation, SC/ST facilities, Central Government Health Schemes, Prevention of food adulteration, establishment of food and drug testing laboratories, L.R.S. Institute of Tuberculosis and Respiratory Diseases, National Rural Health Mission, etc. In March 1950, the Government of India had set up a Planning Commission to promote a rapid rise in the standard of living of the people by efficient exploitation of the resources of the country, increasing production and offering opportunities to all for employment in the service of community.

PLANNING COMMISSION

Health, being an important contributory factor to national development, the Planning Commission gave due importance to health and established a separate Division in the Planning Commission for the formulation of the health programs to be included in the nations Five Year Plans. A Bureau of Planning was also constituted in 1965 in the Union Health Ministry to secure better coordination between the Center and State Governments. For purposes of planning, the health sector has been divided into the following subsectors:

- Control of communicable diseases
- Medical education, training and research
- Medical care including hospitals, dispensaries and primary health centers
- Public health services
- Family Planning Indigenous system of medicine

NATIONAL HEALTH COMMITTEES

The strategies of health planning were provided mainly by the constitution of India (1950), the national development council, the planning commission general advisory boards and consultative committees the ministry of health and welfare and legislature. The committees an commissions appointed from time to time played an important role in formulation of health policies.

The health care measures formulated and implementation in the successive 5-year plans have been based on the approaches recommended by the health committees constituted by the government of India. The Alma-Ata declaration on primary health care and the National Health policy of the government gave a new direction to health planning in India.

National Planning Committee (1938)

In 1938, Indian National Congress headed by Netaji Subhash Chandra Bose, set up a national planning committee (NPC) and Subsequent Sub-committees under the chairmanship of Jawaharlal Nehru. The NPC had many problems due to lack of data and statistics, lack of cooperation from the British Government of India, lack of real interest in all Indian planning on the provincial governments.

BHORE COMMITTEE (1946)

In 1943, the Government of India appointed a Committee as the Bhore Committee or the health survey and development committee with Sir, Joseph Bhore as Chairman. Its aim was to survey the existing position regarding the health conditions and health organization in the committee which had among its members some of the pioneers of the health, met regularly for 2 years and submitted in 1946 its famous report which runs into 4 volumes.

Important Recommendations

Nutrition of the people: They pointed out the main defects of he average Indian diet results from the insufficiency of proteins, mineral salts and vitamins. They also recommend special measures to increase the production of food rich in proteins. Also prevention of food adulteration and improvement of the quality of the food.

Health education: Bhore committee suggested that health education to school children on hygiene should begin at the earliest. The doctors, the nurses, the midwife and in fact every health worker will discharge his or her duties and by educating the persons with whom they deal with regard to prevention of disease and the promotion of positive health.

Physical examination: Committee that there is great dearth of suitable and qualified teachers for imparting instructions in this subject. Also physical training program for the community with emphasis on national games and exercises.

Health services for mothers and children: At the head quarters of each primary unit and in place where 30 bed hospitals are located the service for mothers.

> **BHORE COMMITTEE 1946**
> - Health Survey and Development Committee—1943
> - Sir Joseph William Bhore—Chairman
> - To survey the existing position regarding the health conditions and health organization in the country
> - Emphasis on integration of curative and preventive medicine at all levels

Health services of the school children: The school teachers who have to carry or certain health duties require careful training and continuous supervision. They have to conduct health education programs. In each primary unit, the male medical officer should take charge of the school health services.

Occupational heath including industrial health: The committee recommended that the industrial health organization should form an integral part of the provincial health department and government.

Health services for certain important diseases: Bhore's committee studied the existing legal and administrative provisions to deal with communicable diseases and suggested certain measures for controlling communicable diseases.

Environmental hygiene: An essential part of the campaign for promoting public health was to improve man's physical environment. The committee's main recommendations were improvement in village and town planning.

Vital statistics: The committee recommended administrative organization at the center, organization at provincial headquarters and district organization. Another recommendation is provision of training facilities for statistics.

Professional education: The main objective of the committee during his period was the provision of adequate and suitably trained staff to enable the plan of health work effectively.

Drug and medical requisites: They recommended our universities should undertake research with a view to produce life saving drug in this country.

MUDALIAR COMMITTEE (1962)

In 1959, the government of India appointed another committee known as "health survey and planning committee" popularly known Mudaliar committee after the name of its chairman Dr. A.L. Mudaliar. The Mudaliar committee found the quality of services provided by the primary health centers inadequate and advised strengthening of the existing primary health centers before new centers were established.

> **Health Survey and Planning Committee**
> **Mudaliar Committee, 1961**
>
> ❖ **Recommendations:** Training in Ayurveda and other indigenous systems should be in the Shudha in place of the integrated system and syllabus and courses should be left to experts in these systems.
> ❖ Chairs of Indian system of medicine should be established in all Medical Colleges.
> ❖ After 3–4 years training in Ayurveda graduate should be trained in preventive medicine, OBG and principles of surgery ... so that their services can be utilized in the health services.
> ❖ Research in indigenous systems should be done in Central Institute of Medicine and Modern Medical Colleges.
> ❖ Postgraduate training should be available to medical men from both systems... and the integration of the two systems of medicine will eventually come about as a result of the labors of such scientific worker.
> ❖ Separate councils of research and sufficient financial support for training in indigenous systems.

(*Source:* Community Health Cell-1993)

Important Recommendations

- Strengthening of the district hospital with specialist services to serve as central base of regional services.
- Regional organizations in each state between the head quarters organizations in each state between the head quarters organization and the district in change of a regional deputy or assistant directors—each to supervise 2 or 3 district medical and health officers.
- Each primary health center not to be served more than 40,000 populations.
- To improve the quality of healthcare provided by the primary health centers.
- Integration of medical and health services as recommended by the Bhore committee.
- Constitution of All India Health Service on the pattern on Indian Administrative Service.

CHADAH COMMITTEE (1963)

In 1963, special committee on the preparation entry by the National malaria Eradication of India, under the chairmanship of Dr. Ms. Chandha.

> **Chadah Committee, 1963**
>
> ❖ National malaria eradication programme responsibility of general health services, i.e., PHC at block level
> ❖ Monthly home visits by basic health worker for vigilance operations of Malaria
> ❖ One basic health worker/10,000 population
> ❖ Basic health worker also called multipurpose worker, entrusted to look after duties like vital statistics, family planning, etc.

Important Recommendations

- Appointing a basic health worker per 10,000 populations later make it one worker per 5,000 population. Along with malaria, vital statistics and family planning work also should be looked for.
- Vigilance operation in respect of the National Malaria Eradication Programme should be the responsibility of the general health services, e.g., PHC.
- The vigilance operation should be done through monthly home visits by basic health worker (Junior Health assistant Male)
- Family planning health assistant should be responsibility to supervise the worker of 3–4 basic health workers.

MUKHERJEE COMMITTEE (1965)

A committee was appointed by the Government of India during 1965 to review the strategy of family planning, under the chairmanship of Shri Mukherjee.

Important Recommendations

- To have separate staff for the family planning duties only.
- The family planning assistants were to undertake family planning duties only.
- The basic health worker was to utilize for purposes other than family planning.
- To delink the malaria activities from family planning so that the latter would receive undivided attention of its staff.

MUKERJI COMMITTEE (1966)

The Central council of health held in Bangalore in 1966. The Central Council recommended examining the difficulties of the maintenance phase of malaria and other mass programs like family planning, smallpox, leprosy, trachoma, etc., due to paucity of funds under the chairmanship of the Union health secretary Shri Mukerji.

Important Recommendations

- Basic health service should be provided at the block level.
- Basic health services should be strengthening from block level right up to Central level.

JUNGALWALA COMMITTEE

The Central Council of Health at its meeting held in Srinagar in 1964, taking note of the importance and urgency of integration of health services and elimination of private practice by Government doctors, appointed a committee known as the "Committee on Integration of health services" under the chairmanship of Dr. N. Jungalwala, Director, National Institute of Health Administration and Education, New Delhi.

Important Recommendations

- **Integrated health service** should be unified approach for all problems instead of a segmented approach for different problems. The medical care of the sick and conventional public health program functioning under a single administrator.

- **The committee recommended** integration from the highest to the lowest in the services, organization and personnel—unified cadre, common seniority, recognition of extra qualifications, equal pay for equal work, special pay for specialized work, no private practice and good service conditions.

KARTAR SINGH COMMITTEE (1973)

The Government of India constituted a committee in 1972 known as "The committee on multipurpose workers under health and family planning" under the Chairmanship of Kartar Singh, additional secretary, ministry of health and family planning.

> **Kartar Singh Committee, 1973**
> - The committee on Multipurpose Workers under Health and Family Planning'
> - ANM to be replaced by 'Female Health Worker' and basic health workers, malaria surveillance workers, vaccinators, etc., to be replaced by 'Male Health Worker'
> - One PHC for 50,000 population
> - Each PHC should be divided into 16 subcenters which caters to 3,000–3,500 population
> - Each subcenter to be staffed by a team of one male and one female health worker
> - Doctors in charge of PHC should have overall charge of all supervisors and health workers in his area.

Important Recommendations

- The present auxiliary nurse midwives to be replaced by the newly designed female health worker and the present day basic health worker, malaria surveillance, vaccinators, health education assistants (Trachoma) and the family planning health assistants to be redesignated as male health worker.
- The program for having multipurpose worker to be first introduced in areas where malaria is in maintenance phase and smallpox has been controlled and later to other areas as malaria passes into maintenance phase or smallpox is controlled.
- For purpose of coverage there should be divided into 16 subdivisions each having a population of about 3000 to 3,500 depending upon topography and means of communication.
- Each subcenter to be staffed by a team of one male and female health worker.
- There should be a male health supervisor to supervise the work of 3 to 4 male health worker and a female supervisor to supervise the work of 4 female health workers.
- The present day health visitors to be designated as female health supervisors.
- The doctor in charge of a primary health center should have the overall charge of all the supervisors and health workers in his area. The recommendations of the Kartar Singh committee were accepted by the Government of India and implemented in a phased manner during the fifth five year plan.

SHRIVASTAV COMMITTEE (1975)

- Step should be taken to create bands of paraprofessional or semi-professional health workers from the community itself to provide simple, protective preventive and curative services which are needed by the community.
- Health workers should be trained and equipped to give simple specified remedies for day to day illness.
- The primary health center should provide with an additional doctor and a nurse to look after the maternal and child health services.
- Development of a "Referral services complex" by establishing proper linkage between PHC and higher level referral services.
- Establishment of medical and health education commission for planning and implementing the referrals needed in health and medical education on the lines of the university grants commission.

> **Shrivastav Committee, 1975**
> - 'Group on Medical Education and Support Manpower'
> - Creation of bands of Para- and semi-professional health workers from within the community itself
> - Development of a 'Referral Services Complex'
> - Establishment of a Medical and Health Education Commission for planning and implementing the reforms needed in health and medical education
> - Recommends one male and female health worker for 5,000 population
> - Health assistant should be located at the subcenter, not at the PHC.

RURAL HEALTH SCHEME (1977)

The most important recommendations the Shrivastava committee was that the primary healthcare should be provided within the community itself through specially trained workers to that the health of the people is placed in hands of the people themselves. The basic recommendations of the committee were accepted by the Government in 1977, which led to the launching of the Rural Health Scheme,. The program of training of the community health workers was initiated during 1977–1978.

The rural health scheme steps were initiated involvement of medical colleges in the total healthcare of selected PHCs with the objective of reorienting medical education to the needs of rural people. Control of various communicable diseases programs, in order to make them unipurpose workers. This plan of action was adopted by the joint meeting of the Central Council of Health and Central Family Planning Council held in New Delhi in April 1976.

> **NRHM—National Rural Health Mission**
>
> The key features of NRHM include:
> - Making health delivery system fully functional and accountable to the community convergence of National Health Program at all levels of health system
> - Improved management through capacity building
> - Involvement of community
> - Monitoring progress against standards
> - Flexible financing for optimum fund utilization
> - Inter-sectoral coordination for financial enhancement
>
> **Objectives of NRHM**
> - Reduction in maternal and child mortality
> - Universal access to affordable and quality health care services
> - Prevention and control of communicable and non-communicable diseases
> - Access to integrated comprehensive primary healthcare
> - Population stabilization
> - Promotion of healthy lifestyles

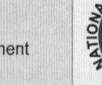

BAJAJ COMMITTEE (1986–87)

The Ministry of Health and Family Welfare Government of India following the adoption of the National Policy on education, 1986, set up a committee on Health Manpower Planning, Production and Management in 1986 under the chairmanship of prof. J.S. Bajaj committee professor of medicine, All India Institute of Medical Sciences, New Delhi.

Important Recommendations

- To formulate a national policy on Education in health services.
- To prepare curriculum for school teachers which should constitute a holistic approach including social, moral, health and physical education?
- To utilize the services of Indian system of medicine, e.g., homeopathy.
- Continuing education program for the health personnel.
- Health service statistics need to be improved in quality.
- Health manpower requirements for nursing personnel.

NATIONAL HEALTH POLICIES

National health policy in India was not framed and announced until 1983. The ministry of health and family welfare evolved a national health policy in 1983 keeping in view the national commitment to attain the goal of health for all by 2000 AD. The policy lays stress on the preventive promotive, public health and rehabilitation aspects of healthcare.

The health policy is supported by components of wider socioeconomic policies addressed towards the reduction of regional disparities, fuller employment, elementary education, integrated rural development, population control, welfare of women and children, etc.

Elements of Health Policy

- A greater awareness of health problems and means to sole these by the communities.
- Supply of safe drinking water and basic sanitation using technologies that the people can afford.
- Reduction of existing imbalance in health services by concentrating on the rural heath infrastructure.
- Establishment of a dynamic health management information system to support health planning and health program implementation.
- Provision of legislative support for health programe protection and promotion.
- Concerted actions to combat widespread malnutrition.
- Research for alternative methods of healthcare delivery and low cost health technologies.
- Greater coordination of different system of medicine.

National Health Policies (1983-2002)

- **National Health Policy (1983)**—To attain the objectives "Health for all by 2000 AD", the union ministry of health and welfare formulated National health policy in 1983.
- **National Health Policy (2000)**—Ministry of health and family welfare has declared new population policy on 15th February 2000 amending the policies declared earlier. New demographic objectives are defined in this policy.
- **National Health Policy (2002)**—It has been formulated and accepted by Central Government in September 2002. It emphasizes the importance of "Health for all by the year 2000 AD" through the universal provision of comprehensive primary healthcare services.

Objectives of National Health Policy

- The need to establish comprehensive primary healthcare services within the reach of population even in the remotest areas of the country.
- The need to view health and human development as vital component of overall integrated socioeconomic development.
- Decentralized system of healthcare delivery with maximum community and individual self-reliance and participation.

PLANNING COMMISSION OF INDIA

The Constitution of India came into force in 1950 and India became republic in common wealth. The planning commission was set up by the government of India. The Government of India set up a planning commission in 1950 to make an assessment of the maternal capital and human resource of the country and to draft developmental plans for the most effective utilization of these resources.

In 1957, the planning commission was provided with a perspective planning division which makes projections into the future over periods of 20 to 25 years. Planning commission is essentially an advisory body to the government. It has neither constitutional nor even statutory authority. It assists the government in formulating five year plans through the active involvement of various ministries and their technical departments both at the center and states.

Functions of Planning Commission

- Make an assessment of the maternal, capital human resources of the country including technical personnel and investigate the possibilities of augmenting such of these resources as found to be deficient in relation to the nation's requirements.

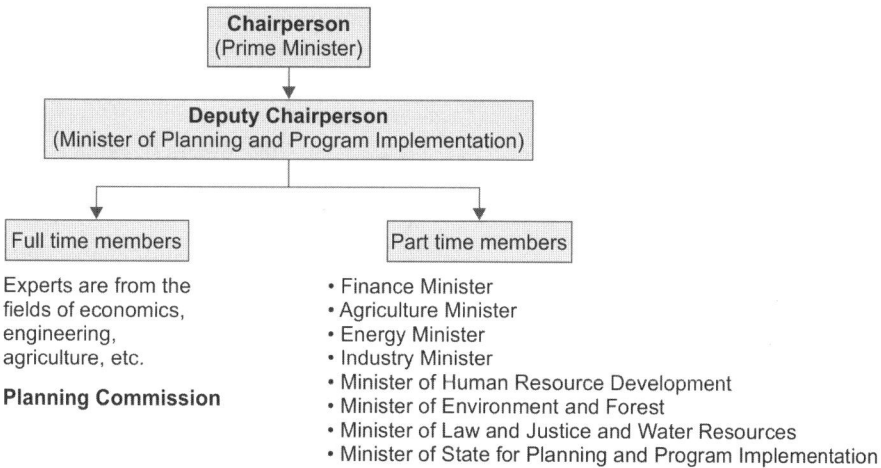

Fig. 12.3: Members of planning committee of India.

- Formulate a plan for the most effective and balanced utilization of the country's resources.
- On determination of priorities define the stages in which the plan should be carried out and propose the allocation of resources for due completion of each stage.
- Indicate the factors which are tending to retard economical development and determine the condition which in view of the current social and political situation should be established for the successful execution of the plan.

Branches of Planning Commission

- **General branches**—General branches either carry out studies related to the plan as a whole or coordinate the work of the various subject branches. There are altogether ten general branches in planning commission to name the few such as statistics and survey, resources and scientific research, information and publicity.
- **Subject branches**—Subject branches are altogether twelve in number. These are agriculture, community development and cooperation local works, irrigation and power oil and mineral village and small industries, large scale industries, transport and communication education health housing and social welfare.
- **Housekeeping branches**—The main housekeeping branches are administration and general coordination.

Advisory bodies: The staff of a planning commission includes administrators, technical officers and a complement of secretarial and other subordinate's personnel. The planning commission consists of a chairman, deputy chairman and 5 members. The planning commission works through 3 major divisions—program advisors, general secretariat and technical division which are responsible for scrutinizing and analyzing various schemes and projects to incorporated in five year plans **(Fig. 12.3)**.

Planning Commission and Five Year Plan

Planning commission also reviews from time to time the progress made in various directions and makes recommendations to the government on problems and policies relevant for the pursuit of rapid and balanced economic development. The five-year plans were conceived to rebuild rural India, recognizing health is an important contributing factor in the utilization of manpower and the uplifting of the economic conditions of the country.

NATIONAL DEVELOPMENT COUNCIL AND HEALTH (NDC)

The National Development Council was established on 6th August 1952 by the cabinet resolution on the basis of suggestions of planning commission.

The Members of NDC

National Development Council headed by the Prime Minister and Chief Minister members of the commission comprise its members but its meetings are attended by others as per requirement of the agenda items. These members from Central and State governments, eminent, economist, Governor, Reserve Bank of India.

Functions of Advisory Body

- To review the working of the national plan from time to time.
- To consider important questions of social and economic policy effecting national development.
- To recommend measures for the achievements of the aims and targets set out in the plan.

FIVE YEAR PLAN AND HEALTH

The five year plan was conceived to rebuild rural India to lay the foundations of industrial progress and secure the balanced development of all parts of the country. Recognizing health is an important contributing factor in the utilization of manpower and the uplifting of the economic conditions of the country **(Fig. 12.4)**.

Soon after Independence the country's health requirements and the type of healthcare services and delivery system, etc. were determined by holding of conferences by Prime minister with health minister in 1947, 1948 and 1950

Chapter 12: Health Planning in India

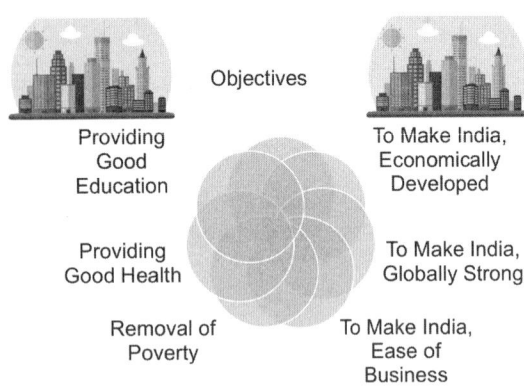

Fig. 12.4: Five year plans.

and by studying and discussing the Bhore committee report. As a result some important changes took place in the health administration of India.

In 1950, planning commission was constituted to help government to plan out integrated development plan for the entire country within the available resource for a defined period of five years for its socioeconomic progress. The government of India and the planning commission give considerable importance of health in five year plans.

Objectives of Five Year Plans

- Control or eradication of major communicable diseases, deficiency and chronic diseases.
- Development of health manpower resources.
- Improvement of environmental sanitation.
- Strengthening of basic health services through the establishment of PHCs and subcenters.
- Population control.

FIVE-YEAR PLANS IN INDIA	
Plan	Year
First Plan	1951–1956
Second Plan	1956–1961
Third Plan	1961–1966
Three Annual Plans	1966–1969
Fourth Plan	1969–1974
Fifth Plan	1974–1979
Sixth Plan	1980–1985
Seventh Plan	1985–1990
Eighth Plan	1992–1997
Ninth Plan	1997–2002
Tenth Plan	2002–2007
Eleventh Plan	2007–2012
Twelfth Plan	2012–2017

FIRST FIVE YEAR PLAN (1951–56)

The first five-year plan increase in the production of food and raw materials was the major objectives. The first five-year plan was a modest beginning towards the development of healthcare facilities. Primary health centers were established on the recommendations of the Bhore committee, albeit with significant departures both in terms of increased population coverage and decreased staff strength. The central council of health was constituted (1952).

A Seven Point Priorities of First Five Year Plan

1. Provision of water supply and sanitation.
2. Control of malaria.
3. Preventive healthcare of the rural population through health units.
4. Health services for mother and children.
5. Education and training in healthcare.
6. Self sufficiency in drugs and equipment.
7. Family planning and population control.

The National Health Programmes Introduced

- National Malaria Control Programme (1953)
- National Family Planning Programme (1953)
- National Leprosy Control Programme (1954)
- National Water Supply and Sanitation Programme (1954)
- National Filaria Control Programme (1955)
- The prevention of food and adulteration Act was passed by the Parliament in 1954.
- Contributory health service scheme was also introduced in 1954.

Objectives

- The net domestic product went up by 15%. The monsoon was good and there were relatively high crop yields, boosting exchange reserves and the per capita income, which increased by 8%.
- National income increased more than the per capita income due to rapid population growth.
- Many irrigation projects were initiated during this period, including the Bhakra Dam and Hirakud Dam.
- The World Health Organization, with the Indian government, addressed children's health and reduced infant mortality, indirectly contributing to population growth.

SECOND FIVE YEAR PLAN (1956–61)

The second five year plan was to expand existing health services to brig them within the reach of all people so as to promote progressive improvement of nation's health.

The development of health infrastructure and the implementation of national health programs initiated in the first plan continued in the second plan period. The National Malaria Control Programme was switched over to National Malaria Eradication Programme in 1958.

Institutions Established during Second Five Year Plan

- Central health education bureau (1956)
- Indian Medical Council (1956)
- Indian tuberculosis Institute (1959)

THIRD FIVE YEAR PLAN

The main objectives of the health and family planning program of the third five year plan is to expand health service to about progressive improvement in the health of the people by ensuring certain level of physical well-being and to create favorable condition for achieving greater efficiency and productivity.

Increased emphasis has laid on preventive public health services. Specific programs have been formulated in the 3rd plan for the improvement of environmental sanitation especially rural and urban water supply, control of communicable diseases, organization of institutional facilities for health services, training of medical and health personnel and provision of services such as maternal and child welfare, health education and nutrition.

Priorities

- Safe water supply in villages and sanitation especially the drainage program in the urban areas.
- Expansion of institutional facilities to promote accessibility especially in the rural areas.
- Eradication of malaria and control of various other communicable diseases.
- Family planning and other supporting services for improving health status of people.
- Development of manpower.

National Health Programs Introduced

- National Smallpox Eradication Programme-1962
- National Goiter Control Programme-1962
- District Tuberculosis Control Programme-1962
- School Health Programme-1962
- National Trachoma Control Programme-1963
- Applied Nutritional Programme-1963
- The institutions established were:
  - Central Bureau of Health Intelligence-1961
  - Central Family Planning Institute-1961
  - National Institute of communicable diseases-1963
  - National Institute of Health administration and Education-1964.

FOURTH FIVE YEAR PLAN

During the fourth five year plan, efforts were made to strengthen the primary health center complex in the rural areas for understanding preventive and curative health services and for ensuring the maintenance of the communicable diseases and eradication programs.

Objectives for Fourth Five Year Plan

- Mudaliar committee report acted as the basis for 4th five year plan.
- The objectives were to provide an effective base for health services in rural areas by strengthening the primary health services.
- Strengthening of sub-divisional and district hospitals to provide effective referral services from primary health services.
- Expansion of the medical and nursing education and training of paramedical personnel to meet the minimum technical manpower requirements.

Priorities

- Family planning program.
- Strengthening of primary health centers.
- Strengthening of subdivisional and district hospitals.
- Intensification of control programs.
- Expansion of medical and nursing education training.

Health Issued Occurred during Fourth Five Year Plan

- Chittaranjan mobile hospitals 1970.
- Postpartum family planning program 1970.
- Medical termination of pregnancy facility 1971.
- Multipurpose health workers scheme 1973.
- National program for minimum needs 1973.

FIFTH FIVE YEAR PLAN

The fifth five year plan was implemented to rebuild rural India, to lay the foundations of industrial progress and to secure the balanced development of all parts of the country. Five year plans are a mechanism to bring about uniformity in the policy formulation in programs of national importance.

The primary objective during the fifth five year plan has been to provide at least the minimum public health facilities integrated with family planning and nutritional for vulnerable groups especially children, pregnant women and feeding mothers.

The specific objectives are:
- Increasing accessibility of health services in rural areas.
- Correcting the regional imbalance.
- Further development of referral services by removing deficiencies in district and subdivisional.
- Intensification of the control and eradication of communicable diseases especially malaria and smallpox.
- Qualitative improvement in the education and training of health personnel by converting workers to multipurpose workers.
- Development of referral services by providing specialists attention to common diseases in the rural areas.

Programs Introduced during Fifth Five Year Plan

- Rural health scheme-1977
- Integrate child development scheme-1975
- Community health workers scheme-1977
- The National Malaria eradication program strategy was replaced by modified plan of operation (1977)
- 20 pointed program 1975.
- National program for prevention of blindness (1976)
- Reorientation of Medical education scheme 1977.

- Expanded program of Immunization 1978.
- A new population policy was introduced in 1976.
- The child marriage restraint Act 1978.
- National program for control of blindness was launched in 1976.

SIXTH FIVE YEAR PLAN

During the sixth five year plan the world health assembly endorsed the Declaration of "Alma Ata" or primary healthcare (1979) and Government of India adopted the goal of Health for all by 2000 AD in 1981 and accordingly revised the minimum needs program to reinforce the healthcare infrastructure.

Main Objectives

- A progressive reduction in the incidence of poverty and unemployment.
- To set up the rate of growth of Indian economy.
- Promoting policies for controlling the population growth through voluntary acceptance of small family norm.
- To improve the quality of life of people in general through a minimum needs program.

Priorities of Sixth Five Year Plan

- Rural health services.
- Control of communicable and other diseases.
- Development of rural and urban hospitals/dispensaries.
- Improvement in medical and training.
- Medical research.
- Drug control and prevention of food education.
- Population control and family welfare including MCH.
- Water supply and sanitation.

Programs Introduced

- National health policy was approved 1983.
- The international drinking water and sanitation decade was launched 1981.
- Leprosy control program was switched over to Leprosy Eradication program.
- Guinea worm eradication program introduced 1983.

SEVENTH FIVE YEAR PLAN

The guiding principles of Indian planning are provided by the basic objectives of growth, modernization, self-reliance and social justice. Within this framework, the seventh plan seeks to emphasize policies and programs which will accelerate the growth in food grains production, increasing employment opportunities and raise productivity.

Priorities

- Health Services in rural, tribal and hilly areas under minimum need program.
- Medical education and training.
- Control of emergency health problems especially I the area of noncommunicable diseases.
- MCH and family welfare.
- Medical Research.
- Safe water supply and sanitation.
- Standardization, integration and application of Indian system of medicine.

Programs Introduced

- Expanded program of immunization was converted into universal immunization program 1985.
- National Diabetes Control Programme 1987.
- National AIDS Control Programme 1987.
- The New 20 point program 1987.
- The Control of acute respiratory infection program 1990.

EIGHTH FIVE YEAR PLAN

The objective of the eighth five year plan have been formulated as par of the long-term strategy, which seeks by the year 2000 to virtually eliminate poverty, illiteracy, achieve almost full employment, secure satisfaction of the basic need of food, clothing and shelter and provide health for all.

Priorities of Eighth Five Year Plan

- Developing rural health infrastructure.
- Medical education and training.
- Control of communicable diseases.
- Strengthening of health services.
- Medical research.
- Universal immunization.
- MCH and family welfare.
- Safe water and sanitation.

Programs Introduced

- Child survival and safe motherhood program (CSSM).
- CSSM was converted into reproductive and child health program.
- Revised Rational Drug policy 1995.
- Revised TB control program 1997.
- Infant feeding and infant foods 1992.
- Rights to persons with disabilities 1995.

NINTH FIVE YEAR PLAN (1977–2002)

The ninth five year plan is unique in a way that although the plan commenced on 1st April 1997, but still the formal 9th plan document finally received all the necessary clearance and was started only on 9th February 1999.

The approach of during ninth five year plan to improve the quality of the primary healthcare to increase the accessibility and to enhance quality care in urban and rural primary health centers. The existing healthcare infrastructure at primary, secondary and tertiary care setting are to be strengthened and referral linkage improved.

Priorities

- Control communicable and non-communicable diseases.
- Efficient primary healthcare system as part of basic healthcare services to optimize accessibility and quality care.
- Strengthening and existing infrastructure.
- Improvement of referral linkages.
- Development of human resources, meeting increasing demands of nurses in specialty and super specialty areas.
- Strengthening of existing national vertical programs.
- Disaster and emergency management.
- Strengthening of health research.
- Involvement of practitioners from indigenous system of medicine.
- Intersector coordination.

Programs Introduced

- Conversion of pulse polio immunization program into intensive pulse polio immunization program (1999).
- National population policy 2000.
- National health policy 2002.

TENTH FIVE YEAR PLAN (2002–2007)

During the tenth five year plan, efforts will be further intensified to improve the health status of the population by optimizing coverage and quality of care be identifying and rectifying the critical gaps in infrastructure, manpower, equipment, essential diagnostic reagents and drugs.

The approach during the tenth five year plan will be to improve access to an enhance the quality of primary healthcare in urban and rural areas by providing an optimally functioning primary healthcare system as a part of Basic minimum services and to improve the efficiency of existing healthcare system.

Target of Tenth Five Year Plan

- Reduction of poverty ratio by 5% points by 2007, and by 15% points by 2012.
- All children in school by 2003, all children to complete 5 years of schooling by 2007.
- Reduction in gender gaps in literacy and wage rates by at least 50% by 2007.
- Reduction in the decadal rate of population growth between 2001 and 2011 to 16.2%.
- Increase in literacy rate to 75% with the plan period.
- Reduction of infant mortality rate to 45 per 1,000 live births by 2007 and to 28 by 2012.
- Reduction of maternal mortality ratio to 2 per 1,000 live births by 2007 and to 1 by 2012.
- All villages to have sustained access to potable drinking water within the plan period.

ELEVENTH FIVE YEAR PLAN (2007–2012)

The health of a nation is an essential component of development, vital to the nation's economic growth and internal stability. Assuring a minimal level of healthcare to the population is a critical constituent of the development process.

Main Goals

- Reducing Maternal Mortality Ratio (MMR) to 1 per 100 live births
- Reducing Infant Mortality Rate (IMR) to 28 per live births.
- Reducing Total Fertility Rate (TFR) to 2.1.
- Providing clean drinking water for all by 2009 and ensuring no slip-backs.
- Reducing malnutrition among children of age group 0–3 to half its present level.
- Reducing anemia among women and girls by 50%.

Thrust areas: The thrust areas to be pursued during the Eleventh Five Year Plan are summarized below:
- Improving health equity
- NRHM
- NUHMA
- Adopting a system—centric approach rather than a diseases-centric approach
- Strengthening health system through upgradation of infrastructure and Public Private Partnership.
- Converging all programs and not allowing vertical structures below district level under different programs.

Increasing Survival

- Reducing maternal mortality and improving child sex ratio through gender responsive healthcare.
- Reducing infant and child mortality through IMNCI.
- Taking full advantages of local enterprises for solving local health problems.
- Integrating AYUSH in health system.
- Training the TBAs to make them SBAs.
- Propagating low cost and indigenous technology.
- Preventing indebtedness due to expenditure on health/ protecting the poor from health insurance.
- Creating mechanisms for health insurance.
- Health insurance for the unorganized sector.

Decentralizing Governance

- Increasing the role of NGOs, and civil society.
- Creating and empowering health committees at various levels.
- Establishing e-Health.
- Adapting IT for governance.
- Increasing role of telemedicine.

Increasing Focus on Health Human Resources

- Improving medical, paramedical, nursing, and dental educational and availability.
- Re-orienting AYUSH education and utilization.
- Reintroducing licentiate course in medicine.
- Focusing on excluded/neglected areas.
- Taking care of the older persons.

- Reducing disability and integrating disabled.
- Providing kind mental health services.
- Providing oral health services.

Enhancing Efforts at Diseases

- Reversing trend of major diseases.
- Launching new initiatives (Rabies, Fluorosis, and Leptospirosis).
- Providing focus to health system and biomedical research.
- Focusing on conditions specific to our country.
- Making research accountable.
- Translating research into application for improving health.
- Understanding social determinants of health behavior, risk taking behavior, and healthcare seeking behavior.

COMMUNITY DEVELOPMENT AND HEALTH

A beginning was made in India in 1952 during the first five year plan to involve the rural population in the process of planning their own welfare measures. A program known as the community development program was launched on 2nd October 1952 for the all-round development of the rural areas, where nearly 80% of India's populations live.

Community development is a process which is designed to promote better living of the whole community with the active participation by the community itself along with governmental efforts. The community development program is India was born as part of the Nation's five year plan. This is a method to facilitate social, economic and cultural progress of the rural people though a multi-disciplinary approach of availing the manpower, material, leadership another resources of the community itself.

The community development program was to involve the rural population in the process of planning their own welfare measures. It was hailed as a program of the people, for the people, by the people to exterminate the triple enemies. Poverty, ill health and ignorance. Under this program the rural areas of the country have been organized into community development blocks, each block comprising of approximately 100 villages and a population of one lakh.

Community Development

- Community development approach is linked to the Holistic Concept of Health.
- Create a model for the wall which identifies Holistic Health using these headings:
  - Mental health
  - Physical health
  - Emotional health
  - Social health
  - Spiritual health
  - Societal health
- Ensure you give examples of what each of them mean.
- Any activity which improves any of the aspects of health outlined in your model will contribute to the promotion of health.

Activities of Community Development Program

- Interpretation of the heath needs of villages to the authorities responsible for planning and implementing the health program.
- Improvement of agriculture.
- Improvement of establishment of primary health centers and subcenters.
- Improvement of housing through self help.
- Social welfare and training in rural arts.
- Crafts and industries to local people.

PLANNING PROCESS IN COMMUNITY HEALTH NURSING

Planning is a process of making decisions in the present to affect future outcomes. The planning sets the future framework to guide the future behavior of an organization. Planning is one of the major functions of administration (**Fig. 12.5**).

Definition

Planning is a continuous process of making present entrepreneurial decisions systematically and with the best possible knowledge of their futurity, organizing systematically that effort needed to carry out these decisions and measuring the results of the decisions against expectations through systematic feedback.

Planning is a process of analyzing and understanding a system, formulating its goals and objectives assessing it capabilities, designing alternative course of actions or plans for the purpose of achieving these goals and objectives, evaluating the effectiveness of these plan, choosing the preferred plan, initiating necessary actions arrive at optical relationship between the plan and systems.

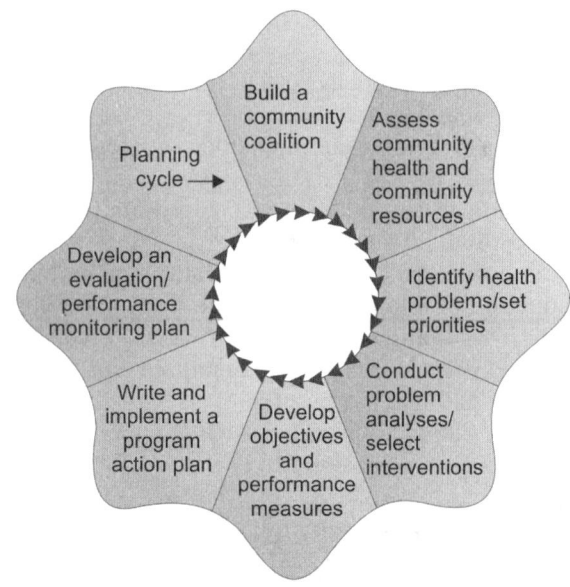

Fig. 12.5: Planning process in community health nursing.

Health Planning

- National health planning is the orderly process of defining community health problems, identifying unmet needs and surveying the resources to meet them, establishing priority goals that are realistic and feasible and projecting administrative action to accomplish the purpose of the program–WHO.
- Health planning is an aid to political and administrative authorities to decide how health services can be modernized and improved to provide affective decent healthcare to the community. The planning of community health services means the careful analysis, intelligent interpretation and orderly development of these activities, in accordance with modern knowledge, techniques and experience to meet the health needs of a nation within its resources.

Objectives of Community Health Planning

- To clarify the nature of existing health problems within the social, cultural, economic and political context.
- To clarify inter-relationships between the health sector its components and various social and economic factor.
- To identify national objectives, as far as possible, in quantifiable terms.
- To identify new and existing program areas.
- To help elaborate alternative strategies and to produce feasible programs for choice by decision-making.
- To define mechanism for the formulation and implementation of projects and to suggest procedures as a long-term goal, for a rational allocation of resource in the field of health.
- To identify program areas suitable for external assistance.

Community Health Planning Levels (Fig. 12.6)

- **Central level:** At central level authorities will laid down the directional planning often called policy making is concerned with setting to framework of an intent philosophy within which the program will function. For the health plan administrative capacity at the central level is generally vested in planning committee in the ministry of health.
- **Intermediate level:** At intermediate level authorities will lay down the administrative planning. Administrative planning is concern with overall implementation of the policies development and with the mobilization and co-operation of the personnel and material available in the administrative unit for the effectuation of the service.
- **Peripheral level:** The operational level is carried out at peripheral level. It is concerned with actual delivery of the services to the public. In general this responsibility is one of the field rather than office staff, although supervisory, consultative and administrative staffs serve in an advisory and to some extent in a controlling capacity.

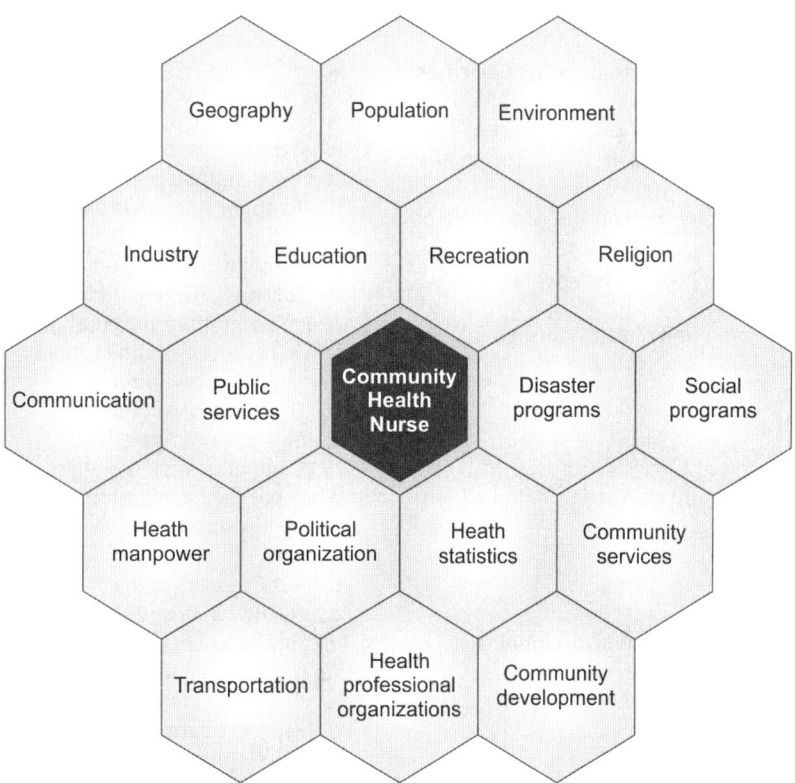

Fig. 12.6: Community health services sectors.

CONCLUSION

India has grown up in health and education sectors. Many health programs have been coordinated to precede good status of health and health organization. For this many health committees are responsible to produce different health planning according to the need of public. The National health policy also pointed out the need for establishing comprehensive primary healthcare services to reach the population in the remotest areas of the country, the need to view health and human development as a vital component of overall, integrated. Socioeconomic development, decentralized system of healthcare delivery with maximum community and individual self-reliance and participation.

BIBLIOGRAPHY

1. Gulani KK. Community Health Nursing: Principles and Practices. 1st edition Delhi: Kumar Publishing House; 2008.
2. Kumari Neelam. Essentials of Community Health Nursing, 1st Edition. Jalandhar: PV Books: Jalandhar; 2011.
3. Lucita M. Public Health and Community Health Nursing in the New Millennium. 1st edition Chennai: B.I. Publications (P) Ltd. 2006.
4. Park K. Essentials of Community Health Nursing, 4th Edition. Jabalpur: Banarasidas Bhanot Publisher; 2004.
5. Swarnkar K. Community Health Nursing, 2nd Edition. Indore: N.R. Brother; 2008.

REVIEW QUESTIONS

Long Essays

1. Define health planning. Explain the purposes, steps and objectives of health planning.
2. Define planning cycle. Explain the steps of planning cycle.
3. Define national health committees. Explain Bhore committee recommendations.
4. Enumerate national health policies. Explain the objectives of national health policy.
5. Describe planning commission of India. Explain the functions of planning commission.
6. Define planning process in community health nursing. Explain community health planning levels.

Short Essays

1. Elements of plan.
2. Cross-sectoral goals related to health.
3. Health planning steps.
4. Constrains of health planning.
5. Health planning in India.
6. Planning commission.
7. Health survey and planning committee mudaliar committee.
8. Jungalwala committee recommendations.
9. Kartar Singh committee recommendations.
10. Rural health scheme.
11. National development council and health (NDC).
12. Five Year Plan and health.
13. Community development and health.
14. Objectives of community health planning.

Short Answers

1. Health planning.
2. Policy.
3. National development planning.
4. Define national health planning.
5. Health finance.
6. Health infrastructure and human resource.
7. Health management information.
8. Branches of planning commission.
9. Functions of advisory body.
10. Objectives of five year plans.
11. Community development.

Multiple Choice Questions

1. What was the Mudaliar Committee's recommendation?
    a. To strengthen primary health centers and district hospitals
    b. To appoint separate assistants to undertake family planning duties
    c. To initiate the program of training community health workers
    d. To focus on integrated health services
2. Who chaired the committee that studied the arrangements necessary for the maintenance phase of the National Malaria Eradication Programme?
    a. Mudaliar committee
    b. Dr MS Chadah
    c. Mukerji committee
    d. Kartar Singh committee
3. What did the Mukerji committee recommend in 1965?
    a. To strengthen primary health centers and district hospitals
    b. To appoint separate assistants to undertake family planning duties
    c. To initiate the program of training community health workers
    d. To focus on integrated health services
4. What did the Central Council of Health recommend in 1966?
    a. To strengthen primary health centers and district hospitals
    b. To appoint separate assistants to undertake family planning duties
    c. To initiate the program of training community health workers
    d. To focus on integrated health services
5. Which committee talked about integrated health services for providing better health facilities in 1967?
    a. Mudaliar committee
    b. Dr MS Chadah committee
    c. Mukerji committee
    d. Committee on integration of health services
6. What was the big milestone in the field of health?
    a. Appointment of social workers to support health social work part
    b. Rural health scheme
    c. Health for all by 2000 AD.
    d. Appointment of psychiatric social workers
7. What was the focus of the Five Year Plans in health programs?
    a. Control or eradication of major communicable diseases
    b. Establishment of primary health centers and subcenters
    c. Development of health manpower resources
    d. All of the above

8. What is the Central Council of Health?
    a. A council set up by the government to provide coordinated and concerted action between the center and the state in the implementation of all the programs and measures pertaining to the health of the nation
    b. A department of the Ministry of Health and Family Welfare created in 1964
    c. An apex body in health systems at the state level
    d. A directorate that works as the principal advisor to the Union Ministry in both medical and public health matters

9. What was the need for a social worker in the health setting?
    a. To provide curative services
    b. To provide preventive services
    c. To provide rehabilitation services
    d. All of the above

10. What has professional social work in India been rooted in?
    a. The welfare approaches in India
    b. The development of health systems and families in India
    c. The health initiatives in India
    d. All of the above

ANSWERS

| 1. a | 2. b | 3. b | 4. a | 5. d | 6. c | 7. d | 8. a | 9. c | 10. d | | |

Specialized Community Health Services and Nurse's Role

LEARNING OBJECTIVES

1. Reproductive and child health (RCH)
2. National Health Mission (rural/urban)
3. Janani Shishu Suraksha Karyakaram (JSSK)
4. Emergency ambulance services
5. Government health insurance schemes
6. School health services
7. Occupational health nursing (including healthcare providers)
8. Geriatric nursing
9. Care of differently abled—Physical and mental
10. Rehabilitation nursing

TERMINOLOGY

Maternity care: Complete care of the infant, laboring and newly delivered women and her newborn also includes pre-pregnancy counseling, infertility counseling and parenting education.

Postpartum period: Period after women gives birth until her recovery six weeks later, when all of the reproductive changes, which occur over a nine month pregnancy, return to the prepregnant stage.

Labor: A process that involves a series of integrated uterine contractions that occur over time and work to propel the fetus from the birth canal relies on the uterine muscles and cervical compliance.

Family centered care: The maternity delivery system that emphasize professional quality healthcare of the total family unit, utilizes a combined nursery and postpartum nursing staff to form one mother-baby dyad.

Congenital: Refers to condition that is present at birth, regardless of cause. Congenital defects may result from a verity of cause including genetic factors, chromosomal factors, and disease affecting the mother or drugs taken by the mother, the cause of most congenital defects is unknown.

APGAR: A five part scoring system to assess newborns at one minute and five minutes after birth regarding heart rate, respiratory effort, muscle tone, reflex irritability and color.

Abortion: The termination of pregnancy by expulsion of the products of conception prior to viability, which is less than 28 weeks of gestation. The international acceptance is either 20 weeks or fetus weighing 500 gm.

Reproductive health: People live the ability to reproduce and regulate their futility, women are able to go through pregnancy and child birth safely, the outcome of pregnancies is successful in terms of maternal and infant survival and well being and couples are able to have sexual relations free of fear of pregnancy and of contracting diseases.

Maternal child health service: It refers to a package of integrated services, designed to promote the health and nutritional status of mothers and children and ensure the birth of a healthy infant to every expected mother.

School: School is defined as educational institutions groups of people pursue defined studies at defined level, receive instructions from one or more teachers frequently interact with other officers and employees such as principal, various supervisors/instructors, maintenance staffs, etc., usually household in a single building.

School health services: School health services refer to need based comprehensive services rendered to pupils, teachers and other personnel in the school to promote and protect their health, prevent and control diseases and maintain their health.

Measurement: It is the objective process of determining capacity, quality or dimension of an object, phenomenon, or outcome.

Standard: It is the desired quality, quantity or level of performance that is established as a criterion against which workers performance will be measured.

School nurse: A registered nurse charged with the healthcare of school-age children and school personal in an educational setting.

School health: It is a part of community health service through which comprehensive care of the health and well-being of children throughout the school years is taken care of.

School health program: It refers to all school activities/procedures that contribute to initiation, understanding, maintenance and improvements of the health of pupils and school personal including health services, health education and heartfelt school living.

School health team: The school health team may comprise a minimum of three members, the doctor in charge, a primary school healthcare functionary and trained teacher of the school.

School health committee: It is coordinating body that is charged with the overall responsibility of smooth functioning of the school health program. It is a committee consisting of members representing various fields of interest.

Evaluation: It is an ongoing activity that begins at the first identification of the needed for a program process throughout the planning and implementing phases and extends well beyond the length of the program itself.

Occupational health nursing: It is the application of nursing principles in conserving the health of worker in all occupations. It involves prevention, recognition and treatment of illness and injury and requires special skill and knowledge in the field of health, education and counseling, environmental health, rehabilitation and human relations.

Occupational health program: It is an intensive health program planned to take of the worker and his family program planned to take of the worker and his family to promote the general health and welfare of the worker by providing a good and safe working environment.

Occupational health nurse: Registered nurse employed in a work setting who focuses of the health and well being of people in the work place.

Occupational health: It is an art and science of conserving and promoting the health and efficiency of individuals at their work place during and throughout the course of their employment.

Ergonomics: It is the science and art of fitting the job to the work place.

Occupational accident: An injury caused by an accident to an employee in the work place.

Occupational disability: A condition in with a worker is unable to perform a job properly because of an occupational disease or a work place accident.

Occupational disease: An illness due to performing a certain job, usually from contact with disease or from performing certain action repeatedly.

Occupational medicine: Medicine that deals with the prevention, treatment and diagnosis of medical problems relating to work and to the health of worker in different types of work places and jobs.

Rehabilitation: According to WHO, Rehabilitation is combined and coordinated use of the medical, social, educational and vocational measures for training and retraining the individual to the highest possible level of functional ability.

Disability: Disability is the total lack of, or restricted, ability to perform an activity in the manner or in the range considered to be normal for human being. Disability may be temporary or permanent. It may be visual, auditory, learning, speech, musculoskeletal, mental or sexual.

Impairment: Any loss or abnormality psychological, physiological, anatomical structure or functions. For example, missing limb, paralysis after polio, mental retardation, etc.

Handicap: Disadvantage for a given individual resulting from impairment or a disability that limits or prevents the fulfillment of a role that is normal for that individual.

Accidentology: It can be defined as science, which includes all aspects of accidents. It involves types of accident, occurrence of accidents, characteristics and extent of accidents, prevention and safety measures.

Mental retardation: Mental retardation means a condition of arrested or incomplete development of mind of a person which is specially characterized by subnormal intelligence.

Hospice care: A system of comprehensive care that provides support and assistance to clients and families affected by terminal illness. Providing respectful, non-invasive care, pain symptom control and emotional, physical, physiologic and spiritual support.

Trauma: Physical injury caused by violent or disruptive action or poisonous substances.

Disability indicates: It includes incidence and prevalence of causes who are not able to perform full range of activities because of same inherited or acquired problems.

Tertiary level prevention: It includes all those measures which help in minimizing, suffering, reducing or limiting the impairments and disabilities. For example, medical rehabilitation, vocational, social, and psychological rehabilitation.

REPRODUCTIVE AND CHILD HEALTH (RCH)

Reproductive and child health (RCH) program is a comprehensive sector wide flagship program, under the umbrella of the Government of India's (GoI) National Health Mission (NHM), to deliver the RCH targets for reduction of maternal and infant mortality and total fertility rates. RCH program aims to reduce social and geographical disparities in access to and utilization of quality reproductive, maternal, newborn, child and adolescent health services. Launched in April 2005 in partnership with the State governments, RCH is consistent with Government of India's National Population Policy-2000, the National Health Policy-2001 and the Millennium Development Goals. Six key components of the

RCH program are Maternal Health, Child Health, Nutrition, Family Planning, Adolescent Health (AH) and PCPNDT.

Evolution of Maternal and Child Health Services

Mothers and children not only constitute a large group, but they are also vulnerable or special risk group. The risk is connected with child bearing in the case of women and growth, development and survival in the case of infants and children. A pregnant woman is a dyad a unit of two individuals consisting of the mother and the fetus.

Maternal child health services are directed towards mothers and children under nutrition to attain total well-being of the children within the framework of family and community. Every aspect of community health programs in India has marked effects on the health of infants and children.

Global observations show that in developed regions maternal mortality ratio averages at 30 per 100,000 live births. In developing regions the figure is 480 for the same number of live births. The problems affecting the health of mother and child are multifactorial. The present strategy is to provide mother and child health services as an integrated package of "essential healthcare".

Maternal and child health services were first organized in India in 1921 by a committee of "**The lady Chelmsford League**" which collected funds for child welfare and established demonstration services on an all India basis. Other voluntary agencies took up this work and in 1932 the Indian Red Cross Society established a maternal child welfare bureau **(Fig. 13.1)**.

- 1921—The maternal and child health services started by lady Chelmsford league.
- 1931—The maternal and child health bureau was established by Indian Red Cross Society.
- The Victoria memorial scholarship fund was established and provided to the trainees.
- It was again the Madras state which first attempted to replace dais by the better qualified personnel, such as midwives and nurse midwives.
- 1938—The maternal morbidity and mortality cause were investigated in Indian Research fund Association. Sri AL Ambedkar was the key person of this committee. Investigation revealed that the Institutional midwifery services were limited.
- 1946—The Bhore committee stated in his report that India was having the problem of high maternal and infant mortality.
- 1954—First five year plan continued. Central Drug Research Institute was started at Lucknow BCG vaccine was introduced.
- 1960—School health committee was formed.
- 1971—Medical termination of pregnancy (MTP) bill was passed by the parliament and it came into force in that year itself.
- 1975—Integrated child development scheme (CDS) was launched in India.
- 1979—A healthy child – a safe future
- 1984—Children's health – Tomorrow's wealth—WHO theme.
- 1985—Universal immunization program was launched.
- 1987—Immunization- A chance for every child—WHO theme.
- A world wide safe motherhood "campaign" was launched by the World Bank.
- 1992—Child survival and safe motherhood program (SSM) was launched on 20th August.
- Safe motherhood Initiative (SMI)
- Infant food Act 1992 came into force (Regulation of production supply and distribution)
- 1995 ICDS renamed as integrated mother and child Development Services (IMCD)
- 1996—Pulse polio immunization (PPI), the largest single day public health event took place on the 9th December 1995 and 20th January 1996.
- 1997—Family Welfare program made target free from 1st April 1996.
- Prenatal Diagnostic Techniques Act 1994 came into force from 1996. (Regulation and prevention).

Milestone in MCH Care

- 1880—Establishment of Training of Dais in Amritsar
- 1902—1st Midwifery Act to Promote Safe Delivery
- 1930—Setting up of Advisory Committee on Maternal Mortality.
- 1946—Bhore Committee Recommendation on Comprehensive and Integrated Health care
- 1952—Primary Health Center Network and Family Planning Program
- 1956—MCH Centers Become Integral Part of PHCS
- 1961—Department of Family Planning Created
- 1971—MTP Act
- 1974—Family Planning Services Incorporated in MCH Care
- 1977—Renaming Family Planning to Family Welfare
- 1978—Expanded Program on Immunization
- 1985—Universal Immunization Program
- 1992—Child Survival and Safe Motherhood Program
- 1997—RCH Program Phase-1 (15.10. 1997)
- 2005—RCH Program Phase-2 (01-04-2005)

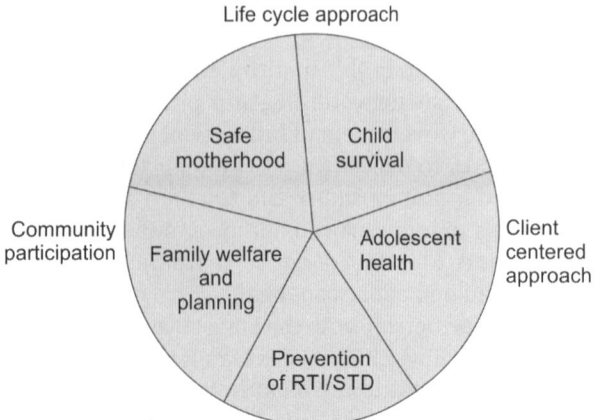

Fig. 13.1: Maternal and child health services.

Maternal and Child Health Development Stages

Maternal Stages

- **Prepregnant stage:** It refers to nonpregnant time during the mother's reproductive period. The optimum level of health of the mother prior to pregnancy is essential.
- **Pregnant stage:** It refers to antenatal/prenatal period. It begins with fertilization of mature ovum by the fusion of spermatozoa in the fallopian tube.
- **Labor and delivery stage:** It refers to intranatal period. Full term normal delivery occurs after nine months or 40 weeks.
- **Puerperium stage:** It refers to postnatal period. This period starts after the birth of child and expulsion of placenta. It lasts up to six weeks.
- **Interconception stage:** It starts after six weeks of postnatal period.

Child Health Stages

- **Early fetal stage**: It starts from first 20 weeks of pregnancy is the early period of fetal growth and development. During this period, the fetus is not capable of surviving outside the womb. It is being reported that 10% of all pregnancies get aborted spontaneously before 20 weeks of gestation.
- **Late fetal stage:** It starts from second 20 weeks is the period of late fetal development. The baby born between 28 weeks to 37 weeks is called as preterm baby. The fetus born dead after 28 weeks of gestation and weighing 1,000 gm is said to be stillborn.
- **Infancy and preschool stage:** Infancy is the period from birth to the first birthday. Infancy is the time of rapid growth and development. As the child grows, the organs also grow and mature in their functions. The preschool period extends from first birthday to fifth birthday. The child continues to grow and develop physically, mentally, emotionally and socially.

Mother and Child–One Unit

Mother and child health refers to a package of comprehensive healthcare services, which are developed to meet promotive, curative, rehabilitative needs of pregnant women before during and after delivery and of infants a preschool children from birth to five years. Components of MCH are explained in **Figure 13.2**. Various reasons for considering mothers and children, as the most vulnerable group of the society, as one unit for providing health services are as follows:

- Since conception the development of fetus (280 days) takes place in the mother's womb and receives all nutrition and oxygen from the mother.
- Healthy mother begets a healthy baby. Healthy child is closely related to maternal health.
- Certain diseases of the mother during pregnancy are likely to have their impacts upon the fetus.
- After birth, child depends upon the mother for feeding protection, love, security and prenatal and social development.

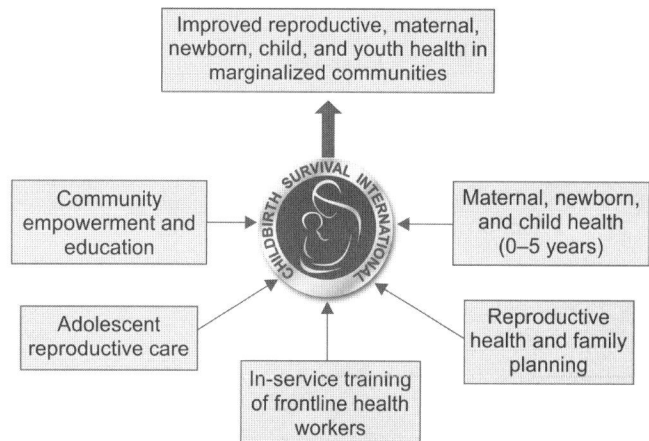

Fig. 13.2: Components MCH care.

- Child learns many self care tasks from the mother. The mother is also the first teacher of the child.

Review of Reproductive Health

Reproduction refers to the ability to reproduce is one of the properties in human being. The reproductive organs of the male and the female differ anatomically and physiologically. The female produces egg cell or ovum which is fertilized by the germ cell or spermatozoa produced by the male.

The resultant zygote embeds itself in the wall of the uterus in the female, where it grows and develops until the mature baby is born after a gestation period of 40 weeks. The function of the female reproductive system is therefore to form the ovum and if it is fertilized, to nurture it until it is born.

Female Reproductive System (Fig. 13.3)

External Genitalia

- **Labia majora:** These are the two large folds of skin which form the boundaries of the vulva. They are composed of skin fibrous tissue and fat and they contain large number of sebaceous glands in the medial layer of the folds. At puberty hair grows on the mons pubis and on the lateral aspect of the labia majora.
- **Labia minora:** These are two small folds of skin containing numerous sebaceous glands which lie between the labia majora. Anteriorly they are divided into two parts, one stretching in front of the clitoris to form the prepuce, the other passing behind it to form frenulum. The area between the labia minora is called the vestibule.
- **Clitoris:** It corresponds to the penis in the male and contains erectile tissue. It is attached to the symphysis pubis by a suspensory ligament and lies between the prepuce and frenulum.
- **Hymen:** The Hymen is a thin layer of mucous membrane which partially occludes the opening of the vagina.
- **Greater vestibular glands:** The greater vestibular glands lies in the labia majora, one on each side near the vaginal opening. They are about the size of a small pea and have ducts about 2 cm long which open into the vestibule. The glands secrete mucous which lubricates the vulva.

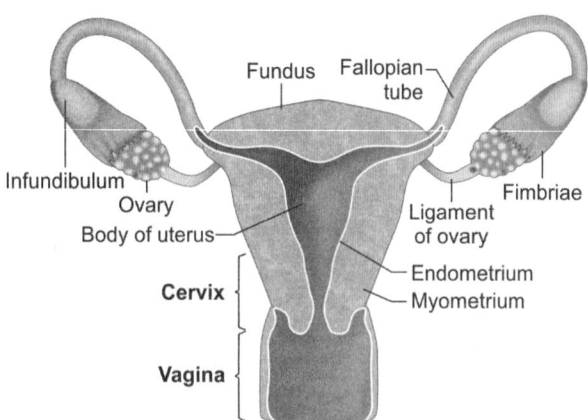

Fig. 13.3: Parts of female reproductive system.

Internal Organs

- **Vagina:** It is a fibro muscular tube connecting the internal and external organs of generation. It runs obliquely upwards and backwards at an angle of approximately 45 degree. In the adult, the anterior wall of vagina measures about 7.5 cm and the posterior wall about 9 cm. Vagina has three layers of tissue—areolar and elastic tissue, smooth muscle tissue and stratified squamous epithelium.
- **Uterus:** It is hallow muscular organ shaped like a pear which is flattened anteroposteriorly. It lies in the pelvic cavity between the urinary bladder and the rectum and its position is one of the ante version and ante flexion. The uterus is about 7.5 cm long, 5 cm wide and its walls are about 2.5 cm thick. It weighs from 30 to 40 gram. The uterus is described in three parts—the fundus, the body and cervix. The walls of the uterus are composed of three layers of tissues—Perimetrium, myometrium and endometrium.
- **Uterus supported** with surrounding organs the muscles of the pelvic floor and ligaments derived from folds peritoneum and connective tissues which suspend it from the walls of the cavity. After puberty the uterus goes through a regular cycle of changes which prepares it to receive nourish and protect a fertilized ovum. It provides the environment for the growing fetus during the 40 weeks gestation period, at the end of which the baby is born.
- **The uterine tube:** It lies one on each side of the uterus in the upper free border of the broad ligament. They are about 10 cm long and extend laterally form the wall of the uterus to penetrate the posterior wall of the broad ligament opening into the peritoneal cavity near the ovaries. They are described in three parts—the uterine, isthmus and ampulla's. The infundibulum is a dilated trumpet like portion opening into the peritoneal cavity.
- **The end of the tube has finger like projections** called fimbriae, one of which is longer than the others and is called the ovarian fimbria. The function of uterine tubes is to convey the ovum from the ovary to the uterus. Fertilization of the ovum usually takes place in the uterine tube.
- **Ovaries:** The ovaries are the female gonads or sex gland. They lie in a shallow fossa on the lateral walls on the pelvis. The size of the ovaries varies in different individuals. Their length is between 2.5 cm and 3.5 cm, their breadth is about 2 cm and they are about 1 cm thick. The ovaries are formed by two distinct layers of tissue the medulla and the cortex.

Factors Influences

- **Puberty:** It is the age at which the internal reproductive organs reach maturity. The age which the internal reproductive organs reach maturity. The age of puberty varies between 10 and 14 years and a number of physical and psychological changes take place at this time.
- **Menstrual cycle:** It includes a series of events which occur about every 28 days throughout the entire child bearing period of about 35 years. The menstrual cycle is described as having three phase—the proliferative phase 14 days the secretary phase 10 days and the menstrual phase is 4 days.
- **Menopause (climacteric):** It is the name given to the time when the processes which occur at puberty are reserved. The ovaries gradually become less responsive to the FSH ad LH from the anterior pituitary.
- **Breasts or mammary gland:** Are accessory glands of the female reproductive system. In the female the breast are quite small until puberty. Thereafter they grow and develop under the influence of estrogen and progesterone. The mammary glands consist of the following tissues such as—Glandular tissue, fibrous tissue and fatty or adipose tissue. The mammary glands are active only during pregnancy and after the birth of a baby when they produce milk.
- **Maternal and child health/Reproductive and child health services:**
    - **Maternal and child health services** are directed towards and children in order to maintain total well being of the child within the framework of the family and the community. Every aspect of community health programs in India has marked effects on the health and welfare of expectant mothers and particularly of infants and children.
- **New maternal and child healthcare** (MCH) which now also being described as reproductive and child health (RCH). Reproductive child health can be defined as a state in which "people have the ability to reproduce and regulate their fertility, women ability to reproduce and regulate their fertility; women are able to go through pregnancy and child birth safety.

Menstrual Hygiene

Menstrual cycle: Menstrual cycle refers mainly to changes in the uterus and ovaries, which recur cyclically from the tie of the menarche to the menopause. Length of cycle measured from the onset of a period of uterine bleeding to the onset of the next period of bleeding, mean cycle length is 28 days with a range of 21 to 45 days **(Fig. 13.4)**.

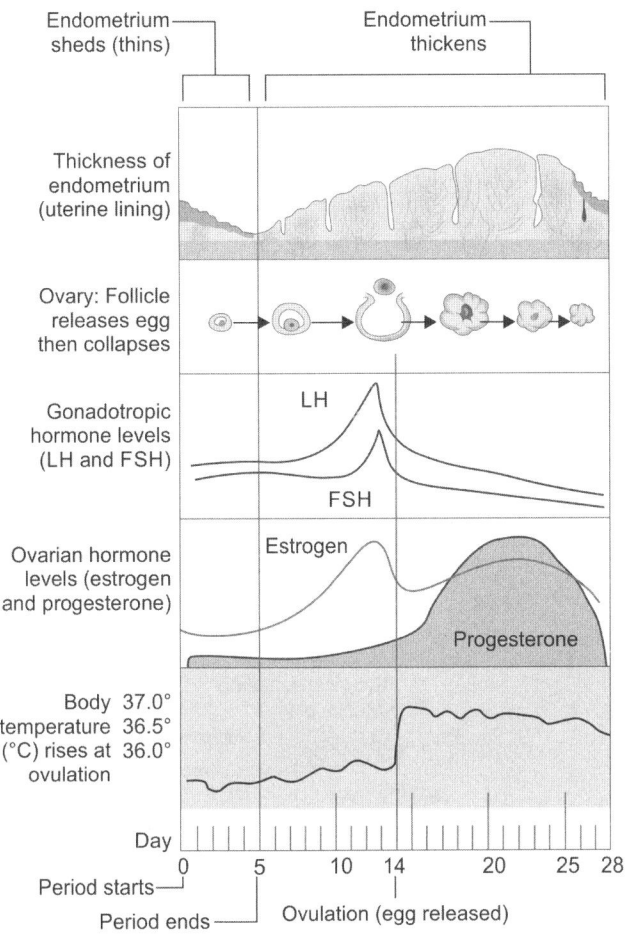

Fig. 13.4: Menstrual cycle.

Menstrual Hygiene

Menstrual hygiene is defined as "sympathetic, emotional and hygienic care given during menstruation. Menstruation is commonly called a period, menstrual flow; it consists of blood, mucus, endometrial fragments and vaginal epithelial cells. It is usually dark red and has characteristics odor and contains 60 to 150 mL of fluid. Menstrual hygiene consists of 60 to 150 mL of fluid genital area, sanitary napkins, personal hygiene diet and exercise.

- **Care of sanitary napkins:** Selection of pads should be proper size, length and quality. Pads are not usually washed after usage but they are disposed. The best method of disposal is burning.
- **Care of cotton cloths:** Use of clean cotton clothes during menstruation, wash the clothes immediately in cold water. Wash the menstrual cloth or undergarment with soap and antiseptic lotion, dry it in sun. Never use soiled pads or clothes.
- **Personal hygiene:** Menstrual fluid usually has very little odor until it contacts bacteria on the skin or in the air. Daily bathing or showering is adequate to control the odor. Bathing is done in hot water or warm water.
- **Dietary pattern:** Making dietary adjustments, starting about 14 days before a period may help some women with premenstrual syndrome. Avoid red meats, dairy products, and saturated fat and commercial junk foods. Include plenty of grains, fruits and vegetables.
- **Exercise:** Exercise is very important in maintaining good health. Vigorous exercise can cause menstrual irregularity.

Menstrual symptoms: Premonitory symptoms of menstruation such as pelvic discomfort, backache, fullness of the breasts or mastalgia occurs just before menstruation. If these premonitory symptoms are predominant, these grouped into a syndrome called "premenstrual syndrome".

Menstrual Education

Sympathetic and careful handling of the young girls experiencing first menstruation is on paramount importance.

- Menstrual hygiene should be done by the mother or teacher explaining the physiological and other associated changes during period.
- The girls should continue with their normal activities.
- The daily bath should be suspended.
- The girls should use clean sanitary napkins during menstruation which must be changed frequently.

Phases of Menstrual Cycle

- **First phase (menstrual or ischemic stage):** Characterized by shedding of spongiosum endometrium with the discharge exiting through the vagina.
- **Second phase (follicular ovary or proliferative):** Endometrium regenerates and thickness in preparation for possible implantation. At the same time, a single dominant follicle develops from a cohort of maturing follicles and approaches full maturation under influence of estradiol, which being produced by the ovarian follicles
- **Third phase and secondary (endometrium):** Begins after ovulation and is a relatively finite time period of about 12 to 14 days. Under continuing LH secretion, a temporary endocrine gland is formed (corpus luteum) from the ruptured follicle. The corpus luteum becomes nonfunctional 10 to 12 days after ovulation, progesterone and estrogen blood level drops, the negative feedback effect of estrogen of FSH ceases and the first phase begins again.

Changes in Pregnancy

Pregnancy is a normal physiologic process that affects all body systems and result in both objective and subjective changes; it is a stressful time requiring many adaptations and may lead to minor discomforts (**Fig. 13.5**).

Figure 13.6 shows the weekly changes of pregnancy.

Endocrine

- **Endocrine**—During pregnancy the chorion of the placenta secretes a hormone, hCG that maintains the corpus luteum, the continuation of progesterone and estrogen secretion from the corpus luteum maintains the pregnancy during the early weeks of development, presence of hCG hormone is an indicator of pregnancy.

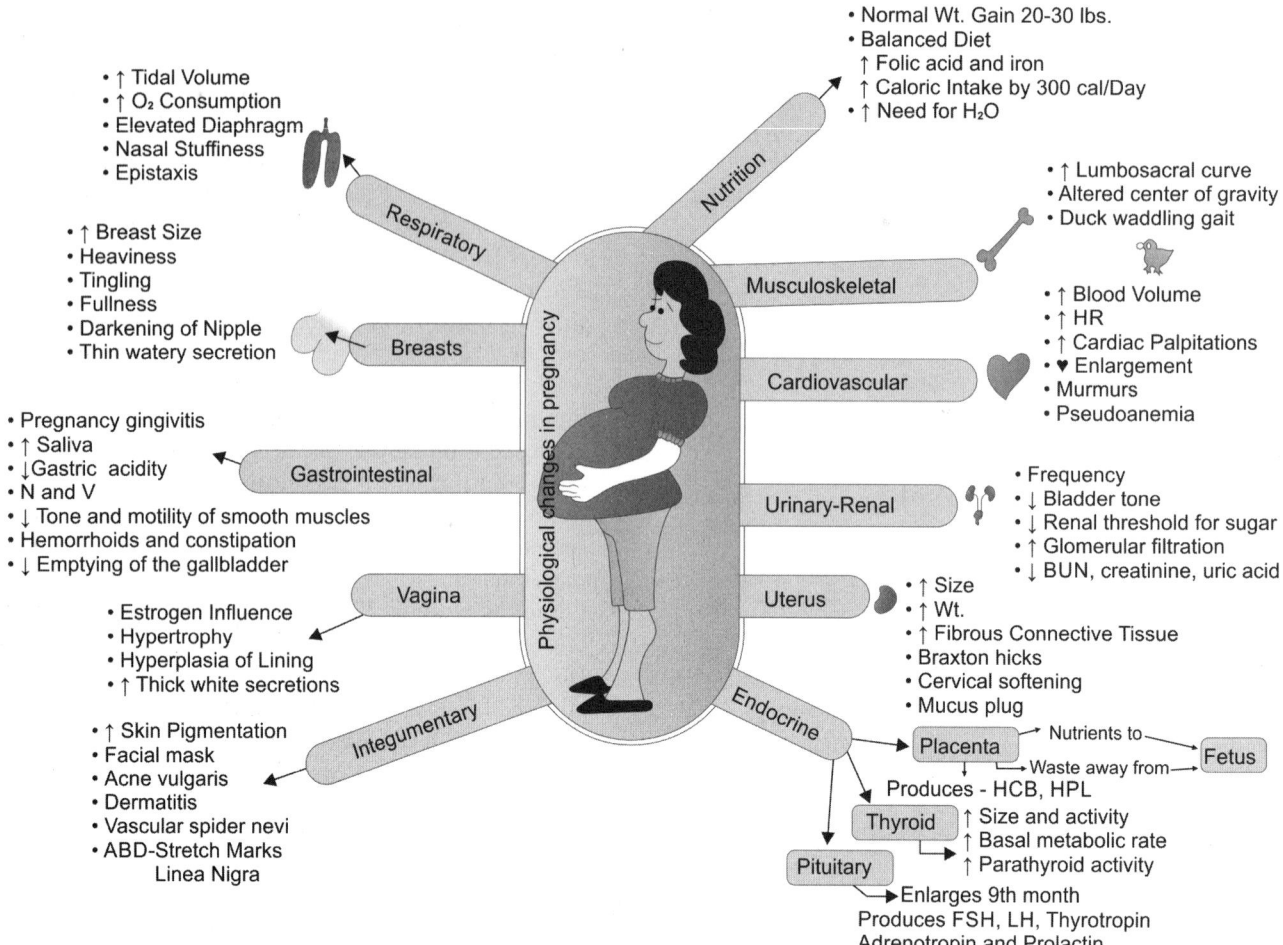

Fig. 13.5: Physiological changes during pregnancy.

Estrogen ad progesterone increase and continue to be secreted from the placenta during the last 6 months of pregnancy, progesterone acts to inhibit uterine contractions, which might occur as the result of the uterus stretching as the fetus grows. Thyroid activity is increased; human placental lactogen (hpL) is increased. Estriol levels increased.

Reproductive Changes

- **Amenorrhea occurs** because the corpus luteum persists, and ovulation is inhibited by high levels of circulating estrogen and progesterone.
- **Breast changes** such as fullness, tingling, soreness and darkness of the areolae and nipples occur along with an increase in hormonal levels.
- **Leucorrhea** is increased as hormonal levels rise, and the increased acidity is a protection from bacterial invasion.
- **Changes in the uterus** are circulatory, hormonal and related to fetal growth.
- **Goodell's sign:** Softening of the cervix
- **Hegar's sign:** Softening of lower uterine segment
- **Chadwick's sign:** Purplish hue to the cervix and vaginal mucosa.
- **Uterus** enlarges in size.
- **Changes in position of the uterus:** First trimester uterus is in pelvic cavity, second and third trimester uterus is in abdominal cavity.

Gastrointestinal Changes

- **Reduction in gastric motility** and relaxation of esophageal sphincter result from hormonal changes causing nausea and vomiting (morning sickness) and pyrosis (heart burn).
- **Elevated estrogen** levels cause excessive salivation (ptyalism).
- **Hyperemia** and softening of gums with accompanying hyperacidity of oral secretions result in non-specific gingivitis, precipitate gallstones.
- **Food craving** may occur, only significant if substance craved is unusual (pica) for example day, starch dirt.
- **Heart burn** (pyrosis) occurs because of delayed emptying time of stomach and reflex of gastric acid contents into esophagus.
- **Constipation** is caused by hypoperistalsis.

Excretory Changes

Weight of uterus on bladder in early and late pregnancy causes urinary frequency.

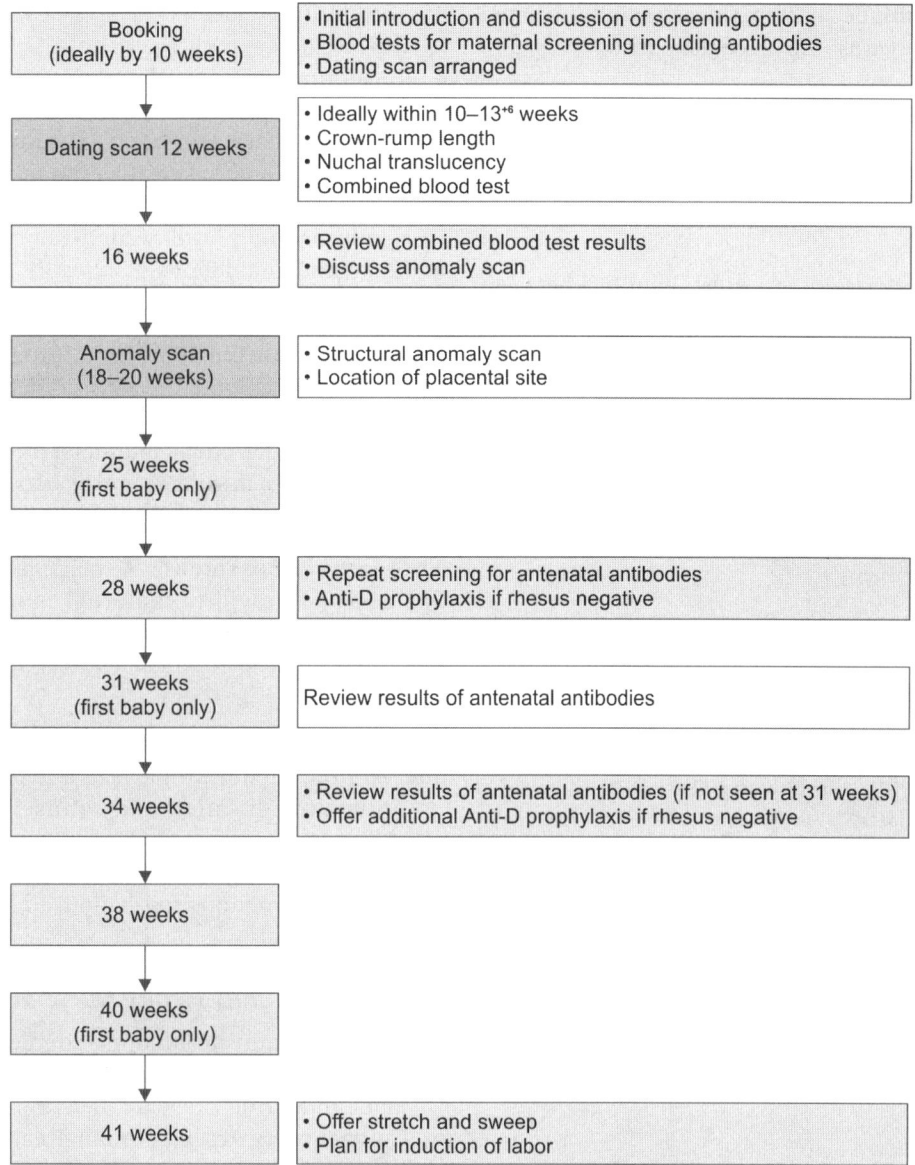

Fig. 13.6: Weekly changes of pregnancy.

- **Bladder tone** is reduced by effects of hormones on smooth muscles.
- **Asymptomatic** bacteria can occur and must be treated aggressively, if ascending infections occur they may cause premature labor.
- **Increased urinary output** results in lowered specific gravity.
- **Increased excretion** of sugar caused by lowered renal threshold.
- **Pressure** of enlarging uterus causes dilatation of right ureter and kidney.

Circulatory Changes

- **Physiologic anemia** occurs as a result of the hemodilution of the blood, there is a 45 % to 50% increase blood volume expansion, which is about 75% plasma and 25% red blood cells, the imbalance between the plasma and RBCs leads to a reduced hematocrit. Blood volume is increased to meet the needs of the mother and developing fetus.
- **Cardiac output** increases 25% to 50% peaking at 28 to 32 weeks.
- **Heart rate** increases 10 to 15 beats per minute in the latter half of pregnancy.
- **Palpation** occurs in early months from sympathetic nervous stimulation and in later months from increased thoracic pressure because of enlarged uterus.
- **Blood pressure** may drop slightly in second trimester.
- **Supine hypotension** syndrome (vena cava syndrome) in supine position weight of enlarged uterus obstructs vena cava, which decreases blood return to heart, decreased cardiac output ensures with hypotension light headedness, faintness and palpations.
- **White blood cells**, fibrinogen and other clotting factors increase.
- **Varicose veins** of legs, vulva and perianal area may occur.
- **Edema** of extremities common in the last 6 weeks of pregnancy because of stasis of blood.

- **If Thrombophlebitis** occurs heparin may be administered because it does not cross the placental barrier.

Respiratory Changes

- **Respiratory changes:** During the third trimester pressure of enlarged uterus on the diaphragm and lungs may cause dyspnea that subside when lightening occurs at about 38 weeks.
- **Oxygen consumption** is increased by about 15% between the 16th and 40th weeks, although there may be only a slight increase in vital capacity during pregnancy, tidal volume increases because of an expansion of thoracic cavity.
- **Hyperventilation** occurs because of mother's need to blow of increased CO_2 transferred to her from fetus.
- **Nasal congestion** occurs as a response to increased estrogen level.

Integumentary Changes

- **Excretion of wastes** through the skin causes diaphoresis
- **Skin changes**—darkening of the areolae, darkening patches on the face (melasma, formerly chloasma), linea alba becomes nigra of the abdomen and legs caused by skin stretching as pregnancy advances erythematous changes on the palms and face in some women.

Skeletal Changes

- **Softening** of all ligaments and joints, especially symphysis and sacroiliac joint caused by increased hormonal action of estrogens and relaxin.
- **Leg cramps** may occur from an imbalance of calcium (hypocalcemia) in the body and from pressure of the gravid uterus on nerves supplying lower extremities.

Emotional Changes

- **Ambivalence** about pregnancy and parenting
- **Acceptable of biologic** fact of pregnancy usually occurs during first trimester.
- **Acceptance** of growing fetus as distinct from self, usually occurs during second trimester.
- **Preparation for birth** usually occurs during third trimester.
- **Mood swings**
- **Increase** or decreased in sexual desire.
- **Anxiety** related to birth and adult responsibility.

Antenatal entenatal care began as a social service in Paris in 1788 for women who had committed the double inconvenience of being pregnant and destitute. Antenatal care to be provided to pregnant women to help them tide over the period of pregnancy successfully and to ensure a healthy pregnancy outcome.

Objectives

- To maintain the health and well-being of pregnant women and their fetuses through the period of pregnancy.
- To identify risk factors and apply appropriate measures of intervention as early as possible.
- To identify complications of pregnancy and institute immediate remedial measures including referral care.
- To impart health education to women on pregnancy and child birth, and to sensitize them on the desirability of family planning, fertility control and breastfeeding of family planning, fertility control and breast feeding.
- To lay the foundations of a healthy pregnancy outcome and good mother child relationship.

Antenatal examination: Examining mother to record height, weight, blood pressure and to rule out anemia, jaundice, edema, varicosities, breast tumors, nipple deformities, hydramnios, multifetal pregnancy, anteversion or retroversion of the uterus and also to observe the height of fundus and presentation, position and attitude of fetus.

Antenatal assessment: Assessing maternal risk on the basis of gravidity maternal age, maternal weight, pregnancy weight gain, previous obstetric experience and accordingly placing mothers in low risk class for appropriate management.

Antenatal care and attention: The care provided for risk intervention, anemia prophylaxis and tetanus prophylaxis.

Antenatal education and counseling provided about diet (**Fig. 13.7**), work, exercise, travel, smoking drinking, bathing, clothing, chemotherapy, family planning, breastfeeding, mental preparation, active participation and warning signals.

Role of Community Health Nurse at Antenatal

- The community health nurse should assist the parents in understanding the anatomy and physiology of pregnancy, labor and birth.
- Contact every expected mother early in pregnancy and help her to seek adequate medical supervision.
- Teach mother to monitor visual disturbances, edema of face, epigastric pain, signs of infection, burning on

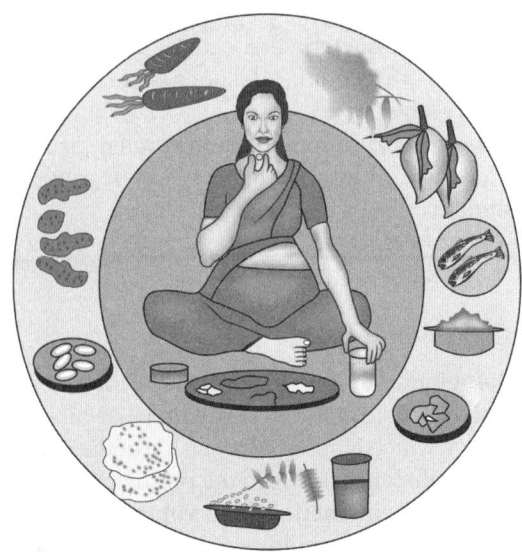

Fig. 13.7: Dietary management during pregnancy.

urination, any vaginal discharge and absence of or decrease in fetal movements after initial presence.
- Respond to mother's questions about bathing, douching, work, sex, exercise, etc.
- Help parents discuss and explore feeling related to child bearing and rearing.
- Prepare mother for physical work of labor through the use of relaxation and breathing exercises for the various phases of labor.
- Teach the mother to avoid over the counter or prescription drugs without checking with her care provider because many drugs considered harmless may be teratogenic to the developing fetus.
- Teach the mother the importance of adequate fluid intake and moderate exercise to promote circulation and prevent stasis.
- Demonstrating and teaching to mother and relatives on several aspects of maternity care.
- The community health nurse acting is a liaison between the hospital, health center, clinic and home in referring mothers to appropriate agency for safe delivery, when indicated.
- Maintaining adequate records all mother in her area and recording relevant information adequately on follow-up visits.
- Training midwives and dais and participating in training programs for nurses, midwives village health nurses (health worker F/M).

Intranatal Care

Child birth is a normal physiological process but complications may arise. The need for effective intranatal care is therefore indispensable, even if the delivery is going to be a normal one. The emphasis is on the cleanliness. It entails clean hands and finger nails, a clean surface for delivery, clean cutting and care of the cord and keeping the birth canal clean by avoiding harmful practices **(Fig. 13.8)**.

Aims of Good Intranatal Care
- Thorough asepsis
- Delivery with minimum injury to the infant and mother.
- Readiness to deal with complications such as prolonged labor, antepartum hemorrhage, convulsions, malpresentations prolapse of the cord, etc.

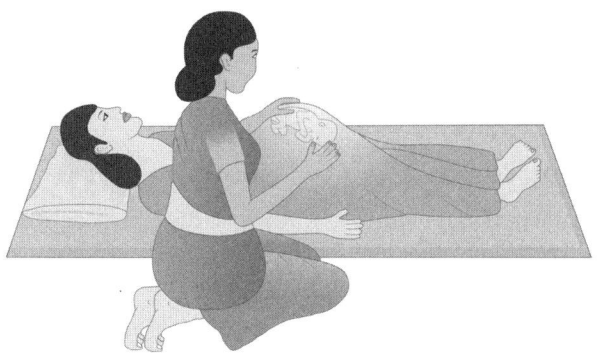

Fig. 13.8: Intranatal care.

- Care of the baby at delivery—resuscitation, care of the cord, care of the eyes, etc.

Objectives of Intranatal Care
- To maintain the health and well-being of pregnant women and their off springs during the intranatal period.
- To keep the women in labor under close observation and avoid interference with the natural process of delivery unless there is a valid reason to do so.
- To encourage and support women in labor and extend personal attention to them.
- To ensure a safe delivery; outcome in the form of healthy mothers healthy babies.

Intranatal examination:
- Examining mother to rule out any rise in temperature and blood pressure intrauterine bleeding and maternal distress.
- Examining fetuses for observing heart rate, fetal movements and color of the liquor.

Intranatal assessment: Assessing birth weight and also the apgar score of the newborn on the basis of heart rate, muscle tone respiratory effort, response to nasal stimulation and cyanosis, if any undertaking the follow-up action.

Intranatal care and attention: Provided for prevention of infection birth canal, establishment of respiration of the newborn prevention of heat loss, care of the eyes and cutting the umbilical cord.

Intranatal Education and Counseling

Provided on the desirability of colostrums feeding bonding personal hygiene, etc.

Role of the Nurse in Intranatal Care
- The community health nurse should inspect perineum for any laceration or tear watch for bleeding.
- Clean the mother, napkin, demonstrates the perineal care.
- Place the mother comfortably on the bed after delivery and provide some hot drink (coffee or tea).
- Provide the instructions to family such as watch for bleeding in the mother as well cord bleeding in baby, to give normal diet to the mother, report to the health authorities about the birth.

Postnatal Care

Care of the mother (and the newborn) after delivery is known as postnatal or postpartal care or puerperium. Puerperium is a 6 week period following birth in which the reproductive organs undergo physical and physiological changes a process called involution **(Fig. 13.9)**.

Objectives of Postpartal Care
- To prevent complications of postpartal period.
- To provide care for the rapid restoration of the mother to optimum health.
- To provide family planning services.

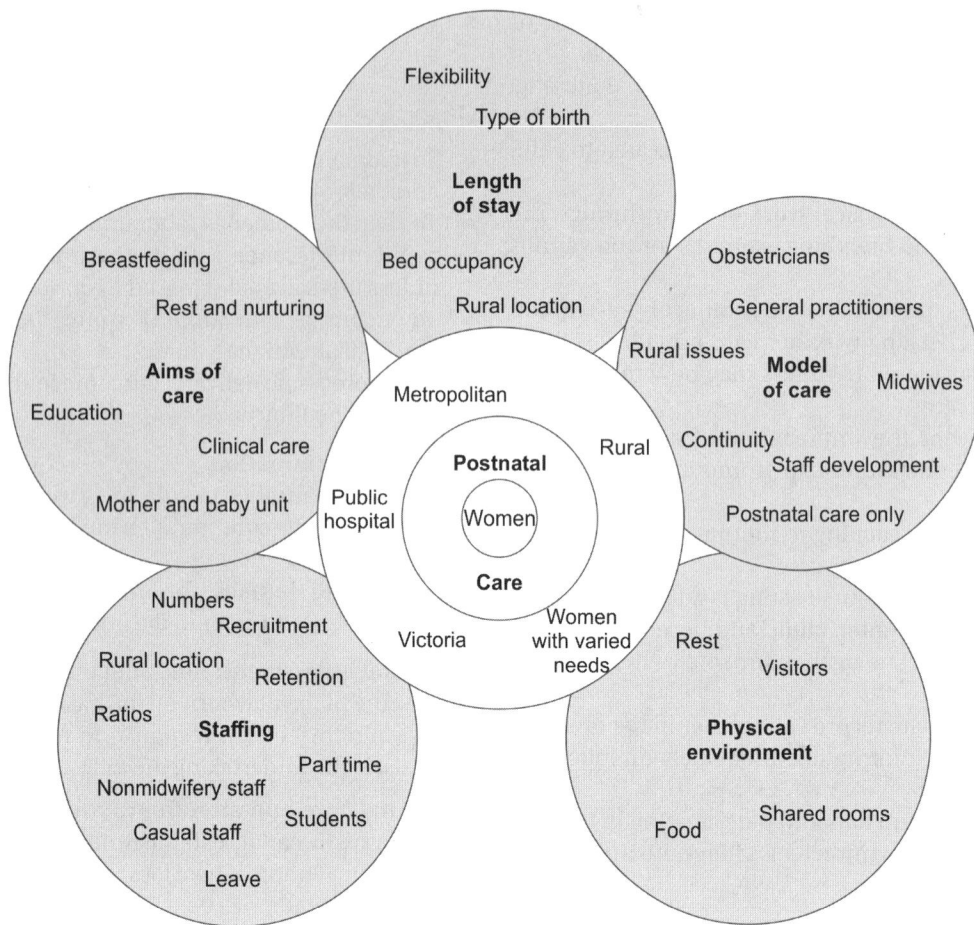

Fig. 13.9: Postnatal care.

- To check adequacy of breastfeeding.
- To provide basic health education to mother/family.

Postnatal examination: Examining postnatal mother to rule out any fever, tachycardia, laceration, and erosion of cervix, rectocele, cystocele, displacement of uterus and inflammatory swellings in the abdomen, examining the neonates to rule out birth injuries, congenital defects and low birth weight.

Postnatal assessment: Assessing weight changes of the neonates and the nature and extent of birth injuries and congenital defects. Assessing the temperature and pulse rate of the mothers.

Postnatal care and attention: Provide for the care of the perineum, care of the breast, prevention of infection, early ambulation, immunization and psychological support to mothers. Also provided for prevention of infection and care of the cord stump of newborns. Postnatal education and counseling includes breastfeeding, dietary intake, danger signals and family planning.

Complications of Postnatal Period

- **Puerperal sepsis**—This is infection of the genital tract within 3 weeks after delivery. This is accompanied by rise in temperature and pulse rate, foul smelling lochia, pain and tenderness in lower abdomen, etc. this can be prevented by attention to asepsis before and after delivery.
- **Thrombophlebitis:** This is an infection of the vein of the legs, frequently associated with varicose vein. The leg may become tender, pale and swollen.
- **Secondary hemorrhage:** Bleeding from vagina anytime from 6 hours after delivery to the end of the puerperium (6 weeks) is called secondary hemorrhage and may be due to retained placenta or membranes.
- **Others**—Urinary tract infection and mastitis, etc.

Role of Nurse in Postnatal Care

- Care during postpartum period to the mother—enquire and observe her condition generally and with reference to sleep, diet, after the pain subsides. Check vital signs, inspect perineum for discharge and inspect breast and nipples.
- Care of newborn is an interwoven activity along with the care to mother. It involves taking body temperature, checking skin, color, eyes, bowel movements, urination, watching the cry, checking the sleeping and feeding.

Neonatal Care

Neonatal period is defined as birth up to the first 28 days of life. First week (7 days) of life is called early neonatal period. Late neonatal period extends from 7th day to less than 28th day of life.

Early neonatal care is the first week of life is the most crucial period in the life of an infant. The risk of death is the greatest during the first 24–48 hours after birth.

Item	0	1	2
Appear	Totally cyanotic	Acrocyanosis (blue distally)	All pink
Pulse	None	<100	>100
Grimace bulb to nares	No reaction	Grimace	Cough, sneeze
Activity	Limp	Some flexion	Active motion
Resp	None	Weak cry	Strong cry

Objectives of early neonatal care
- Maintenance of body temperature
- Establishment and maintenance of cardiorespiratory function.
- Avoidance of infection
- Establishment of satisfactory feeding regimen.
- Early detection and treatment of congenital and acquired disorders, especially infections.

Immediate Care

- **Clearing the airway:** Establishment and maintenance of cardiorespiratory function is the most important thing the moment of baby is born. To help establish breathing, the airway should be cleared of mucus and other secretions.
- **APGAR score:** It is taken at 1 minute and again at 5 minutes after birth. It requires immediate and careful observation of the heart rate, respiration, muscle tone, reflex response and color of the infant.
  A score below 5 needs prompt action APGAR score at 5 minutes of age are subjected to a high risk of complications and death during the neonatal period.
- **Care of the cord:** Umbilical cord should be cut and tied when it has stopped pulsating. Care must be taken to prevent tetanus of the newborn by using properly sterilized instruments and cord ties. The cord should be kept dry as possible **(Fig. 13.10)**.
- **Care of the eyes:** Before the eyes are open the lid margin of the newborn should be cleaned with sterile wet swabs. One for each eye from inner to outside. Instill a drop of freshly prepared silver nitrate solution 1% to prevent gonococcal conjunctivitis.
- **Care of the skin:** First bathing may be delayed for 12–24 hours after birth to avoid cooling the body temperature.
- **Maintenance of body temperature**: Newborn has little thermal control and can lose body heat quickly. The normal body temperature of a newborn is between 36.5 to 37.5 °C. It is important that immediately after birth the child is quickly dried with a clean for skin to skin contact and breastfeeding.
- **Breastfeeding:** Breastfeeding should be initiated within an hour of birth instead of waiting several hours as is often customary. The first milk which is called "Colostrum" is the most suitable food for the baby during this early period because it contains a high concentration of protein and other nutrient the baby needs **(Fig. 13.11)**.

Neonatal Examination

- **First examination** is made soon after birth and preferably in the delivery room.
  - To ascertain in the baby has not suffered injuries during the birth process.
  - To detect malfunctions especially those requiring urgent treatment.
  - To assess maturity.
- **Second examination** should be done preferably by a pediatrician within 24 hours after birth. It is a detailed systematic examination from head to food. It includes body size, temperature, skin, cardiovascular activities neurobehavioral activities head and face, abdomen, limb and joints, spine and external genitalia.

Infant Care

Infant (1 month to 1 year) growth and development is rapid and enables maturation to unfold in a relatively short time. Health status is based on the infant's ability to adapt to these rapid changes. As a healthcare providers, the nurse must have an understanding of these changes to ensure the infant his or her family maintain an optimal health.

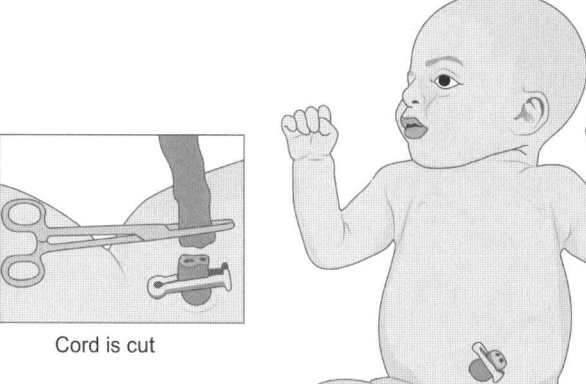

Fig. 13.10: Cord cutting technique.

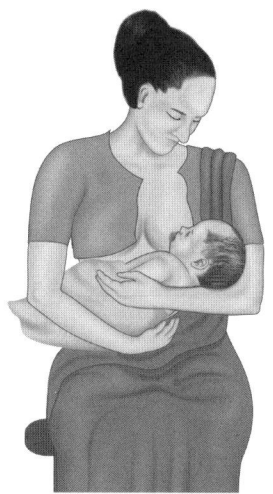
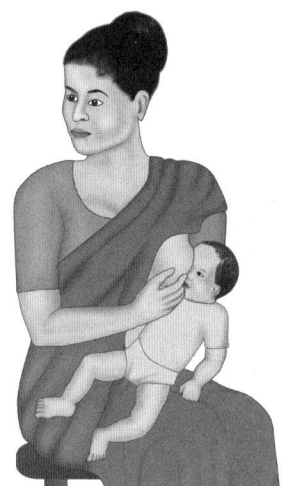

Fig. 13.11: Breastfeeding technique.

Physiological Developments

- **Height and weight:** Height increases during the first 6 months by approximately 1inch per month. The rate of growth in height slows to approximately 0.5 inches per month by 12 months of age. The weight gains 1.5. ib per month or 5–7 oz per week. By 12 months of age, the infant's birth weight will have tripled. Checking height (anthropometric measurement) is depicted in **Figure 13.12**.
- **Head growth:** The size of the head changes rapidly during infancy, reflecting rapid brain growth. By the age of 12 months the infant's brain will be two thirds the size of a adult brain. During first 6 months, the head circumference will increase by approximately 0.5 inches per month.
- **Motor development:** Motor development is related to physical, cognitive and social development, which provides the infant with the means and freedom to explore the environment. Gross motor development is the ability to use large muscle groups to maintain balance and postural control or locomotion. Fine motor development is the ability to coordinate hand eye movement in an orderly and progressive manner.
- **Health screening:** Health screening provides the opportunity to assess for detect any problems the infant may have and includes test to detect phenylketonuria (PKU), iron deficiency anemia, lead poisoning and hypothyroidism. The infant's health screening actually begins immediately after birth with the first APGAR scoring and physical examination. The screening visits typically include health assessment, physical examination, growth indicators, anticipatory guidance, parental concerns and administration of scheduled immunizations.

A Role of a Nurse in Infant Care

- **The community health nurse** can be instrumental in providing information related to development, nutrition, elimination, hygiene, safety, immunization **(Fig. 13.13)** and play. The nurse should provide information about possible reactions the infant might experience after receiving the immunizations.
- **Feeding of infants:** A child who is breastfed has greater chances of survival than a child artificially fed. Prolonged breastfeeding does protect the infant from early malnutrition and some infections. Artificial feeding given the babies suffers with prolonged illness or death of the mother.
- **Weaning** is not sudden withdrawal of child from the breastfed. It is a gradual process starting around the age of 4–5 months because the mother's milk alone is not sufficient to sustain growth beyond 4–5 months. It should be supplemented by suitable foods rich in protein and other nutrients. The community health nurse should clearly explain to the mother and family.

Care of Under Fives

Rights of the child: To meet the special need of the child the general assembly of the United Nations adopted on 20th November 1959, the declaration of the Rights of the child. India was a signatory to this declaration.

- Right to develop in an atmosphere of affection and security and whenever possible in the care and under the responsibility of his/her parents.
- Right to enjoy the benefits of social security including nutrition, housing and medical care.
- Right to free education.
- Right to full opportunity for play and recreation.
- Right to a name and nationality.
- Right to special care if handicapped.
- Right to be among the first to receive protection and relief in times of disaster.
- Right to learn to be a useful member of society and to develop in a healthy and normal manner and in conditions of freedom and dignity.
- Right to bring up in a spirit of understanding brotherhood.
- Right to enjoy these rights, regardless of race, color sex, religion, social and national origin.

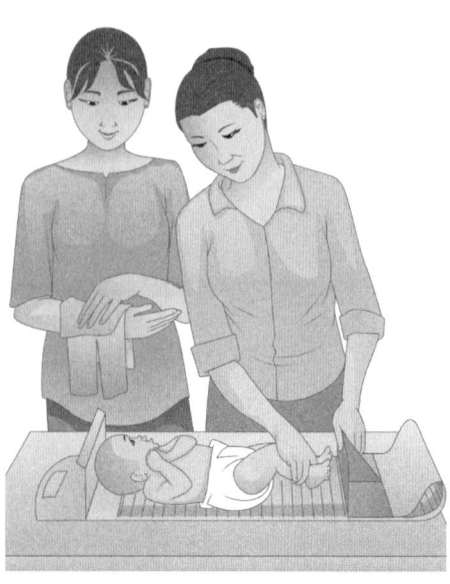

Fig. 13.12: Checking height (anthropometric measurement).

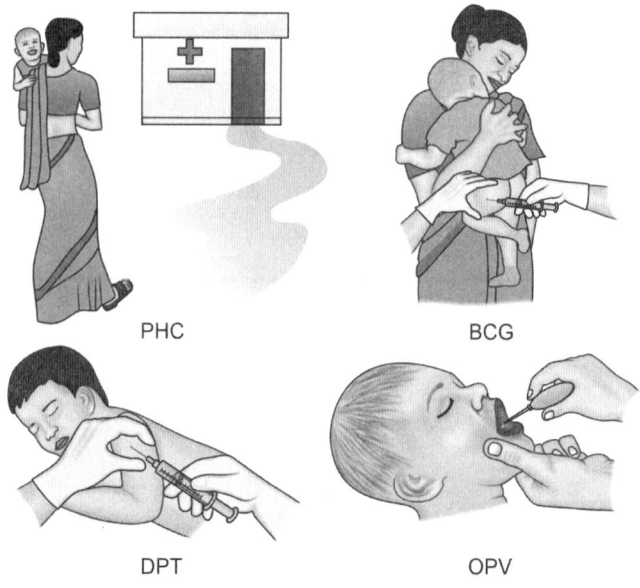

Fig. 13.13: Administration of vaccination for infant.

Under Five's Clinic

The under five's clinic or well baby clinics combines the concepts of prevention, treatment, health supervision, nutritional surveillance and education into a system of comprehensive healthcare within the resources available in the country, making use of non-professional auxiliaries, thus making the service not only economical but also available to a larger proportion of children in the community. Under five clinics must provide for courteous reception of mother and children, with enthusiasm and zeal on the part of each member of the team.

Aims of Under Five Clinics (Fig. 13.14)

- **Care in illness:** The basic philosophy of the "under five's" clinic to give nurses effective training and responsibility for handling the child healthcare service. The illness care for children will comprise of diagnosis and treatment, X-ray and laboratory services and referral services.
- **Preventive care:** The preventive care gives on the bases of immunization, nutritional surveillance, health checkups, oral rehydration, family planning and health education.
- **Growth monitoring:** For under five clinic to weigh the child periodically at monthly intervals during the first year, every 2 months during the second year and every 3 months thereafter up to the age of 5 to 6 years. The growth curve will help the health worker to detect early onset of growth failure.

Objectives of Under Five Clinics

- The prevention of malnutrition, pertussis, tuberculosis, poliomyelitis, diphtheria, tetanus and measles.
- The supervision of the health of all children upon the age of five.
- The education of parents to promote health and family planning.
- The provision of simple treatment for diarrhea, with or without dehydration, pneumonia, skin conditions and other common disorders.

Role of a Nurse in Under Five's Clinic

- Treating minor illness
- Referring the more seriously ill children.
- Instructing about feeding, nutrition and hygiene.
- Encouraging child spacing and family planning.
- Maintaining the children's weight cards, e.g., road to good health cards.
- Being alert in every in which the effectiveness of the service can be improved.

Physical Facilities for a Children's Clinic

- Outside compound—playground for children waiting to be served including swings slides and sand box are needed. These facilities may be provided by the community volunteer group or by the health committee.
- Waiting room should include a reception table and the record. The area should include child health posters, display exhibits and plays are for the children.
- Weighing and measuring should be provided in a separate area if possible or it may be part of the waiting room.
- Isolation area for children with signs and symptoms of illness is essential for every child health clinic.

Growth Monitoring

The growth chart or 'road to health 'chart' first designed by David Morley and later modified by WHO. It is visible display of the child's physical growth and development. It is designed primarily for the longitudinal follow-up of a child.

Uses of Growth Chart

- Growth monitoring which is of great value in child healthcare.
- It is used as diagnostic tool for identifying "high risk children"
- It helps planning and policy making in relation to child healthcare at the local and central levels.
- Educational tool for the mother to participate more actively in growth monitoring.
- It helps the health worker on the type of intervention that is needed. It will help to make referrals easier.
- It provides a good method to evaluate the impact of a program or of special interventions for improving child growth and development.
- It is used as tool for teaching for example, the importance of adequate feeding.

Alternative Methods of Growth Monitoring

The growth chart or road to health chart is described as a passport to child healthcare. The Road to health chart helps to identify "at a glance". It also provided on the card to record important events such as immunization, birth history and if any treatment given.

Growth charting is only one method of growth monitoring; there are other indications such as height for age, weight for height and arm circumference.

Child Health Problems

- **Low birth weight:** International agreement low birth weight has been defined as a birth weight of less than

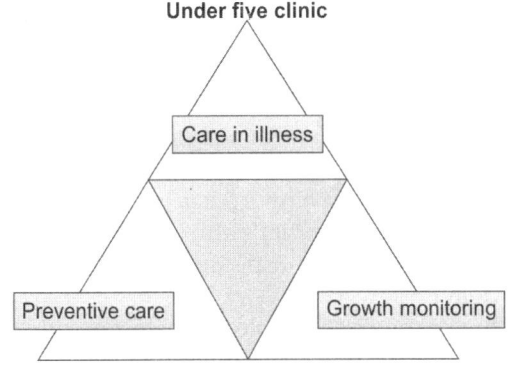

Fig. 13.14: Symbol of under five clinic.

2.5 kg the measurement being taken preferably within the first hour of life, before significant postnatal weight loss has occurred. There are two main groups of low birth weight babies those born prematurely (short gestation) and those with fetal growth retardation.

- **Malnutrition:** Malnutrition makes the child more susceptible to infection. Undernourished children do not grow to their full potential of physical and mental abilities. Malnutrition in infancy and childhood leads to stunted growth. Micronutrient malnutrition refers to a group of condition caused by deficiency of essential vitamins and minerals.
- **Infectious and parasitic disease:** The leading childhood diseases are diarrhea, respiratory infections, measles, pertussis, polio, neonatal tetanus, tuberculosis and diphtheria. Parasitic diseases such as eruptive fevers, poliomyelitis, malaria, intestinal parasites such as ascariasis, hook worm giardiasis and amoebiasis, etc. which are common because of poor environmental sanitation and paucity of portable drinking water.
- **Accidents and poisoning:** Children and young adolescents are particularly vulnerable to domestic accidents—including falls, burns, poisoning and drowning. Accidents among children are home accidents and traffic accidents.
- **Other factors affecting child health:** Child health is affected by various factors—behavioral problems, maternal health, family environment, socioeconomic circumstances, environment and social support and healthcare.

Breastfeeding

Breast milk is the most desirable method of feeding an infant. Breast milk is the natural food which a mother produces soon after her baby is born. It is the best milk for the baby and uniquely suited to the nutritional need for the newborn and the young infant. A rural Indian mother usually produces about 600 mL of milk per day during the first months, equal to the amount same as four glasses of milk. As child grows older the production of milk reduces in the mother, viz. 600 mL or 200 ounces (1–2 years), and 425 mL or 14 ounces (2 to 3 years).

- Start immediately after birth even before the placenta is out.
- Encourage "Baby friendly policy" in all the institutional deliveries.
- Feed on demand during the day as well as at night.
- Exclusive breastfeeding up to six months.
- Feed should be given every 2–3 hours at least 7 times per day.
- Do not stop breastfeeding if the baby or the mother is sick.
- Record birth weight immediately after birth.
- For home deliveries birth weight should be taken within 48 hours.

Main advantages of breast milk are as follows:
- It is a safe, clean, hygienic, cheap and ready for use and at body temperature.

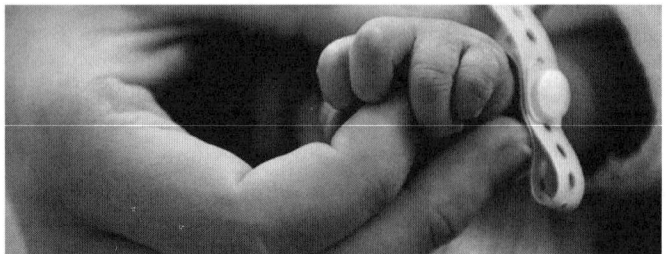

Fig. 13.15: Maternal and child health bond.

- It provides full nutritional requirement and promotes optimal growth.
- It helps in building up a strong psycho-emotional bond **(Fig. 13.15)** between the mother and the child which brings a great deal of satisfaction and happiness to both.
- It is usually supplied in enough quantity, more so by the mother has good diet and is well prepared during the prenatal period for breastfeeding.
- The anti-infective qualities of breast milk make it especially valuable in reducing the risk of illness in the baby.
- It is believed to give some degree of protection against a new conception occurring during a short period after delivery.

The mothers breasts secrete a yellowish fluid, during first two days after child is born, called "colostrums." It is very Food for the child. It contains a very high concentration of agents which protects the baby from infections and also contains many nutrients and plenty of vitamins A.

Breastfeeding is essential because it reduces gastrointestinal diseases to a minimum and during the first three months, provides complete requirements for the baby. It is not contraindicated, if not only on exceptional circumstances, such or when mother is seriously ill or no production of milk in the mother's breast.

All mothers should be encouraged to breastfeed their infants. The average baby likes to feed every three hours up to the age of two months and the every four hours. Underweight babies may be fed every two to three hours. Babies should be fed when hungry and not necessarily be kept on a strict feeding schedule. But allow an interval of at least six hours, fix rest during night. And the length of time for every feeding 5–10 minutes at each breast. After feeding, mother should burp the infant.

Procedures for Breastfeeding

- Make mother comfortable in a sitting position **(Fig. 13.16)**.
- Wash hands, mothers and attendant, needs.
- Clean one breast with moistened cotton ball starting with the nipple and wiping outward in a circular motion.
- Put the baby on the mother's arm (which may be resting or a pillow) with baby's head slightly higher than the rest of his body).
- Raise breast and direct nipple into baby's mouth.
- When she nurses (feeds) for 5 minutes, change baby to other breast.

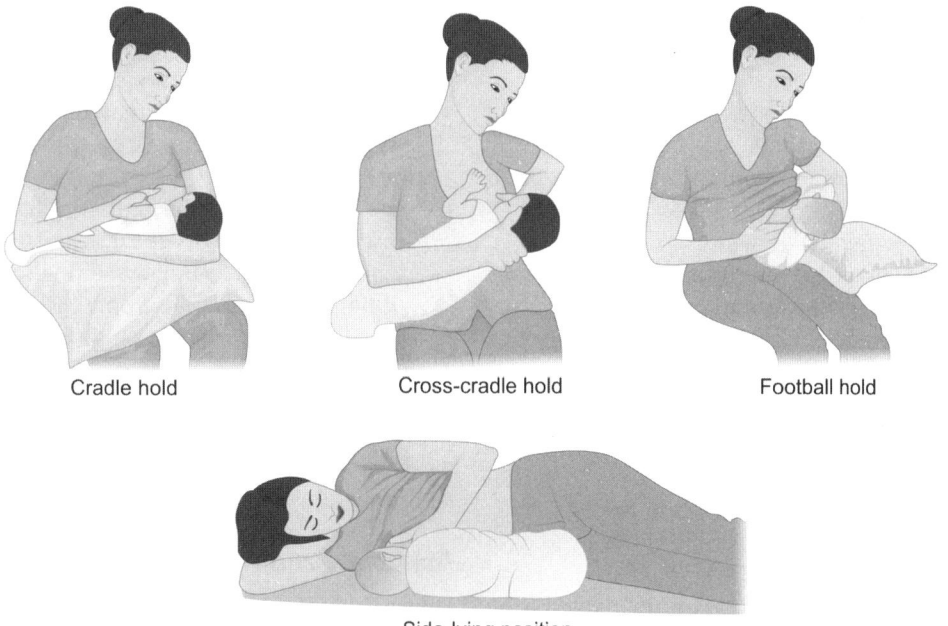

Fig. 13.16: Breastfeeding techniques and position.

- Repeat the same procedures for this breast.
- Remove baby from the breast where he has been nurse for ten minutes.
- Cleanse the mother's nipple with moistened cotton balls using a separate cotton ball for each breast.
- Hold the baby over left shoulder and pat him gently on the back to relaxe any air bubbles.

Nurse has to Take Certain Steps to Increase the Breast Milk of a Mother

- Encourage mother to have three substantial meals each day which are adequate in protein and vitamins A and B.
- Encourage minimum fluid intake into 1.5 liters daily.
- Reassure the mother, tell her that she has the ability to breastfeed her baby and help her to reduce any feelings of anxiety.
- Encourage the mother to change to more frequent feedings, as more frequent feedings will increase the total supply of breast milk.
- Recommend more rest and sleep.
- Advise manual expression for five minutes after each feeding to give extra-stimulation to the breast. Ask her to use following method:
  - Lift the breast by placing the fingers of the right hand under it and thumb above, grasping the outer border of the primary areola (darkened ring around nipple).
  - With a deep inward compressing movement squeeze the reservoir about thirty times per minutes, moving the areola but not the fingers. Avoid touching the nipples, the milk should flow from the breast in a steady stream, collect in a cup or bowl.

And the community health nurse has got the responsibility to teach the mother for procedure for breast care as follows:

Instruct the mother to prevent cracked nipples after birth of her baby by:
- Not allowing the baby to suck for longer than three to five minutes every three hours during the first two days after birth.
- Ensuring that the baby has "fixed" properly on the areola behind the nipple to avoid bruising the nipple with his gums.
- Not pulling the baby off the breast when he has finished sucking, instead press the baby's cheeks and depress his lower jaw to avoid trauma to the nipple, or lift the outer border of his upper lip to break the suction.
- Drying the nipples thoroughly after each feeding.
- Not allowing the baby to sleep at the breast.

Instruct mother to treat tender or cracked nipples by:
- Taking baby off the breast for 24 hours and manually expressing the breast milk into a sterile cup and feeding milk to baby with a tea spoon.
- Using a nipple shield for 28–72 hours if nipple is cracked.
- Applying one drop of gentian violet 1% to the cracked nipple twice daily.

Ten steps to successful breastfeeding:
Every facility providing maternity services and care for newborn infants should:
1. Have a written breastfeeding policy that is routinely communicated to all healthcare staff.
2. Train all healthcare staff in skills necessary to implement this policy.
3. Inform all pregnant women about the benefits and management of breastfeeding.
4. Help mothers initiate breastfeeding within half an hour of birth.

5. Show mothers how to breastfeed and how to maintain lactation even if they should be separate from their infants.
6. Give newborn infants no food or drink other than breast milk, unless medically indicated.
7. Practice rooming-in-allow mothers and infants to remain together-24 hours.
8. Encourage breastfeeding on demand.
9. Give no artificial teats or pacifiers (also called dummies or soothers) to breastfeeding infants.
10. Foster the establishment of breastfeeding support groups and refer mothers to them on discharge from the hospital or clinic.

Principles of Breastfeeding

- Breastfeeding should be initiated within the first half-hour after birth, and should not be unduly delayed as is often customary.
- Colostrums is the most suitable food for the baby during the first few days after birth because it contains a high concentration of nutrients and anti-infective substances. The baby should not be deprived of it because of customs, traditions and ignorance.
- The baby should be allowed to suckle from both the breasts during each feeding—starting with 3 minutes on each breast and gradually increasing the time.
- It is desirable to feed the baby "on demand", it helps the baby to gain weight. It is neither necessary nor desirable to train a baby to "feed by the clock".
- The intervals between feeds vary between 1 to 4 hours. Babies have different rhythms of feeding. Every child develops its own demand for feeding.
- An interval of 6 hours during night should be encouraged. This rest at night is important both for the mother and baby.
- The mother should be taught to give the baby a full feed so that her breasts are emptied.
- The mother should be instructed to feed the baby even when the child is ill.
- A baby should be fed for as long as possible—at least for one year.
- When the baby is 4 to 6 months old, breast milk alone will not be sufficient to sustain growth. Additional foods should be given (supplementary feeding).
- Weigh the child every month and plot the weight on a growth chart. This is known as "growth monitoring". With adequate nutrition, the child's weight will continue to increase within the 2 reference curves.

Problems in Breastfeeding

- Emotional worry, shock or anxiety can stop the flow of milk. Emotional problems can interfere with the "let down" reflex.
- Flat nipples: most common in women who are having their first baby. Teach the mother to squeeze her nipples and pull them gently. She should do this for several minutes every day.
- Engorged (swollen) breasts
- Sometimes a mother's breasts make more milk than her baby needs. Prevent and treat this condition by emptying the breasts regularly.
- Sore or cracked nipples: This may happen when the baby sucks very hard. Sometimes the soreness may develop into a crack. To prevent sore nipples, keep the skin soft by rubbing the areola and nipple with an antiseptic cream.
- Painful tender breasts this may be due to infection. It calls for appropriate treatment with antibiotics.
- The baby may have a blocked nose and be unable to suck properly.
- The baby may be having respiratory infection.
- Congenital defects such as hare-lip or cleft palate.

Artificial Feeding

How to identify that Breast Milk is not enough for the infant?
- No weight gain or stationary weight.
- Cries soon after feeding.
- Constipation.
- Often falls sick.

What is the Solution for Insufficient Breast Milk?
The solution depends on the age of the infant.
- If it occurs within 3 months, start on artificial milk or formula feeds.
- After 3 months, give artificial milk and/or semisolids / solid diet.

Types of Milk

- Cow's milk.
- Milk powder (Dried whole milk)—the fat content of fluid is adjusted to 3.5% and the milk is evaporated with extreme rapidity to powder from by spray, freeze; or roller drying.
- Condensed milk—contains 60% carbohydrates, low in protein, useful in short-term feeding when a high caloric diet is desired.
- Acid milk—prepared by adding lactic acid or lime drop by drop, when milk is boiled and in the process of cooling.
- Skimmed milk.

Quantity of Formula

The quantity of formula depends upon the individuals' child, and varies on different days and at different times.

Dilution: Depends upon the source and age of the infants.
Disadvantages of artificial feeding
- **Contamination:** Artificial needs are often contaminated with bacteria, especially if the mother uses a feeding bottle which she does not clean and boil properly.
- Animal milk does not contain living white cells and antibodies to protect the baby against infections. Artificially-fed babies fall ill more often with diarrhea and respiratory infections.

Age of infant	Artificial feeding	Frequency
0–2 weeks	Cow's milk dilution 1:1	3 hourly
2–4 weeks	2:1 (2 parts of milk to 1 part of water)	3 hourly
1–3 months	3:1	4 hourly (If the baby demands 3 hourly needs to be adjusted)
3–6 months	Undiluted cows milk	4 hourly

- Animal milk may not contain enough vitamins for a baby.
- The iron from animal milk is not absorbed as completely as the iron from human milk.
- An artificially-fed baby may develop anemia.
- Animal milk contains too much salt, which may result fri fits. Animal milk also contains excessive calcium and phosphates, which may cause tetany, i.e., twitching.
- Animal milk contains more saturated fatty acids and does not contain enough for the essential fatty acids, which are vital for proper growth and development.
- Animal milk contains too much casein, which is difficult for a baby's immature kidneys to excrete.
- Animal milk is more difficult to digest, as it does not contain the enzyme lipase, which helps digest the fat.
- Babies fed on animal milk may develop allergies.
- Animal milk is expensive and the family might not be able to afford it. Any supplement started before the baby is four months of age increases the risk of infection and even death.

Supplementary Feeding

The supplementary feeding also should be encouraged in the third or fourth month, and when this is done, care should be taken in the preparation of the food for the baby because of the danger of infection through contaminated foodstuffs, water and utensils. Same care should be taken in artificial feeding if it is necessary.

Infancy is a crucial period of rapid growth and development. Since infants grow very fast, they require extra-energy, which necessitates substantial increase in nutritional needs. In the past, the well neonate was not fed until 4 to 12 hours, after birth to allow for adjustment to extrauterine life. Now early feedings are standard for the well-full term infant, for the following reasons:

- During the first period of reactivity, the neonate is alert and eager to feed, making this an ideal time to start breastfeeding.
- Early feeding stimulates early passage of meconium which reduces enterohepatic circulation and later bilirubin elevations.
- Early ingestion of colostrums coats the gastrointestinal tract with secretory IgE and other immune factors which may give protection against gastroenteritis.
- In infants gastrointestinal tract is also colonized with friendly organisms, allowing less opportunity for pathogens to proliferate.
- Early feedings may lessen the chance of hypoglycemia, because the act of feeding stimulates glycogen secretion and therefore glycolysis.

Supplying essential nutrients to an infant is done primarily through breastfeeding. Breast milk is recommended by many health professionals as the preferred and method of feeding and infant in the first six months of life. The requirements of the infants are divided into 2 stages, i.e., 0–6 months and 6–12 months. The requirement of the energy (kcal), iron and vitamin B are expressed in terms of Kg. The following table will show the RDI of Indian infants (ICMR 1990).

The nurse has to calculate the energy for protein requirement as follows. First find out the age of the infant (in months) and expected body weight of the infant at that particular age. Having base on the age and expected weight of the infant calculate the nutrient need for the particular infant by using RDI. For example, an infant aged 5 months and expected weight 6 kg, requires energy and protein as follows:

Total energy requirement = RDI for energy × Expected weight = $108 \times 6 = 648$ kcal.

Total protein requirement = RDI for protein × Expected weight = $2.05 \times 6 = 12.3$ grams.

Always use the expected body weight of an infant at that particular age to calculate energy or protein needs and advise the locally available protein resources and their preparation according to age of the child.

Weaning

As stated earlier, weaning is a process of gradual and progressive transfer of the baby from breast milk to the family diet. It does not mean discontinuing to breastfeeding.

A baby can be successfully weaned when it can grasp with both hands, reach and sit well. Babies often lose interest in breastfeeding after 7 to 8 months. Others will continue longer. Weaning is not sudden withdrawal of child from the breast. It is gradual process starting around the age of 4–5 months, because the mother's milk alone is not sufficient to sustain growth beyond 4–5 months.

Depending on the age of the infant, liquid, semisolid or solid supplement can be served to the infant as follows:

Birth to 12 months (only weight)		Preschool children (weight and height)	
Age height (cm)	Weight (kg)	Age	Weight (kg)
At birth	3 kg	1 year	9	74
2 months	5 kg	2 years	11	84
5 months	6 kg	3 years	13.5	93
8 months	8 kg	4 years	15	100
10 months	8.5 kg	5 years	17	106
12 months	9 kg			

It should be supplemented by suitable foods rich in protein and other nutrients. These are called "supplementary foods." Supplementary feeding is gradual process which begins from the moment other foods (like liquid. semisolid or solid food preparation) are started and continues till the time the child is completely taken off the breast about 12 months to 18 months.

At 4–6 months, juices, soups or other milk substitutes such as cow's, buffalo's or goat's milk which are the common liquid supplement can be given to infants. About 5–75 mL of juice or soup can be fed at one time. if cow's milk, first 4 weeks 2:1 (water: milk): 2–3 months 3:1 (milk: water), diluted milk and by six months whole milk can be given.

At 5–6 months onwards the semi solid supplement can be started, i.e. a soft, thin, liquid porridge made from staple-food (cereal, potato) and given with milk.

By 8 months the infants starts teething. Now is the time to give:

- **Chopped, lumpy (thick) foods:** Foods which were earlier boiled, mashed and served, may now be boiled and cut into small pieces before being served. Pieces of boiled vegetables (potato. carrots), cooked chapatti or grams of rice can be given.
- **Crunchy foods:** Like biscuits, pieces of toasters or any other such food which the infant can chew will help in teething.
- When the staple, i.e., the cereal has more foods added to it, (protein source plus vitamin and mineral source), similarly we use the terms 'kichri' in north India and 'Pongal' in south India.

By 9 to 10 months, an infant can eat everything cooked at home but without adding spices. The following should be adhered to:

- Food need not be mashed but should be soft,
- Feed about half cup, 5–6 time a day,
- Continue breastfeeding.

By 12 to 18 months an infant:

- Can eat everything cooked in the family,
- Need about half the amount the mother eat daily,
- Feed 4 to 5 times a day,
- Continue breastfeeding at night.

While feeding infants, some vital points to be convinced and advised to their mothers are as follows:

The mother should be advised that along with supplementary foods, continue breastfeeding at least until the baby is one year old. If breast milk is ceased, then the child may switch on to the following:

- Advise the mother to provide plenty of fluids to the infants with frequent intervals.
- Advise the mother not to:
  - Give bottle feeding
  - Give egg or egg containing food to the baby before six months.
  - Add anything to the milk in the bottle.
  - Give too much sugar or sweets to the baby as too much sugar causes tooth decay and may make baby fat.
  - Give whole nuts (peanuts, cashew nuts) as the baby may choke. Finely chopped nuts can be given.
  - Serve the skin or the seed of the fruits or vegetable to the baby.
  - Leave the baby alone while feeding.
- Advise the mother or anybody, to wash hands before cooking and serving the food to the baby.

Maternal and Child Health Program

Maternal and Child Health Objectives

- Reduce fetal and infant death.
- Increase proportion of pregnant women who receive early and adequate prenatal care.
- Increase the proportion of pregnant women, who attend a series of prepared childbirth classes.
- Reduce preterm births.
- Increase abstinence from alcohol, cigarettes and illicit drugs among pregnant women.
- Increase the percentage of health full-term infants who are put down to sleep on their back.
- Increase the proportion of mothers who breastfeed their babies.

Objectives of MCH Programs

- To give expert advice to the couples to plan their families.
- To identify "high risk" cases can give them special attention.
- To provide health supervision for antenatal mothers.
- To give skilled assistance at the time of child birth and during puerperium.
- To supervise trained dais, community health volunteers and community health workers.
- To impart useful knowledge on desirable health practices which mother should carry out during pregnancy, labor and during puerperium.
- Encourage the deliveries by trained workers in the safe and clean environment.
- Prevent communicable and non-communicable diseases.
- Educate the mother to improve their own and children's health.

Aims of MCH Services

- To pay attention on stability in population, safe childhood and health of children.
- To pay special attention to the health of women, boys, girls, protection from sexually transmitted diseases, antenatal, intranatal, and postnatal mothers.
- To have safe pregnancies is successful in terms of safe motherhood, safe child and good health.
- To provide sound reproductive health for men and women and also safe control of their reproduction activities.
- To have effective control on maternal morbidity and mortality.

Components of Reproductive and Child Health

- Family planning services
- Child survival and safe motherhood program (CSSM)
- Prevention or management of STD and AIDS
- Providing counseling, information and communication services on health.
- Referral services.
- Growth monitoring and nutritional education.

Importance of MCH Services

- Mother and child are considered as one unit.
- Mother and child are "special Risk group" or vulnerable group or dependent or weaker group of community.
- Most of the problems of maternal and child health are preventable.
- Effective maternal and child health protects from infant morbidity and mortality.
- To maintain the health and well-being of pregnant women.
- To identify risk factors and complications arises during pregnancy.

Major MCH Problems

- **Nutritional anemia:** Anemia is a condition in which concentration of hemoglobin the red blood cells is reduced. Hemoglobin is essential for life. It carries oxygen to all parts of the body. Anemia during pregnancy leads to 20% of all maternal deaths, 3 times greater risk of premature delivery and low birth weight babies. Anemia can retard physical and mental development of the child.
- **Infection:** The common infection causes are urinary tract infection, reproductive tract infection, STD and other common problems. Urinary tract infection causes frequent burning micturition due to *E. coli*, reproductive tract infection/STD caused by bacterial, viral and protozoan, infection occur due to unsafe deliveries and abortion or IVP insertions. Other common problems are toxoplasmosis, rubella; cytomegalovirus and Herpes simplex are common in pregnancy.
- **Uncontrolled reproduction:** Uncontrolled reproduction has been very well recognized by LBW, severe anemia, abortion, APH, high mortality and perinatal utilization of MCH and family welfare services, MTP sterilization, Health education and family welfare counseling.

National Health Mission MCH Services

Improving Maternal Health is one of the Sustainable Development Goal and a vital component towards achieving Continuum of Care. Gujarat has made considerable progress over the last decade in Maternal and Child Health by providing accessible qualitative health services especially for rural areas, outreached areas and the poor. Maternal Mortality Ratio (MMR) of Gujarat has reduced from 172 per 1 lakh live births in year 2001–2003 to 70 per 1 lakh live births in year 2017–2019 (SRS).

Services to Pregnant Women

- All pregnancies are registered either by community health workers or at health facilities.
- All registered pregnant women are provided three antenatal check-up which also include Blood Pressure measurement and ruling out any complications, high risk factors
- The pregnant women are given two doses of Td vaccines.
- The pregnant women are also provided Iron Folic Acid supplementation, Albendazole and Calcium Supplementation as per guidelines.

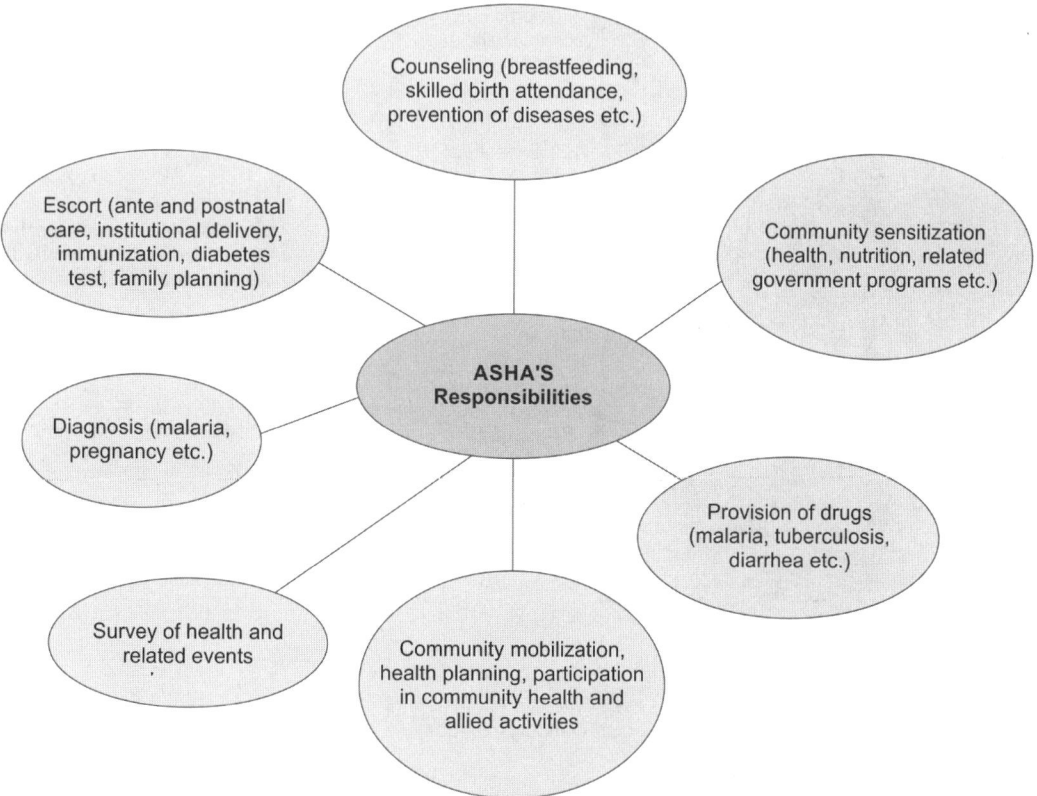

Fig. 13.17: Duties and responsibilities of ASHA worker.

- Institutional deliveries are encouraged by all stakeholders, in unavoidable circumstances deliveries by trained personnel in safe and hygienic surroundings are ensured.
- In case of complication referrals are made either to First Referral Units or higher health facility as per the requirement for Management of obstetric emergencies.
- Spacing of at least three years between children is encouraged.
- Antenatal and postnatal checkups are restructured across the state.

Surakshit Matritva Aashwasan (SUMAN) (Fig. 13.18)

- To expedite the reduction in maternal mortality, the government of India has framed "SUMAN"—a comprehensive, multipronged policy to assured free cost service delivery at public health institutes for pregnant women, postnatal mothers and sick infants.
- SUMAN is an initiative of the government to ensure qualitative maternal and infant health services without any OOPE for health.
- To make further decline in mortality rates and to achieve SDG targets; all pregnant women are provided a minimum package of antenatal care services (including investigations and drugs), identification and line-listing of high risk pregnancies based on obstetric/medical history and existing clinical services are being carried out.
- The SUMAN initiative was launched on 10th October 2019, at the 13th conclave of the Central Council of Ministers, wherein the GoI and the State Governments collectively committed to achieve zero preventable maternal and newborn deaths in the country and providing service assurance for maternal and newborn care services.

Pradhan Mantri Surakshit Matritva Abhiyan (PMSMA) (Fig. 13.19)

- To reduce Maternal Mortality ratio and to ensure qualitative Maternal Health services, various programs and schemes have been implemented in State.
- Pradhan Mantri Surakshit Matritva Abhiyan have been implemented since 9th June 2016 across state to ensure early identification and prompt treatment of high risk pregnant women of 2nd/3rd trimesters under guidance of specialist.
- Across state 9th of every month/Pradhan Mantri Surakshit Matritva Abhiyan clinic has been organized at every Public Health Institute.
- Under this campaign essential Antenatal care and other necessary health services has been provided by specialist at every Public Health Institute at 09th of every month.

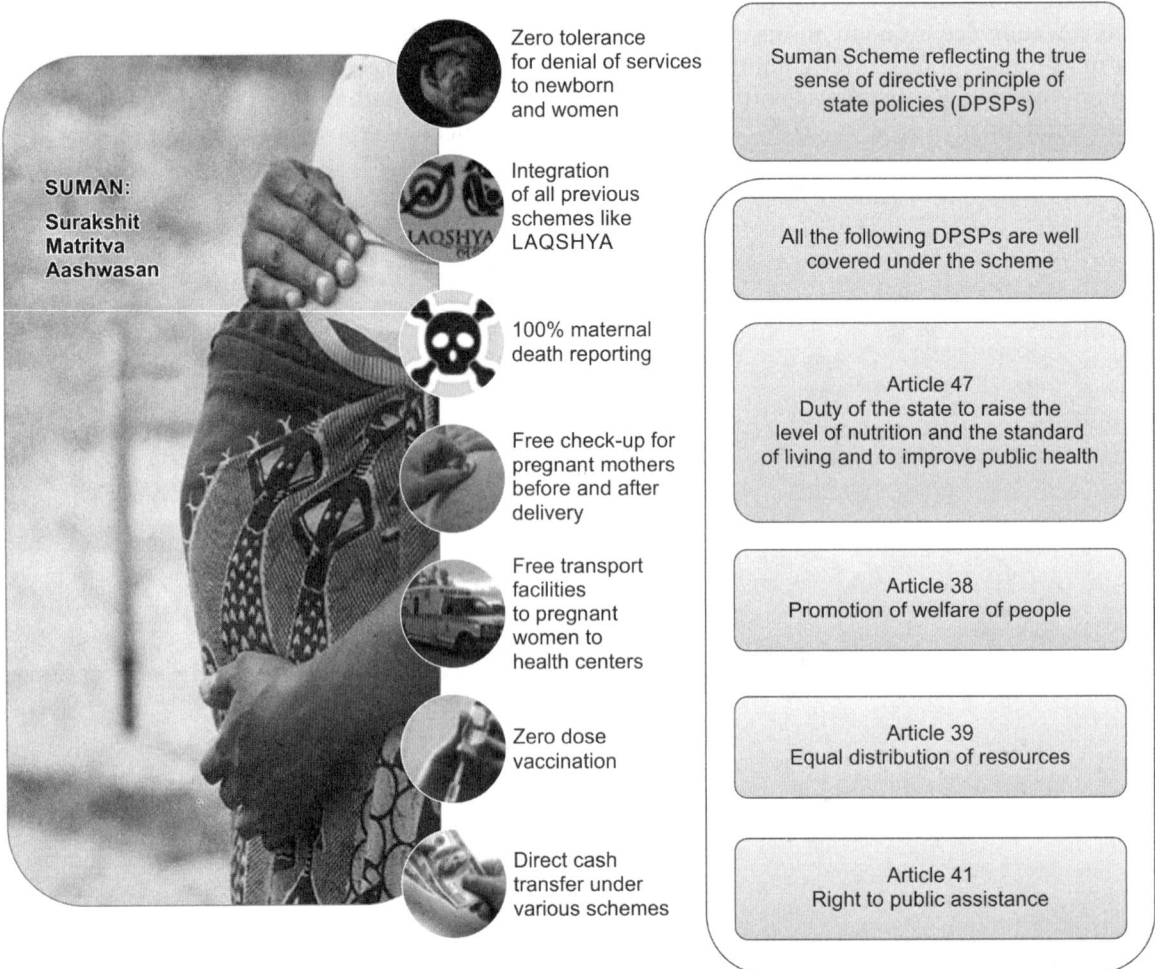

Fig. 13.18: Surakshit Matritva Aashwasan (SUMAN).

Chapter 13: Specialized Community Health Services and Nurse's Role

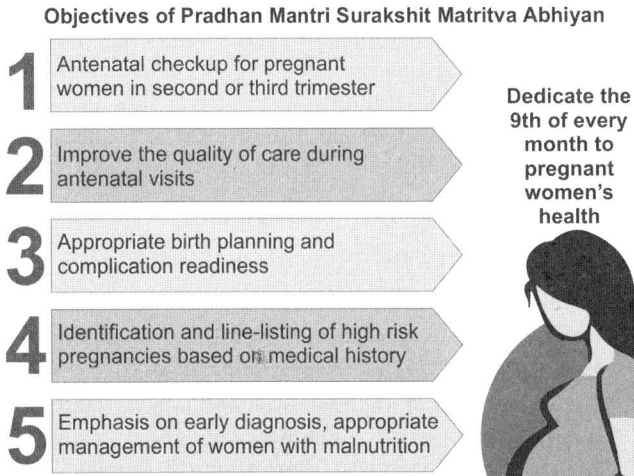

Fig. 13.19: Pradhan Mantri Surakshit Matritva Abhiyan.

- In the 31st July 2016 episode of "Man ki Baat" Hon'ble Prime Minister has appealed to private sector obstetricians/physicians to volunteer their services for this program.
- Pradhan Mantri Surakshit Matritva Abhiyan is being monitored by web portal, under PMSMA specialist/physician can do registration by self for volunteer services.
- Pradhan Mantri Surakshit Matritva Abhiyan clinic has been organized at all Community Health center, Sub-district Hospital, District Hospital and Medical College Hospitals.
- All essential Antenatal examinations, check up, Hemoglobin, Urine, Routine Blood Sugar, Malaria, HIV, Blood grouping, etc. essential laboratory services is also ensured, even if required USG services has also been provided to all pregnant women.
- Pradhan Mantri Surakshit Matritva Abhiyan ensures essential examination of pregnant women and early identification of pregnant women with high risk factors and also ensures necessary medical check-up, treatment and laboratory investigations under guidance of specialist. If it is required than pregnant women is also referred for essential medical check-up and treatment to higher level public health institutes. All these services has been provided free of cost to all pregnant women at all public health institutes.
- More than 16 lakh pregnant women are examined and out of which total 86,000 High Risk Pregnancy have been identified and given treatment under the campaign.

Extended Pradhan Mantri Surakshit Matritva Abhiyan (e-PMSMA)

- To achieve significant reduction in maternal mortality has incorporated additional antenatal checkups are added to routine ANC checkups for High Risk Pregnancies (HRPs) in Extended Pradhan Mantri Surakshit Matritva Abhiyan.
- This new initiative includes Additional 3 ANCs of HRPs by either specialists or MBBS doctor under PMSMA, Additional PMSMA day—a fixed-day for assured, comprehensive qualitative ANC service apart from existing 9th of every month under PMSMA and Conditional incentives for HRPs and ASHAs.
- The pregnant women are also entitled get Free Drug and Consumables, Free Diagnostic services, Free provision of Blood Transfusion, Free transportation service from Home to Health Institutions, between facilities in case of referral and drop back to home and Exemption from all kind of user charges at public health institutes (as a part of JSSK).

Janani Suraksha Yojana

- This scheme is implemented from December 2005. The benefit of this scheme is given to those pregnant women who are from BPL/SC/ST families regardless of age and number of children for delivery in Government/GIA institutions.
- Pregnant women are paid an incentive of ₹ 700 (Rural Beneficiaries) and ₹ 600 (Urban Beneficiaries) before 8–12 weeks of delivery.

Janani Shishu Suraksha Karyakram (JSSK)

Janani Shishu Suraksha Karyakram is an initiative of Government of India and Government of Gujarat to assure completely free and cashless services to pregnant women including normal deliveries and cesarean operations, postnatal women up to 42 days and sick Infants (up to 1 year after birth) in Government health institutions. JSSK Entitlements are as follows:

- Free and zero expense Delivery and Cesarean Section
- Free Drug and Consumables
- Free Diagnostic services
- Free Diet during stay in the health institutions
- Free provision of Blood Transfusion
- Free transportation service from Home to Health Institutions, between facilities in case of referral and drop back to home
- Exemption from all kind of user charges.

Referral Transport

- **Referral transport from home to health facility:** EMRI Ambulance Services (108-Ambulance Service) are currently available throughout Gujarat through the toll free number 108, which is controlled by state level call center. The pre-hospitalization emergency care provided by EMRI is free and the patient is admitted to a hospital of her or his choice.
- **Interfacility transfer:** The free interfacility Transfer is provided by state owned CHC ambulances and by PHC vehicles and 108.
- **Informed referral services:** All efforts put in making FRUs functional can help survive the pregnant mother or a child in case of emergency is dependent on timely and intelligent referral. State has envisioned having robust established Referral System through 108 and PHIs own fleet of ambulances.

Chiranjeevi Yojana

The Health and Family Welfare Department has initiated a scheme involving private sector specialists in providing services related to safe delivery, primarily for socio-economically weaker sections, which is named as Chiranjeevi Yojana.

- The scheme was launched on pilot basis in December 2005. In the initial stage, this scheme is made operational in five most under served, tribal, desert and bordering districts i.e. Kutch, Banaskanta, Sabarkanta, Panchamahals and Dahod as a pilot project in the State.
- The beneficiaries are the mothers from BPL, since 26/03/2007 APL-Non Income Tax Paying families are also incorporated in beneficiary criteria.
- The Initial package of ₹ 1,85,000 for 100 deliveries, which was modified by Govt. Resolution No.: FPW/102013/73/B-1 dated 29/07/2013, now revised package of 100 deliveries is ₹ 3, 80,000.
- In Chiranjeevi Yojana, there is provision of ₹ 2500/- per Cesarean Section if enrolled Private gynecologists conduct Cesarean Section in Government health facility.
- The package also includes ₹ 200/- for transportation of the pregnant mother Chiranjeevi Yojana has so far served to more than 13.8 lakh pregnant mothers.

Benefits

This scheme empowers the poor in several ways:

- It provides them entitlement for free delivery care in private sector.
- It provides immediate access to Emergency Obstetric Care (EmOC) when needed.
- Reduction in out of pocket expenditure.
- It also provides them choice of several providers nearby from which they can choose from..
- It also shows that it is possible to develop large scale partnership with private sector to provide skilled birth attendance and EmOC to poor women at a relatively small expenditure.
- The Chiranjeevi scheme is now linked with Emergency Management and Research Institute (EMRI) services for elimination of transportation time delay. EMRI is providing free ambulance services to all sections of the society in entire Gujarat state.

Screening of Dental Diseases During Pregnancy (SDDDP)

- Many women make their first antenatal visit with the pregnancy already compromised or at risk from use of tobacco (smoke or smokeless), inappropriate nutrition, anemia and poor dental health.
- There is an increase in research evidence suggesting associations between periodontal disease and adverse pregnancy outcomes that includes preterm birth, low birth weight, early pregnancy loss and preeclampsia. Preeclampsia and preterm births are major causes of maternal and perinatal morbidity and mortality.
- Minimum four dental checkups during antenatal period (1st Visit within 12 weeks, 2nd visit Between 14 to 26 weeks, 3rd visit Between 28 and 34 weeks, 4th visit Between 36 weeks and term).
- Inclusion of screening for dental diseases and management as a part of PMSMA, Extended PMSMA and JSSK.

Collaborative Framework for Management of Tuberculosis in Pregnant Women

- TB in pregnancy can have serious and sequential effects: repeated reproductive failure, fetal ill-health, preterm delivery, and TB of the newborns and infants, leading to high maternal and perinatal morbidity and mortality.
- TB in pregnancy is considered as a high risk factor during pregnancy. The risk of activation of latent TB infection is also higher during pregnancy as a result of the immunological changes.
- The main objective of the initiative is to ensure symptomatic screening (cough more than two weeks, fever more than two weeks, perspiration at night, weight loss or no adequate weight gain, Extrapulmonary symptoms—localized swellings/lumps in the body—lymph node) of each pregnant women during every antenatal check-up and to create systems that support and empower pregnant women with TB to access care and to be delivered at FRU/ higher facility only.

Mamta Ghar

- Mamta Ghar is the key element to 'bridge the geographical gap' in obstetric care between rural areas, with poor access to facilities.
- The purpose of Mamta Ghar is to provide a setting where high-risk women or women from remote areas can be accommodated during the last 7–10 days of pregnancy or even more if needed near a hospital where Obstetric and Newborn care facilities are available, as well additional emphasis is put on education and counseling regarding pregnancy, delivery and care of the newborn infant and family.

Strengthening of FRUs

The state has taken various steps like phase wise strengthening of FRUs is carrying out by fulfilling the Gaps pertaining to in Human Resource, equipment, blood transfusion services, Facility Based Newborn Care etc. in order to improve status of maternal health services by strengthening First Referral Units (FRUs). As per the need, the state has designated and operationalized District hospitals (DH), Sub-district hospitals (SDH) and Community Health Center as FRUs to ensure comprehensive obstetric neonatal care services.

Respectful Maternal Care

Respectful Maternal Care promotes Respect for beliefs, traditions and culture, Empowerment of the woman and her family to become active participants in healthcare, Continuous support during labor, Choice of companion during labor and birth, The right to information and privacy, Freedom of movement during labor, Choice of position during birth, Good communication between client and provider, Support of the mother-baby pair, Improvement of working conditions and respectful and collaborative relationships among all cadres of health workers and Prevention of disrespect and abuse and institutional violence against woman.

Birth Companion during Pregnancy ('Mamata Sakhi')

To improve the quality of maternal and newborn care, birth companionship is a key component of providing respectful maternity care. The birth companion provides informational support and bridge communication gaps between clinical staff and woman. Companions also provide encouragement and emotional support to women to remain mobile during labor and help women feel in control and build their confidence through praise, reassurance, and continuous physical presence.

Strengthening Referral Services

Maternal Mortality ratio of the state decreased from 87 per one lakh live births (SRS 2015–17) to 75 per one lakh live births (SRS 2016–18). Similarly, improvement has been documented in trend of institutional deliveries, 99% of reported deliveries are institutional deliveries. However, to ensure further marked reduction in the maternal and neonatal mortality and to improve qualitative perinatal health services across the state.

Mapping of Each Public Health Facility with a Tertiary Level Health Facility

- Medical College Hospital (MCH) carried out across the state. The special drive for the informed referral 'SMART' (Streamline Management and Appropriate Referral in Time) services is ensured by active involvement of various stakeholders since November 2020.
- The key components of the drive includes establishment of referral linkages, ensuring pre-referral stabilization, informed referral, post referral follow-up, mentoring for area specific issues.

Obstetric ICU: Obstetric ICU is an intervention for providing tertiary level critical MCH services. Total 12 Obs-ICUs are functional out of approved 20 across the state to ensure intensive care to critical antenatal and postnatal mothers.

NATIONAL HEALTH MISSION (RURAL/URBAN)

The National Health Mission (NHM) encompasses its two Sub-Missions, The National Rural Health Mission (NRHM) and The National Urban Health Mission (NUHM) **(Fig. 13.20)**. The main programmatic components include Health System Strengthening, Reproductive-Maternal-Neonatal-Child and Adolescent Health (RMNCH+A), and Communicable and Non-communicable Diseases. The NHM envisages achievement of universal access to equitable, affordable and quality healthcare services that are accountable and responsive to people's needs. Continuation of the National Health Mission—with effect from 1st April 2017 to 31st March 2020 has been approved by Cabinet in its meeting dated 21.03.2018.

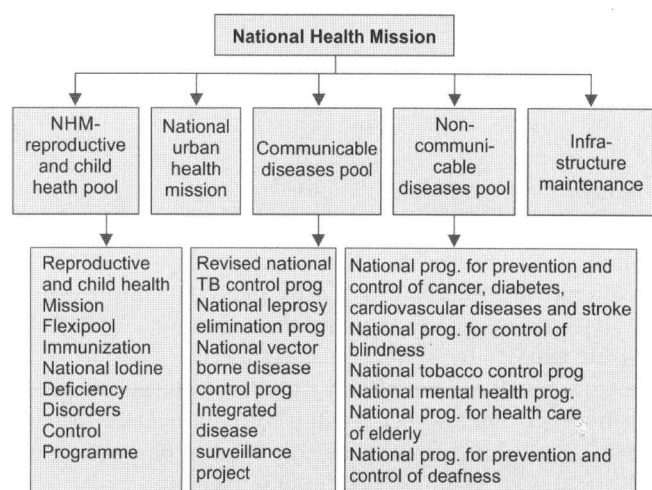

Fig. 13.20: National health mission.

Six Financing Components

1. NRHM-RCH Flexipool,
2. NUHM Flexipool,
3. Flexible pool for Communicable disease,
4. Flexible pool for noncommunicable disease including Injury and Trauma,
5. Infrastructure Maintenance and
6. Family Welfare Central Sector component.

Goals

Outcomes for NHM in the 12th Plan are synonymous with those of the 11th Plan and are part of the overall vision. Specific goals for the states will be based on existing levels, capacity, and context. State specific innovations would be encouraged. Process and outcome indicators will be developed to reflect equity, quality, efficiency, and responsiveness. Targets for communicable and non-communicable diseases will be set at state level based on local epidemiological patterns and taking into account the financing available for each of these conditions. The endeavor would be to ensure the achievement of indicators as follows:

- Reduce MMR to 1/1000 live births
- Reduce IMR to 25/1000 live births
- Reduce TFR to 2.1
- Prevention and reduction of anemia in women aged 15–49 years
- Prevent and reduce mortality and morbidity from communicable, noncommunicable; injuries and emerging diseases
- Reduce household out-of-pocket expenditure on total healthcare expenditure
- Reduce annual incidence and mortality from Tuberculosis by half
- Reduce the prevalence of Leprosy to <1/10,000 population and incidence to zero in all districts

- Annual Malaria Incidence to be <1/1,000
- Less than 1% microfilaria prevalence in all districts
- Kala-azar Elimination by 2015, <1 case per 10,000 population in all blocks.

National Rural Health Mission

The National Rural Health Mission (NRHM) was launched by the Hon'ble Prime Minister on 12th April 2005, to provide accessible, affordable and quality healthcare to the rural population, especially the vulnerable groups. The Union Cabinet vide its decision dated 1st May 2013, has approved the launch of National Urban Health Mission (NUHM) as a Sub-mission of an over-arching National Health Mission (NHM), with National Rural Health Mission being the other Sub-mission of National Health Mission.

National Health Mission (NHM)

The National Health Mission aims for attainment of universal access to equitable, affordable and quality healthcare services, accountable and responsive to people's needs, with effective inter-sectoral convergent action to address the wider social determinants of health **(Fig. 13.21)**.

Under NHM, support to States/UTs is provided for five key programmatic components:
- Health Systems Strengthening including infrastructure, human resource, drugs and equipment, ambulances, MMUs, ASHAs etc. under National Rural Health Mission and National Urban Health Mission.
- Reproductive, Maternal, Newborn, Child and Adolescent Health Services (RMNCH + A)
- Communicable Disease Control Programs
- Noncommunicable Diseases Control Program interventions upto District Hospital level
- Infrastructure Maintenance—to support salary of ANMs and LHVs etc.

Vision of the Mission

- To provide effective healthcare to rural population throughout the country with special focus on 18 states, which have weak public health indicators and/or weak infrastructure.
- 18 special focus states are Arunachal Pradesh, Assam, Bihar, Chhattisgarh, Himachal Pradesh, Jharkhand, Jammu and Kashmir, Manipur, Mizoram, Meghalaya, Madhya Pradesh, Nagaland, Orissa, Rajasthan, Sikkim, Tripura, Uttaranchal and Uttar Pradesh.
- To rise public spending on health from 0.9% GDP to 2–3% of GDP, with improved arrangement for community financing and risk pooling.

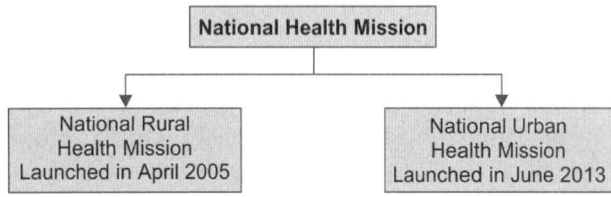

Fig. 13.21: Types of national health mission.

- To undertake architectural correction of the health system to enable it to effectively handle increased allocations and promote policies that strengthen public health management and service delivery in the country.
- To revitalize local health traditions and mainstream AYUSH into the public health system.
- Effective integration of health concerns through decentralized management at district, with determinants of health like sanitation and hygiene, nutrition, safe drinking water, gender and social concerns.
- Address inter-state and inter-district disparities.
- Time bound goals and report publicly on progress.
- To improve access to rural people, especially poor women and children to equitable, affordable, accountable and effective primary healthcare.

Objectives of the Mission

- Reduction in child and maternal mortality
- Universal access to public services for food and nutrition, sanitation and hygiene and universal access to public healthcare services with emphasis on services addressing women's and children's health and universal immunization
- Prevention and control of communicable and non-communicable diseases, including locally endemic diseases.
- Access to integrated comprehensive primary healthcare.
- Population stabilization, gender and demographic balance.
- Revitalize local health traditions and mainstream AYUSH.
- Promotion of healthy lifestyles.

The expected outcomes from the mission as reflected in statistical data are:
- IMR reduced to 30/1,000 live births by 2012.
- Maternal Mortality reduced to 100/100,000 live births by 2012.
- TFR reduced to 2.1 by 2012.
- Malaria mortality reduction rate—50% up to 2010, additional 10% by 2012.
- Kala-azar mortality reduction rate—100% by 2010 and sustaining elimination until 2012.
- Filaria/Microfilaria reduction rate—70% by 2010, 80% by 2012 and elimination by 2015.
- Dengue mortality reduction rate—50% by 2010 and sustaining at that level until 2012.
- Cataract operations-increasing to 46 lakhs until 2012.
- Leprosy prevalence rate—reduce from 1.8 per 10,000 in 2005 to less that 1 per 10,000 thereafter.
- Tuberculosis DOTS series—maintain 85% cure rate through entire Mission Period and also sustain planned case detection rate.
- Upgrading all Community Health Centers to Indian Public Health Standards.
- Increase utilization of First Referral units from bed occupancy by referred cases of less than 20% to over 75%.
- Engaging 4,00,000 female Accredited Social Health Activists (ASHAs).

Approaches of NRHM is depicted in **Figure 13.22**.

Chapter 13: Specialized Community Health Services and Nurse's Role

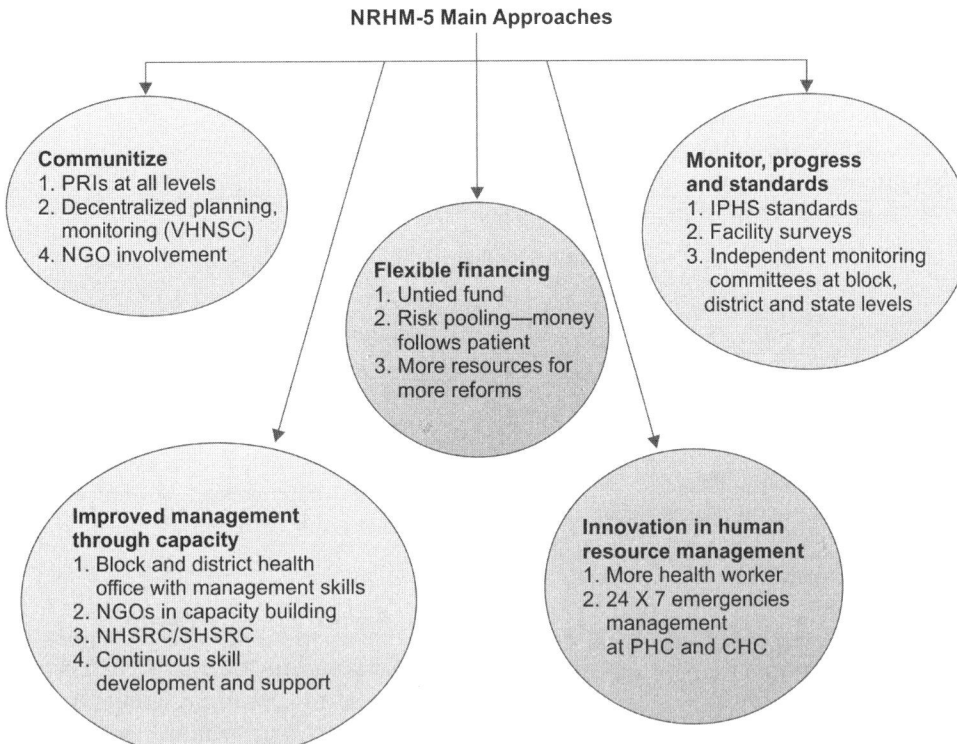

Fig. 13.22: Approaches of NRHM.

Expected Outcomes at Community Level

- Availability of trained community level worker at village level, with a drug kit for generic ailments.
- Health Day at Anganwadi level on a fixed day/month for provision of immunization, ante/post natal checkups and services related to mother and child healthcare, including nutrition.
- Availability of generic drugs for common ailments at sub-Center and Hospital level.
- Access to good hospital care through assured availability of doctors, drugs and quality services at PHC/CHC level and assured referral-transport-communication systems to reach these facilities in time.
- Improved access to universal immunization through induction of Auto Disabled Syringes, alternate vaccine delivery and improved mobilization services under the program.
- Improved facilities for institutional deliveries through provision of referral transport, escort and improved hospital care subsidized under the Janani Suraksha Yojana (JSY) for the below poverty line families.
- Availability of assured healthcare at reduced financial risk through pilots of Community Health Insurance under the Mission.
- Availability of safe drinking water.
- Provision of household toilets.
- Improved outreach services to medically under-served remote areas through mobile medical units.
- Increase awareness about preventive health including nutrition.

Core Strategies of the Mission

- Train and enhance capacity of Panchayati Raj Institutions (PRIs) to own, control and manage public health services.
- Promote access to improved healthcare at household level through the female health activist (ASHA).
- Health Plan for each village through Village Health Committee of the Panchayat.
- Strengthening sub-center through better human resource development, clear quality standards, better community support and an untied fund to enable local planning and action and more Multi-Purpose Workers (MPWs).
- Strengthening existing (PHCs) through better staffing and human resource development policy, clear quality standards, better community support and an untied fund to enable the local management committee to achieve these standards.
- Provision of 30–50 bedded CHC per lakh population for improved curative care to a normative standard. (IPHS defining personnel, equipment and management standards, its decentralized administration by a hospital management committee and the provision of adequate funds and powers to enable these committees to reach desired levels).
- Preparation and implementation of an inter-sector District Health Plan prepared by the District Health Mission, including drinking water, sanitation, hygiene and nutrition.
- Integrating vertical Health and Family Welfare programs at National, State, District and Block levels.
- Technical support to National, State and District Health Mission, for public health management.

- Strengthening capacities for data collection, assessment and review for evidence-based planning, monitoring and supervision.
- Formulation of transparent policies for deployment and career development of human resource for health.
- Developing capacities for preventive healthcare at all levels for promoting healthy lifestyle, reduction in consumption of tobacco and alcohol, etc.
- Promoting non-profit sector particularly in underserved areas.

Supplementary Strategies of the Mission

- Regulation for private sector including the informal Rural Medical Practitioners (RMP) to ensure availability of quality service to citizens at reasonable cost.
- Promotion of public private partnerships for achieving public health goals.
- Mainstreaming AYUSH—revitalizing local health traditions.
- Reorienting medical education to support rural health issues including regulation of medical care and medical ethics.
- Effective and visible risk pooling and social health insurance to provide health security to the poor by ensuring accessible, affordable, accountable and good quality hospital care.

National Urban Health Mission

The National Urban Health Mission (NUHM) as a sub-mission of National Health Mission (NHM) has been approved by the Cabinet on 1st May 2013. NUHM envisages to meet healthcare needs of the urban population with the focus on urban poor, by making available to them essential primary healthcare services and reducing their out of pocket expenses for treatment. This will be achieved by strengthening the existing healthcare service delivery system, targeting the people living in slums and converging with various schemes relating to wider determinants of health like drinking water, sanitation, school education, etc. implemented by the Ministries of Urban Development, Housing and Urban Poverty Alleviation, Human Resource Development and Women and Child Development.

Goals

- Need based city specific urban healthcare system to meet the diverse healthcare needs of the urban poor and other vulnerable sections.
- Institutional mechanism and management systems to meet the health-related challenges of a rapidly growing urban population.
- Partnership with community and local bodies for a more proactive involvement in planning, implementation, and monitoring of health activities.
- Availability of resources for providing essential primary healthcare to urban poor.
- Partnerships with NGOs, for profit and not for profit health service providers and other stakeholders.

Health Condition of the Urban Poor

- U5MR of 72.7 against urban average of 51.9
- 46% under-weight children among urban poor—urban average—32.8%.
- 46.8% women with no education; urban average 19.3%.
- 44.4% institutional deliveries; urban average—67.5%.
- 71.4% anemic among urban poor; urban average—62.9%
- 18.5% urban poor have access to piped water supply; urban average—50%.
- 60% miss total immunization before completing one year.
- Poor environmental condition with high population density—lung diseases, TB, etc.
- Poor access to safe water and sanitation—water-borne diseases, diarrhea and dysentery
- High incidence of vector borne diseases among urban poor.

Urban Primary Health Center

- In order to provide comprehensive primary healthcare services, the National Urban Health Mission aims to establish Urban Primary Healthcare Centers, not as a stand-alone health facility, but as a hub of preventive, promotive and basic curative healthcare for its catchment population.
- Within its catchment area, the UPHC is responsible for providing the primary healthcare and public health needs of the population. The U-PHC is located preferably closer to slum or similar habitations.
- The hours of operation may be such so as to enable the urban working population to conveniently access the UPHC services. States may opt for any suitable timing, providing 8 hours of services, which are convenient to the community.
- It is recommended that the UPHC operates preferably from 12 noon to 8 PM or in dual shifts (i.e., 8 AM to 12 PM and 4 PM to 8 PM); dual shift timing of UPHC could be flexible with the ability to be modified according to the catchment communities.
- The package of services envisaged at UPHC inclusive of preventive, promotive, curative, rehabilitative and palliative care. Further, in order to strengthen comprehensive primary healthcare across the country through "Ayushman Bharat-HWCs", states are upgrading their primary healthcare centers as health and wellness centers (HWCs).

Urban Community Health Centers

Urban Community Health Center (U-CHC) is set up as a referral facility for every 4-5 U-PHCs. The U-CHC caters to a population of 2,50,000 to 5 Lakhs. For the metro cities, UCHCs may be established for every 5 lakh population with 100 beds. In addition to primary healthcare facilities, it provides inpatient services, medical care, surgical facilities and institutional delivery facilities. It is a 30–50 bedded facility.

Urban—Health and Wellness Centers

In order to ensure delivery of Comprehensive Primary Healthcare (CPHC) services, existing U-PHCs would be converted to Health and Wellness Centers (HWC). Services could also be provided/complemented through outreach services, Mobile Medical Units, health camps, home visits and community-based interaction, but the principle should be a seamless continuum of care that ensures equity, quality, universality and no financial hardship.

Benefits of NUHM

The significance of NUHM is therefore undeniable in the Indian urban context. Urban people eligible for this mission can therefore avail following benefits while handling their healthcare expenses.
- Marginalized sections of this population can avail of cost-effective healthcare services.
- It helps prevent the spread of diseases with health thrust on social determinants, including vector control, sanitation and clean drinking water.
- It has increased disease awareness among the target audience and influenced them to visit government health centers for regular check-ups.
- The community groups maintain effective communication with the population to inform them about the services, availability of beds, procedures, etc.
- Existing institutional structures and arrangements are designed to suit city-specific needs under NUHM.

JANANI SURAKSHA YOJANA

Janani Suraksha Yojana (JSY) is a safe motherhood intervention under the National Health Mission. It is one of the largest conditional schemes in the world and is being implemented with the objective of reducing maternal and neonatal mortality by promoting institutional delivery among pregnant women. Launched on 12th April 2005, JSY is being implemented in all States and Union Territories (UTs), with a special focus on Low Performing States (LPS). JSY is a centrally sponsored scheme, which integrates cash assistance with delivery and post-delivery care using Accredited Social Health Activist (ASHA) as an effective link between the government and pregnant women **(Fig. 13.23)**.

Background on JSY
- About 56,000 women in India die every year due to pregnancy related complications.
- Similarly, every year more than 13 lakh infants die within 1 year of the birth and out of these approximately 2/3rd of the infant deaths take place within the first four weeks of life.
- Out of these, approximately 75% of the deaths take place within a week of the birth and a majority of these occur in the first two days after birth.
- In order to reduce the maternal and infant mortality, reproductive and child health.
- Program under the National Health Mission is being implemented to promote institutional deliveries so that skilled attendance at birth is available and women and new born can be saved from pregnancy related deaths.
- Several initiatives have been launched by the Ministry of Health and Family Welfare (MoHFW) including Janani Suraksha Yojana (JSY) a key intervention that has resulted in phenomenal growth in institutional deliveries.

Concept of JSY
- Janani Suraksha Yojana is a safe motherhood intervention under the National Rural Health Mission (NHM) **(Fig. 13.24)**.
- The scheme is under implementation in all states and Union Territories (UTs), with a special focus on Low Performing States (LPS).
- Janani Suraksha Yojana was launched in April 2005 by modifying the National Maternity Benefit Scheme (NMBS).
- The NMBS came into effect in August 1995 as one of the components of the National Social Assistance Program (NSAP).
- The scheme was transferred from the Ministry of Rural Development to the Department of Health and Family Welfare during the year 2001–02.

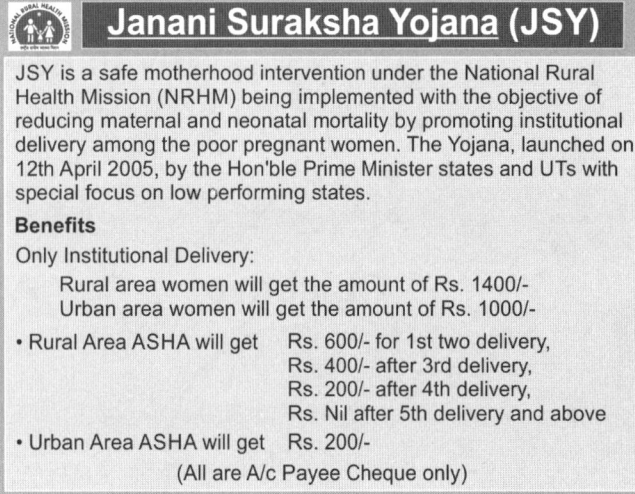

Fig. 13.23: Janani Suraksha Yojana benefits.

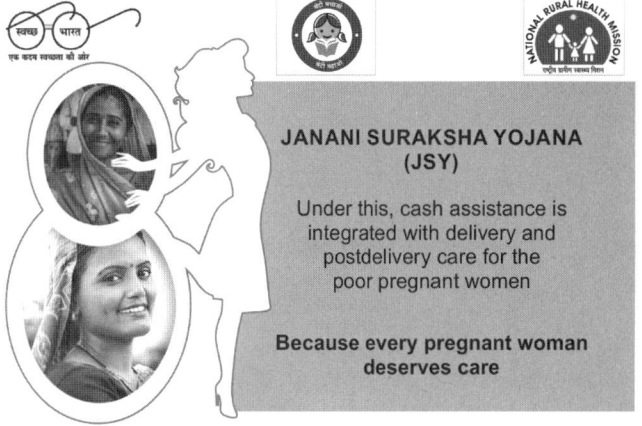

Fig. 13.24: Janani Suraksha Yojana (JSY).

- The NMBS provides for financial assistance of ₹ 500/- per birth up to two live births to the pregnant women who have attained 19 years of age and belong to the below poverty line (BPL) households.
- When JSY was launched the financial assistance of ₹ 500/- which was available uniformly throughout the country to BPL pregnant women under NMBS, was replaced by graded scale of assistance based on the categorization of States as well as whether beneficiary was from rural/urban area.
- States were classified into Low Performing States and High Performing States on the basis of institutional delivery rate, i.e., states having institutional delivery 25% or less were termed as Low Performing States (LPS) and those which have institutional delivery rate more than 25% were classified as High Performing States (HPS).
- Accordingly, eight erstwhile EAG states namely Uttar Pradesh, Uttarakhand, Madhya Pradesh, Chhattisgarh, Bihar, Jharkhand, Rajasthan, Odisha and the states of Assam and Jammu and Kashmir were classified as Low Performing States.
- The remaining States were grouped into High Performing States.

Objectives of the JSY

The main objective of JSY is to reduce maternal and neonatal mortality by promoting institutional delivery for making available medical care during pregnancy, delivery and post delivery period **(Fig. 13.25)**.

Certificates Required for Availing JSY Benefits

- BPL certificate.
- SC/ST Certificate.
- ANC Registration in a Government Health Institution. (MCP Card)
- Bank Account Number and AADHAR Card Number should be filled in MCP Card.
- If an expectant mother does not have a BPL certificate but the Pradhan of Gram Panchayat where she resides certifies that she belongs to an economically weak/poor family, it will be sufficient to give her JSY benefits.

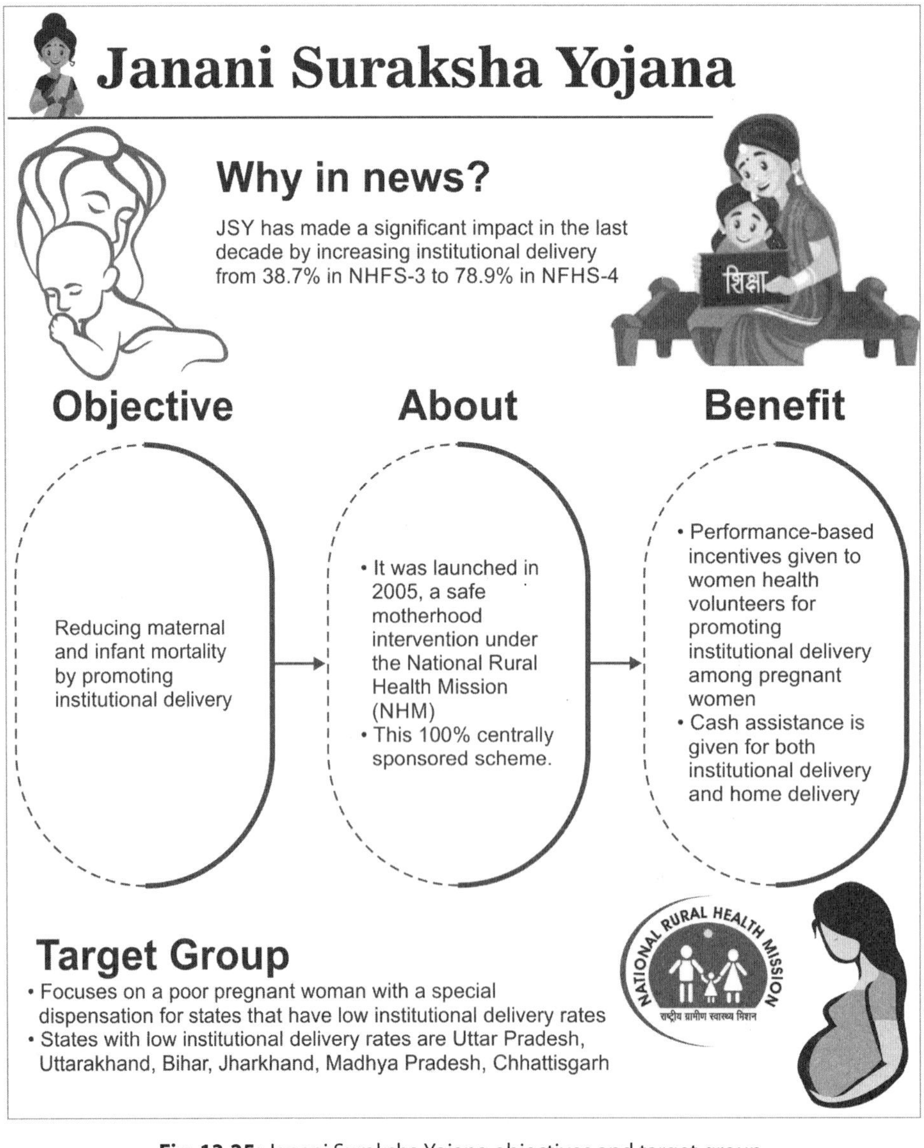

Fig. 13.25: Janani Suraksha Yojana objectives and target group.

In all such cases, where the JSY beneficiaries produce a certificate/document required to make the payment to JSY beneficiary which is signed by the Pradhan of the Gram Panchayat the same shall be accepted without insisting that a Magistrate should issue the certificate.

Important Features of JSY

The scheme focuses on poor pregnant woman with a special dispensation for states that have low institutional delivery rates, namely, the states of Uttar Pradesh, Uttarakhand, Bihar, Jharkhand, Madhya Pradesh, Chhattisgarh, Assam, Rajasthan, Orissa, and Jammu and Kashmir. While these states have been named Low Performing States (LPS), the remaining states have been named High Performing states (HPS).

Role of ASHA or other link health worker associated with JSY would be to (Fig. 13.17):
- Identify pregnant woman as a beneficiary of the scheme and report or facilitate registration for ANC,
- Assist the pregnant woman to obtain necessary certifications wherever necessary,
- Provide and/or help the women in receiving at least three ANC checkups including TT injections, IFA tablets,
- Identify a functional Government health center or an accredited private health institution for referral and delivery,
- Counsel for institutional delivery,
- Escort the beneficiary women to the pre-determined health center and stay with her till the woman is discharged,
- Arrange to immunize the newborn till the age of 14 weeks,
- Inform about the birth or death of the child or mother to the ANM/MO,
- Postnatal visit within 7 days of delivery to track mother's health after delivery and facilitate in obtaining care, wherever necessary,
- Counsel for initiation of breastfeeding to the newborn within one-hour of delivery and its continuance till 3–6 months and promote family planning.

Target Group and Benefits

- The scheme focuses on poor pregnant woman with a special dispensation for states that have low institutional delivery rates, namely, the states of Uttar Pradesh, Uttarakhand, Bihar, Jharkhand, Madhya Pradesh, Chhattisgarh, Assam, Rajasthan, Orissa, and Jammu and Kashmir.
- While these states have been named Low Performing States (LPS), the remaining states have been named High Performing states (HPS).
- The scheme also provides performance based incentives to women health volunteers known as ASHA (Accredited Social Health Activist) for promoting institutional delivery among pregnant women.
- Under this initiative, eligible pregnant women are entitled to get JSY benefit directly into their bank accounts.

EMERGENCY AMBULANCE SERVICES

An ambulance service team includes technicians and paramedics. They are well-trained in first-aid skills in order to handle cardiac arrests, profuse bleeding, road accidents, crush and fall injuries, and many more. Paramedics determine whether the victim has to be taken to a hospital or can be treated on the emergency situation. Ambulance vans are equipped with pre-hospital emergency machines to give temporary medical assistance as what hospitals can offer? In the digital era, all the industries are grown rapidly like manufacturing industry, business industry, and service industry. The medical sciences are also improved tremendously with advance medical facilities **(Fig. 13.26)**.

Concept of Emergency Ambulance Services

Emergency Response Service is a 24 × 7 emergency service for medical, police and fire emergencies. The service is available for the entire state of Andhra Pradesh, Telangana, Gujarat, Uttarakhand, Goa, Tamil Nadu, Karnataka, Assam, Meghalaya, Madhya Pradesh, Himachal Pradesh, Chhattisgarh, Uttar Pradesh, Rajasthan, Kerala and 2 Union Territories Dadra and Nagar Haveli and Daman and Diu. The main highlights are it is a 24 × 7 emergency service. Toll Free number accessible from landline or mobile Emergency help will reach you in an average of 18 minutes 1-0-8/1-1-2 is dialed for the purposes mentioned below:
- To save a life
- To report a crime in progress
- To report a fire

GVK-EMRI

- GVK EMRI (Emergency Management and Research Institute) is a pioneer in Emergency Management Services in India. As a not-for-profit professional organization operating in the Public Private Partnership (PPP) mode, GVK EMRI is the largest professional Emergency Service Provider in India today.
- GVK EMRI handles medical, police and fire emergencies through the "1-0-8 Emergency service". This is a free

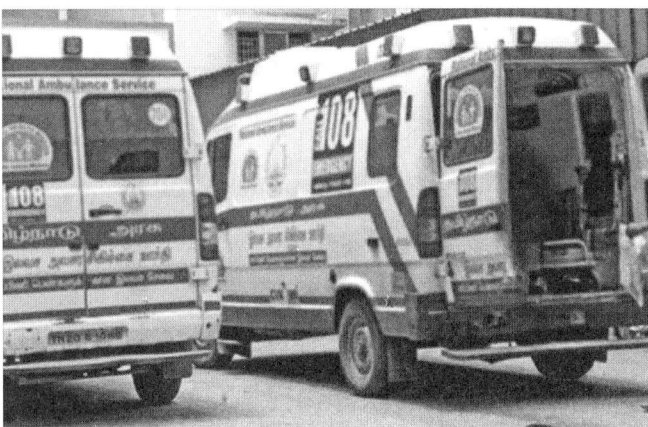

Fig. 13.26: Emergency Ambulance Services.

service delivered through state-of-art emergency call response centers and has over 7016 ambulances including 996 drop back Ambulances across Andhra Pradesh, Gujarat, Uttarakhand, Goa, Tamil Nadu, Karnataka, Assam, Meghalaya, Madhya Pradesh, Himachal Pradesh, Chhattisgarh, Uttar Pradesh, Rajasthan, Kerala and 2 Union Territories Dadra and Nagar Haveli and Daman and Diu.
- With a vision is to respond to 30 million emergencies and save 1 million lives annually, GVK EMRI is set to expand fleet and services set to spread across more states.
- With increased focus on research and analytics, GVK EMRI has plans to significantly enhance the overall emergency management scenario—further reducing individual suffering.

Accessibility of GVK EMRI-108 in India

- Having launched the 108 emergency response service on August 15, 2005, in Hyderabad, GVK EMRI presently provides an integrated emergency service across the state of Andhra Pradesh, with 802 ambulances serving over 3500 emergencies per day.
- GVK EMRI is currently operational in 17 States and union Territories, i.e., Andhra Pradesh, Telangana, Gujarat, Uttarakhand, Goa, Tamil Nadu, Karnataka, Assam, Meghalaya, Madhya Pradesh, Himachal Pradesh, Chhattisgarh, Uttar Pradesh, Rajasthan, Kerala and 2 Union Territories Dadra and Nagar Haveli and Daman and Diu with 7,600+ambulances.
  Ambulances distribution in various states
  - Andhra Pradesh-802
  - Gujarat-671
  - Uttarakhand-245
  - Goa-33
  - Tamil Nadu-638
  - Karnataka–517
  - Assam-899
  - Meghalaya-47
  - Madhya Pradesh-604
  - Himachal Pradesh-174
  - Chhattisgarh-540
  - Uttar Pradesh-1194
  - Rajasthan-592
  - Kerala-43
  - Dadra and Nagar Haveli and Diu and Daman-13 (Included Boat Ambulances).

Volunteers in Case of Emergency (VoICE)

Volunteerism is a major initiative by GVK EMRI to ensure that no emergencies go unreported and unattended. GVK EMRI is keen to enlist the support of volunteers to disseminate knowledge and information about 1-0-8 services. Volunteers can assist in the following areas:
- Reporting emergencies to help those who have no access to a telephone
- Provide assistance to victim till the ambulance arrives
- Accompany victims to the hospital and serve as referral for the unknown
- Transporting the victim to a meeting point where the ambulance will take over or take the victim directly to the hospital in case the ambulance is busy or not available.

Expectations of GVK EMRI

- **As First Respondent:** Provides pre-hospital care to the victim. For instance, if a volunteer is doctor, in case of Medical emergencies, he/she can give pre hospital care before the ambulance reaches to the site.
- **As Attendee:** The Volunteer may accompany the victim in the Ambulance/Hospital.
- **As Pilot (Driver):** The volunteer may extend service to transport the victim by driving the vehicle and render service if the field staff of GVK EMRI in Ambulance are not available due to unavoidable circumstances such as sudden illness and so on.
- **As Vehicle Mechanic:** Provides services for minor / major repairs and servicing of GVK EMRI network vehicles so as to facilitate and keep the field operations intact.

Special Features of the Ambulance and Services

- Ambulances are being monitored through GPRS for deployment to the site.
- Ambulance are getting instruction from highly trained doctor sitting in the control room.
- Ambulance is manned by specially trained Medical Technician and Driver.
- Ambulance has all emergency medicines, which are being given to the patients in the ambulance itself.
- Ambulance is equipped with emergency medical equipment like Collapsible Auto Loading Stretcher, Scoops Stretcher, Spine Board, Oxygen Manifold System, Airway related equipment, Automatic BP apparatus.
- Ambulance is equipped with rescue tools for extraction of patient from accident vehicles with electrocution Kit
- Ambulance and control room simultaneously interact with the nearest hospital where the patient to be taken.

GOVERNMENT HEALTH INSURANCE SCHEMES

Every government has a responsibility towards its citizens to provide affordable and accessible healthcare to whoever requires it. And to make this possible, governments launch many different health insurance services so that the common citizen can use these facilities when they need it the most. Similarly, the Indian government has also launched a variety of health insurance schemes that have low premiums and offer a significant sum insured in the hope to make good healthcare available to all.

Definition

A government health insurance scheme is a health insurance policy sponsored by a state or the central government. The aim of such schemes is to offer affordable health insurance to the common man and improve healthcare facilities in different strata of society.

Features and Benefits of Government Health Insurance Schemes

The features and benefits of government health insurance schemes are given below:
- Government health insurance schemes are offered at a low price
- With this policy, BPL families can also avail of insurance benefits
- The policy ensures coverage for the poor people
- The policy includes treatment in both private and government hospitals for better healthcare.

Need of Health Insurance in India

More than 100 crore people in the country don't have any kind of health insurance which can cover them against any health issue. Keeping this in mind, the Government of India has launched different health insurance schemes which are affordable and provide a moderately good cover against any medical emergency. National health insurance schemes are basically health programs initiated by government for making health facilities accessible for poor and destitute class. Government has launched some health insurance schemes like Rashtriya Swasthya Bima Yojana, Central Government Health Scheme, Employee's State Insurance Scheme, Universal Health Insurance Scheme, Janashree Bima Yojana and Aam Aadmi Bima Yojana.

Types of Government Health Insurance Scheme

Read ahead to know more about the several health insurance schemes by the Government of India:

Ayushman Bharat Yojana

- Ayushman Bharat is a universal health insurance scheme of the Ministry of Health and Family Welfare, Government of India. PMJAY was launched to provide free healthcare services to more than 40% population of the country. The scheme offers a health cover of ₹ 5 Lakh **(Fig. 13.27)**.
- In this scheme, it covers medicines, diagnostic expenses, medical treatment, and pre-hospitalization costs. The poorest families of India can benefit from this healthcare scheme.

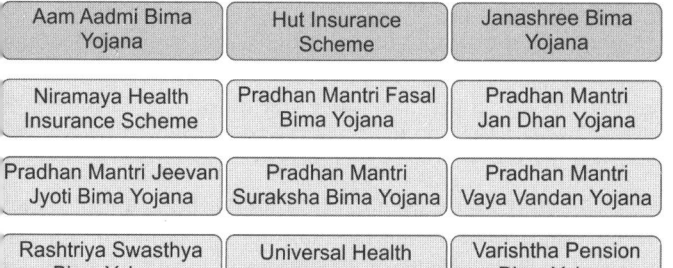

Fig. 13.27: Ayushman Bharat Yojana.

Pradhan Mantri Suraksha Bima Yojana

- Pradhan Mantri Suraksha Bima Yojana aims to provide accident insurance cover to the people of India. People in the age group of 18 years to 70 years who have an account in a bank can avail benefit from this scheme.
- This policy provides an annual cover of ₹ 2 lakh for total disability and death cover and ₹ 1 lakh for partial disability.
- The policy premium gets automatically debited from the policyholder's bank account.

Aam Aadmi Bima Yojana (AABY)

- This is one of the latest National Health Insurance schemes having been established in the year 2007, October. It basically covers individuals from the age of 18 years-59 years. AABY insurance scheme is tailored for all those citizens living in the upcountry and in the rural areas.
- It also covers the landless citizens who are tenants living both in urban and rural areas. It also includes giving scholarships to underprivileged children.
- Basically, the head of the family or the earning member is the one protected by this scheme.
- The premium of 200 rupees per annum is shared equally by the state and the central government.
- Upon a natural death, the family is compensated at 30000 rupees. However, upon death caused by a permanent disability, the family is compensated at 75,000 rupees.

Central Government Health Scheme (CGHS)

- This scheme was started in the year 1954 and provides comprehensive healthcare facilities for central government officials and pensioners residing in cities. Operations of this scheme take place in cities such as Kolkata, Mumbai, Lucknow, Delphi, Nagpur, and Pune.
- The people covered by this scheme are required to be residing in India. This is a National Health Company Online Renewal Program that includes the privilege of health education to the beneficiaries.
- This scheme has the following main components: All dispensary related services including domiciliary care. In addition, the beneficiaries of this scheme have the privilege of being hospitalized each and every time they fall ill.
- On the other hand, whenever you have an X-ray or laboratory examination requirements, they would be provided free under this particular scheme.
- The most important advantage of this National Health Insurance scheme is that it provides free specialists consultations both at hospital level and dispensaries.

Employment State Insurance Scheme

- This is a multidimensional National Health insurance scheme due to the fact that it provides social security as well as socioeconomic protection to all workers in India.

In addition, it provides the same privileges those who depend on workers protected under this scheme.
- This insurance scheme commences upon the first day of insurable employment to each and every worker. They are provided with full medical care insurance for themselves and their families as well.
- On the other hand, those covered under this scheme (which is basically workers) are also entitled to a wide range of cash benefits. They include cash in times of physical distress such as sickness or even when one might become disabled may it be temporal or permanent.
- In addition, for any woman who would lose the capacity to earn or dependents of persons injured during occupational accidents, they are entitled to a monthly pension commonly referred to as dependents benefits.
- This scheme is not applicable to each and every person or company. It is only applicable to all permanent factories employing more than ten employees. Recently, the scheme has been extended to various businesses including shops, restaurants, road and motor transports and newspaper entities that employ more than 20 people.

Janashree Bima Yojana

- Janashree Bima Yojana is designed for individuals in the poor category who are within the age group of 18–59 years.
- The scheme includes special features like Women SHG Groups and Shiksha Sahyog Yojana. At present there are 45 occupational groups under this scheme.

Chief Minister's Comprehensive Insurance Scheme

- Chief Minister's Comprehensive Insurance Scheme is a Tamil Nadu state government scheme.
- It was launched in association with the United India Insurance Company Ltd.
- It is a family floater policy that was designed to provide quality healthcare services to people. This scheme covers more than a thousand medical procedures.
- In this policy, you can claim for hospitalization expenses up to ₹ 5 lakh. The beneficiary can select from both private and government hospitals under this scheme.
- Tamil Nadu residents with an annual income of lesser than ₹ 75,000 per year are eligible to enroll under this scheme.

Universal Health Insurance Scheme (UHIS)

- This type of scheme was implemented to help the families who live below the poverty line. It covers the medical expenses of each and every member of the family. In case of death due to an accident, there is a cover that is provided.
- The main drivers of the Universal Health Insurance Scheme are basically the four public sector general insurance companies who have been doing this with an aim of improving healthcare to the underprivileged and especially the economically disabled citizen in India.
- Once a family member is hospitalized, this scheme may facilitate the medical expenses of up to 30,000 rupees. However, when the earning head of the family is admitted to the hospital, the Universal health insurance scheme compensates a total of 50 rupees daily for a maximum of 15 days.
- We can therefore say that this insurance scheme is designed for families below the poverty line.

West Bengal Health Scheme

- The Government of West Bengal launched this scheme for its employees in the year 2008. It is also available for the pensioners.
- This coverage is provided on both individual and family floater basis up to a sum insured of ₹ 1 lakh.
- The policy covers OPD treatment and medical surgeries as per the policy terms and conditions.

Yeshasvini Health Insurance Scheme

- The Karnataka State Government promotes the Yeshasvini Health Insurance Scheme.
- This scheme is useful for peasants and farmers and who are associated with a cooperative society.
- This health insurance scheme covers more than 800 medical procedures such as Neurology, Orthopedic, Angioplasty, etc.
- Cooperative societies help the farmers to get enrolled in the Yeshasvini Health Insurance Scheme.
- The beneficiaries can avail of healthcare services through network hospitals, and coverage benefits are extendible to the beneficiary's family members.

Mahatma Jyotirao Phule Jan Arogya Yojana

- The Government of Maharashtra introduced this health insurance policy for the benefit of people in the state around.
- The scheme is going to be helpful for below the poverty line and was targeted at the farmers in Maharashtra.
- The policy offers a family health cover of up to ₹ 1.5 lakh for specified illnesses. The best part about this policy is that there is no waiting period, and it is claimable after the first day itself, unless it is specifically mentioned in the policy terms.

Mukhyamantri Amrutum Yojana

- Mukhyamantri Amrutum Yojana was initiated by the Gujarat government in the year 2012 for the benefit of the poor people living in Gujarat.
- People who are in the lower middle-income group and below the poverty line are eligible to enroll under the scheme.
- It is family floater health insurance policy that provides coverage up to ₹ 3 lakh per family. The policyholder can avail of medical treatment from private and government hospitals, as well as trust-run hospitals.

Karunya Health Scheme

- In 2012, the Kerala Government had launched this scheme to provide health cover for listed chronic illnesses.
- It is a Critical Illness plan for the poor and covers major diseases such as kidney, cancer, cardiovascular illnesses, etc.
- People who are below the poverty line can enroll themselves in this scheme. The beneficiary needs to provide a copy of the Income Certificate and Aadhaar Card for the same.

Telangana State Government Employees and Journalists Health Scheme

- Telangana Government launched this scheme for its journalists and employees. It is beneficial for the employed, retired, and pensioners.
- In this scheme, the beneficiary can avail of cashless treatment in the hospitals that are registered. The beneficiaries do not have to rush to arrange funds for emergency medical expenses.

Dr YSR Aarogyasri Healthcare Trust

Four health welfare schemes were launched by the Andhra Pradesh Government along with the Dr YSR Aarogyasri Trust. These schemes offer medical cover to different people and help them at the time of a medical emergency. The schemes are given below:
- Dr YSR Aarogyasri scheme for the welfare of the poor
- Arogya Raksha scheme is for Above the Poverty Line (APL)
- Working Journalist Health Scheme that provides cashless treatment cover for specified procedures
- Employee Health Scheme provides health cover to the state government employees.

SCHOOL HEALTH SERVICES

School health services are an important aspect of community health. Attainment of health is one of the major aims of education. To achieve this goal educators have to design and implement school health programs comprising school health education, school health service and healthful school living.

Any comprehensive school health program should consist of procedures activities designed to protect and promote the well-being of students and school personnel. These procedures and activities include those organized in school health services, providing a healthful environment and health education.

A developing country like India is in dire need of improvement in every detail in respect of education both qualitative and quantitative. Government of India has given an important place to school health services five year plans and the 20 point program. In the Indian context, two reports of Bhore committee and mudaliar committee offer valuable information and suggestions for health planners.

The school health service is an economical any powerful means of raising the health of the communities. It is a personal health service. It has grown from the narrow concept of medical examination of children to the more comprehensive care of health and well-being of school going children.

Relevance of School Health Services

- **Sizeable population segment:** School children represent more than 25% of total Indian population.
- **Crucial phase of development:** School children pass through a continuous process of physical, mental, social and emotional development.
- **Group living experience:** Within the school premises, the children are exposed for the first time, to a group living experience outside their homes.
- **Crowded living conditions:** Student population is a created community exposed to contact borne respiratory and mucocutaneous infections.
- **Controlled population group:** School children constitute a controlled population group well organized and well disciplined.
- **Impressionable age period:** School age is an impressionable period sensitive to all kinds of influences and motivations, a period when healthy habits and practices can be in grained in the lifestyle of students and injurious attitudes, habits, urges and practices can be weeded out.
- **Willing for change:** School children have a clean mind free of misbelieves, prejudice and superstitions. They are eager to learn quickly and experience a change in their behavior and outlook. This ready to change attitude of school children facilitates their involvement in variety of health promoting activities.
- **Useful community link:** School children represent a useful connecting link between the school and the surrounding population. They carry the massages picked up from schools to their families.
- **Valuable national asset:** There is no denying the fact that a child is the "father of man". In other words, the school children are the future generation and a valuable national resource.

Development of School Health Services in India

- 1909—The beginning of school health service in India.
- 1944—The Central Advisory Board of Education recommended that there should be separate program of school health services under the administrative control of education department.
- 1946—The Bhore Committee reported that school health services were practically nonexistent in India and where they existed, they were in an under developed state.
- 1953—The Secondary Education Committee emphasized the need for medical examination of pupils and school feeding programs.
- 1955—The Central Health Council viewed with concern directed the state Governments to take immediate steps to establish a student.
- 1957—Planned approach to strengthening of School Health Services was initiated in 1957 when child education—nutrition education committee and WHO assisted school health education project were set up.

- 1960—The Government of Indian constituted a school health committee to assess the standards of health and nutrition of school and children suggest ways and means to improve them.
- 1961—During five years plan, many state governments have provided for school health and school feeding programs.
- 1977—Centrally sponsored National Health Scheme was started that services could reach to children studying in primary schools in remote rural backward hilly and tribal areas.

  The scheme was implemented in selected Primary Health Centers where two or more physicians were available and PHC which were located in remote, tribal backward and hilly areas. The scheme was fully financed by the Central Government.
- 1979—The National School Health Program was handed over to state governments.
- The states like Andhra Pradesh, Kerala, Tamil Nadu, Sikkim, Maharashtra, Gujarat, Pondicherry, Goa, Delhi, Punjab and Haryana had covered comprehensive school health service scheme successfully.
- Gujarat was the first state which had appointed district level health inspectors for the implementation of scheme.
- Pondicherry was pioneer for covering all the students from class upto college level.
- Mid-day meals was also introduced in many of these states of India, ministry of health and family welfare to study the progress of school health program functioning in various states of the country and to propose comprehensive school health model which can be tried out.
- 1981—Task Force was established by the government of India, ministry of health and family welfare to study the progress of school health program functioning in various states of the country and to propose comprehensive school health model which can be tried out.
- 1982—Task Force Committee submitted that only 14 out of 22 states had put in efforts to set up school health program from their own health budgets but the performance was not up to the standards.
- The pilot project was taken up in 1982 by the Ministry of Health and Family Welfare in 25 blocks of 17 states and union territories. The project was financially supported by Swedish International Development Agency (SIDA).
- 1984-85—The pilot project was extended to 75 more blocks covering four more states making the total number of 100 blocks (100 PHCs).
- 1988—The evaluation of intensive pilot project and extended program was done by National Institute of Health and Family Welfare (NIHFW).
- 1989—The Central Health Educational Bureau Directorate General of Health Services had launched an intensive school health education project. The project envisaged to benefit about 10,00,000 primary school children in 100 blocks of 10 states.

Bhore Committee Recommendations (1960)

- Children between the age of 5-14 years form ¼ of India's total population. The socioeconomic progress of the nation depends upon their care and development.
- The growth of the child physically, emotionally and socially is rapid during this stage. Therefore, there is a great need for health supervision.
- 25 million children of the age group 6-11 years in rural areas out of 40 million should be covered by physical check up by the end of third five year plan period.
- 1962-63 school health service may be provided through primary health centers and then to increase the coverage gradually.
- School health program for children at this age are very receptive to new knowledge.

School Health Scheme Major Components (1982) (Fig. 13.28)

- Observation and screening of students for defects and deviations from normal health, height, weight vision, screening and treatment of minor ailments by teachers.
- Regular annual medical examination of students and their immunization.
- Identification of sick children and their referral to specialties.
- Maintenance of cumulative health records for each student in the school.
- Health education of students to include desirable health knowledge, attitude and practices.

Aims of Central Health Education Bureau (1989)

The main aim of the project was to improve health and nutrition status of primary school children. Innovative measures such as "child to child" and "youth to child" approaches were used to reach message from children to other members of the family.

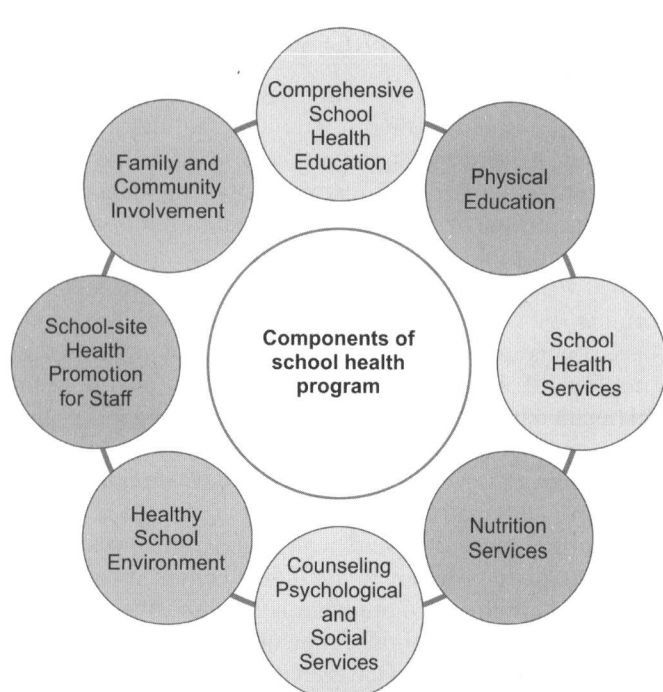

Fig. 13.28: School Health Program Components.

School Health Services

Definitions

- School is defined as an educational institution where groups of pupils pursue defined studies at defined levels, receive instructions from one or more teachers, and frequently interact with other officers and employees such as principal, various supervisors/instructors, and maintenance staff, etc. usually housed in a single building.
- School health services referred to need based comprehensive services rendered to pupils, teachers and other personnel in the school to promote and protect their health, control diseases and maintain the health.
- School health is a part of community health program through which comprehensive care of the health and well-being of children throughout the school years is taken care of.
- School health service is part of educational program through which changes are brought about in knowledge skills and behavior for a healthy living.
- School health program refers to all school activities/procedures that contribute to initiation understanding, maintenance and improvement of the health of pupils and school personnel, including health services health education and heartfelt school living.

Nature of School Health Program

- School health program is an integral part of community health. It is that phase of community health and family health service that promotes the well-being of the child and his education for healthful living.
- School health program can be a powerful influence for shaping health behavior. There is a unique opportunity to promote, maintain and improve health and well-being since teachers reach most people early in life where attitudes and values are most readily developed.
- School Health Service is a personal health service. It stresses the role of the child as a "change agent" for community. A child has greater capacity to observe, learn, experiment and then transfer knowledge to others.
- School health helps in formation of health habits and practices of healthful living throughout school life are very important during the formative period of one's life continuous practice and experience will help and individual to lead a healthy life.
- School Health Program helps the younger generation become healthy and useful citizens who will be able to perform their role effectively for the welfare of themselves, their families the community at large and country as a whole.

Objectives of School Health Programs (Fig. 13.29)

- To increase health awareness in children to a level where they can treat health as a valuable personal family, community and national asset.
- To educate and guide the school children and prompt them to adopt health giving habits and healthy lifestyle and give up injurious habits practices and urges that can undermine their health.
- To facilitate early diagnosis and prompt treatment of diseases in school children and arrest their propagation if communicable.
- To promote interest of students in individual and community health activities and to use them as "change agents" in various areas of public health significance.
- To work towards a total personality development of school children in all dimensions physical, mental, social, moral and emotional treating them as a valuable national asset and useful community resources.

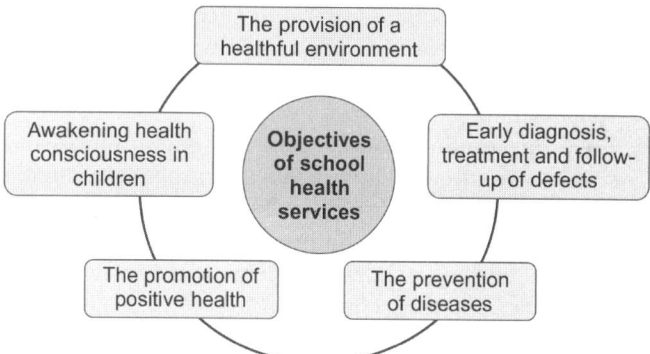

Fig. 13.29: School health service objectives.

Importance/Scope of Community Health Program (Fig. 13.30)

- **Growth and development:** School life is the state of physical and mental growth and intense development of the children.
- **Socioeconomic development:** One fourth of the India's population is comprised of children between 5 to 14 years of age. Social and economic development of the nation is possible only through care and development of this group.

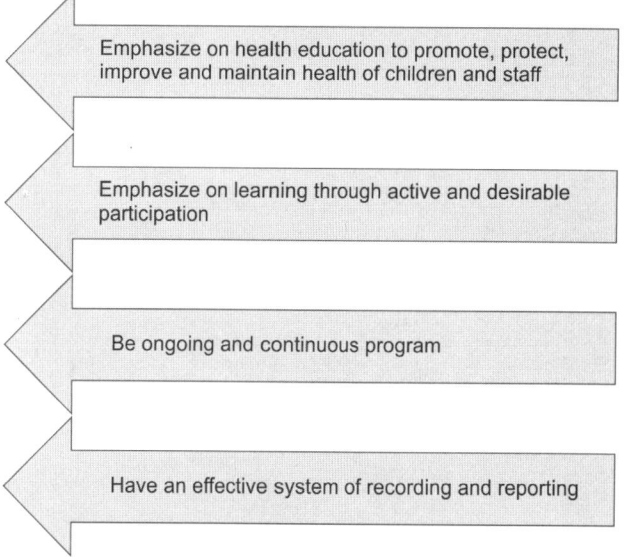

Fig. 13.30: Importance/scope of community health program.

- **Socialization:** School is another social group the child gets after family. They get much experience through this social life. Contribution of school is vital in the socialization of children.
- **Easy implementation:** School going children form a specific age group, otherwise called controlled population. They are within the easy reach for the implementation.
- **Early detection and diagnosis:** Infectious diseases, physical and mental disorders can be detected at early stage in school going children.
- **Adaptability:** School going children have the ability to quickly adopt and acquire new knowledge therefore school children can be used for giving effective health education to children and to develop healthy habits in them.

Principles of School Health Programs

- It is based on health needs of school children.
- It is an ongoing and continuous program.
- It emphasizes on learning through active and desirable participation.
- It emphasizes on promotive and preventive aspects.
- It should be well planned in coordination with school, health personnel, parents and community people.
- It emphasizes on learning through active and desirable participation.
- It has an effective system of record keeping and reporting.

Health Problems of School Children

Health Service must be based on the local health problems of the school child, the culture of the community and the available resource in terms of money, material and manpower. Health problems of school children vary from one place to another, survey carried out in India indicate that the main emphasis will fall one of the following categories:
- Malnutrition—anemia, protein calorie malnutrition vitamin deficiencies, etc.
- Infectious diseases
- Intestinal parasites
- Disease of skin, eyes and ear
- Dental caries.

School Health Preventive and Promotive Services

The components of school health services include all those aspects which help achieve its aim and objectives. The service need to be comprehensive in nature and include all elements of promotive, preventive, therapeutic and rehabilitative care **(Fig. 13.31)**.

- **Health appraisal:** Health appraisal should cover not only the student but also the teacher and other school personnel. Health appraisal consists of periodic medical examination and observation of children by the class teacher **(Fig. 13. 32)**.

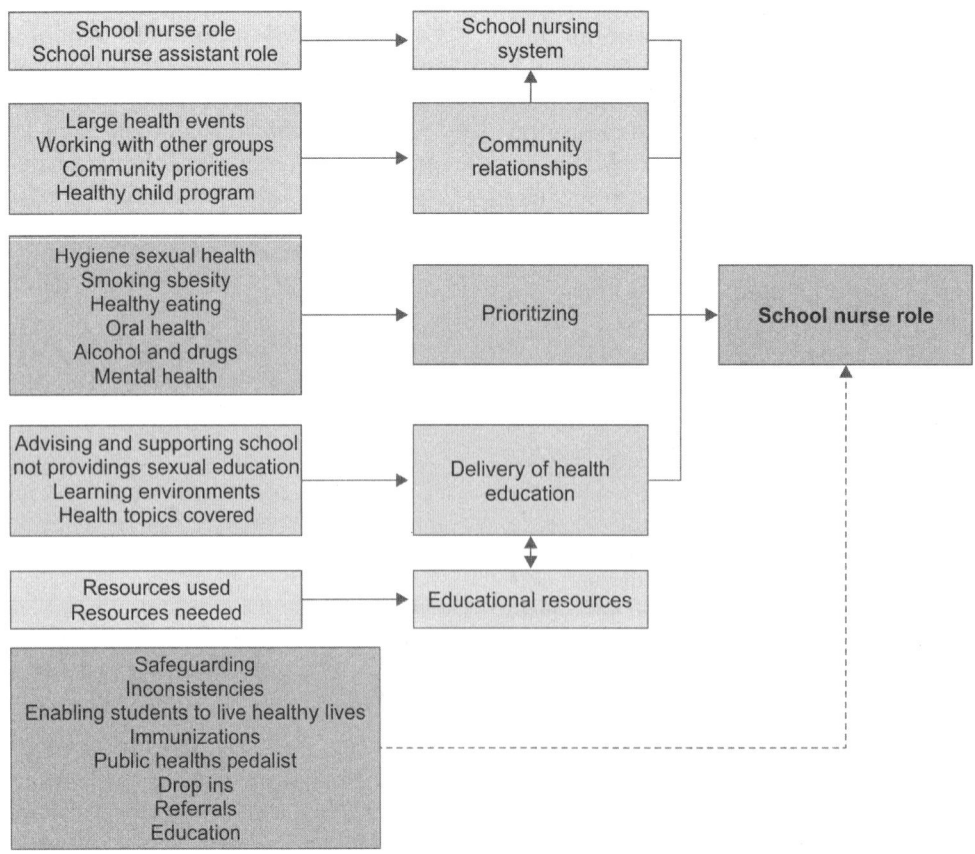

Fig. 13.31: School health preventive and promotive services.

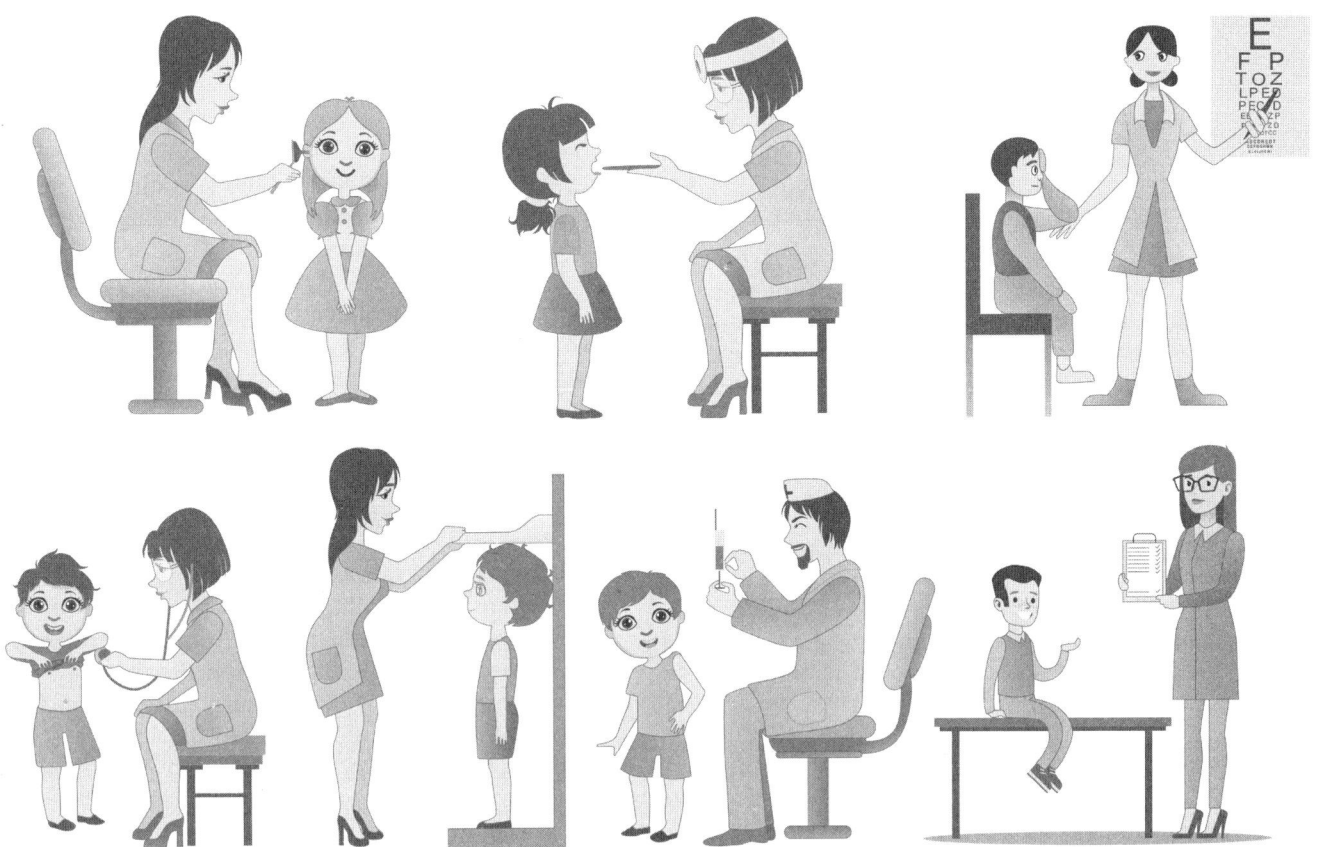

Fig. 13.32: Periodic medical examination of school children.

- **Remedial measures and follow-up:** Medical examinations are not an end in themselves. They should be followed by appropriate treatment and follow-up. Special clinics should be conducted exclusively for school children at primary health centers.
- **Prevention of communicable disease:** Protection of all school going children against preventable disease by immunization according to the national immunization schedule.
- **Healthful school environment:** The school building site and equipment are part of the environment in which the child grows and develops healthful school environment therefore is necessary for the best emotional, social and personal health of the pupils, e.g., as regards safe drinking water, sanitation accident prevention, food hygiene, etc.
- **Nutritional services:** Good nutrition is very essential not only for optimal health. Growth and development of the school child but also for his/her educational achievement. A nutritious mid-day meal for children in the school is considered a practical solution to combat malnutrition in children.
- **First-aid and emergency:** The school must have an arrangement for providing first aid and emergency care to children who get injured or sick at the school. So all the teachers should receive adequate training during teacher training program or in service training programs to prepare them to carry out this obligation.
- **Mental health:** The mental health of the child affects his physical health and the learning process. Juvenile delinquency, maladjustment and drug addiction are becoming problems among school children. They need to plan and organize well balanced curricular, co-curricular and extracurricular activities so that students are not over burdened and have sufficient relaxation and recreation etc.
- **Dental health:** Dental caries and periodontal disease are the two common dental diseases in India. A school health program should have provision for dental examination, at least once a year.
- **Eye health services:** Schools should be responsible for the early detection of refractive errors, treatment of squint and amblyopia and detection and treatment of eye infection such as trachoma.
- **Health education:** Health education is very important for school children. It creates awareness, makes them knowledge regarding health matter, develops motivation and promotes change in health behavior and health attitudes in them. Therefore health education is considered as one of the crucial and key element of school health services. Health education content areas include personal hygiene, environmental health, nutrition, prevention and control of communicable and non-communicable diseases.
- **Education of handicapped children:** The ultimate so that the child will be able to reach his maximum potential to lead as normal a life as possible to become as independent as possible and to become a production and self-supporting member of society.

Chapter 13: Specialized Community Health Services and Nurse's Role

- **School health records:** It is essential to maintain complete, accurate and continuous health records of school children. Such health records will be useful for providing need based healthcare and guidance to children. It will also help evaluate the school health services and assist further development and improvement of health services considered to school children.

School Health Nurse

School health is a team function. The team should be comprised of medical officer, school health nurse and auxiliary health workers, teachers, parents, students and representative from the community. Practice components for each principle in the framework for 21st century school nursing practice is depicted in **Table 13.1**.

- Each member of the team has on important role and accordingly the functions and responsibilities to carry on.
- The school health nurse is responsible for comprehensive services which include major emphasis of preventive promotive and personal care of the child, health education of children, parents, school teachers and community.
- The school health nurse also helps and asserts in early diagnosis, treatment, prevention of complications and rehabilitation.
- She also performs managerial and supervisory functions. She also performs all these functions by making use of nursing process involving teachers, students and their parents, community leaders, etc., she has many roles to play in school health program.
- The American Nurses Association official statement of functions and qualifications for school health nurse listed 20 functions and qualifications for school health nurse listed 20 functions, which are grouped under the general responsibilities areas of assessment, planning, implementation, evaluation and research.

Responsibilities of Nurse School Health

- **Health promotion and specific protection:** Health promotion and specific protection refers to primary prevention. The activities include immunization, nutritional supplementation (mid day meal), health education, providing guidance and counseling programs, consultation to teachers, examination of school environments and involving community participation to eliminate safety hazards in the community.
- **Early diagnosis and treatment:** Early diagnosis and treatment refer to secondary level prevention. It includes regular and periodical health appraisal, notifying parents about health appraisal results, making referrals for further investigation follow-up, of referred cases, counseling of students, dispensing medicines as prescribed, providing first aid, and teaching family members, Auxiliary nurse midwife/multipurpose health worker to perform special treatment or procedures.
- **Prevention of complications and rehabilitations:** This is tertiary level of prevention. It includes eliminating risk factors responsible for particular conditions, health education of students, their parents and teachers, helping parents/family to meet special nutritional needs and financial help to deal with chronic and handicapping conditions.
- **Other functions of a school health nurse includes:** Maintenance of health records, assisting, supervising and guiding of auxiliary nurse midwives/multipurpose health workers, management of school health and clinic, holding conferences with teachers students and parents, participate in health committee or health council and participate in-service education of teachers on health matters.

Role of Nurse in School Health Services

- **Initiation and implementation:** Beginning and implementation of school health service is the responsibility of community health nurse. Before initiating school health services, the nurse should collect complete information about school administration, number of students and teachers, available resources,

TABLE 13.1: Practice components for each principle in the framework for 21st century school nursing practice.

Care coordination	Leadership
➢ Case management ➢ Chronic disease management ➢ Collaborative communication ➢ Direct care ➢ Motivational interviewing/counseling ➢ Nursing delegation ➢ Student care plans ➢ Student-centered care ➢ Student self-empowerment ➢ Transition planning	➢ Advocacy ➢ Change agents ➢ Education reform ➢ Funding and reimbursement ➢ Healthcare reform ➢ Lifelong learner ➢ Models of practice ➢ Technology ➢ Professionalism ➢ Systems-level leadership
Public health	**Quality improvement**
➢ Access to care ➢ Cultural competency ➢ Health equity ➢ Healthy people 2020 ➢ Levels of prevention ➢ Outreach ➢ Population-based care ➢ Social determinants of health ➢ Surveillance	➢ Data collection evaluation ➢ Quality improvement cycle ➢ Research ➢ Uniform data set
Standards of practice	
➢ Clinical competence ➢ Clinical guidelines ➢ Critical thinking ➢ NASN position statements ➢ Nurse practice acts ➢ Evidence-based practice ➢ Code of ethics ➢ Scope and standards of practice	

school environment, facilities of entertainment and sports, etc.
- **Liaison activities:** The main role of school health nurse is to establish liaison between the school, home and the community. The school health nurse also interacts, involve and coordinate with governmental or nongovernmental national or international health agencies.
- **Coordination:** The school health nurse takes up the responsibility of coordination between doctors, teachers, parent's local leadership, NGOs and voluntary organizations, etc.
- **Evaluation:** The school health nurse evaluate school health services on the basis of different fats, documents and information. She also provides feedback on these services of her basis of her knowledge and experience.
- **Training and guidance:** School health nurse plays an important role in training of teachers about daily checkup, maintaining health records and providing first aid. She contributes effectively in developing healthy habits in children.
- **Active participation:** In organizing health check up, providing treatment, immunization programs, nutritional programs, maintaining school health records good environmental at school and providing follow-up services.

School Visit and Community Health Nurse

School health services and health education are included among other things in the basic services of a primary health center. As long as we do not have a separate school health service wing, this program forms a routine activity of the primary health center. The primary health center has to play attention to the following services and activities in the school.
- Medical inspection of school
- Treatment of defects
- Sanitation of school environment
- Control of communicable diseases
- Health education
- School lunch

Medical inspection should be conducted at least three times during the school carrier of each pupil, i.e., at school entrance in the fourth standard and again before leaving the school. School for making arrangements for medical inspection, immunization activities and for taking measures for the improvement of environmental sanitation. The public health nurse can effectively carry out health education programs in schools involving parents and community leaders.

Role of Nurse in Community Health Programs

- Identification of schools available in area
- Preparation of tentative plan
- Submission of plan of action
- Ensure supplies of vaccines and drugs
- Prior permission from CEO/HM
- Implementation as per plan of action with team
- Screening of children
- Treatment of minor ailments
- Immunization and health education
- Supervision of mid-day meals
- Referral services and follow-up
- Formation of health committee
- Recording and submission of school health report.

School Health Team

The school health team may comprise a minimum of three members, the doctor in charge, a primary healthcare functionary and a trained teacher of the school.

Doctor-in Charge

- WHO is the leader of the team, is a medical officer of the nearest health facility, a primary health center or a dispensary.
- He is responsible for the overall healthcare of the school children in which he is assisted by the other two members of the team.
- He guides and advises the school athletics and health education. He also offers advice on school outreach programs for promotion of community health.
- The doctor in-charge runs a weekly school clinic in his health facility exclusively for the treatment and advice of cases referred to him from the school.
- He conducts investigation of deserving cases and arranges for referral care of the children in special need.

Trained School Teacher

- He/she is responsible for the continuity of the school health program under the guidance of the doctor in charge.
- He conducts health monitoring of students every day to check their personal hygiene and identify cases needing medical consultation and treatment.
- He provides first aid care and refers cases to the nearest health facility for further action.
- He assists the doctor in anthropometry of children and their subsequent growth monitoring.
- He participates actively in the school meal program and holds the change of school garden, school kitchen and perhaps school athletics.
- He is actively involved in health education of children through frequent health talks. He carries out school health service records and reports in an important duty of the program teacher.

Primary Healthcare Functionary

- Preferably a female health supervisor working in the nearby a female supervisor working in the nearby primary health center.
- She visits the school frequently and serves as a connecting link between the school and the doctor-in charge.
- She provides follow-up of deserving cases under the instructions of the doctor.
- She supports the program teacher in technical areas such as identification of students having defective vision, defective hearing, orodental problems and various forms of malnutrition.

- She provides assistance in anthropometric measurement of children, and overseas school sanitation.
- She takes active part in the control of epidemic and endemic diseases and carries out immunization of school children besides conducting disinfection and disinfection of school building.
- She also extends control activities of endemic diseases to school children as envisaged under national health programs.

School Health Committee

The ministry of education appointed a school health committee under the chairmanship of Smt. Renuka Ray in 1960 to assess the present standard of health and nutrition of school children and suggest ways and means of improving them. In 1963, Government of India constituted the National School health council, it was reconstituted in 1966 to carry out the recommendations of Renuka Ray committee, 1962-63 as part of minimum needs program, mid-day meals Programs for rage group 6-11 was introduced to school children for 200 days in a year.

Areas of School Health Services

- School meal
- Preschool child
- School health education
- School environment
- Training and research
- School health administration
  - Health appraisal of school children and school personnel.
  - Remedial measures and follow-up
  - Prevention of communicable diseases
  - Healthful school environment
  - Nutritional services
  - First-aid and emergency care
  - Mental health
  - Dental health
  - Eye health
  - Health education
  - Education of handicapped children.
  - Proper maintenance and use of school health records.

Five Years Plan and School Health Recommendations

- **Third five year plan:** On 12th June 1959, the Government of India appointed another popularly known as the Mudaliar Committee to survey the progress made in the field of health.

  Mudaliar Committee recommendations are the each directorate of health services should have a bureau of school health services to plan and initiate activities of the government, the local bodies and the voluntary organizations. It also helps to establish close liaison with the education departments in the states.

  General hygiene and sanitation in school premises should be improved. Every school must have a source of wholesome water supply, sanitary facilities, regular and proper cleaning up the classrooms and the school campus. Production of birth and vaccination certificate should be made compulsory for admission in schools. School staff should actively assist in inoculation of pupils at the time of an epidemic. School health services should be looked after by the primary health center in the area.

- **Fourth five year plan: The fourth five year plan** and Kartar Singh committee was from 1969 to 1974. During fourth five year plan, there is a nationwide need for a school health program, ministries of health and education will jointly implement the program with the help of teachers, parents, students and social worker.

  The school health committee had this program be developed rapidly with a view to improve nutritional standards and to inculcate sound dietary habits. Provision for continuing the program started during third year plan was given. It was expected to get local support from non-official and voluntary agencies such as panchayats, local bodies.

  The program for the improvement in health of school children includes the immunization against preventable disease and scientific health education for students and teachers about clean water supply, sanitary latrines, and hygienic surroundings. It is proposed to provide facilities to school children and college student at the time of their admission.

- **School health committee at school level:** School health committee is a coordinating body that is charged with the overall responsibility of smooth functioning of the school health program. It is a committee consisting of the school health program. It is a committee consisting of members representing various fields of interest. Besides the principal teacher of the school health committee may include representatives from parents and school children and some selected community leaders and officers of health related departments whose cooperation is necessary for the optimum functioning of the school health program.

  School health committee should meet frequently to oversee the program operation, evaluate its performance and identity impediments, if any and attempt their removal for ensuring uninterrupted functioning of the program. The committee should provide moral and material support to the school health team to make it optimally functional.

School Health Policies

Policies governing the school health programs should be done drawn by the representatives committee. Policies must be understood equally well by teachers, nurse and other school personnel. The following policies may be used as a guide to develop more specific policies for individual schools.

- The school health program should be a part of the total community health program.
- Community health facilities should provide for the health needs of school age children including preventive therapeutic and rehabilitative measures.

- Health education should be integrated in the regular school program.
- Provision should be made for regular coordinated action between school, home, community and health services.
- Environmental sanitation in the school should receive priority from both school and health authority.
- Every school should provide mid-day meals for children in need of supplementary food.
- Provision should be made for teacher training in the field of health with particular stress on how to teach sanitation, nutrition and personal hygiene to children as part of the regular curriculum.

Steps of Program Planning

The school health nurse should have thorough knowledge of children, of social conditions and customs, of up to date scientific and medical development and her understanding of families and health practices, health habits and health problems place in her in strategic position to initiate and contribute to policy making in planning.

- **Step 1:** Visit each school and communicable with the principal and discover kind of problems, actions taken to treat and prevent. Observe the environmental status and immunization status of the school children.
- **Step 2:** Make a map showing the location of each school in relation to the health center.
- **Step 3:** Organize a school health committee after discuss the school report with supervisor and health director.
- **Step 4:** Make arrangements for a conference to include school principals and teacher, medical officers nurse health visitor social education organizers, block development officers, sanitarians, village level workers, the head of the panchayat and other leading professional and lay members of he school community and parents.
- **Step 5:** At the second meeting of the group the agenda should provide for a report of the school health survey and the appointment of a school health planning committee.
- **Step 6:** Work with the committee and develop a program based on the needs, personnel and facilities available.
- **Step 7:** The proposed plans should include definite realistic goals and estimated target dates.
- **Step 8:** Make a schedule with the help and approval of the school to include work with each school and health committee.
- **Step 9:** Plan an educational program for the school health staff whereby teachers, doctors, nurses, health visitors, sanitarians and midwives will meet regularly.
- **Step 10:** Evaluate the program at the end of the school year and make plans for the following school term.

National School Health Scheme

The fifth five year plan noted serious deficiencies in the system of medical inspection of school children and emphasized the detection and treatment of defects of school children as part of general health services. It was in 1977 that a modest beginning was made to reach the benefits of school health service program to children in primary classes.

A centrally sponsored national school health scheme was operated to provide health services supported by health education to the children primary classes in giving priority to tribal, backward and hilly areas in rural India through a network of selected primary health centers having two doctors in a phased manner.

In 1979, the national school health scheme was transferred along with a few others centrally-sponsored schemes to the state sector leaving only union territories with the central government. The scheme continued in operation in 8 union territories except Delhi and it had own comprehensive school health scheme.

Package of Services under School Health

Recognizing schools as useful platform, Government of India has launched "School Health Program" under Ayushman Bharat to strengthen health promotion and disease prevention intervention. It is a joint initiative of Ministry of Health and Family Welfare and Department of School Education and Literacy, Ministry of Human Resource and Development.

Objectives

- To provide age appropriate information about health and nutrition to the children in schools.
- To promote healthy behaviors among the children that they will inculcate for life.
- To detect and treat diseases early in children and adolescents including identification of malnourished and anemic children with appropriate referrals to PHCs and hospitals.
- To promote use of safe drinking water in schools.
- To promote safe menstrual hygiene practices by girls.
- To promote yoga and meditation through Health and Wellness Ambassadors.
- To encourage research on health, wellness and nutrition for children.

Components of School Health Program

Health Service Provision

- Screening, healthcare and referral: o Screening of general health, assessment of anemia/nutritional status, visual acuity, hearing problems, dental check up, common skin conditions, heart defects, physical disabilities, learning disorders, behavior problems.
- Basic medicine kit to be provided to take care of common ailments prevalent among young school going children.
- Referral Cards for priority services at District/Sub-District hospitals.

Immunization

- As per national schedule
- Fixed day activity
- Coupled with education about the issue
- Micronutrient (Vitamin A and Iron Folic Acid) management:

- Weekly supervised distribution of Iron-Folate tablets coupled with education about the issue
- Vitamin-A as per national schedule.

De-worming

- As per national guidelines
- Biannually supervised schedule
- Prior IEC with intimation to families to bring siblings to school on the fixed day
- Siblings of students also to be covered.

Health Promoting Schools

- Counseling services, promotion of mental well-being.
- Regular practice of Yoga, physical education, health education
- Peer leaders as health educators
- Adolescent health education
  - Linkages with the out of school children
  - Health clubs, health cabinets, health jamborees
- First Aid room/corners or clinics.

Capacity Building of Teachers and Involved Health Personnel

- Monitoring and evaluation
- Mid-day meal

School Health Promotion Activities

- Age appropriate incremental learning for promotion of healthy behavior and prevention of various diseases.
- Delivered through school teachers/Health and Wellness Ambassadors trained in each school.

Health Screening

The screening of children for 30 identified health conditions for early detection, free treatment and management through dedicated RBSK mobile health teams.

Provision of Services

- Provision of IFA and Albendazole tablets by teachers through WIFS and NDD program respectively.
- Provision of sanitary napkins.
- Age appropriate vaccination.

Electronic health records: Electronic health record for each child.

Imparting skills of emergency care: Training of teachers on basic first aid.

Health Screening: Rashtriya Bal Swasthya Karyakram (RBSK) is an important initiative aiming at early identification and early intervention for children from birth to 18 years to cover 4 'D's viz. Defects at birth, Deficiencies, Diseases, Development delays including disability. The 0–6 years' age group will be specifically managed at District Early Intervention Center (DEIC) level while for 6–18 years' age group, management of conditions will be done through existing public health facilities. DEIC will act as referral linkage for both the age groups. Once the child is screened and referred from school, it would be ensured that the necessary treatment/intervention is delivered at zero cost to the family.

Electronic health records: It is envisaged to develop an electronic health record for each student. Student Health Card will include health screening and service access data for each student. Under the RBSK, the screening and referral records of all the school children will be digitalized. The relevant information related to school health activities/will be added to existing electronic records maintained under RBSK.

Upgrading skills in emergency care: A child spends a considerable part of the day in school, which makes it the responsibility of the school to ensure the safety of all children in every possible way during their stay at school. Thus, students and teachers should know the basics of first aid and should be able to respond to emergencies. There should be a first aid box available in each school. The teachers and students will be made aware of the various services available to attend to emergencies like the ambulance, fire brigade, police, closest health facility, etc. Sessions on basic first aid will be taken up and linkages with local disaster response teams will be made, to build the capacity of school teachers and children to respond to emergencies.

Implementation

- A National level coordination committee under the co-chairmanship of MoHFW and MHRD is responsible for policy formulation, technical support, planning of the program establishing monitoring systems and reviewing progress on program preparedness.
- At the State level, Coordination Committee will be constituted under the co-chairpersonship of Principal Secretary(s) Health and Education with Secretaries of Women and Child Development, drinking water and sanitation, Panchayati Raj and other relevant department as members.
- A District Level Coordination Committee should be led by District Magistrate with Civil Surgeons/CMHOs, District Education Officer, District Institute of Education and Training officer; District ICDS Program Manager, and representatives from other departments and development partners as members if so desired.
- At Block Level, Coordination Committee is constituted under the chairpersonship of Sub-Divisional Magistrate (SDM) with BMO, Block Education Officer, Block Development Officer (BDO), selected principals and representatives from other relevant departments as members.

Role of School Health Nurse

The National Association of Nurses Defines School Nursing as: A specialized practice of professional nursing that advances the well-being, academic success and lifelong achievements of students to that end, school nurses facilitate positive student responses to normal development, promote health and safety, intervene with actual and potential health problem, provide case management services and actively collaborate with others to build students and family capacity for adaptation, self-management, self-advocacy and learning (Fig. 13.33).

Role of Nurse in Planning

- The team should be comprised of medical officer, school health nurse and auxiliary health workers, teachers, parents, students and representative from the community.
- Each member of the team has on important role and accordingly the functions and responsibilities to carry on.
- The school health nurse is responsible for comprehensive services which include major emphasis of preventive promotive and personal care of the child, health education of children, parents, school teachers and community.
- The school health nurse also helps and asserts in early diagnosis, treatment, prevention of complications and rehabilitation.
- She also performs managerial and supervisory functions. She also performs all these functions by making use of nursing process involving teachers, students and their parents, community leaders, etc. she has many roles to play in school health program.

Roles of the School Health Nurse

- **Health promotion and special protection:**
  - Immunization
  - Nutrition
  - Health education
  - Develop positive attitude towards school health
  - Healthful environment
  - Community participation
- **Early diagnosis and treatment:**
  - Health appraisal
  - Parent notification
  - Referral services
  - Follow-up care
  - Home visit
  - Counseling services—students, parents and teachers.
  - Treating and de-worming
  - Health education
  - First Aid and emergency services, demonstration of first Aid.
- **Prevention of complication and rehabilitation:**
  - Prevention of acute condition
  - Promotion of adjustment in chronic conditions
  - Help in prevention of learning disabilities.
- **Other functions:**
  - School record
  - Preparation of appraisal report
  - Supervision of ANM
  - School health clinic
  - Meeting with teachers and parents
  - Participation in team/committee
  - In-service education to teacher.

School Health Policies, Programs and Scheme

The health and well-being of children and youth must be a fundamental value of society. Urgent health and social problems have underscored the need for collaboration among families, schools, agencies, communities and governments in taking a comprehensive approach to school-based health promotion.

Comprehensive School Health Approach

A comprehensive school health approach includes a broad spectrum of activities and services which take place in schools and their surrounding communities that enable children and youth to enhance their health, develop to their fullest potential and establish productive and satisfying relationships in their present and future lives. The goals of a comprehensive approach are to:
- Promote health and wellness.
- Prevent specific diseases, disorders and injury.
- Prevent high risk social behaviors.
- Intervene to assist children and youth who are in need or at risk.
- Help support those who are already exhibiting special healthcare needs.
- Promote positive health and safety behaviors.

School Health Policies

Policies governing the school health programs should be done drawn by the representatives committee. Policies must be understood equally well by teachers, nurse and other school personnel. The following policies may be used as a guide to develop more specific policies for individual schools:
- The school health program should be a part of the total community health program.
- Community health facilities should provide for the health needs of school age children including preventive therapeutic and rehabilitative measures.

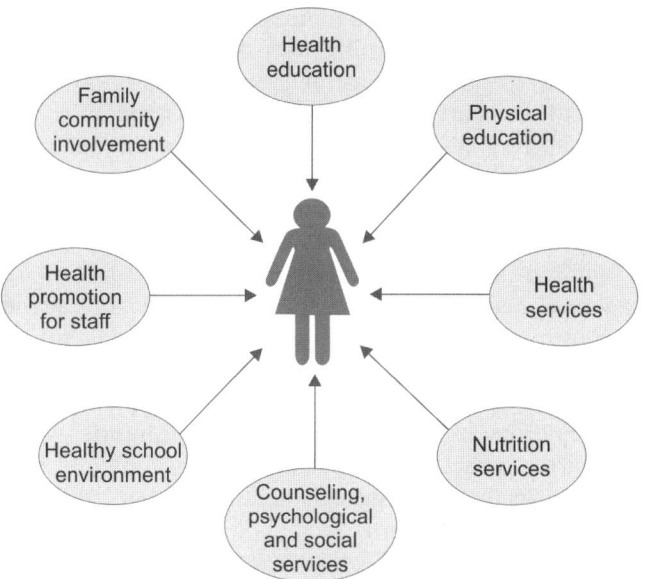

Fig. 13.33: Role of school health nurse.

- Health education should be integrated in the regular school program.
- Provision should be made for regular coordinated action between school, home, community and health services.
- Environmental sanitation in the school should receive priority from both school and health authority.
- Every school should provide mid-day meals for children for children in need of supplementary food.
- Provision should be made for teacher training in the field of health with particular stress on how to teach sanitation, nutrition and personal hygiene to children as part of the regular curriculum.

Steps of Program Planning

The school health nurse should have thorough knowledge of children, of social conditions and customs, of up to date scientific and medical development and her understanding of families and health practices, health habits and health problems place in her in strategic position to initiate and contribute to policy making in planning.

- **Step 1:** Visit each school and communicable with the principal and discover kind of problems, actions taken to treat and prevent. Observe the environmental status and immunization status of the school children.
- **Step 2:** Make a map showing the location of each school in relation to the health center.
- **Step 3:** Organize a school health committee after discuss the school report with supervisor and health director.
- **Step 4:** Make arrangements for a conference to include school principals and teacher, medical officers nurse health visitor social education organizers, block development officers, sanitarians, village level workers, the head of the panchayat and other leading professional and lay members of the school community and parents.
- **Step 5:** At the second meeting of the group the agenda should provide for a report of the school health survey and the appointment of a school health planning committee.
- **Step 6:** Work with the committee and develop a program based on the needs, personnel and facilities available.
- **Step 7:** The proposed plans should include definite realistic goals and estimated target dates.
- **Step 8:** Make a schedule with the help and approval of the school to include work with each school and health committee.
- **Step 9:** Plan an educational program for the school health staff whereby teachers, doctors, nurses, health visitors, sanitarians and midwives will meet regularly.
- **Step 10:** Evaluate the program at the end of the school year and make plans for the following school term.

Integration of School and Community Health Activities

School can be one of the primary sites through which children and youth learn about the factors that influence their health. It also can be the site that provides or coordinates some or all of the needed healthcare services. It has been said that youth are one-third of our population and all of our future **(Fig. 13.34)**.

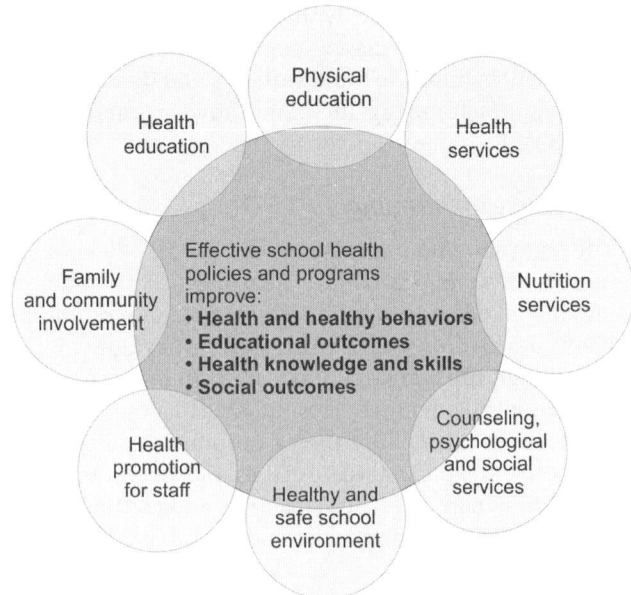

Fig. 13.34: Integration of school and community health activities.

Goals and objectives: The goals and objectives of the school-community component of comprehensive school health are clear, based on assessed needs and stated in terms of intended outcomes.

Program Components

- An interdisciplinary/interagency school health coordinating council that includes school staff, families who represent all segments of the community, students and community resource personnel is organized at the community level to coordinate programs among agencies that promote the health and safety of youth.
- Interdisciplinary school health teams (committees) that include teachers, families, students, school nurses, physicians, health educators, school psychologists, coaches, social workers/counselors and community resource personnel are organized at the school level to address priority school health and safety issues that interfere with the learning process.
- Interdisciplinary school health teams and the interdisciplinary/interagency coordinating council achieve identified goals by implementing the program planning model (assessment; planning; setting of goals, objectives and strategies; implementation; and evaluation).
- A systematic means for sharing information and resources and coordinating programs is established
- Periodic meetings of the interdisciplinary/interagency coordinating council are held to assess needs, initiate recommendations and evaluate programs.
- Integrated efforts to eliminate illegal use of alcohol and other drugs, use of tobacco, motor vehicle injuries, sports injuries, sexually transmitted diseases, suicide, child abuse, violence, teen pregnancies and other health and safety-related concerns are implemented.
- Evaluations are conducted at least annually to assess the level of satisfaction with the comprehensive school health program.

- Continuing education programs are offered for families and community members.
- Efforts are made to encourage family and other community member attendance and involvement with school and academic programs (e.g., health education, child care, evening meetings, and coordination with other school activities).
- A two-way communication system is established between school and homes to encourage maximum involvement in areas of mutual interest.
- Families, after receiving the results of health-related fitness tests, encourage their child to complete an individualized activity plan.
- Programs are provided to assist families and community members in building communication and other family skills, as well as understanding child growth and development.

The school nurse typically provides population-based primary prevention and healthcare services, including
- Physical and mental health assessment and referral for care;
- Development and implementation of healthcare plans for students with special healthcare needs;
- Health counseling;
- Mandated screenings, such as vision, hearing, and immunization status;
- Monitoring the presence of infectious conditions among students and enforcing public health precautions to prevent spread of infections and infestations;
- Skilled nursing services for students with complex healthcare needs; case management of students with chronic and special healthcare needs;
- Outreach to students and their families;
- Interpretation of the healthcare needs of students to school personnel;
- Development and implementation of emergency care plans and provision of emergency care and first aid;
- Serving as liaison for the school, parents, and community health agencies;
- Collaboration with other school professionals-particularly counselors, psychologists, and social workers-to address the health, developmental, and educational needs of students; and
- For nurse practitioners only, the provision of primary care, including prescribing medications when allowed under the State Nurse Practice Act.

MAINTENANCE OF SCHOOL HEALTH RECORDS

Schools are required to keep certain health-related records about all students, including immunization information, growth, vision testing and hearing screening findings, attendance data, preschool health screening, and TB screening information. In addition, many schools provide medical services to individual students. These medical services generate health records (**Fig. 13.35**).

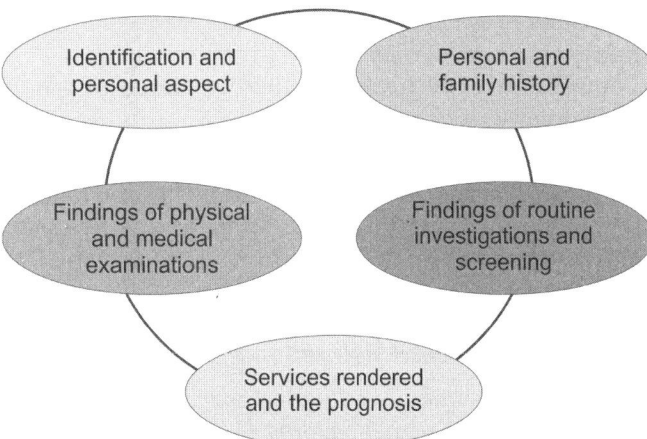

Fig. 13.35: Health record informations.

School Health Record
- A cumulative health record of each student should be maintained. Such records should contain:
    - Identifying data—name, date of birth, parent's name, address, etc.
    - Past health history.
    - Record of finding of physical examination and screening tests and record of service provided.
- Purposes:
    - To maintain cumulative information on the health aspect of school children.
    - To analyzing and evaluating school health program and providing a useful link between the home, school and community.

Types of Registers
- Minor ailments register
- Health record register
- Medical camp register
- Health education class registers
- Observance of important health days registers
- Health club activity registers
- Stock register

Need of Health Records
- It is important to note that any health records that the school receives from outside providers will most likely be considered school health records.
- This means they may be reviewed by teachers and other school officials who have a legitimate educational interest in the information.
- It is also possible that teachers and officials from schools where your child seeks, to or intends to enroll, may also have access to the information.

Essentials of School Health Records
- Essential to maintain complete, accurate and continuous health record of school children.

- Useful in providing need based healthcare and guidance to children evaluate the school health services.
- Assist in future development.
- Improvement of health services rendered to school children.

Health record should include information on: Identification and personal aspect, personal and family history, findings of routine investigations and screening, services rendered and the prognosis and findings of physical and medical examinations.

School Health Record Maintenance

Health records shall be maintained for each child. These records shall be kept in the school building where the child attends school and shall be available to the school nurse at all times. Records shall be transferred with the child when he moves from one school to another or from one district to another.

- The designated nodal officers looking after adolescent program at the State, District and Block levels will be responsible for recording and reporting of the activities.
- Health and Wellness Ambassadors will record the progress of each class every month in a prescribed format.
- The principal or Health and Wellness Ambassadors will compile the reported class data into the School reporting format every month and submit to Block Resource Center of education department by 7th of next month.
- The nodal officer at Block Resource Center will share the compiled reports of all schools from respective blocks to the Block Medical Officer by 10th of next month.
- Block Adolescent Health Coordinators will ensure the coordination between the two departments. He or she will ensure reporting of block level report on the e-MIS by 15th of next month.
- The District Nodal officer or District Level Adolescent Health Counselor (if in position) will compile data of all blocks and submit the duly signed compiled report to the State Nodal Officer under Health Department. He or She will also ensure the sharing of reports with the District Education Officer.
- The State Nodal officer will compile the reports of all the districts in the State level format and submit the duly signed report to Adolescent Health Division at MoHFW.

OCCUPATIONAL HEALTH NURSING (INCLUDING HEALTHCARE PROVIDERS)

- Occupational health broadly defined in the occupational health and safety encyclopedia as being concerned with physical, mental and social well being of man in relation to his work and working environment his adjustment to work and adjustment of work to man.
- Occupational health is the promotion and maintenance of the highest degree of physical, mental and social well-being of the workers in all occupations (WHO 1953).

Aims of Occupational Health

- Promote and maintain highest degree of physical, mental and social well-being of workers in all occupations;
- Prevent among workers all departures from Health caused by their working condition;
- Protect workers in their employment from risks resulting from factors adverse to health; and,
- Place and maintain the worker in an occupational environment adapted to his physiological and psychological capacity.
- Prediction of health outcomes!

Objectives of Occupational Health (Fig. 13.36)

- To identify and bring under control at the work place all chemical, physical, mechanical, biological and

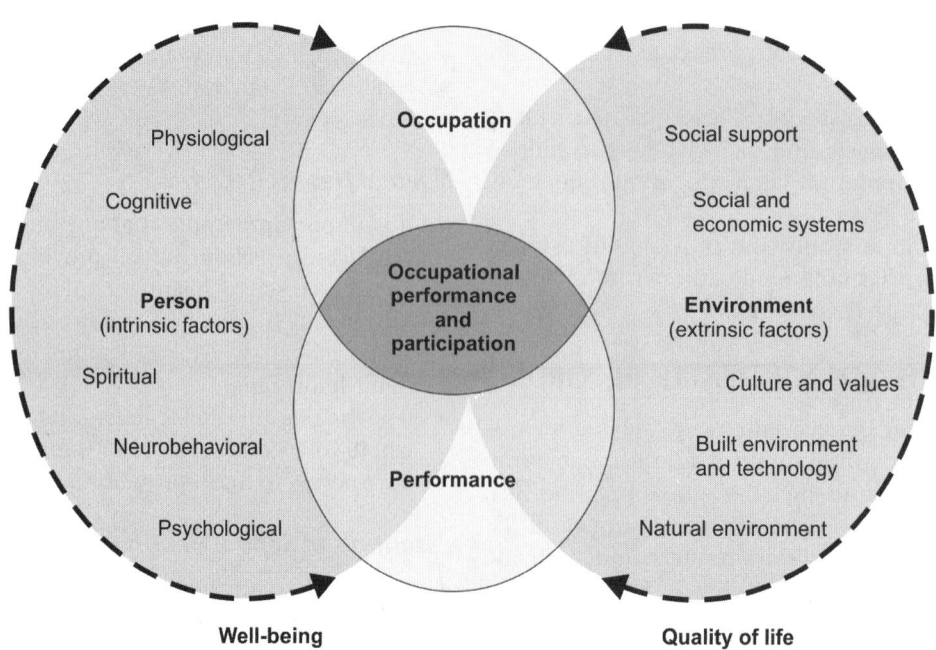

Fig. 13.36: Occupational environment.

psychological agents that are known to be or suspected of being hazards.
- To ensure that physical and mental demands imposed on people at work by their respective jobs are properly matched with their individual physiological agents that are known to be or suspected of being hazardous.
- To provide effective measures to protect those who are especially vulnerable to adverse working conditions and also to raise their level of resistance.
- To discover and improve work situations that may contribute to the overall ill health of workers in order to ensure that the burden of general illness in different occupational groups is not increased over community level.
- To educate management and workers to fulfill their responsibilities relevant to health protection and promotion.
- To carry out comprehensive in plant health Programs dealing with man's total health.
- Identification and improvement which implies identifying the hazardous agent and instituting measures of control to improve the working environment.
- It also involves protection of the vulnerable by offering sheltered placement.
- Education and motivation which applies to workers as well as to industrial management that both the parties are persuaded to fulfill their responsibilities in the sphere of occupational health.
- Holistic healthcare which amounts to the provision of total healthcare service to workers which is comprehensive enough to answer all their health needs.

Occupational Environment

- **Internal occupational environment:** It is the conventional industrial setting in which service of industrial workers are utilized in the industrialized countries of the world. The workers in the industrial settings are exposed to a variety of physical, chemical biological and psychological hazards and to a host of stress factors which may originate from the work, the worker or the work environment.
- **External occupational environment:** It is an extra industrial and extra institutional environment that exists in the world outside. It includes the occupational environment of farmers, sailors, sheep herders, construction workers, rangers, and a wide variety of departmental field workers. They are exposed to intense cold, intense heat, high humidity, besides the hazards caused by chemical, mechanical and biological agents leading to injuries, accidents and disease of various types.
- **Residential environment:** Though, it is not a component of occupational environment, it has a close association with the occupational environment. A congenial and comfortable residential environment has a favorable effect on industrial environments also interact with the community around. Diseases endemic in the community enter the factory environment mainly through the agency of the workers residing in the area.

Developmental of Occupational Health in India

- 1911—Provision for weekly holidays for all the workers and prohibited the employment of women and children below 9 years in the factories.
- 1934—Factories Act provision for appointment of factory inspectors, prevention of accidents and maintenance of sanitary conditions.
- 1946—Bhore Committee reported emphasized the need for investigation of occupational diseases and development of departments for teaching and research in occupational health.
- 1948—The Employees State Insurance Act which was enacted, to provide beneficial step towards social security for factory workers. The Act alleviates economic and physical suffering by providing benefits in cash and kind during sickness, maternity and occupational injury.
- 1960—Central Labor Institute was established in Bombay to study the various aspects of occupational health. Three regional institutes have been established in India at Kanpur, Calcutta and Chennai.
- 1973—For the first time, public attention drawn to working conditions in factories. It was major more who reported on factory conditions in Bombay and mentioned especially about the working conditions of women and children works.
- 1981—Indian Factories Act was enacted; the act prescribed working hours, holidays and employment of young men and women and prohibited the employment of women and children below 9 years in the factories.

Occupational Health and Research Institute Activities

There are five research institutes in the country which are focusing their activities towards occupational health.
1. The Central Mining and Research Station, Dhanbad under the Control of Scientific and Industrial Research (CSIR).
2. The Industrial Toxicology Research Center, Lucknow, under the CSIR.
3. Occupational Health Research Institute, Ahmadabad under the Indian Council of Medical Research.
4. National Environment Engineering Research Institute at Nagpur.
5. The All India Institute of Hygiene and Public Health, Calcutta.

Five Year Plans and Occupational Health

- Bhore committee recommended that the Industrial Health Service should be an integral part of the proposed National Health Service and should be administered centrally by the ministry of health. The work of the industrial organization should be integrated with the work of the general health services in each local area under the national health scheme.
- The industrial health services will consist of medical and paramedical personnel. Their report emphasizes the importance of establishing departments of industrial health in the medical institutions and universities.

- Bhore Committee recommended that the Industrial Health Organization should form and integral part of the provisional health departments and that should work in close association with the provisional government. The Central Government funds should be utilized for developing higher level of general health service for industrial workers.

Bhore Committee Recommendations of Occupational Health

- Training in First aid
- Crèches
- Maternity benefits
- Employment of women in coal mines.
- 45 hours of work in a week or 8 hours a day for 5 days for 5 hours a day with one day interval and mid-day meal break for not less than one hour.
- Accidents—compensation in case of accident should be payable to all notifiable accidents cases from the day of disablement and the seven days of waiting period should be abolished. There should be a provision for the proper treatment and rehabilitation of injured persons.
- There should be a proper registers for sickness and injury should be maintained in every industrial establishment.
- An enquiry into the prevalence of occupational disease should be done. Department of industrial medicine should study about occupational diseases and industrial research while teaching in medical institutions.
- Adequate number of women doctors should be employed in the proposed industrial health services.
- Preparation of housing schemes for the population.
- Food for workers—systematic nutritional survey should be undertaken by provisional governments. Canteens in the industries should provide balanced diet at reasonable cost.
- The employers should encourage workers to observe regular meal hours. Municipal by-laws regarding the protection of food require strengthening enforcement.
- Every canteen, food shop, tea shop and kitchen should be protected from flies. There should be strict supervision over the food supplies inside the factory.

Committee Recommendation on Industrial Hygiene

- Control of humidity and temperature
- Air ventilation
- Protection against the inhalation of poisonous or toxic gases, dust or other impurities.
- Washing facilities
- Drinking water facilities
- Bathing arrangements
- Urinals and latrines
- Clock room
- Special clothing
- Protective equipment
- Rest shelters
- Pre-employment and medical examination of adult employees.

Occupational Health Services

Definition

The joint committee of ILO/WHO on occupational health, held in 1950 for the first time gave the following statements about occupational health. The general aims of occupational health should be the promotion and maintenance of highest degree of physical, mental and social well-being of workers in all occupations, the prevention among workers of departures from health caused by their working conditions the protection of workers in their respective employments from risks resulting from factors adverse to health, the placing and maintenance of the workers in an occupational environment adopted to their physiological and psychological needs (**Fig. 13.37**).

Occupational Health Nursing

- The application of nursing principles in conserving the health of worker in all occupations. It involves prevention recognition and treatment of illness and injury, and requires special skills and knowledge in the fields of health, education and counseling environmental health, rehabilitation and human relations"—American Association of Occupational Health Nurses.
- "Occupational Health Nursing is the application of nursing and public health philosophy and skills to the relationship of people to their occupations for the purpose of prevention of disease and injury and the promotion of optimal health, productivity and social adjustments— Brown and Page.
- Occupational health nursing practice in the especially of practice thus provides for and delivers healthcare services to workers and workers population. The practice focuses on promotion, protection and restoration of workers health within the context of a safe and healthy work environment.

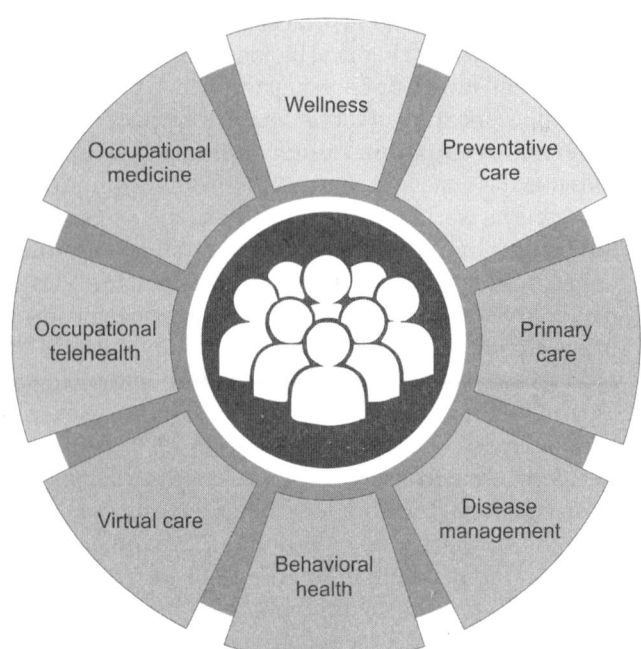

Fig. 13.37: Occupational health services.

Concept of Occupational Health

- The Occupational Health Program is an intensive health program planned to take of the worker and his family to promote the general health and welfare of the workers by providing a good and safe working environment.
- Occupational health implies not only health protection but also health promotion, emergency care, wide range preventive curative services, rehabilitative services, a concept which includes everything that can apply to promote the health and working capacity of worker.
- Ergonomics is a well recognized discipline and constitutes an integral part of any advanced occupational health service. The application of ergonomics has made a significant contribution to reducing industrial accidents and to the overall health and efficiency of the workers.
- Occupational health is the health science which is related to human work, work-place and work-environment **(Fig. 13.38)**. Occupational health is entirely preventive medicine. The chief objective of occupational health is the safety of workers in all occupations from injuries and disease and to improve their health status.
- Occupational health is an important branch of community health. Industrial hygiene means industrial health which involves industrial accidents, industrial toxicology, industrial hazards and industrial rehabilitation.

Aims of Occupational Health Services

- The promotion and maintenance of highest degree of physical, mental and social well-being of workers in all occupations.
- To contribute towards the workers physical and mental adjustments and particularly the adaptation of the work to the workers and their assignments to jobs for which they are suited.
- To contribute to the establishment and maintenance of physical and mental well-being of the workers.
- To provide effective services to workers who are incapacitated for any reasons to rehabilitate them as soon as possible.

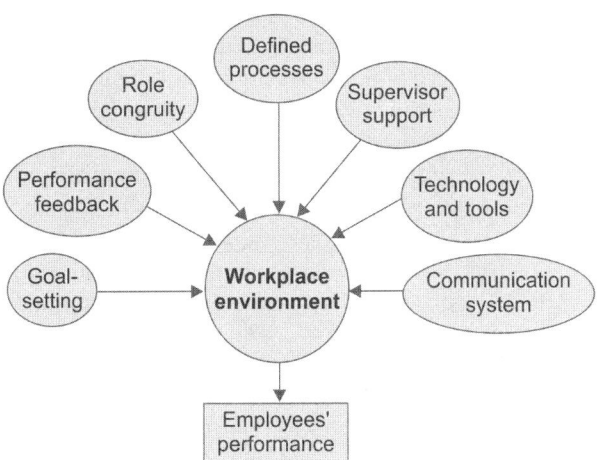

Fig. 13.38: Work place environment.

- Provide effective services to workers who are incapacitated for any reasons to rehabilitate them as soon as possible.

Scope of Occupational Health Services

- **Health promotion measures:** Preplacement, pre-employment examination, job training and continuing education, periodical health checkups, health education and counseling provision of wholesome environment, provision of welfare facilities, and suitable working hours.
- **Health protection measures:** Immunization agent specific infective agent, using protective devices like shoes and masks, using ear plugs, etc. Protection against chemical agents, specific engineering devices and health education.
- **Early diagnosis and treatment:** It is very essential for arresting the disease early recovery, regaining health, preventing any disabilities, etc. The medical services are provided by ESI Corporation for the workers as well as for the family members.
- **Disability limitation and rehabilitation:** Early diagnosis and prompt treatment, recertification of conditions responsible for occupational health problems. In case if the worker is handicapped he or she should be given suitable alternative job and other benefits.

Objectives of Occupational Health Services

- To improve human efficiency in his work by applying ergonomics (human engineering)
- To promote and maintain the highest degree of positive health and welfare of workers in all occupations.
- To provide a self-occupational environment in order to safeguard the health of the workers and to set up industrial production.
- To protect from factors adverse to health during their employment.
- To assist the injured and disabled for rehabilitation.
- To ensure that physical and psychological demands imposed on workers by their respective job are properly matched with their individual anatomical, physical and psychological needs, capabilities and limitations.
- To educate workers to promote and maintain their health.
- To provide care during emergencies.
- To promote general health and welfare of the worker by providing a good and safe working environment.

Health Problems Due to Industrialization

- Air pollution
- Water pollution
- Soil pollution
- Shortage of houses
- Communicable diseases
- Mental health problems
- Accidents
- Social problems like alcoholism, drug addiction, gambling, prostitution, juvenile delinquency.
- High morbidity and mortality from certain diseases, e.g., chronic bronchitis and lung cancer.

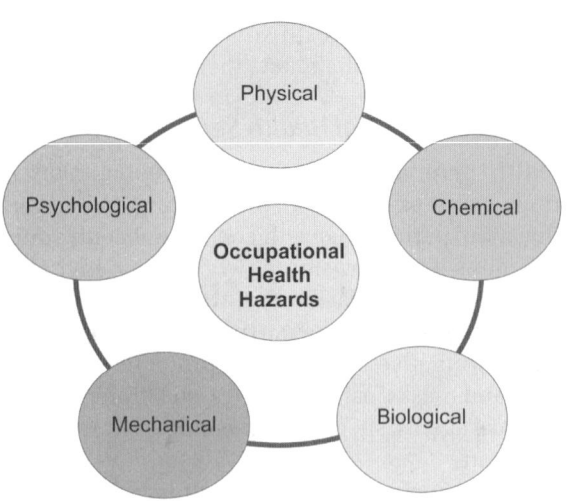

Fig. 13.39: Occupational health hazards.

Occupational Hazards

Currently occupational environment in the industrialized world is challenging health and safety of man. The risk associated with modern occupation necessitates the adaptation of man to industrial environment on the one hand and his protection from the risks on the other. The occupational hazards safety measures are depicted in **Figure 13.40**. These risks referred to occupational hazards threaten the physical, mental social and psychological health of workers. Occupational hazards are classified as physical, chemical and biological **(Fig. 13.39)**. Sources and health risks of occupational health hazards are depicted in **Figure 13.41**.

Physical Hazards and Health (Fig. 13.42)

- **High temperature:** Occupational exposure to extremely high temperature is experienced by construction workers, bakers, blacksmiths, and dry cleaners are allowed under high temperature in tropical climate. Workers toiling under high temperature may suffer from heat cramps, heat exhaustion or heat strokes.
    - *Heat cramps:* Caused when workers lose fluids and electrolytes from their bodies due to excessive sweating. Cramps develop in limbs and abdomen the pain in the lower limbs starts characteristically from calf muscles.
    - *Heat exhaustion:* There is peripheral vasodilatation leading to circulatory collapse. It may be associated with mild manifestations like headache, fatigue and dizziness.
    - *Heat stroke:* Extreme form of heat stress which results unconsciousness without any prodromal symptoms.
- **Low temperature:** Extreme low temperature in outdoor workers in cold northern regions of the world. Disease associates with cold stress are chilblains, trench foot and frost bite.
    - *Chilblains:* Caused by prolonged cooling of the body chilblains are superficial lesions without any associated vascular changes.
    - *Trench foot:* It is usually observed in army personnel working in extremely cold temperatures. The clinical picture of trench foot is an expression of the underlining vascular changes namely vasoconstriction followed by vasodilatation.
    - *Frost bite:* It involves actual freezing of tissues usually preceded by exposure to cold dry air at subzero temperatures. Frost bite commonly affects peripheral parts of the body like arms, nose, cheeks and digits.
- **Low pressure:** Exposure to low pressure results in the appearance of a group of clinical manifestations referred to as decompression sickness or caisson disease.
    - *Caisson*—is a chamber placed deep down in a sea, where from water has been drained out by air under high pressure to provide room for construction workers. Caisson disease appears in deep sea altitude in unpressurized planes.
    - *Decompression sickness*—movement from high pressure to low pressure area results in decompression sickness.
- **Vibration:** Exposure to vibration hazard occurs while using vibratory tools. Vibration sickness starts with an initial phase associated with tingling of fingers, accompanied by numbness and followed by episodes of blanching of finger tips the fingers turn white due to underlying vasospasm.
- **Nonionizing radiation:** Occupational exposure to external sources of non-ionizing radiation occurs among farmers, ranchers sailors mountaineers sheep herders and construction workers.
    - *Infra red radiation*—exposure may occur from natural source, i.e., sunlight or from manmade source. The radiation causes thermal damage to eyes and skin. In the eyes, it causes injury to cornea, iris or lens and in the skin produces acute skin burns associated with hyperpigmentation.
    - *Ultraviolet radiation*—skin exposed to ultra violet radiation develops erythema, sunburn and tanning associated with migration of melanin pigmentation. Ultraviolet radiation produces photokeratitis and conjunctivitis. Repeated exposure to ultrasound is

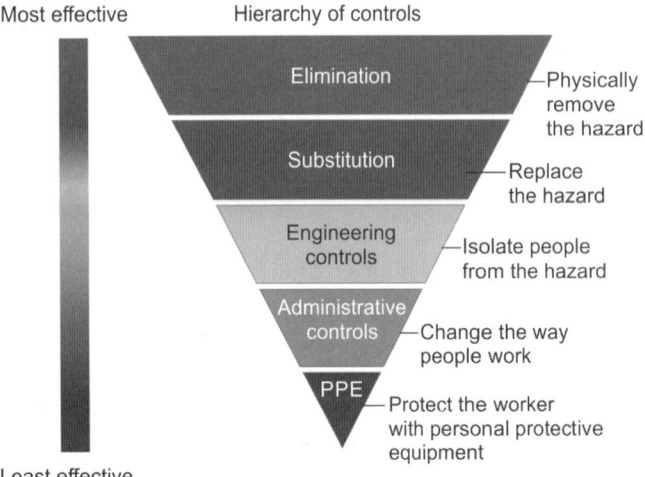

Fig. 13.40: Occupational hazard safety measures.

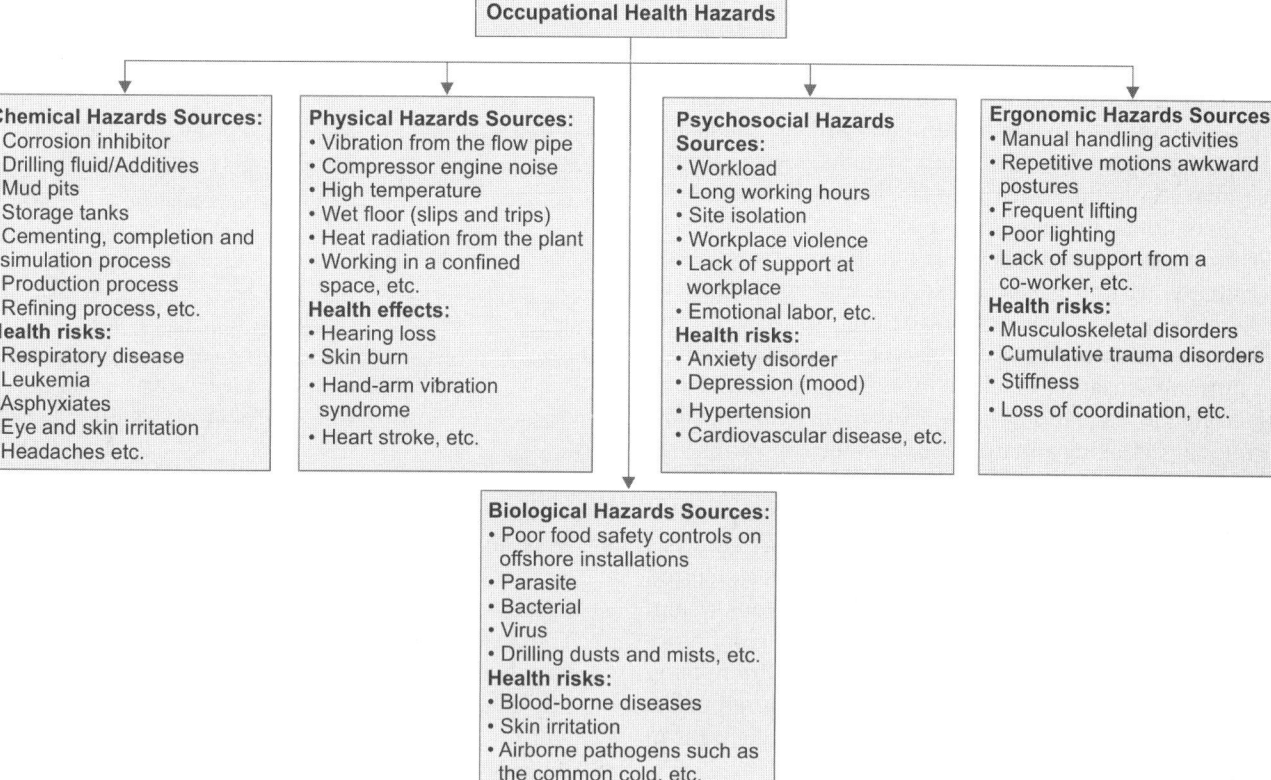

Fig. 13.41: Sources and health risks of occupational health hazards.

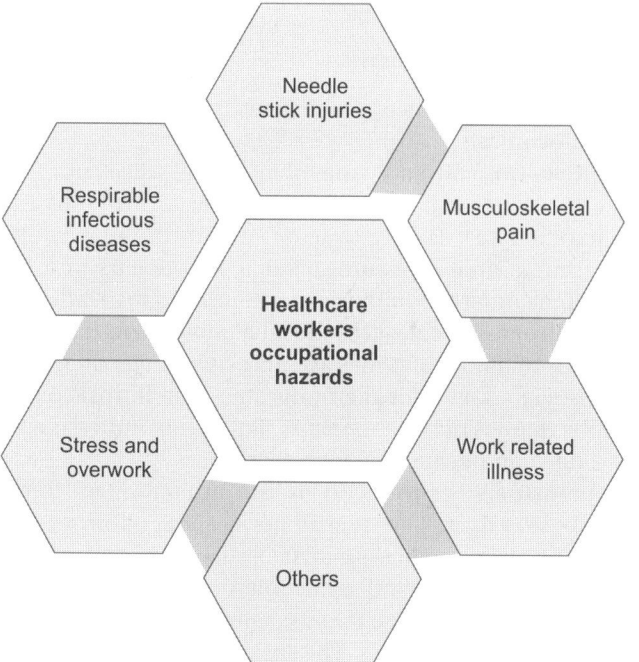

Fig. 13.42: Occupational hazards for health worker.

associated with premalignant lesions like actinic keratosis, keratocanthoma and Hutchin's melanoma.
- *Microwave injuries*—microwave generates intense heat in deeper tissues exposed to the radiation causing localized damage. The damage caused includes corneal injuries, lens opacities frank cataract and retinal damage. Testicular damage associated with decreased sperm count.
- *Laser injuries*—exposure to laser results in corneal retinal and cutaneous burns. The injuries occur among field construction workers who use lasers to obtain alignment among field construction workers who use lasers to obtain alignment of dams, tunnels pipes, etc. or who use laser beams for cutting hard metals and diamonds.

Prevention and Control of Physical Hazards

- **Personal protection:** Warm clothing can afford protection from low temperature hazards and light clothing from high temperature hazards. Periodic salt drinks administered to workers engaged in high temperature zones, prevent the development of heat cramps.
- **Case management:** Acute emergencies are of immediate concern, the nature of their management varies with the physical agent responsible and also with the degree of damage caused. Accordingly heat stroke is managed by immediate reduction of core body temperature preferably by immersion in an ice water tank.

Chemical Hazards and Health

Chemical hazards threatening the health of workers in various occupational setting may be conveniently discussed in relation to gases, dusts and aerosols that serve as their etiological agents. The chemical agents are harmful to skin, respiratory system and gastrointestinal system.

- **Gases:** Gases those are harmful to humans causes damage by their asphyxiant, irritant, toxic or narcotizing action and hydrogen sulfide and hydrogen cyanide. Carbon monoxide produces anoxia hydrogen sulphate is an irritant by causing inflammation of eye, nose and respiratory passages. Hydrogen cyanide arrests internal cellular respiration which leads to histotoxic anoxia even oxygenation of blood remains normal.

  Irritant gases—ammonia sulfur dioxide and chlorine are principal irritant gases. These gases affect the mucus membrane of eyes, nose and throat and invade the respiratory tract as well as lung parenchyma. They produce a burning sensation in all the affected areas followed by lacrimation, salivation, chemosis, conjunctivitis, rhinitis, coughing, choking and dyspnea. Extreme exposures may be pulmonary edema.

  Toxic agents—arsine and stibine are important toxic gases which invade the red blood cells causing hemolysis hemolytic anemia, hemoglobinuria and associated complications. Stibine invades the central nervous system causing cerebral edema and depression of the respiratory center. Exposure to these gases produces increasing weakness, severe low back pain and dark-colored urine. Arsine exposure lends characteristic garlic like odor to breath.

  Inert gases—like nitrogen, methane and carbon dioxide also cause asphyxia by diluting the quantity of oxygen in the air and thereby producing anoxic anoxia. Exposure to excess of methane carries an added stimulates the respiratory centers and causes headache tinnitus and visual disturbances. Carbon dioxide exposure happens mostly in mines, tunnels, vauts, cellars, tanks, cisterns, caissons, etc.

- **Dust:** The fate of dust particles deposited in the respiratory system is decided by their inherent nature. Accordingly particles may be identified as organic and inorganic soluble and insoluble and inert and fibrogenic. Fibrogenic reaction is initiated, leading to pneumoconiosis, pneumoconioses as a group of occupational lung diseases is subdivided into three subgroups.

Main process	Passible chemical hazards
Cleaning	Hydrogen peroxide, sulfuric acid, phosphoric acid, nitric add, hydrofluoric acid, hydrochloric acid, isopropyl alcohol, acetone and ammonia
Oxidation and diffusion	Diborane and phosphine
Ion implantation	Phosphine, arsine, and boron trifluoride
Lithography	TMAH, cyclopentanone, isopropanol, ethylene glycol, and butyl acetate
Wet etching	Sulfuric acid, hydrofluoric acid, nitric acid, phosphoric acid, ammonia, and hydrogen peroxide
Dry etching	Sulphur hexafluoride, hydrogen chloride, and chlorine
Chemical vapor deposition	Hydrogen chloride, fluoride, silane, phosphine, arsine, diborane, chlorine trifluoride, ammonia, chlorine, and nitrogen oxides
Chemical mechanical polishing	Ammonia, hydrofluoric acid, hydrogen peroxide, and potassium hydroxide
Metalization	Copper, ammonia, hydrofluoric acid, sulfuric acid, nitric acid, fluoride, and hydrogen peroxide
Public auxiliary facilities	Hydrochloric acid, sulfuric acid, sodium hydroxide, ammonia, fluoride, hydrogen fluoride, chlorine, isopropyl alcohol, acetone, ozone, carbon monoxide, carbon dioxide, methane and MACHs

Minor pneumoconiosis: Byssinosis and bagassosis are two important examples of minor pneumoconiosis.

- **Byssinosis** is also referred as "Monday fever" or Monday sickness characterized by cough, dyspnea and fever. Byssinosis is caused by the inhalation of cotton dust. The dust initiated an allergic response in the respiratory tract leading to brochospasm and edema of respiratory mucosa. Prolonged exposure to cotton dust ends in emphysema.
- **Bagassosis** is caused by the inhalation of dust containing fibrous residue of sugar cane, called bagasse. The bagasse dust blocks the bronchioles resulting in acute bronchiolitis and bronchopneumonia.

Major Pneumoconiosis

Silicosis, anthracosis and abestosis are example of major pneumoconiosis.

- **Silicosis** is caused by the inhalation of silica containing dust which gives rise to nodular fibrosis of lung parenchyma usually concentrated in the upper lobes. Occupational exposure to silica dust occurs in mines, tunnels, quarries, foundries, potteries and soap industries.
- **Anthracosis** is caused by the inhalation of coal dust which leads to diffuse and massive fibrosis of lung parenchyma associated with focal emphysema. The fibrosis usually precipitates right heart failure. Pulmonary tuberculosis is a rare complication of anthracosis.
- **Asbestosis** is produced by the inhalation of fibrous asbestos dust. The dust fibers get lodged in terminal bronchioles. Asbestos dust is also generated during asbestos spaying and textile operation using asbestos as a fire proof material. It causes progressive dyspnea, dry cough and weight loss. The sputum when produced may contain characteristics asbestosis bodies.

Benign Pneumoconiosis

Siderosis and stannosis are two well known examples of benign pneumoconiosis caused by the inhalation of iron and tin particles. The lung may get loaded with dust after prolonged exposure. The lung may get loaded with dust after prolonged exposure. There are obviously no complaints.

Complications like super added infection or cancer have not been reported in benign pneumoconiosis.

Aerosols: Aerosols of various types are released in metal processing industries. Among the aerosols, dusts are released by the disintegration of metals like copper, cobalt, chromium and beryllium. Inhalation of aerosols by workers results in metal intoxication manifested by metal fume fever, pulmonary disease and systematic diseases affecting various organs of the body.

Group A intoxications—are provided by chromium, beryllium and nickel aerosols. Chromium produces lesions in skin and respiratory tract. Chromium dust causes perforation of nasal septum and lung cancer. Beryllium exposure causes dermal and pulmonary lesions. Beryllium dermatitis is an edematous papulovesicular eruption mainly appearing on exposed areas of skin. The eruption is associated with inching and a burning sensation. Exposure to nickel results in respiratory and skin lesions. Lesion includes airway irritation and cancer, nasal cancer is much more frequent than respiratory tract.

Group B intoxications—examples of group B intoxication are seen in the course of exposure of lead, mercury and manganese or aerosol. Exposure to lead poisoning referred to as lead encephalopathy include delirium, coma, convulsions, mental dullness, transient paresis and toxic psychosis. Chronic exposure results in poor memory, poor concentration, headache, transitory deafness and trembling.

Exposure to mercury occurs in industries manufacturing thermometers, manometers, fluorescent tube lights and electric goods of various types. Mercurial erythrism is a type of personality disorder characterized by the loss of self control and self confidence. Mercurial tremors which usually start peripherally from fingers, lips, eyelids and tongue eventually prorogues to involve arms and legs which restricts walking considerably.

Exposure to manganese fumes occurs in industries dealing with manganese and manganese containing a alloys. The intoxication of manganese produces neurological and pulmonary manifestations. Involvement of central nervous system leads to a disease resembling Parkinsonism. The symptoms of nonspecific initially comprising of headache, fatigue irritability and impaired memory.

Measures of Prevention and Control of Chemical Hazards

- **Personal protection**—makes afford to protection from inhalations of dusts, respirators prevent inhalation of noxious agents dust and other type of aerosols. Use of eye shields, gloves and protective clothing prevents contact with injurious chemical agents.
- **Case management**—acute emergencies due to exposure to noxious gases need immediate resuscitation by various means such as artificial respiration, oxygen inhalation rest and warmth. Antinodes like BAL (dimercaprol) and EDTA have an important place in the management of metal poisoning. Intoxication caused by accidental ingestion of a chemical substance may be managed by gastric lavage, emetics, antidotes and various other measures.
- **Health education**—health education motivates workers to observe personal hygiene and apply various precautionary measures to avert hazardous effects of chemical agents. It promotes the use of personal protective device that disallow direct contact of worker with injurious chemical agents.

Biological Hazards and Occupational Health

Workers occupied in industries dealing with infected animals and infected animal material like hides and skins are exposed to a host of zoonotic diseases of viral, bacterial protozoal and metazoal origin. Workers engaged in field areas suffer from a variety of environmental-infective diseases which may be dust-borne, soil-borne, water borne or vector-borne.

Diseases of Environmental Origin

- **Schistosomiasis**—Occupation hazard of agriculture workers who are exposed to contaminated water containing swimming larvae (cercariae) of the parasites of *Schistosoma* species releasing by snails. Man is the principal reservoir of *Schistosoma mansoni* and *S. haematobium* causes painless terminal haematuria, pulmonary hypertension and cor pulmonale.
- **Coccidioidomycosis**—The disease initially resembles an acute febrile illness characterized by chills, cough, and chest pain. Skin lesions of coccidioidomycosis include erythema nodosum and erythema multiforme.
- **Blastomycosis**—The disease exists in respiratory and cutaneous forms. The respiratory form presents as upper respiratory tract infection characterized by fever, cough and purulent sputum eventually leading to weight loss and cachexia. The cutaneous form of the disease starts as a papulae which appears at the site of the entry.
- **Histoplasmosis:** It is transmitted by inhalation of air borne spores of histoplasma capsulatum which is a fungus that grows on soil rich in organic matter. It starts as a mild respiratory illness associated with fever, cough chest pain and malaise. The disease eventually results in splenomegaly and lymphadenopathy.
- **Nocardiosis:** The disease as a localized lesion (mycetoma) at the site of the entry. It spreads by hematogeous route including the brain and the meninges.

Diseases of Zoonotic Origin

- **Leptospirosis:** The infected animals that serve as reservoirs are cattle, dogs, hogs, rats and mice. The leptospires penetrate skin or mucous membrane of the host who initially develops fever, chills, headache, and vomiting and malaise. The disease may eventually lead to myalgia, conjunctivitis, meningeal irritation and jaundice which may progress to hemorrhage anemia, renal insufficiency, and hemorrhage in skin and mucous membranes.

- **Psittacosis:** Psittacosis or parrot fever is a disease of poultry raisers, duck and turkey raisers, poultry dressers, pet shop keepers, pigeon keepers and zoo attendants. Psittacosis is an acute infectious disease characterized by fever, headache, cough, pneumonia and several systemic manifestations.
- **Q fever:** It is an air-born disease of wild and domestic animals caused by *Coxiella burnetii*. Q fever is acute febrile influenza like illness characterized by sudden onsets, chills, sweats, headache, myalgia and weakness. The disease may also lead to pneumonia associated with mild cough, scanty sputum and chest pain.
- **Anthrax:** Caused by *Bacillus anthracis*. It transmitted by contact with infected animals or contaminated animal material and inhalation of infected dust. The clinical features are skin lesion with cellulites (malignant pustule) severe pneumonia (wool sorter's disease)
- **Tularemia:** Caused by *Pasteurella tularensis*. The disease transmitted by direct contact with infected animals or infected animal materials. The clinical features are cutaneous ulcers, lymphadenitis fever, chills and prostration.

Prevention and Control of Biological Hazards

- **Personal protection:** Use of foot wear evades larval invasion of skin and disallows entry to various helminthic disease agents to which workers are exposed in the field. The use of gloves, overalls and overalls protects workers handling infected animals or their infected products.
- **Public health measures:** Filling of ditches, improvement of drainage and reclamation of swamps and low lying areas can control larval invasion of field workers. Sanitary disposal of night soil and provision of piped water may be exposed in the field. Immunization of animals against vaccine preventable diseases.
- **Health education:** Health education promotes the awareness of workers on the nature of biological hazards to which they are exposed while working inside the industries or outside in the fields. It motivates worker participation in the control of zoonotic and environmental diseases **(Fig. 13.43)**.

Mechanical and Psychosocial Hazards

Mechanical Hazards

Mechanical hazards refer to mechanical agents. About 10% of accidents in industry are due to mechanical cause such as protruding or moving parts of machinery. These may cause variety of accidents which may result in partial or permanent disabilities.

Psychosocial Hazards

- **Psychosocial hazards** refer to psychosocial agents, these are various human related factors which are there in work environment and influence the health of workers. These include human relationships among workers themselves, among workers and the authority, job security, conditions of employment, working for long hours in some posture, etc.
- **Due to frustrations** at work or at home and lack of job satisfaction which leads to physical symptoms such as headache, mental ill health and organic disease. Occupational disease creates absenteeism of the worker. Therefore to promote economic progress through better production the health of workers in industries requires high priority.

Health Acts and Occupational Health Services

- **Factories Act:** The Factories Act was passed in the country in the year 1948 with a view to protect and promote the health, safety and welfare of workers employed in factories.
- **Administrative profile:** The Act extends to cover all the factories in the whole of India including the state of Jammu and Kashmir. For the purpose of the act, a factory means an establishment **(Fig. 13.44)**.
  - In which 10 or more workers have been employed during the preceding 12 months in a manufacturing process operated on power.
  - In which 20 or more workers have been employed during preceding 12 months in a manufacturing process, operated without power.

Appointment and Employment

- The state governments are also empowered to appoint "chief Inspectors" invested with powers of inspection throughout their state territories.
- The state government can also appoint "additional chief inspectors", joint chief inspectors and deputy chief inspectors where and when necessary.
- The state government are also empowered to appoint qualified medical practitioners as certifying surgeons for purposes of the act.
- The state governments is empowered to enforce registration and licensing of factories and also grant permission for the establishment of new factories or extension of old ones.

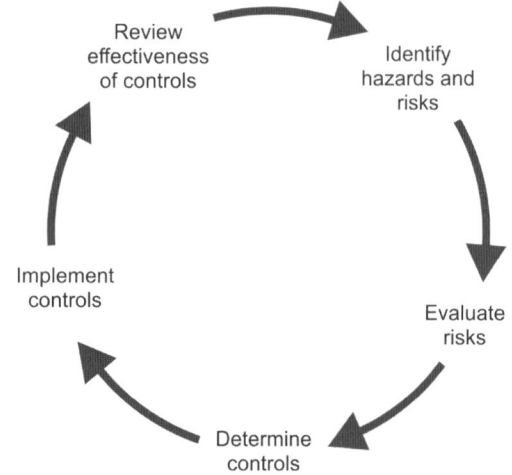

Fig. 13.43: Prevention and control of hazards.

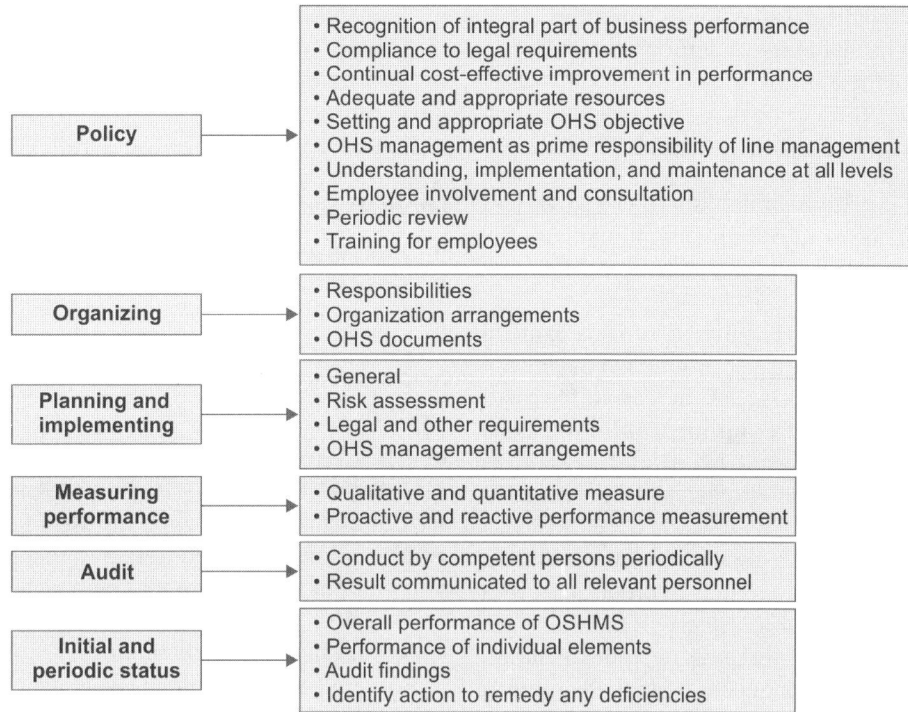

Fig. 13.44: Administrative measures of occupational hazards.

Provision of Industrial Workers

- **Employment provision:** In terms of age of workers, hours of work, intervals of rest and entitlement to leave with wages.
- **Welfare provisions:** Involving enclosure and fencing of plants and dangerous machine parts, inbuilt safety, provisions and safety exits for escape.
- **Sanitary provisions**—Involving ventilations, illumination, latrines, urinals, drinking water points, cleaning and disposal arrangements.

ESI Act (Employees State Insurance Act)

The ESI of 1948 covered all powers using factories other than seasonal factories wherein 20 or more persons were employed. It proved to be a very beneficial step towards social security of factory workers. The act alleviates economic and physical suffering by providing benefits in cash and kind during sickness, maternity and occupational injury.

Benefits of ESI Act

- **Medical benefits**—implying comprehensive medical care including outpatient, inpatient domiciliary investigational and MCH services.
- **Sickness benefits**—implying periodical payments to workers during pregnancy and pregnancy related disorders.
- **Maternity benefits**—implying periodical payments to workers disabled as a result of an employment injury.
- **Dependent's benefit**—implying periodical payments to the dependent of a deceased worker.
- **Disablement benefit**—benefit for temporary disablement is paid at the rate about 75% of the wages for the education of disablement. For permanent total disablement, the payment is made at the same rate for the whole life in the form of pension and at a proportional rate incase of permanent partial disablement.
- **Funeral benefits**—the maximum amount of ₹ 1,000 for funeral expenses is given to the eldest surviving member on death of insured worker.
- **Rehabilitation benefits**—ensured workers who require artificial limbs are provided with artificial limbs and also the cash allowance equivalent to the sickness benefit rate at the time when they are admitted for provision/replacement of artificial limbs.

ESI—Pattern of Financial Support

- The employer pays 4.75 percentages of total wages.
- The employee contributes 1.75% of his/her wage.
- The state government shares 7/8th of the total expenditure on medical care.
- The ESI corporation shares 7/8th of a total expenditure on medical care.
- As far the central government is concerned it supports 2/3 of the administrative expenditure.

ESI—Administrative Members

- Minister of labor—chairperson
- The secretary—ministry of labor—Vice chairperson
- Representatives of central government—5 members
- Representatives from the states—one from each state.
- Representatives from union territories—one member from each.
- Representatives of employees—5 members
- Representatives of employers—5 members

- Representatives of medical profession—2 members
- Representatives of parliament—3 members
- Director General of the ESI.

ILO and WHO Recommendations

The committee on occupational health by ILO and WHO I 1953 recommended. The promotion and maintenance of the highest degree of physical, mental and social well-being of the workers in all occupations.

- **Nutrition:** The industries are required to provide canteen facilities when there are more than 250 employees with the provision of balanced diet and snacks at reasonable costs.
- **Prevention and control of communicable diseases:** Adequate and periodic immunization program is required to protect the employees against the preventable communicable diseases.
- **Environmental sanitation:** The environmental sanitation requires to be established adequately in order to prevent and control the communicable disease. It includes safe and sufficient water supply, food hygiene, toilet facilities, wastage and garbage disposal, general plant cleanliness, floor space, adequate lighting and ventilation protection against hazards and housing.
- **Maternity benefit:** Women workers should have the privilege of availing 6 weeks leave prior to and 6 weeks after the delivery with full wages.
- **First aid:** There should be a small dispensary to provide first aid and emergency medical care.
- **Creche:** A crèche should be provided in factories where more than 30 women workers are employed.
- **Mental health:** The goal of mental health in the industry is to promote health and happiness to the employee and his family.
- **Health education:** It is an important health promotional activity and an integral part of total health program of the industry.

Occupational Health in India

The national government has recognized the need for protecting the health of the workers. The government department of labor and health and the board of mines maintain vigilance over health and working conditions of industrial workers.

Occupational State Health Policy

- The state shall in particular, direct its policy towards securing that the health and strength of the workers, man, women, and the tender age of the children are not abused, and that citizens are not forced by economic necessity to enter avocations unsuited to their strength.
- The state shall make provision for securing just and humane conditions of work.

Important Reports on Occupational Health

- Adarkar's Report of Health Insurance for Industrial Workers (1945)
- Report of Health Survey and Development Committee (1946)
- Report of Health of the Industrial Workers (Thomas Bedford 1946)
- Report on the Health of Workers in Plantation (Jones 1947).

Legal Aspects on Occupational Health

- Administration of Factory Act (1948)
- Coal Mines Labor Welfare Act (1947)
- ESI Act (1948)

National Level Research Institutes on Occupational Health

- The Central Mining and Research Station, Dhanbad.
- Industrial Toxicology Research Center, Lucknow.
- Council of Scientific and Industrial Research (CSIR)
- Occupational Health Research Institute, Ahmadabad.
- National Environmental Engineering Research Institute, Nagpur
- Indian Institute of Technology, Kanpur,
- The All India Institute of Hygiene and Public Health.
- Occupational Health Division in ICMR.

Activities of Labor Institutes

For scientific study of the various aspects of occupational health, particularly the "human factor" in industry the central Labor institute was set up in Mumbai in 1960. Three Regional Labor Institutes at Kanpur, Kolkata and Chennai have also been set up. These institutes are dealing with a variety of activities important in the field of safety and health.

- A museum of industrial health, safety and welfare.
- Industrial hygiene laboratory
- Training section
- Library cum information center
- Industrial psychology
- Occupational physiology

Occupational Health Nursing

Occupational health is concerned with health in its relation to work and the working environment, practice of occupational health as a specialty calls for specialized knowledge from any disciplines. Occupational health implies not only health protection but also health promotion, emergency care, wide range of preventive curative services and rehabilitative services.

Industrial nursing requires specialized knowledge and skill which means they need proper additional training. Occupational health is the additional training. Occupational health is the entirely preventive medicine. The chief objective of occupational health is the safety of workers in all occupations from injuries and diseases and to improve their health status.

History of Occupation Health Nursing

The history of occupational health nursing is very ancient. In 1888 in America, group of Coal-Mine Company had appointed a occupational health nurse started taking place of doctors in factories. In this way the first occupational health nurse has become the root pillar of modern occupational health nursing.

Definition: Occupational health nursing is the application of nursing practice and public health procedures for the purpose of conversing, promoting and restoring the health of individuals and groups through their places of employment.

Components of Occupational Health Nursing

- To carry out significant, positive health programs
- To provide therapeutic service for the workers.
- To establish meaningful interpersonal relationship between herself and the workers to identity problem sand workout solutions together.
- To ensure that her nursing activities are compatible with the management policy and the healthcare system.

Beneficiaries of Occupational Health Nursing

- **Individual-Labors/employee:** Occupational health nurse has to provide healthcare to skilled—unskilled trained untrained new or old, all types of works. The occupational untrained nurse has her primary responsibility towards workers to promote, protect and preserve their health.
- **Employee's group**—Occupational health nurse has responsibility towards her employees to protect the company from adverse effects of work process and hazardous substances on workers.
- **Managerial personnel:** The community health nurse has to give feedback regarding the health of workers. This includes informing the health limits of worker related to work, giving information regarding health hazards and helping the management to identify the health problem of the workers.
- **The company** gets direct or indirect benefit from the occupational health nurse.

Tools of Occupational Health Nursing

- **Data collection:** It includes not only the workers chief complaint but also information about unhealthy behaviors. The nurse is also required to specifically document the individual job duties and any work related physical and psychological complaints.
- **Health survey:** Health surveys are investigations to identify the frequency, distribution and the determinants of health related events or state in the community. Health surveys help in knowing the community and making diagnosis. The health surveys can be general health survey and special or specific health surveys.
- **Surveillance:** Surveillance means supervision or close observation especially on suspected person. Epidemiologically surveillance means close vigilance on occurrence and distribution of diseases and health related problems, population dynamics, community behavior and environmental processes resulting in increased risk of ill health in the community.
- **Health education:** Health education is a process that informs, motivates and helps people to adopt and maintain healthy practices and lifestyles, advocates environmental processes dynamics, community behavior and environmental processes resulting in increased risk of ill health in the community.
- **Evaluation:** Evaluation measures the achievement of intended goals and objectives by comparing with actual outcomes. Evaluation is an ongoing process. Evaluation is both qualitative and quantitative. Evaluation is formative and summative. It determines the strengths and weakness of the program.

Occupational Health Nurse

Educational preparations: Occupational health nursing is one of the extensive and specialized branching of nursing. It is essential to include various aspects of occupational health nursing in nursing curriculum.

- Epidemiology and toxicology
- Occupational health problems
- Occupational hazards and diseases
- Industrial hygiene
- Industrial security
- Industrial health programs
- Preparation of industrial budget
- Occupational rehabilitations
- Work evaluation technique.

Roles of Occupation Health Nurse

- Nurse practitioner
- Nurse educator
- Health administrator/manager
- Counselor.

Functions of Occupational Health Nurse

- Assistance in general administration, maintenance and arrangements of health facilities in the plant.
- Emergency and primary treatment of accidents and illness based on standing orders from physicians.
- Arranging follow-up treatments, where indicated, including health supervision of employees returning to work after illness.
- Assistance in general preventive health measures in the plant.
- Health education and counseling for employees.
- Assistance in supervision of factory hygiene and accident prevention.
- Advice on specific health question to management and workers.
- Maintenance of records and statistics.
- Co-operation with and referral of workers to general community agencies for help as and when necessary.

- Participation in a health surveillance program that includes the assessment and recording of the health status of employees.
- Participation in the environmental control program the aims to work related.
- Counseling and crisis intervention for those individuals experiencing work related problems and health promotion through specific health education and screening Programs.

Specific Areas and Activities of Occupational Health Nurse

- Shop floor healthcare—field health survey practice
- Occupational medicine—clinical practice
- Occupational Hygiene—working environment hazards monitoring
- Health supervision of worker—surveillance of health.
- Health education and counseling.
- Occupational health services—administration.

Occupational Healthcare Team

Occupational healthcare team changes according to circumstances. In addition to people employed in industries, outside agencies also can contribute to the healthcare of workers.

Members of Occupational Healthcare Team

- Occupational healthcare team
- Physiotherapist
- Specialist doctor
- Industrial manager
- Supervisor
- Shift in charge
- Rehabilitation specialist
- Labor welfare officer
- Labor union representative
- Representative of voluntary organizations.

Major Activities of Occupational Healthcare Team

- Emergency situation
- Disaster management services
- Worker's education program.

GERIATRIC NURSING

An elderly person needs to feel safe, remain close to other people and believe that his life continues to be meaningful. Meeting his emotional needs can help him avoid depression. Signs that he lacks sufficient support may include difficulty in sleeping, a poor appetite or an inability to concentrate, points out the American Association of Retired Persons. Emotional care for a senior should include steps designed to deal with vulnerability, loneliness, boredom and isolation (**Figs. 13.45 and 13.46**).

Concept of Geriatrics

- The phenomenon of population ageing has become a major concern for the policy makers all over the world, for both developed and developing countries, during last two decades.
- The elderly population (aged 60 years or above) account for 7.4% of total population in India in 2001. (Males 7.1% while for females 7.8%).
- The old-age dependency ratio climbed from 10.9% in 1961 to 13.1% in 2001.
- Among females it was 13.8% and males 12.5%.
- In view of the increasing need for intervention in area of old age welfare, Ministry of Social Justice and Empowerment, Government of India adopted 'National Policy on Older Persons', 1999.
- Policy provides broad guidelines to State Governments for taking action for welfare of older persons by devising their own policies and plan of action.
- To ensure well-being of senior citizens and improve quality of their lives through providing specific facilities, concessions, relief, services and helping them cope up with problems associated with old age.

Definition

Gerontological nursing is the specialty of nursing pertaining to older adults. Gerontological nurses work in collaboration

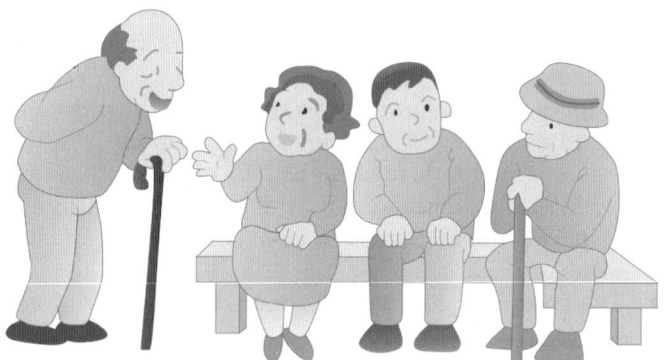

Fig. 13.45: Geriatric care.

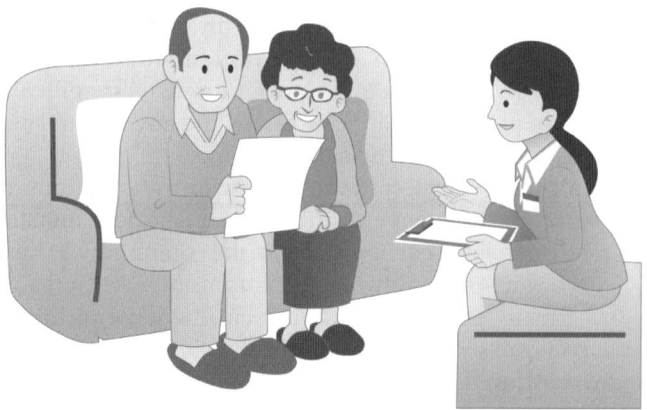

Fig. 13.46: Geriatric nursing assessment.

with older adults, their families, and communities to support healthy aging, maximum functioning, and quality of life.
- **Geriatrics:** It is a branch of medicine which deals with problems of old age.
- **Gerontology:** Science which deals with processes of ageing.
- **Preventive geriatrics:** It is a branch of Geriatrics which deals with prevention and control of disability and improving the quality of life of the aged people.

Geriatric Care

Geriatric Nurses help elderly patients. These older adults are at greater risk of injuries and diseases like osteoporosis, Alzheimer's and cancer, which is why Geriatric Nurses focus on preventative care.

Goals of Geriatric Care

- Provide a safe and supportive environment.
- Restore and maintain the highest possible level of functional capacity.
- Preserve individual autonomy.
- Maximize quality of life.
- Provide comfort and dignity for disabled and ill.
- Stabilize and delay progression of chronic diseases.
- Prevent acute medical illnesses, early detection and treatment.

They also help patients, and their families, cope with certain medical conditions that develop later in life. As a Geriatric Nurse, you can work in nursing homes, with home healthcare services and in hospice facilities taking care of bedridden patients, those with impaired mental ability, and for patients who are in pain.

When working with their patients, a geriatric nurse will:
- Assess the patient's mental status and cognitive (thinking) skills
- Understand patient's acute and chronic health issues
- Discuss common health concerns, such as falls, incontinence, changing sleep patterns and sexual issues
- Organize medications
- Educate the patient about personal safety and disease prevention
- Explain and recommend adjustments to the patient's medication regimen to ensure adherence
- Link the patient with local resources as needed

Many older people have health conditions that do not require hospitalization, but must be treated with medication, changes in diet, use of special equipment (such as a blood sugar monitor or walker), daily exercises or other adaptations. Geriatric nurses help design and explain these healthcare regimens to patients and their families. They often function as "case managers," linking families with community resources to help them care for elderly members **(Figs. 13.47 and 13.48)**.

Geriatric Nurse

Geriatric nursing is a nursing sub-field which involves caring for older adults **(Fig. 13.49)**.

The standards and scope of geriatric nursing practice were originally developed in 1969 by the American Nurses Association. It was revised in 1976 and again in 1987.

Goals of Geriatric Nursing

- Promoting and maintaining functional status
- Helping to use their strengths to achieve optimal independence.

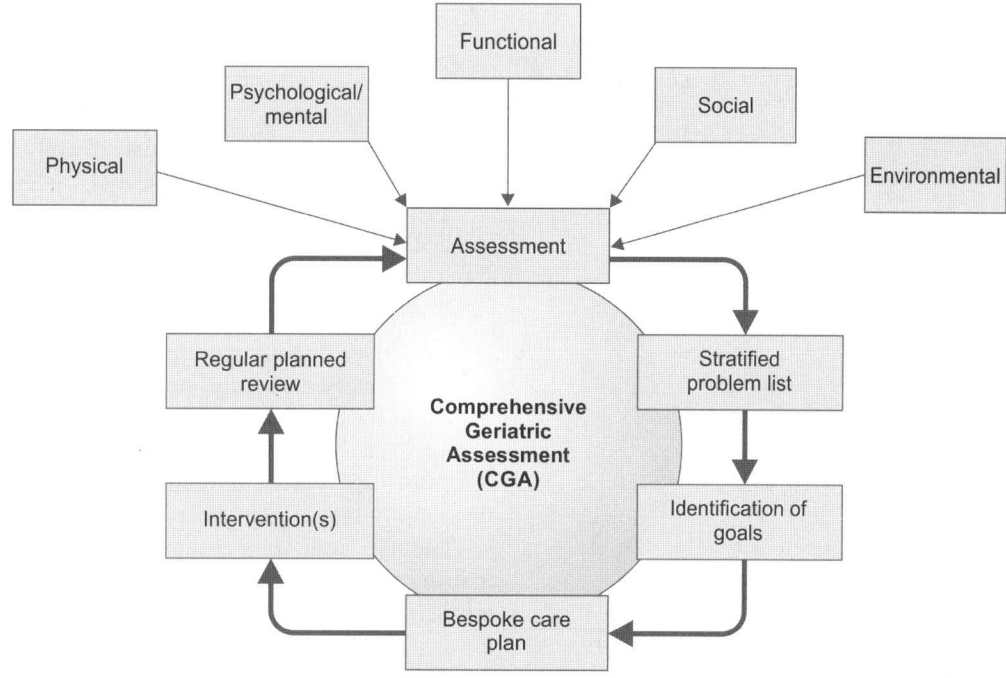

Fig. 13.47: Assisting mobility for geriatric patients.

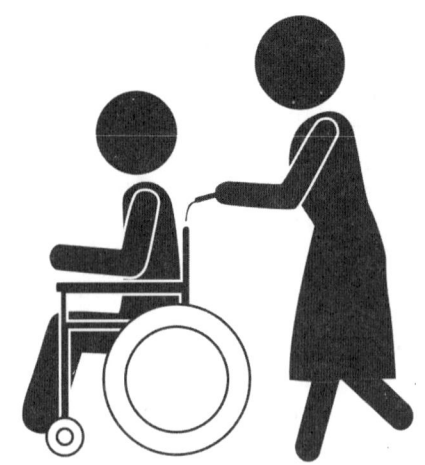

Fig. 13.48: Comprehensive geriatric assessment.

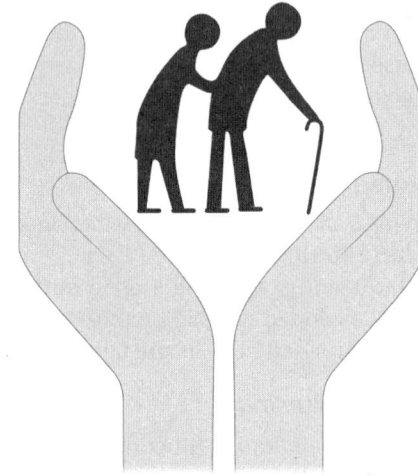

Fig. 13.49: Geriatric nursing care.

- Maintain dignity and maximum autonomy despite physical, social, and psychological losses.
- Long-term care for elderly patients.
- Use current scientific knowledge to solve clinical problems.
- Collaborate with the interdisciplinary team members.
- Provide a holistic approach to care.

Characteristics of a Geriatric Nurse

- Provide basic nursing services
- Offers emotional support to patients
- Good observer
- Coordinator
- Emotionally strong
- Advocate
- Hard worker
- Cope with the challenges
- Provide home-based care

Theories of Aging

There are many theories about the mechanisms of age related changes, and they are mutually exclusive, no one theory is sufficiently able to explain the process of aging, and they often contradict one another **(Fig. 13.50)**.

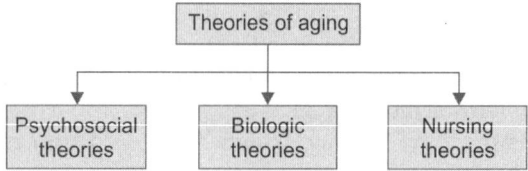

Fig. 13.50: Types of aging theories.

Disengagement Theory

- Refers to an inevitable process in which many of the relationships between a person and other members of society are severed and those remaining are altered in quality.
- Withdrawal may be initiated by the aging person or by society, and may be partial or total.
- It was observed that older people are less involved with life than they were as younger adults.
- As people age they experience greater distance from society and they develop new types of relationships with society.
- In America there is evidence that society forces withdrawal on older people whether or not they want it.
- Some suggest that this theory does not consider the large number of older people who do not withdraw from society.
- This theory is recognized as the 1st formal theory that attempted to explain the process of growing older.

Activity Theory

- Is another theory that describes the psychosocial aging process.
- Activity theory emphasizes the importance of ongoing social activity.
- This theory suggests that a person's self-concept is related to the roles held by that person, i.e., retiring may not be so harmful if the person actively maintains other roles, such as familial roles, recreational roles, volunteer and community roles.
- To maintain a positive sense of self the person must substitute new roles for those that are lost because of age. And studies show that the type of activity does matter, just as it does with younger people.

Neuroendocrine Theory

First proposed by Professor Vladimir Dilman and Ward Dean MD, this theory elaborates on wear and tear by focusing on the neuroendocrine system. This system is a complicated network of biochemicals that governs the release of hormones which are altered by the walnut sized gland called the hypothalamus located in the brain **(Fig. 13.51)**.

The hypothalamus controls various chain-reactions to instruct other organs and glands to release their hormones etc. The hypothalamus also responds to the body hormone levels as a guide to the overall hormonal activity. But as we grow older the hypothalamus loses it precision regulatory ability and the receptors which uptake individual hormones become less sensitive to them. Accordingly, as we age the

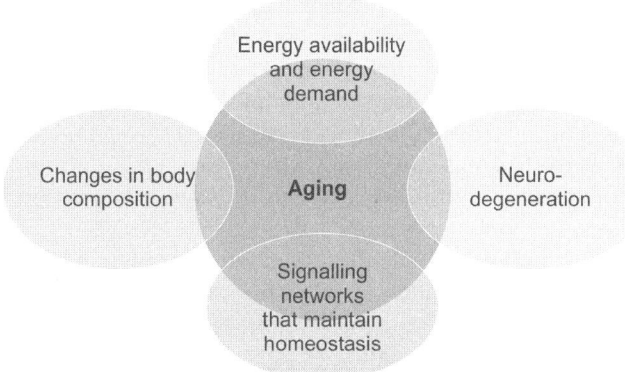

Fig. 13.51: Neuroendocrine theory of aging.

secretion of many hormones declines and their effectiveness (compared unit to unit) is also reduced due to the receptors downgrading

Free Radical Theory

- This now very famous theory of aging was developed by Denham Harman MD at the University of Nebraska in 1956. The term free radical describes any molecule that has a free electron, and this property makes it react with healthy molecules in a destructive way.
- Because the free radical molecule has an extra electron it creates an extra negative charge. This unbalanced energy makes the free radical bind itself to another balanced molecule as it tries to steal electrons. In so doing, the balanced molecule becomes unbalanced and thus a free radical itself.
- It is known that diet, lifestyle, drugs (e.g. tobacco and alcohol) and radiation etc., are all accelerators of free radical production within the body.

Membrane Theory of Aging

The membrane theory of aging was first described by Professor Imre Zs.-Nagy of Hungary. According to this theory it is the age-related changes of the cells ability to transfer chemicals, heat and electrical processes that impair it.

As we grow older the cell membrane becomes less lipid (less watery and more solid). This impedes its efficiency to conduct normal function and in particular there is a toxic accumulation.

Mitochondrial Decline Theory

The mitochondria are the power producing organelles found in every cell of every organ. Their primary job is to create Adenosine Triphosphate (ATP) and they do so in the various energy cycles that involve nutrients such as Acetyl-L-Carnitine, CoQ10 (Idebenone), NADH and some B vitamins etc.

Enhancement and protection of the mitochondria is an essential part of preventing and slowing aging. Enhancement can be achieved with the above mention nutrients, as well as ATP supplements themselves.

Cross-linking Theory

The Cross-linking Theory of Aging is also referred to as the Glycosylation Theory of Aging. In this theory it is the binding of glucose (simple sugars) to protein, (a process that occurs under the presence of oxygen) that causes various problems.

Once this binding has occurred the protein becomes impaired and is unable to perform as efficiently. Living a longer life is going to lead to the increased possibility of oxygen meeting glucose and protein and known cross-linking disorders include senile cataract and the appearance of tough, leathery and yellow skin.

Physiological Changes in Old

Physiological functions wane when people getting old. When we take care of the elderly, we should take heed to these changes. Here are some examples **(Fig. 13.52)**.

Vision: In general, old people have a poorer vision. Some even have cataract or glaucoma.

Hearing: The elderly would have a lessened hearing ability. When you need to talk loudly to them, avoid shouting.

Touch: The peripheral sense of some diabetes and under-nutrited patients drops much.

Skin: The layer of subcutaneous fat in the elderly is thinner than young people. Their skin also loses elasticity due to dehydration. When moving the body of the elderly, beware of injuring their skin. Keep them warm during winter time.

Endocrine: Elderly people easily get tired or even sick due to diminished endocrine function and decreased metabolism. Be patient when dealing with these elderly.

Renal: Owing to decreased functioning of the renal system, old people may have problems such as incontinence, frequent urination, etc. Assist them if they need toileting and, be patient with them.

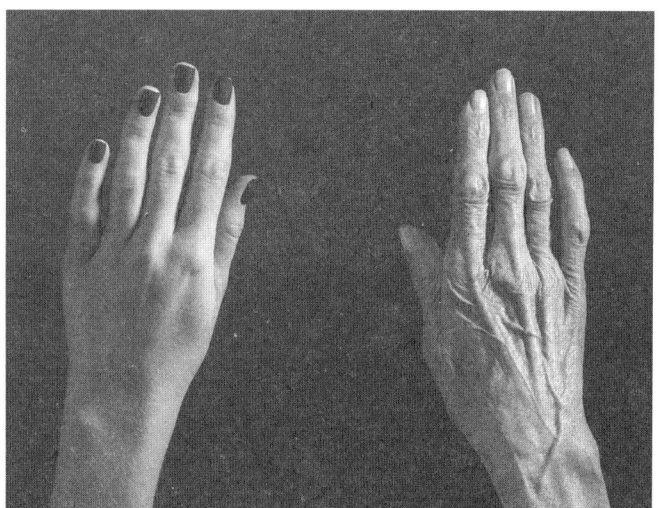

Fig. 13.52: Physiological changes in old.

Musculoskeletal: Obvious changes such as general weakness could easily be seen in this kind of patients. Assist them to move about if necessary. Yet, if the condition is safe while the elderly is able to move by himself/herself, simply let them go ahead. Be patient with their slower motion.

Emotional Care of Old Age (Fig. 13.53)

- **Security:** A senior citizen may feel fearful and nervous, especially if she lives alone or has mobility: problems. Support a positive outlook with practical measures to guard against intruders. Arrange for the installation of additional locks or chains and a spy-hole in the door, so she can see who is calling before she opens the door. An emergency call button could reduce her fear of failing to get help should she fall or become unwell.
- **Connection:** Help senior citizens to maintain contact with their friends and family. Encourage visits from younger family members and use the telephone to maintain regular communication. An elderly person may find Internet access helpful when family or friends are unable to offer frequent visits, but he could need help in learning to use the technology. Use photos, books and music to help him remember happy life events and involve him in important family occasions such as marriages or new babies to help him know that he continues to be an important member of the family.
- **Community:** Maintaining links with her community can support an elderly person's feeling of connection with the world beyond her family. Arrange transport to local events, church services or shopping trips. Contact organizations in the area that may be able to offer visits or send newsletters that support her interests. Make sure she is able to manage the controls of her television or radio and that she knows how to access local channels so that she can continue to enjoy involvement with her neighborhood.
- **Leisure:** Take time to listen carefully to an elderly person. Help him continue to take responsibility for himself by discussing his needs and tailoring any interventions you make to his preferences, whether he loves ball games or prefers reading. Help him overcome any obstacles to his leisure activities that aging might cause. For example, try large print books or different spectacles to overcome visual problems that prevent him from enjoying his favorite authors. Maintain his dignity, whether he lives at home or in a care facility. Ensure he has access to his own clean clothes and that any false teeth or other prosthetics fit securely so he can feel comfortable.
- **Planning:** Look ahead to anticipate the future needs of a senior. Her circumstances will change over time and new difficulties can arise with her physical, emotional or sensory abilities. These can damage her emotional well-being. A sudden loss of the capacity to wash or dress independently needs urgent action to provide her with personal care. Watch for any deterioration in her mood and be prepared to involve health providers.. Make sure she takes any medication exactly as prescribed. Sorting her tablets into the correct daily dose can help overcome a senior's fear of making mistake.

Themes	Categories	Subcategories
Daily living	Problems and needs	Eating
		Cooking
		Grooming
		Housekeeping
		Bathroom usage
	Psychological care	Privacy
		Safety
Social engagement	Participation in social activities	Social events in elderly home
		Special events
		Visit with family members
	Physical activities	Exercise
		Indoor activities
		Outdoor activities
Technology	Adaptability with technology	Devices
		Robots
		Security cameras

Common Health Problems in Old Age

Older adults are among the fastest growing age groups, and the first "baby boomers" (adults born between 1946 and 1964) will turn 65 in 2011. More than 37 million people in this group (60%) will manage more than 1 chronic condition by 2030. Older adults are at high risk for developing chronic illnesses and related disabilities. These chronic conditions include: Diabetes mellitus, Arthritis, Congestive heart failure, Dementia **(Fig. 13.54)**.

- **Heart disease:** In this disease, the blood to the heart is decreased due to the narrowing of the cardiac vessels which supply blood to it. This narrowing is due to atherosclerosis in which fat deposits accumulate on the walls of the blood vessels and narrowing it. The causes of this are high blood pressure, high cholesterol occurring due to high intake of animal fat, cigarette smoking, diabetes mellitus, obesity, inactivity, stress and hereditary factor.
- **High blood pressure** is the most common ailment in almost 90% of the old people. A small rise in BP also should never be neglected and lifestyle changes had to

Fig. 13.53: Emotional care of old age.

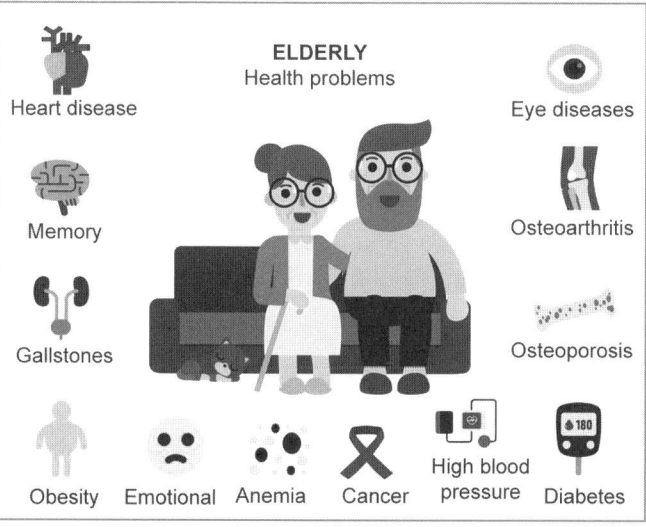

Fig. 13.54: Common health problems in old age.

be adapted. The preventive measures are weight control, daily physical activity, treatment for diabetes, less salt intake and saturated fat, and promoting more intake of fruits and vegetable. Fruits rich in potassium like bananas and oranges, food high in calcium are advisable.

- **Hypotension or low BP:** This is characterized by dizziness and fainting from exertion after a period of long inactivity and also it is due to anemia. This is more severe after sitting or lying down for a longer time-postural hypotension or suddenly standing after which the person loses his balance and fall to the ground. Hypotension is not in itself dangerous but can increase the risk of falls.
- **Stroke or cerebrovascular accident (CVA):** When the heart tissue suffer from lack of nourishment due to poor blood supply, there is a disruption of blood flow to the brain tissue and death of brain cells. The impaired brain tissue circulation is called cerebrovascular disease.
- **Cancer:** The second most common chronic disease in older people is the cancer. This greater risk of cancer in older people is due to their effects of slow acting carcinogen, prolonged development time "necessary for growth to be observable, extended pre-exposure time and failing immune capacity in old age.
  Certain diet and lifestyle factors may also cause cancer in old age. Diagnosing cancer in old age is often more difficult than at earlier life, because of the existence of other chronic diseases and because symptoms of cancer, such as weight loss, weakness, etc. may be thought as related to the old age.
- **Rheumatoid arthritis** is the inflammation of the membranes lining, joints and tendons, and is characterized by pain, swelling, bone dislocation and limited range of motion, mostly effecting women and can cause severe crippling. This affects even younger people but common in older people. The symptoms are general malaise, fatigue, loss of weight, fever, joint pain, redness, swelling and stiffness affecting many joints.

Geriatric Nursing Care/Management

- Providing safe and effective care to older people in enhanced care settings in the community requires coordinated and competent care by a skilled work force of healthcare professional, working efficiently together.
- To provide proper assessment and rehabilitation in the community settings.
- To provide an immediate response to the care of acutely ill older.
- To give medical support to all types of home schemes.
- To give increased and coordinated clinical services for the people who are discharged from the hospital.
- To coordinate the work of all healthcare people in the community.
- To provide leadership and advice, and training for all health personnel by the concerned doctors.
- Higher leadership is needed for health promotion designed to promote, healthier aging, and to avoid premature dependency.
- To provide new service for the older people.
- To integrate all services of older people so that it helps older people who have both physical and mental problems. Holistic care **(Fig. 13.55)** is essential in the care of elderly.
- Facilitating the development and quality assurance of enhanced services for old.
- Teaching the healthcare personnel for more advanced and personalized care.
  This knowledge needs to help them to understand the problems of all health and social care of all professionals to a level sufficient to command their trust.
- Basic understanding of public health issues, including local health needs knowledge of national policies for care of older people, and assessment of quality care.
- To give proper care for the old, all necessary equipment should be available. All types of clinical staff required to support the patient care such as, nursing care, physiotherapy, occupational therapy, speech and communication therapy and mental health professionals. All types of medicines required. Proper patient records and its maintenance is required. Adequate support from social services and public health is required. Proper administration and proper assistant with good libraries also is needed.

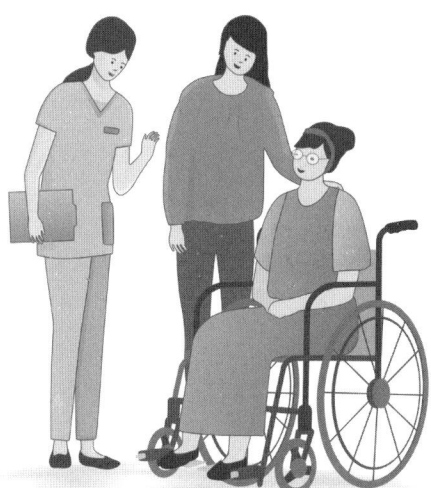

Fig. 13.55: Holistic care of elderly.

Screening area or intervention	Recommendation	Comments
Pancreatic cancer	Recommends against routine screening	–
Peripheral arterial disease	Recommends against routine screening	
Physical activity	Cannot recommend for or against counseling on benefits of physical activity; AAFP recognizes that physical activity is desirable, but cannot recommend for or against	
Prostate cancer	Cannot recommend for or against screening with prostate-specific antigen or digital rectal examination, any screening should be done after discussion with the patient	It is unlikely that any man with a life expectancy of less than 10 years will receive benefit from screening, the large number of false-positive results and unclear benefit of treatment leaves screening controversial
Skin cancer	Cannot recommend for or against screening for, or counseling on, prevention	Most skin cancers are found in older adults, whites have 20 times the risk of blacks and four times the risk of Hispanics of developing skin cancer, by 50 years of age, men have a much higher incidence of and mortality from melanoma than women, these differences become larger with increasing age, by 65 years of age, mortality rates are 25 per 100,000 for men and five per 100,000 for women Update in progress by USPSTF
Suicide risk	Cannot recommend for or against screening in the general population	Suicide risk increases with age in persons older than 65 years; risk factors include depression, alcoholism, chronic illness, divorced marital status, and male sex
Testicular cancer	Recommends against routine screening in asymptomatic adolescents and adults	–
Thyroid cancer	Routine screening by neck palpation or ultrasonography is not recommended in asymptomatic persons	Update in progress by USPSTF
Thyroid disease	Cannot recommend for or against routine screening in asymptomatic adults	–
Tobacco counseling	Strongly recommends screening all adults for tobacco use, medications and brief intervention counseling (less than three minutes) are recommended	
Vaccinations	CDC recommends tetanus toxoid and diphtheria toxoid vaccine for everyone every 10 years, influenza vaccine for everyone each year, and pneumococcal vaccine by 65 years of age	The USPSTF no longer evaluates, but defers to the CDC for all recommendations
Visual impairment (older adults)	Recommends screening for all adults 65 years and older	Update in progress by USPSTF
Vitamin supplements	USPSTF and AAFP cannot recommend for or against vitamins A, C, and E, multivitamins with folic acid; or antioxidants for the prevention of cancer or cardiovascular disease, AAFP recommends against beta-carotene for the prevention of cancer or cardiovascular disease	A three-year RCT of ambulatory men and women older than 65 years showed that 700 IU of vitamin D plus 500 mg of calcium citrate malate daily reduced the odds of falling by 46 percent in ambulatory women, no effect was found in men

AAFP = American Academy of Family Physicians, ADA = American Diabetes Association; CDC = Centers for Disease Control and Prevention, CHD = coronary heart disease, NCEP-ATP III = National Cholesterol Education Program, Adult Treatment Panel III, RCT = randomized controlled trial, USPSTF = U.S. Preventive Services Task Force.

Elderly Abuse

The elderly are the most vulnerable people in our society next to children. When working with the elderly it is important to ensure that they are given dignity and respect, not only for their life experience but for their wisdom.

Types of Elderly Abuse

Physical: Nonaccidental uses of force against an elderly person that results in physical pain, injury, or impairment. Such abuse includes not only physical assaults such as hitting or shoving but the inappropriate use of drugs, restraints, or confinement (**Fig. 13.56**).

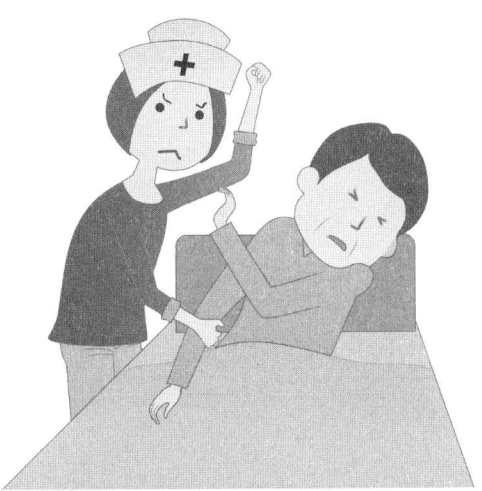

Fig. 13.56: Physical abuse of elderly.

Emotional (Verbal)
- Intimidation through yelling or threats.
- Humiliation and ridicule.
- Habitual blaming or scape-goating.

Psychological (Nonverbal)
- Ignoring the elderly person.
- Isolating an elder from friends or activities.
- Terrorizing or menacing the elderly person.

Neglect: Failure to fulfill a caretaking obligation constitutes more than half of all reported cases of elder abuse. It can be active (intentional) or passive (unintentional, based on factors such as ignorance or denial that an elderly charge needs as much care as he or she does).

Fraud
- Misuse of an elder's personal checks, credit cards, or accounts.
- Steal cash, income checks, or household goods.
- Forge the elder's signature.
- Engage in identity theft.

Scams
- Announcements of a "prize" that the elderly person has won but must pay money to claim.
- Phony charities.
- Investment fraud.

Signs and symptoms: The signs of abuse vary considerably among older people and with the type of harm being experienced. An older person who is being abused may:
- Say she or he is being harmed
- Seem depressed and withdrawn; signs of depression in elders are not getting dressed, not performing basic care of themselves that they are able to do, never going out even if they can, inability to sleep or sleeping too much
- Not accepting invitations to spend time away from their family or a caregiver
- Seem afraid to make their own decisions
- Seem to be hiding something about a caregiver
- Not have any spending money
- Put off going to the doctor
- Feel anxious and fearful
- Try to "run away," leaving their place of residence and not wishing to return.
  Seem to have too many household "accidents".

Any of these potential signs can indicate problems other than abuse or neglect, and none of these "prove" there is harms occurring. The presence of the signs simply indicates that further inquiry may be necessary.

Legal Issues in Elder Care

Growing older will force people to make life care decisions that affect medical and end of life concerns. These decisions about health and medical care are highly sensitive, and they deserve the strongest protection under the law. Therefore, when it comes to a person's healthcare, the law is very strict about who participates in the care related discussions.

These sensitive documents are meant to protect you from someone else making medical decisions on your behalf. The legal forms will give you peace of mind and the guidance to the friends and family members during a medical or financial emergency.

Unfortunately, adults rarely think about their beliefs and preferences regarding end-of-life decisions until a crisis occurs, a time when decision-making is most problematic. By not planning in advance means that a family member might not have access to the information they need, or to act on your behalf.

Preventive Geriatrics

The main objective is to protect, promote and restore the health of elderly people.
- Explaining the biological changes in aging.
- Personal hygiene.
- Regarding smoking, alcohol related diseases.
- Information on CD and NCD specific to old age.
- Availability and utility of health services.
- Over the counter drugs.
- Use of aids like visual, auditory, walking aids, etc.
- Information regarding elderly abuse.

Environmental Modification
- Maintenance of clean housing conditions.
- Need for fresh air, light and ventilation.
- Disposal of waste and human excreta.
- Vector control.
- Prevention of accidents both inside and outside the home.
  - Slip resistant flooring
  - Smooth pathways
  - Hand rails in bathrooms
  - Stairs-landing at short intervals
  - Adequate lighting
  - Contrasting colors

Nutritional Intervention
- Principles of balanced diet
- Food safety
- Food which improve bowel movement.

Life-style and Behavioral Changes
- Physical exercises like yoga and relaxation
- Personal habits like alcohol, smoking and tobacco chewing.

Specific Protection
- Immunization
- Avoidance of injuries and falls
- Vitamin D, calcium supplementation
- Certain food rich with antioxidant property- protect against cancer and degenerative disorders.

Secondary prevention: Screening to identify diseases in the earliest stages, before the onset of signs and symptoms.
- Early diagnosis and treatment–early recognition of CD and NCD, proper treatment, patient compliance and self care.
- Provision of free medical care.
  - **Tertiary prevention:** It seeks to reduce the impact of established disease by eliminating or reducing disability and minimizing suffering.
- Rehabilitation of elderly people with chronic diseases and care for terminal illness.

Rehabilitation—Medical, Vocational, Social and Psychosocial
Measures include:
- Training to increase independence in self care;
- Educational and vocational measures aimed at achieving economic independence;
- Social measures to ensure full integration and acceptance in community.

Medical Rehabilitation
- Appropriate exercise therapy for maintain the range of motion of joints, improving power in weak muscles and strengthening them.
- Restoring function of affected extremity.
- Provision of external appliance, splint or caliper, crutches, wheel chair, etc.
- Relief of pain by means of physical modalities like heat, cold, electricity.
- Bowel/bladder training to achieve continence.

Psychosocial Rehabilitation
- Rehabilitation is never complete unless the psychosocial aspects are duly taken care of.
- Problems—loneliness, anxiety, depression, feeling of insecurity, behavioral disorders, affective disorders, personality disorders, suicidal tendencies, dependence, irritability, malingering, hysteria, etc.
- The clinician's duty is to—explain, reassure, remove problems of the disabled about his disabilities, their effect on work and its possible solutions.

NGOs in Geriatric Care
- NGOs are the first one to bring out the problems of elderly in India.
- Help Age India
- Action for Social Help Assistance
- Center for the Welfare of Aged
- Geriatric Society of India
- Nightingale Medical Trust
- Cheru Resmi Center

Services
- Provision of food
- Day care center
- Old age homes
- Medical and psychiatric care
- Financial assistance-income generation and micro projects.
- Counseling

Geriatric Nursing Process Application
Nursing Assessment
- History
- Physical examination
- Physiological assessment
- Psychological assessment
- Socioeconomic assessment
- Diagnostic assessment

Nursing Diagnosis and Nursing Care
- **Visual changes r/t (related to) age related eye diseases**, i.e macular degeneration, glaucoma, cataract, chronic illnesses like diabetes, hypertension.
  Nursing care
  - Schedule periodic eye exams.
  - Recognize or try to communicate about the problem
  - Watch for behaviors suggesting vision problems
  - Adjust lighting levels
  - Use night lights and large print materials
  - Allow time for the person to adjust to the changes in light
- **Hearing capacity changes r/t age related changes, ear blocked with wax.**
  Nursing care
  - Watch for increased volume with the radio, television, or the person begins speaking loudly.
  - Periodic medical checks for wax build ups in ears.
  - Use hearing aids.
  - Look directly at the person while speaking.
- **Taste and smell: Sensory and perception changes r/t decrease in taste buds.**
  Nursing care
  - Ensure adequate fluids to avoid dehydration.
  - Seasoning may be added. Watch salt.

- Change in taste may be related to a medication or an illness.
- Give feeding through feeding tube in debilitating condition.

- **Skin: Impaired physical mobility r/t joint pain and vision changes.**
  Impaired skin integrity r/t skin thinning and skin diseases.
  Nursing care
  - More susceptible to pressure sores because of decrease in mobility and thinner skin.
  - Use moisturizing lotion.
  - Provide warm clothing for the elderly.
  - Assist with repositioning.
  - Inspect skin on a regular basis.

- **Musculoskeletal System: Risk of Injury r/t sensory perceptual changes and brittle bones.**
  Nursing care
  - Environmental modifications can be made (home safety with non-skid materials in bathtubs to prevent falls, etc).
  - Prevention of fall or injury.
  - Provide adaptive assistive equipment for ambulation.
  - Encourage independence, promote regular exercise (if possible, make it be weight bearing)
  - Proper use of assistive devices addressing the osteoporosis with increasing calcium intake and weight bearing exercises if possible.

CONCLUSION

Gerontological nursing is the specialty of nursing pertaining to older adults. Gerontological nurses work in collaboration with older adults, their families, and communities to support healthy aging, maximum functioning, and quality of life. The branch of nursing concerned with the care of the older population, including promotion of healthy aging as well as prevention, assessment, and management of physiological, pathological, psychological, economic, and sociological problems. Synonym: gerontological nursing.

CARE OF DIFFERENTLY ABLED PHYSICAL AND MENTAL

Handicap develops as the consequence of the disability. It is defined as a disadvantage for a given individual resulting from impairment or a disability that limits and prevents the fulfillment of a role which is normal for that individual, depending on age, sex, social and cultural factors. It is estimated that between 9 and 10% of the population in this country has a disability. People with a disability sometimes have difficulty doing things other people take for granted. However, the greatest challenge facing people with a disability is the misguided view society has long had. Historically people with disabilities have been pitied, ignored, and placed in institutions offering mere custodial care.

Definition

- Handicapped child is one who deviates from normal health status either physically, mentally or socially and requires special care, treatment and education (**Fig. 13.57**).
- According to WHO, the sequence of events leading to disability and handicapped conditions are as follows: Injury or disease, Impairment, Disability, Handicap
- Disability- any physical or mental impairment that limits normal activities, including seeing, hearing, walking, or speaking.
- Challenged person is one who deviated from normal health status either physically, mentally or socially. Children who are affected that way require special care, treatment and education.

The challenged children can be classified as follows:
- Physically challenged children, e.g., blindness, deaf, mute, harelip, cleft palate, crippled—polio, cerebral palsy, heart diseases, road accidents, burns and injuries.
- Psychological challenged—orphans, maternal deprivation, emotional deprivation, and maladjustment.
- Mentally challenged children—feeble minded, mental defect and mental retardation.

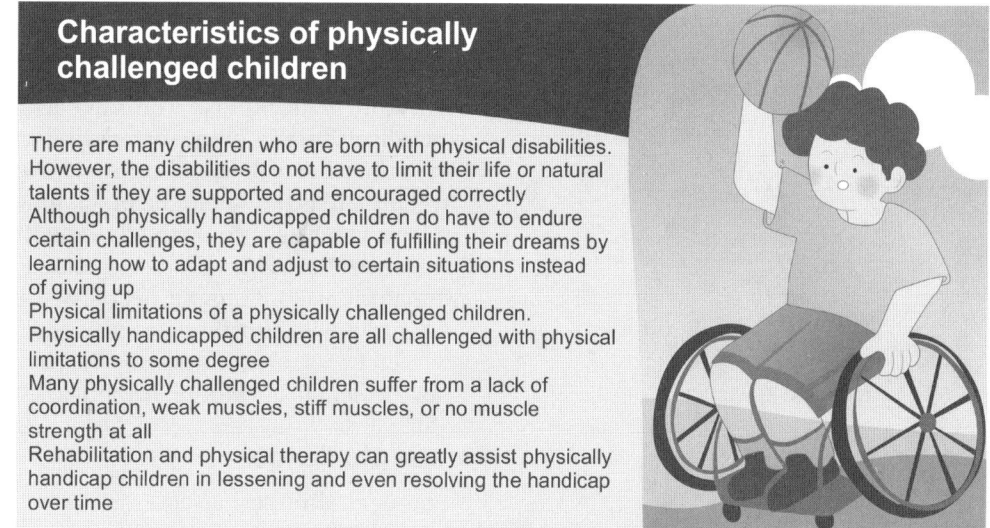

Fig. 13.57: Physically challenged children.

- All these problems may be genetic or due to certain specific diseases, injuries, social factors or nutritional factors.
- From the community point of view it is essential that such children in need of help should be taken care. Parents of such children should also play a major part in planning the care.
- The objective of the care in such situation is to improve the physical condition, prevent further damage and then to help, secure a suitable occupation.

Major Causes

- Malnutrition is another major disability causing factor
- Accidents on the roads and play at home can be another cause
- Genetic disorders and birth defects
- Effects of drugs

The aim of home health nursing is to assist the individual who has a disability and/or chronic illness in restoring, maintaining and promoting his or her maximum health. This includes preventing chronic illness, and disability. The home health nurse is skilled at treating alternations in functional ability, and lifestyle that result from physical disability and chronic illness.

Disability is a form of inequality. An inability to efficiently cope up with the day to day activity can be referred as disability. It is impairment may it be physical, mental, cognitive, sensory or emotional restricting individual in its daily routine. Generally disability is often replaced by the use of the term handicapped or challenged. There are also terms used like differently able than disabled especially in terms of mental disability. We are broadly classifying the disabled as physical and mental disability.

Physical Challenges

- The most common types of physical challenges affect a primary sense or ability to move and get around easily.
- These include sight impairment, hearing impairment, and motor impairment. Physical aids (**Fig. 13.58**) are used in physical disability.

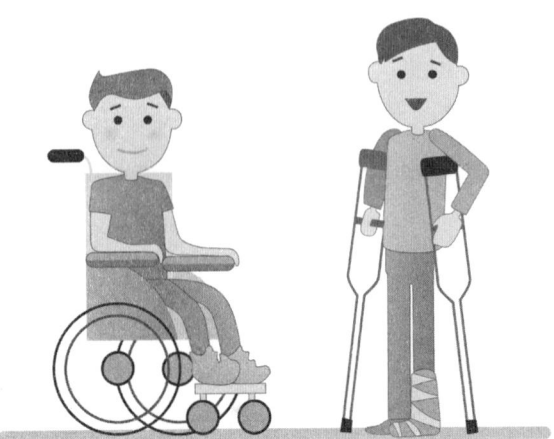

Fig. 13.58: Uses of aids in physical disability.

Sight Impairment

- As with other disabilities, sight impairment can be moderate, as is the case with more than 5 million Americans who are vision impaired, or it can be severe, as with the more than 1 million who are blind. About 10% of people fitting this description are under 20 years old.
- The leading cause of blindness today is from complications due to diabetes. Whereas everyone must take care of their vision and have regular eye examinations, those with diabetes must take special care to have frequent exams in addition to maintaining a special diet.
- Other causes of blindness are macular degeneration, glaucoma, and cataracts. Early diagnosis means that treatment can begin sooner or prevent blindness.

Hearing Impairment

- Hearing impairment affects 20 million Americans. Like blindness, hearing impairment can range from minor to severe.
- Profound deafness—hearing loss so severe that a person affected cannot benefit from mechanical amplification such as a hearing aid.
- Deafness can be inherited or caused by injury or disease. Most hearing impairments are caused by infections, obstructions, or nerve damage. Obstructions may block sound waves traveling to the inner ear. If obstruction is the cause of hearing impairment, the hearing loss may involve only one ear. Obstructions may be due to a buildup of ear wax, bone blockage, or something stuck in the ear
- A person born with abnormal bone growth in the inner ear may have inherited an obstruction that results in impaired hearing or deafness. Surgery can cure many of these cases.
- Nerve damage usually distorts hearing in both ears. Exposure to loud noise can cause nerve damage. It may occur with aging. Hearing impairments from nerve damage and obstruction may be gradual. If your hearing has changed, it may be time for a visit to your doctor or to an audiologist, a specialist in hearing problems.

Motor Impairment

- An injury to the brain or a disorder of the nervous system can affect the body's range of movement and coordination, including that of the hand and eye. Sometimes, especially when there is trauma to the brain, motor impairment of this sort may be accompanied by mental impairment.
- Advances have been made to assist people with motor impairment. For example, people with limb amputations are fitted with prosthetic or artificial limbs. Motorized wheelchairs also allow many people with motor impairment to get around without assistance.

Mental Challenges

- Some challenges affect a person's ability to live independently in society. This is true of the mental challenge called mental retardation—below average intellectual ability from birth to early childhood associated with difficulties in learning and social adaptation.

- Mental retardation affects about 3% of the population.
- The four levels of mental retardation are mild, moderate, severe, and profound. Mildly affected individuals make up about 75% of the mentally retarded population and cannot be outwardly distinguished from non-retarded people.
- Several factors have been isolated as causes of mental retardation. One is heredity. Symptoms of genetic disorders such as Down syndrome, PKU, or Tay-Sachs disease include mental retardation.
- Lifestyle of the mother to be during pregnancy is another factor. Women who use alcohol or other addictive drugs greatly increase the risk that their babies will be born with retardation.
- Yet another preventable risk factor is infection with rubella, or German measles, during pregnancy. Immunization against this disease during childhood or within 3 months of becoming pregnant reduces this risk.

Responsibilities of the Home Health Nurse

- To guide the parent in getting early treatment to prevent further damage and improve the physical condition, e.g., physiotherapy, through which the deformities could be corrected. This knowledge has to be imparted to parents, e.g., as in case of polio.
- To provide occupational therapy. A child who is challenged can be trained to choose any craft according to his ability such as carpentry, painting, cloth weaving or mat weaving.
- **Prosthetics:** To provide guidance in obtaining artificial limbs or a device like an artificial hearing aid.
- **Vocational guidance:** The parent must be educated and convoked that the child can be restored to function as a useful member. Such vocational guidance, as it is called, is given in several schools in India.
  - Occupational and Physical Therapy School at Mumbai
  - Occupational Therapy School at Nagpur
  - All India Institute of Physical Medicine and Rehabilitation, Mumbai
  - Institute of Physical Medicine and Rehabilitation, Christian Medical College and Hospital, Vellore.

  Besides these, there are schools specifically for the deaf and dumb, and for the blind, which are run by private organizations or by government.
- **Preventive activities:** Preventive steps can be adopted to limit the extent of disability. Some disabilities, e.g., due to polio or accidents can be prevented. Adequate nutrition can be maintained, so that mental retardation due to malnutrition can be prevented.
- **Education:** Nurse can arrange for community education on the above aspects to enlighten the people. Specially, in India people associate the mishaps to 'fate' or curse from God. So guiding them in the right way is essential.

Domains of health care quality are explained in **Figure 13.59**.

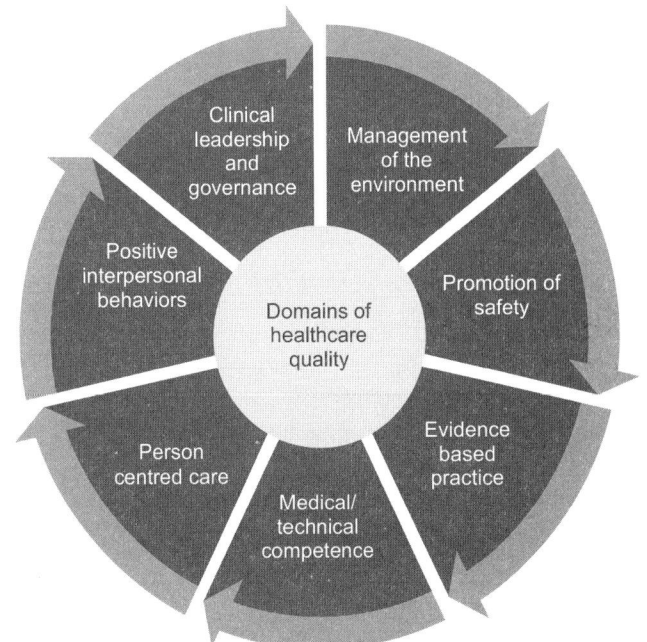

Fig. 13.59: Domains of healthcare quality.

Interdisciplinary Approach in Providing Care to the Disabled by the Home Health Nurse

- Families are often the primary care givers of family members who are disabled. It is important to identify strategies that promote family functioning, stability, growth, and coping.
- Nursing interventions should include assessing the entire family as a unit of care.
- Nurses need to assess their personal feelings, which can inhibit or enhance their ability to function effectively with persons who are disabled.
- Nurses focus on preventive strategies for people who already have potentially disabling conditions to limit the occurrences, impairment and functional limitation.
- Nurses promote self-care, self-management and self-advocacy.
- Nurses provide health education interventions which include teaching clients about their conditions, community resources, self-management, self-care and self-advocacy.
- Nurses assist clients in learning how to find and utilize community resources.

Mental Retardation

Mental retardation is a condition of both clinical and social importance. It is characterized by limitations in performance that result from significant impairments in measured intelligence and adaptive behavior.

Mental retardation is defined as:

- Significantly sub-average general intellectual functioning (IQ below 70)
- Significantly deficit or impairment in adaptive functioning
- Which manifests during the period of development (before 18 years of age).

Types

- Mild mental retardation (IQ 50–70) 85% of the total mental retardation
- Moderate MR (IQ 35–49) 12% of the total MR. Most of them can talk and learn
- Severe MR (IQ 20–34) 7% of the total MR. Only few of them learn to care for themselves completely.

Responsibilities of Home Health Nurse in Care of the Mentally Retarded (Fig. 13.60)

Primary Prevention

- Good antenatal check-up
- Improving socioeconomic status
- Education
- Facilitating research to identify the genetic counseling cause.

Secondary Level

- Early detection of defects and correction
- Prevention of child abuse and sexual abuse.

Tertiary Prevention

- Treatment of physical and psychological problems
- Behavior modification
- Physiotherapy to treat the rehabilitation disability.

Effects of MR on the Family

- Distress
- Depression, guilty feeling
- Over indulgence
- Social problems
- Marital disharmony
- Dissatisfaction about medical and social services

Physical Disability: Visual, Auditory and Orthopedic

A person who is unable to perform normal physical activity in the day to day life due to some impairment is called physically disabled. It is further divided into three types based on the in a particular organ. Those with deformity of vision are called blind or visually disabled. Individuals with problem of hearing come under the category of auditory disabled or dumb. Those with loss or deformity of limbs are called orthopedically disabled. In India, of all the disabled there are around 49% who are blind, 13% are deaf and dumb, 28% has orthopedic disability. Malnutrition, ignorance and inefficient medical faculties are major causes for physical disability in our country.

Visual Disability

A person whose vision is totally or partially lost vision is 6/60 or less are called blind or visually disabled. Blindness is a major disability amongst all forms in India (**Fig. 13.61**).

Deafness/Hearing Impairment

- **Cataract:** In spite of mass awareness programs conducted and easy treatment for cataract, it is one of the major reason for blindness in India. It is associated with old age and can be easily cured with a simple surgery or laser treatment.
- **Glaucoma:** Pressure on the cornea leads to this kind of disease which might lead to partial or complete blindness.
- **Trachoma:** It is a poisonous kind of conjunctivitis that is caused by bacteria. If not treated immediately can cause spread of the disease as well as loss of eye sight?
- **Night blindness and color blindness:** Lack of vitamin A causes night blindness that is loss of vision after sun set and lack of nutrients and genetic disorder can cause color blindness.
- **Accidents:** Eyes are one of the most delicate body organs. Injury of any kind to the cornea or retina can be dangerous to the eyesight.
- **Other diseases:** Hypertension, diabetes or stroke can be the cause for partial or complete blindness.

Treatment

Based on the causes for blindness, it can be treated accordingly. Treating the disease that has caused loss of eye sight like Hypertension, Diabetes or nutritional deficiency can be cured with medication. Timely surgery for cataract can also save the patient from blindness. Cornea transplant are also possible in case of injury or genetic disorder by birth.

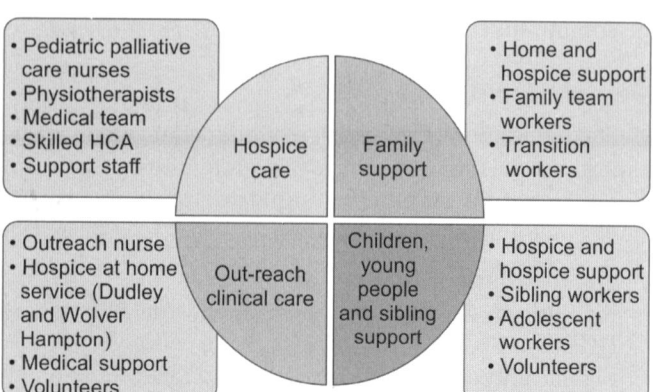

Fig. 13.60: Heathcare team in managing disabled.

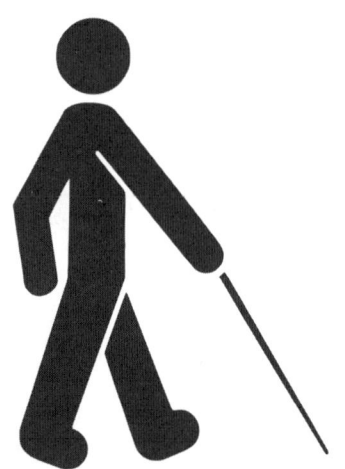

Fig. 13.61: Visually challenged person.

Auditory Disability

A person who is unable to hear a sound of 30 db can be considered as deaf. The person with speech impairment and stammering are considered to be dumb. Those who are deaf by birth are dumb as well as they haven't heard the sounds required to be able to speak and converse. The hearing assessment in shown in **Figure 13.62**.

Types of Deafness

- **Conduction deafness:** Defect in the ear drum or middle ear causes this kind of deafness.
- **Nerve deafness:** If the connecting nerves get damaged or weakened due to old age or other reasons, then nerve deafness can occur. It is caused due to damage to the bacillary membrane.

Causes

- Genetic disorder or hereditary.
- Over dose of antibiotics.
- Inefficient treatment in Jaundice, viral infections can lead to deafness.
- Accidents or severe injury to inner ear, eardrum of nerves of joining ear and brain.

Treatment

Depending on the root cause for deafness, deafness can be controlled or cured in some cases or in case of total loss of hearing are available to enable hearing. Speech therapy in case of stammering or dumbness helps the patient where the Communication can take place through the use of sign language.

Orthopedically Disabled

Inability to use ones hands or legs for motor functioning or loss of limbs can be included into orthopedically disable. Deformity of hands, legs, spinal cord, muscles can all be included in this type of disability. Types of orthopedic imapirement are explained in **Figure 13.63**.

Causes

- **Polio:** The virus of polio damages the limbs and cause paralytic condition in the body. It affects the patient in the childhood. India to a great extent has overcome this

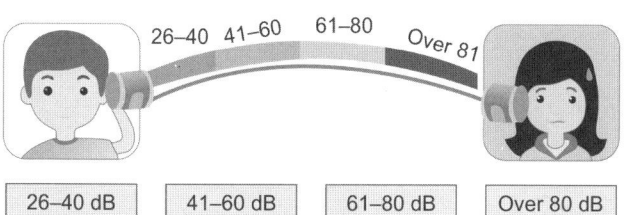

Fig. 13.62: Hearing assessment.

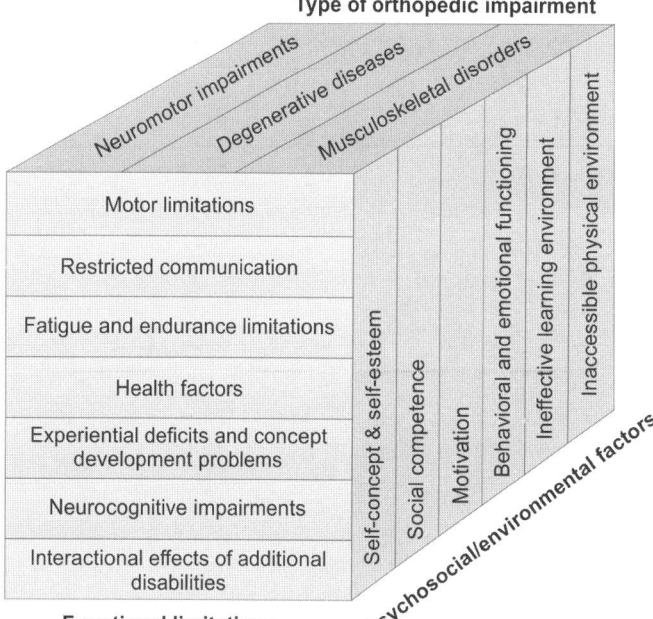

Fig. 13.63: Types of orthopedic impairment.

problem with vaccination. However, there are seldom instances of this disease.
- **Spinal bifida:** Under developed spinal cord or damaged spinal cord lead to spinal bifida. Movement controlled by spinal cord becomes impossible making patient immobile and dependent.
- **Cerebral palsy:** The part of the brain which takes care of motor able activity of a human being if affected adversely or not developed to its optimum level can lead to cerebral palsy.
- **Muscular dystrophy:** Muscle fibers in the body gets weakened then the body gets affected with muscular dystrophy.

Treatment

Regular vaccination should be given for preventing polio. Physiotherapy and occupational therapy can also help patients to be self-reliant in their daily chores. Artificial limb like Jaipur foot helps in movement for those who have lost limbs.

Mental Disability—Levels and Types of Mental Disability

When a person loses the capacity to think independently and rationally, whose intellectual levels are not developed then the person is called mentally disabled. Individuals with an intelligent quotient (IQ) of less than 70 can be considered as a mentally retarded or mentally disabled.

Levels of Mental Retardation

On the basis of the IQ levels of an individual the mental retardation is analyzed at four different levels **(Fig. 13.64)**
- **Mild mental retardation:** An individual whose IQ is between 50–70 is called mild mentally retarded. These children can complete their primary level of education

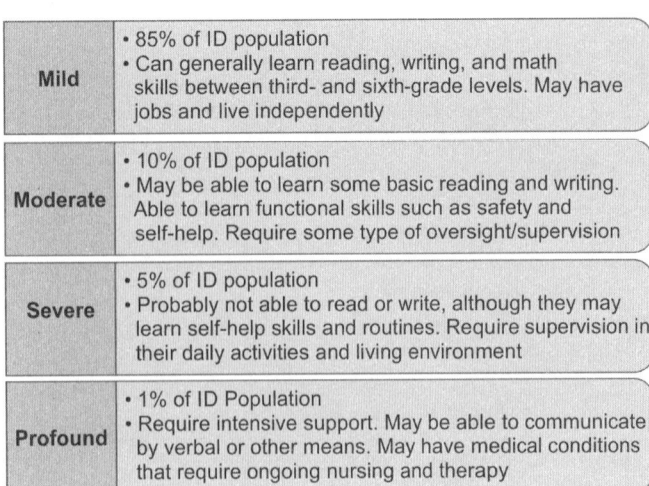

Fig. 13.64: Levels of mental retardation.

comfortably but have problems of concentration and analytical ability is also very low.
- **Moderate mental retardation:** Individual with an IQ between 35–50 is called moderate mentally retarded. They can't take up formal education and needs support of their family members to do their daily chores. They can be made independent with some basic technical skills and can be made self-reliant in their own health and safety.
- **Severe mental retardation:** Persons with an IQ of 20–35 is severely mentally retarded.
- **Profound mental retardation:** Individual with an IQ lower than 20 are profound mentally retarded. They can't be kept at home and need intensive treatment at an asylum or mental hospital.

Types of mental retardation: There are several types of mental retardation or mental disability.
- **Down's syndrome:** It is a genetic disability in which there is a problem in the 21st pair of chromosomes.
- **Autism:** The part of the brain dealing with communication is damaged then it can lead to autism. Eye to eye contact, conversation and sometimes even basic motor abilities get affected.
- **Psychosis and neurosis:** Split personality, hallucination, and schizophrenia are all types of this disorder.

Treatment and Welfare Measures

Psychological counseling, behavioral therapy, occupational therapy can all help the patient to lead a normal like. Special schools and shelter homes provide them skills in art, handicrafts other technical skills that enable them to be self-sufficient and confident. Training in social adjustment through skills for safety, security and hygiene make them more acceptable and adaptable in the family and society. A disabled may it be physical or mental should not be considered as a burden to the family or society. By just giving sympathy is not going to solve their problems. Helping them to be respectable and self-reliant members of the society should be our aim. Providing them with educational and occupational opportunities should be at the helm of all policies and programs by the government. NGOs can play a very constructive role in prevention and cure of disability by joining hands with medical Support.

National Policy for Persons with Disabilities

The Government of India formulated the National Policy for Persons with Disabilities in February 2006 which deals with Physical, Educational and Economic Rehabilitation of persons with disabilities. In addition the policy also focuses upon rehabilitation of women and children with disabilities, barrier free environment, social security, research, etc. The National Policy recognizes that Persons with Disabilities are valuable human resource for the country and seeks to create an environment that provides them equal opportunities, protection of their rights and full participation in society **(Fig. 13.65)**.

Focus of the Policy

The focus of the policy is on the following:

Prevention of Disabilities

- Since disability, in a large number of cases, is preventable, the policy lays a strong emphasis on prevention of disabilities.
- It calls for program for prevention of diseases, which result in disability and the creation of awareness regarding measures to be taken for prevention of disabilities during the period of pregnancy and thereafter to be intensified and their coverage expanded.

Rehabilitation measures: Rehabilitation measures can be classified into three distinct groups:
1. Physical rehabilitation, which includes early detection and intervention, counseling and medical interventions and provision of aids and appliances. It will also include the development of rehabilitation professionals.
2. Educational rehabilitation including vocational education and
3. Economic rehabilitation for a dignified life in society.

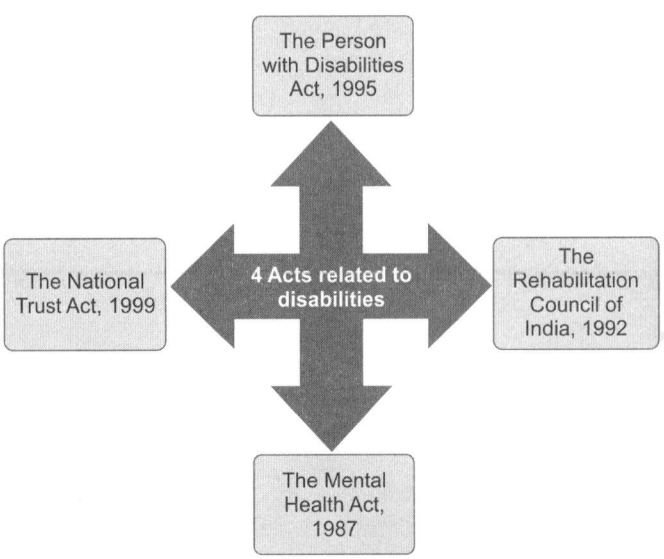

Fig. 13.65: Acts related to disability.

Women with Disabilities

- Women with disabilities require protection against exploitation and abuse. Special programs will be developed for education, employment and providing of other rehabilitation services to women with disabilities keeping in view their special needs.
- Special educational and vocation training facilities will be setup. Programs will be undertaken to rehabilitate abandoned disabled women/girls by encouraging their adoption in families, support to house them and impart them training for gainful employment skills.
- The Government will encourage the projects where representation of women with disabilities is ensured at least to the extent of twenty five percent of total beneficiaries.

Children with Disabilities

Children with disabilities are the most vulnerable group and need special attention. The Government would strive to:
- Ensure right to care, protection and security for children with disabilities;
- Ensure the right to development with dignity and equality creating an enabling environment where children can exercise their rights, enjoy equal opportunities and full participation in accordance with various statutes.
- Ensure inclusion and effective access to education, health, vocational training along with specialized rehabilitation services to children with disabilities.
- Ensure the right to development as well as recognition of special needs and of care, and protection of children with severe disabilities.

Barrier-free Environment

- Barrier-free environment enables people with disabilities to move about safely and freely, and use the facilities within the built environment.
- The goal of barrier free design is to provide an environment that supports the independent functioning of individuals so that they can participate without assistance, in everyday activities.
- Therefore, to the maximum extent possible, buildings/places/transportation systems for public use will be made barrier free.

Issue of Disability Certificates

- The Government of India has notified guidelines for evaluation of the disabilities and procedure for certification.
- The Government will ensure that the persons with disabilities obtain the disability certificates without any difficulty in the shortest possible time by adoption of simple, transparent and client-friendly procedures.

Social Security

- Disabled persons, their families and care givers incur substantial additional expenditure for facilitating activities of daily living, medical care, transportation, assistive devices, etc. Therefore, there is a need to provide them social security by various means.
- Central Government has been providing tax relief to persons with disabilities and their guardians. The State Governments/U.T. Administrations have been providing unemployment allowance or disability pension.
- The State Governments will be encouraged to develop a comprehensive social security policy for persons with disabilities.

Promotion of Nongovernmental Organizations (NGOs)

- The National Policy recognizes the NGO sector as a very important institutional mechanism to provide affordable services to complement the endeavors of the Government.
- The NGO sector is a vibrant and growing one. It has played a significant role in the provisions of services for persons with disabilities.
- Some of the NGOs are also undertaking human resource development and research activities.
- Government has also been actively involving them in policy formulation, planning, implementation, monitoring and has been seeking their advice on various issues relating to persons with disabilities.
- Interaction with NGOs will be enhanced on various disability issues regarding planning, policy formulation and implementation.
- Networking, exchange of information and sharing of good practices amongst NGOs will be encouraged and facilitated.
- Steps will be taken to encourage and accord preference to NGOs working in the underserved and inaccessible areas.
- Reputed NGOs shall also be encouraged to take up projects in such areas.

Collection of Regular Information on Persons with Disabilities

- There is a need for regular collection, compilation and analysis of data relating to socio-economic conditions of persons with disabilities.
- The National Sample Survey Organization has been collecting information on Socio-economic conditions of persons with disabilities on regular basis once in ten years since 1981.
- The Census has also started collection of information on Persons with Disabilities from the Census-2001.
- The National Sample Survey Organization will have to collect the information on persons with disabilities at least once in five years.
- The differences in the definitions adopted by the two agencies will be reconciled.

Research: For improving the quality of life of persons with disabilities, research will be supported on their socio-economic and cultural context, cause of disabilities, early childhood education methodologies, development of user-friendly aids and appliances and all matters connected with disabilities which will significantly alter the quality of their life and civil society's ability to respond to their concerns. Wherever persons with disabilities are subjected to research interventions, their or their family member or caregiver's consent is mandatory.

Sports, Recreation and Cultural Life
- The contribution of sports for its therapeutic and community spirit is undeniable.
- Persons with disabilities have right to access sports, recreation and cultural facilities.
- The Government will take necessary steps to provide them opportunity for participation in various sports, recreation and cultural activities.

Responsibility for Implementation
- The Ministry of Social Justice and Empowerment will be the nodal Ministry to coordinate all matters relating to the implementation of the Policy.
- An inter-ministerial body to coordinate matters relating to implementation of National Policy will be formed. All stakeholders including prominent NGOs, Disabled Peoples Organizations, advocacy groups and family associations of parents/guardians, experts and professionals will also be represented on this body. Similar arrangements will be encouraged at the State and Districts levels. Panchayati Raj Institutions and Urban Local Bodies will be associated in the functioning of the District Disability Rehabilitation Centers' District Level Committees to coordinate the matters relating to the implementation of the policy.
- The Ministries of Home Affairs, Health and Family Welfare, Rural Development, Urban Development, Youth Affairs and Sports, Railways, Science and Technology, Statistics and Program Implementation, Labor, Panchayati Raj and Departments of Elementary Education and Literacy, Secondary and Higher Education, Road Transport and Highways, Public Enterprises, Revenue, Women and Child Development, Information Technology and Personnel and Training will setup necessary mechanism for implementation of the policy. A five-year perspective Plan and annual plans setting targets and financial allocations will be prepared by each Ministry/Department. The annual report of these Ministries/Departments will indicate progress achieved during the year.
- The Chief Commissioner for Disabilities at Central level and State Commissioners at the State level shall play key role in implementation of National Policy, apart from their statutory responsibilities.
- Panchayati Raj Institutions will play a crucial role in the implementation of the National Policy to address local level issues and draw up suitable programs, which will be integrated with the district and State plans. These institutions will include disability related components in their projects.
- Infrastructure created during the course of implementation will be required to be maintained and effectively used for a long period. The community should take a leading role in generating resources within themselves or through mobilization from private sector organizations to maintain the infrastructure and also to meet the running cost. This step will not only reduce the burden on state resources but will also create a greater sense of responsibility among the community and private entrepreneurs.
- Every 5 years a comprehensive review will be done on the implementation of the National Policy. A document indicating status of implementation and a roadmap for five years shall be prepared based on the deliberations in a national level convention. State Governments and Union Territory administrations will be urged to take steps for drawing up State Policy and develop action plan.

Rehabilitation Nursing
- Rehabilitation medicine has emerged in recent years as a medical specialty. It involves disciplines such as physical medicine, occupational therapy, speech, therapy, audiology, psychology, education, social work, vocational guidance and placement services. The wellness perspective of the healthcare industry placed focus on the health of populations rather than just that of individuals.
- The healthcare industry is moving towards healthcare practices that emphasize managing health rather than managing illness. Rehabilitation seeks to assist individuals with restoration of function and maintenance of health and has been described as aiding the individuals to each maximum physical, psychological, educational, vocational, and a vocational, potential consistent with the patients activities and limitations.

Nursing roles in rehabilitation
- Caregiver
- Coordinator
- Educator
- Advocate
- Case Manager
- Leader
- Collaborator
- Facilitator
- Liaison
- Consultant
- Discharge planner
- Researcher
- Counselor
- Coach

- Rehabilitation services may be provided in a variety of settings such as the home outpatient programs, inpatient rehabilitation units, or centers, acute care hospitals and skilled nursing facilities. The setting is selected on the basis of the patients underlying function, potential abilities and individual problems.

Definitions of Rehabilitation
- Rehabilitation defined as the combined and coordinated use of medical, social, educational and vocational measures for training and retraining the individual to the highest possible level of functional ability.
- Rehabilitation is particularly of one who has been ill or injured, so that he may become capable of useful activity.
- Rehabilitation is a creative process that begins with immediate preventive care in the first stage of accident or illness, continued through the restorative phase of care and involves adoption of the whole being to a new life.

- Rehabilitation is the utilization of the existing capacities of the handicapped person, by the combined and coordinated use of social, educational and vocational measures to the optimum level of his functional ability.

Areas of Rehabilitation (Fig. 13.66)

- Medical rehabilitation—restoration of function
- Vocational rehabilitation—restoration of the capacity to earn a livelihood.
- Social rehabilitation—restoration of family and social relationships.
- Psychological rehabilitation—restoration of personal dignity and confidence.

Purpose and Goal of Rehabilitation

- Purpose of rehabilitation is to minimize disability and handicap and help a handicapped person to lead a useful life within his limitations. In other words, to make a disabled person into a "differently able" person.
- The overall goal of Rehabilitative care is to assist an individual to regain the maximal functional status, thereby enhancing the individual's quality of life.
- The intent of the healthcare professional is to promote client's independence and self care thus facilitating him client's resumption of a place in the community.
- The rehabilitative healthcare team supports the client's adoption to or adjustments of the loss of function maximization of the residual functional capacity and return of client to the community.

Types of Rehabilitation

From the point of view of rehabilitation service delivery, the role of nurses in rehabilitation is relevant to all phases and types of rehabilitation care:

- **Acute rehabilitation:** Nurses support basic body functions, such as respiration, cardiovascular functions, skin functions, as well as neuromuscular functions. Nurses take care of adequate nutrition and perform early mobilization and training of self-care functions.
- **Post-acute rehabilitation:** Nursing takes a key role in ensuring mobility and self-care. This includes advice to the patients and their relatives. Nurses also support specific interventions, such as bladder and bowel man agreement, stoma and tracheal cannula management, and the use of assistive and technological devices. Cognitive behavioral treatments that follow 24-h treatment principles need to be backed up and continued by nurses.
- **Nursing homes and geriatric care:** Nursing is in the first line responsible for long-term care. This includes the analysis of functional performance of patients and the capacity to coordinate the various interventions by other rehabilitation professionals. Nursing care itself includes positioning and mobilization, training of self-care functions, nutrition and many other factors.
- **Long-term rehabilitation care:** Depending on the individual needs of a patient and the setting of care, nurses deliver rehabilitation interventions. Nurses support and train body functions, such as bladder and bowel functions, and stoma management; and deliver other interventions.
- **Community-based rehabilitation (CBR) services:** In many cases, nurses are the only professionals who deliver rehabilitation. In this setting, basic rehabilitation interventions are delivered and patients and their families are instructed and trained in managing disability.

Rehabilitation Nurse Job Description

Our growing company is looking to fill the role of rehabilitation nurse. To join our growing team, please review the list of responsibilities and qualifications.

Responsibilities for Rehabilitation Nurse

- Functions as an administrator, educator, and consultant utilizing management theory in collaboration the Deputy Associate Director for Patient Care Service/Nursing Services other services.
- Demonstrates substantial and continuous responsibility for directing and managing an integrated program.
- Clinical supervision and leadership of the unit on a shift-by-shift basis.
- Communication, both verbal and written, with members of the healthcare team, patients, families.
- Customer satisfaction (patients, visitors, physicians and staff).
- Cost effective clinical operations including supply management and clinical utilization.
- Current, recent or previous experience providing patient care for the adolescent, adult and/or geriatric patient in a clinical, academic setting or cardiac rehabilitation setting.
- Care for the patient and have a positive impact on the patients and communities we serve in a fast pace environment.
- Team Leader responsibilities, which include assisting the Nurse Manager to create an environment that promotes personal growth and employee satisfaction.
- Demonstrates evidence of an understanding of the impact on patient injuries and vision loss on families and significant others.

Qualifications for Rehabilitation Nurse

- Ability to work with patients in the Physical, Occupational and speech therapy environments.

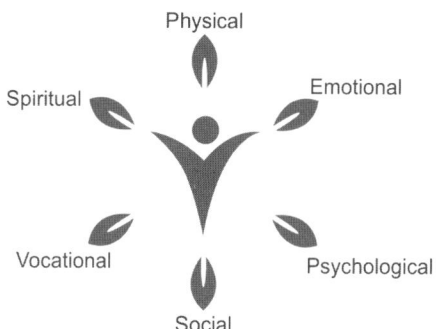

Fig. 13.66: Areas of rehabilitation.

- Individualized learning sessions with Rehabilitation Educator to enhance understanding of rehabilitation nursing.
- Mobility and Safe Patient Handling Training.
- Certificate of Completion in Rehabilitation Nursing Comprehensive Training upon successful completion.
- Chemical Dependency experience preferred.
- Knowledge and skills necessary to provide care and/or interact appropriately to the ages of the patients served by his/her assigned unit as specified below.

Rehabilitative Care Required Conditions

- **Disease conditions:**
  - Heart diseases like coronary artery disease and congestive heart failure.
  - Pulmonary diseases like chronic obstructive pulmonary disease and restrictive lung diseases.
  - Neurological and vascular diseases like Parkinsonism, cerebrovascular accidents and peripheral vascular diseases.
- **Congenital conditions:** Cystic fibrosis, club feet, and heart defects like arteriovenous malformation.
- **Traumatic conditions:** Motor vehicle accident, falls or other injuries particularly involving the spinal cord or the brain.
  Mental and cognitive conditions—drug-induced psychoses, mood disorders like depression, memory loss and dementia for example in Alzheimer's disease.

Gerontological Principles of Rehabilitation

As persons get older, the process of meeting their rehabilitative needs involve a longer, more involved interaction because, in comparison with younger persons.

- Older persons are more prone to nurses and illnesses requiring prolonged and complex restorations.
- Older persons have chronic conditions with unknown origins, extensive therapeutic regimens, and multiple complications of their own, which complicate and slow any recovery or restoration.
- Heal or recovery more slowly because of decrease in perfusion oxygenation, nutrition, skin integrity and tissue integrity.
- The quantity and efficiency of delivery of oxygen, glucose and other nutrients to affected areas is decreased.
- Old person respond less quickly because of sensory deficits, and slower transmission of sensory, motor and neurological impulses. Client's perception, comprehension and mobility are limited; safety and self-care are at risk. Client learning and active participation may be impaired.

Historical Perspectives of Rehabilitation

Initial stage of rehabilitation: Since the opening of the first rehabilitation facility in 1893, rehabilitative care has become an increasingly vital component of the healthcare delivery system. Initially, restorative care services were primarily needed for younger persons who were the victims of traumatic injuries or accidents or for certain debilitating diseases such as polio.

Twentieth century and rehabilitation: Twentieth century advances in the control of infectious diseases, treatment of life-threatening conditions, nutrition, technology and other aspects of healthcare have widened the exposure of rehabilitative care and will continue to do so at an ever increasing place into twenty-first century.

Need of Rehabilitation

- In general, the need of rehabilitative care is directly proportional to longevity. The longer a person lives, the greater the persons chance of experiencing health problems, which create functional problems and require rehabilitation services to maximize the residual functional capacity. Rehabilitative care minimizes the impact of morbidity.
- Before the end of World War II, rehabilitative services are increasing as a segment of the healthcare delivery system. These services were primarily available in association with military services. The social security Act of 1935 was the first attempt to extend rehabilitative services to the American public. Also during that era rehabilitation was viewed solely as a medical specialty and physicians were virtually the only rehabilitative care professionals.

Rehabilitation Council of India Act, 1992

The Act relates to standardization of training courses for rehabilitation professionals, to accreditation of training institutions and of individuals desirous of becoming rehabilitation professionals.

Definitions

- "Handicapped" means a person:
  - Visually handicapped
  - Hearing handicapped
  - Suffering from locomotor disability; or
  - Suffering from mental retardation;
- "Hearing handicapped" means with hearing impairment of 70 decibels and above, in better ear or total loss of hearing in both ears;
- "Locomotor disability" means a person's inability to execute distinctive activities associated with moving both himself and objects from place to place and such inability resulting from affliction of either bones joints muscles or nerves;
- "Mental retardation" means a condition of arrested or incomplete development of mind of person which is specially characterized by sub-normality of intelligence.

Rehabilitation Act

- **Initially,** the inclusion of the nurse on these rehabilitative care teams was limited. A most important event in the United States occurred with the passage of the rehabilitation Act of 1973, which was designed to increase awareness of the need for restorative services and to extend these resources throughout the community.
- **Community rehabilitation:** The goals of rehabilitative care were to return clients to the community and to increase their control of and participation in their care. Subsequent agenda to the act have made physical barrier and discrimination bias against the "disabled" illegal

These changes have further advanced the importance and prevalence of rehabilitative care in the community settings.

- **A freestanding or hospital-associated rehabilitation** center for drug dependency treatment or for physical or emotional rehabilitation is another setting for care. The goal of this type of facility I to help clients reach optimal health so they can become part of the productive community again.
- **With the rehabilitation Act of 1973**, the roles of nursing care rapidly expand. Increasingly, nurses assisted the clients as rehabilitative care managers, care givers and advocates. In 1974, the associations of rehabilitation nurses were formed. Ten years late, the association began to grant credentials to specialists in rehabilitative nursing. Presently rehabilitation nurse practitioners conduct their independent practice also. Solely as a medical specialty and physicians were virtually the only rehabilitative care professionals.

Rehabilitation Services in India

The rehabilitation concept has gained considerable acceptance during the past 50 years. Rehabilitation affects every age group and segment of society. The rehabilitation services depend upon the kind and extent of the disability or impairment. A large number of government departments, NGOs, institutions, voluntary agencies are functioning for disabled/handicapped for their rehabilitation and care.

- Rehabilitation council of India
- Ministry of social Justice and empowerment.
- Ministry of health and family welfare
- All India institutes of physical medicine and rehabilitation
- Regional and district rehabilitation centers
- National institute of mentally handicapped
- National institute for visually handicapped
- National institute for the orthopedically handicapped.

Rehabilitation Theories

- Rehabilitation is an integral part of medical care. It is defined by WHO as the combined and co-ordinate use of medical, social, educational and vocational measures for training or retraining, the individual to the highest possible level of functional ability and enabling the disabled to achieve social integration.
- Theory is an organized, coherent and systematic articulation of a set of statements relating to significant questions in a discipline that are communicated in a meaningful whole. It is a symbolic depiction of aspects of reality that are discovered or invented for describing, explaining, predicting or prescribing responses, events, situations, conditions or relationships.

Rehabilitation and Motivational Theories

- **Safilios-Rothschild** (1970) prepared a classic sociology treatise on three levels of disability and rehabilitation-personal, social and cultural levels. Her concepts of social system in rehabilitation are a multidisciplinary that it is undergoing change to include interdisciplinary or transdisciplinary and community based practice. Her thoughts integrated concepts about spread, stigma and perceptions of disability.
- **Abram Maslow**—according to Maslow a person is motivated to prioritize and direct behavior toward meeting each successive layer of individual needs. Rehabilitation nurses find Maslow's hierarchy helpful for a client is seeking to understand what motivates his or her of self-acceptance of clients in rehabilitation have been examined using Maslow's theory.

Rehabilitation and Wellness Theory

- **Halbert L Dunn (1959):** Introduced the concept of high-level wellness, integrating an individual's maximum potential and holistic balance into definition of health.
- **Richard Eberst:** The theory suggested that a person who would reduced stress and achieve healthy balance must attend to energy among all of six interactive dimensions such as physical, mental, emotional, social, spiritual and vocational.
- **Health belief model:** Health belief model is the product of a group effort of prominent sociologic scientists in the early 1970's who shared the goal "to organize the conceptual, analytical and research skills of the members and to direct them in a coordinates fashion toward the study of crucial problems in understanding preventive health patterns and health maintenance.

Cognitive and Social Learning Theories

- **Albert bandura** a pioneer of behavior modification, found four factors that influence how children learn, when observing others. A child attends to the situation, retains the observation, has a certain capacity to perform the action.
- **Jean Piaget** rehabilitation nurses working with pediatric populations frequently rely on another cognitive. Piaget, assessment of a child's stage of cognitive development provides information about how a child is interacting with environment, as well as guidance for a professional about what learning materials are appropriate for that stage.
- Theories of aging—cognitions are an important but difficult assessment more, especially when a client is very elderly. Among the very old, accurate assessment must distinguish among demented, depression, disorientation, alertness, and communication deficits.
- Stress theories stress and coping are key concepts for rehabilitation nursing. Stress in a complex, dynamic and multidimensional that affects all persons but touches each on differently. According to Selye, the totality of changes induced by stressors is manifested in GAS theory.

Psychosocial Development Theories

- **Erik Erikson's:** Detailed eight stages of individual psychosocial development, each stage with a potential outcome for either successful completion or dysfunctional reworking. In his notion of epigenesist, he maintained that one must successfully complete significant psychosocial development work in one developmental stage before progressing unencumbered to the next.

- **Development and change model:** Developmental model encompass cognitive, motor, bio-psycho-social, (Fig. 13.67) moral, social skills areas in which anticipated developmental patterns or changes may vary widely according to cultural and social expectations.
- **Grounded theory:** It refers to data that are grounded in fact and generate theory from the fact. When no theory exists, and thus no concepts are available to be tested, grounded theory is a method used to search out factors or to relate factors to the research problems.

Rehabilitation and Role Theories

- Integrating Roy's concepts with role theories; Roy dealt role changes related to loss and change when she formulated an adaptation model based on the premise that "man as a biopsychosocial being is interacting constantly with his changing environment".
- Edwin J. Thomas's disability and role theory—Thomas identified five roles related to disability are sick role, functionally limited, helped person, disability co-manager and public relation expert.

Orem's Self-care-deficit Theory

- Orem's theory has been one of the most discussed and used theories in Nursing. The seeds of her theory first published in 1050 in a guide for developing a curriculum for practical nurses.
- Orem proposed three theories there interrelated and have come to consider as one by many of the utilizes. Central to all three theories is that people function and maintain life, health and well-being by caring for themselves.
    - The first theory—'self care deficits' is the most comprehensive and is the core of her ideas. It is a conceptual image of recipients of care as people who are incapable of continuous self-care or independent care due to health-related or health-derived limitations.
    - The second theory—theory of self-care: is based on central idea that a relationship exists between of individuals and groups.
    - The third theory—"the theory of nursing system, describes therapeutic self-care requisites and the action or systems involved in self-care within the context of the contractual and interpersonal relations in human being with self-care deficit.

Rehabilitative Healthcare Team

- Rehabilitation is the restoration of an individual or a part to normal or near normal function after a disabling disease, injury, addiction or prison. The persons who can benefit from rehabilitation service are wide ranging. It includes persons having problems of cancer, orthopedics, respiratory burns, neuromuscular, mental retardation, visual and speech impairment, etc.
- Rehabilitation was an interdisciplinary team approach with a patient/family-centered plan of care and mutual goal setting, in which the patient is an active participant. Rehabilitative healthcare requires an interdisciplinary team approach to ensure the delivery of comprehensive cost effective, non-fragmental quality care. This is composed of a variety of healthcare professionals, the client and the clients family and significant others **(Fig. 13. 68)**.

Definition: Rehabilitation team is defined a group of experts function jointly to provide treatment and the training of the patients to the end the he/she may attain maximal potential for normal living physically, psychologically, socially and vocationally.

Characteristics of Effective Team

- Communication has to be effective, frequent, and documented.
- Collaboration amongst team members must be complete and genuine.
- Conflict resolution among disciplines must be quick.
- Leadership must be determined.

Objectives and Aims of Rehabilitation Team

- To make disabled a useful, self-sufficient and productive member of the society.
- To help the disabled regain functional independence.
- To help the individual develop compensatory abilities in place of disabilities and new functions in place of those lost.
- Provide the disabled person continued motivation and encouragement for participation in social activities.

Rehabilitative Healthcare Team

- Psychiatrist
- Specialists in orthopedics, neurology and other specialties
- Rehabilitative nurse
- Physical therapist
- Occupation therapist
- Speech therapist
- Prosthetist
- Clinical psychologist
- Medical social worker
- Dietitian
- Recreational therapist

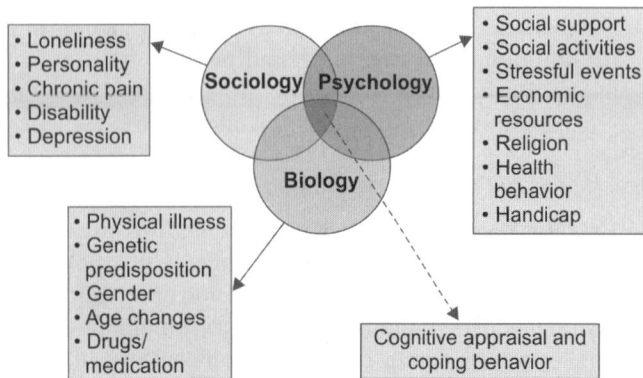

Fig. 13.67: Bio-psychosocial model.

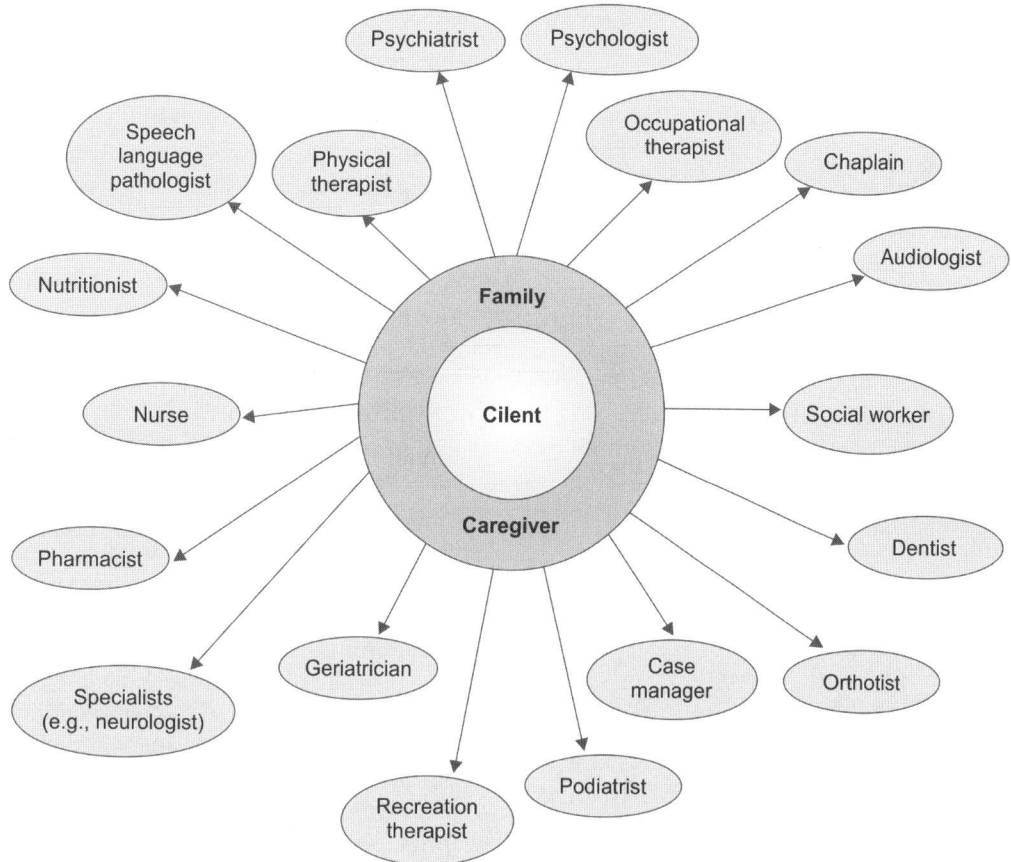

Fig. 13.68: Rehabilitation team.

Role of Rehabilitation Professional

- Rehabilitation professional, whether he is medical, paramedical or non-medical, is seen as a leader, teacher and guide instead of as a health provider. He imparts training, demystifies the rehabilitation concepts, solves specific problems, organizes the set up and generally functions as an advisor.
- It is necessary that each member of rehabilitation team should consider the psychological, biological, social, educational and vocational needs of the disabled/handicapped.

Rehabilitation and Nursing Process

- Rehabilitation is a process of restoring patients or persons to their previous level of health that is to their previous capabilities or to the level that is possible for them. It includes all measures of reducing the impact of disability and handicapping conditions and enables the disabled/handicapped to achieve social integration.
- The nursing process is a problem solving process that addresses community health problems at all aggregate levels and aims to prevent illness and to promote the public health. The rehabilitation goals and purposes are realized through the application of nursing process.

Nursing Assessment

The assessment must focus on the total functional needs of the client. Before the nurse can thoroughly assess the client and family, a pre-assessment phase must take place. This phase involves incorporating information about the client's environment and gradually establishing a nurse-client relationship. The nurse combines information from the referral with an assessment of the client and family in the home. The nurse uses interview, physical assessment and history collection to do this. An assessment usually includes data the following area:

- Physical assessment and history of all body system with emphasis on the present illnesses.
- Psychosocial assessment includes education, ethnicity and social relations.
- Family dynamics—decision making and rituals.
- Spiritual health—life values hope and a sense of community with others.
- Community resources—need for financial assistance and follow-up care.
- Environmental factors housing, transportation and neighborhood.
- Functional limitations—problems resulting in inabilities related to activities of daily living

- Client and family knowledge and attitudes towards illness and health behaviors and the impact on their lifestyles.

Nursing Diagnosis

After collecting data about the client and the home, the home healthcare nurse selects nursing diagnosis. If the nurse has assessed an insufficient number of defining characterizations for a diagnosis, additional information from family or friends may help to confirm a diagnosis. The diagnosis process requires the correct use of assessment skills in revealing the defining characteristics for client problems.

Common nursing diagnosis used is:
- Impaired skin integrity related to physical immobility/pressure.
- Altered nutritional status less than body requirement related to inability to absorb nutrients.
- Self care-deficit related to muscular skeletal impairment.
- Knowledge deficit related to disease and treatment process.
- High risk for complications (infection) related to inadequate acquired immunity.

Planning of Nursing Care

The plan of nursing care identifies nursing diagnosis and established long short-term goals. The nursing diagnosis and goals should be related to the primary disease process, treatment plan, functional limitations, and psychosocial, financial and environmental problems.

Nursing Implementation

Implementation of the plan of care requires close collaboration among clients, family members, restorative healthcare personnel and physicians. The clients are taught how to use special equipment and adaptive aids to improve mobility, coordination and independence where performing activities of daily living. Most procedures can be taught to the client and family.

Concerns of Nurse in Implementation

- Delivery of quality care to the client by meeting and exceeding all standards for care published either the American nurses association or the association of rehabilitation nurses and all criteria for accreditation enforced by either the commission of accreditation of rehabilitation facilities or the joint commission on accreditation of healthcare organizations.
- Accountability for the conduct of the nursing plan of care and the collaboration of the restorative care team.
- Documentation of the nursing plan of care and its implementation to facilitate reimbursement.
- Ultimately, facilitation of clients discharges to independence in care.

Evaluation

Evaluation of outcomes of care is an ongoing process, which is the key to the success of home healthcare. Outcomes of care must be documented for continuity of care, reimbursement, accreditation and research. Evaluation of client response to teaching, treatment and medications results in identification of changes needs in therapy. It also helps identify obstacles that may interfere with the effectiveness of the care plan. Effective, ongoing evaluation of outcomes and thorough follow-up for necessary changes are the most important function of home healthcare personnel.

Rehabilitative Nursing

- Rehabilitative nursing is an important and essential part of comprehensive nursing. The rehabilitation begins when a patient first comes in contact with the healthcare team. A nurse is concerned with facilitating optimal independence for a patient whether the patient is experiencing a short-term illness or a long-term illness or a crippling health problem.
- The rehabilitation nursing applied to all aspects of health. It is the restoration of the handicapped individual to a restoration of the handicapped individual to a future life in the society by solving his physical, mental, social and economic problems. Rehabilitation nursing focuses on the principle that the adult functions independently and is able to meet personal needs as well as the needs of department.

Definition

A rehabilitation nurse is a nursing professional that helps patients suffering from disabling injuries or illnesses live relatively normal and independent lives. This may involve working with them to regain abilities that they lost or gain abilities they may have never had.

Objectives of Rehabilitation Nursing

- To return to those abilities which have been affected by illness to the highest level possible?
- To prevent further disability
- To protect the patient's present abilities.
- To assist the patient to use his existing abilities.

Principles of Rehabilitation

- Rehabilitation should begin during the initial contact with the patient.
- Restoring the patient to independence or the regain his preillness or predisability level of function in a short a time as possible.
- Maximizing independence within the limits of the disability.
- Realize goals based on individual patient assessment and to guide the rehabilitation programs.
- These should be continuous encouragement given for active participation.

- Adequate and appropriate plan should be made to meet activities of daily living.
- Continuous and constant motivation given to establish social independence.
- Self-esteem and dignity of the individual should be respected and supported.

Philosophy of Rehabilitative Nursing

The rehabilitation centers have a philosophy of improving quality of life and facilitating independent self-care the client's full ability. An interdisciplinary healthcare team collaborates to plan and implement care. The role of nurse includes direct care, teaching and counseling.

Scope of Rehabilitation Nurse

Rehabilitation nurses work in a variety of inpatient and outpatient settings:
- Hospitals care for patients with head injuries, orthopedic conditions, multiple body traumas, and more.
- Rehabilitation facilities typically provide outpatient care, which is a next step after hospital care, to focus on speech, physical, and occupational therapy.
- Home health agencies send nurses to patients' homes to help them adjust and learn to use new skills. These rehab nurses are focused on helping patients maintain their independence and preventing a return to the hospital.
- Long-term acute care facilities provide intensive treatment for patients who receive specialized nursing care around the clock.
- Skilled nursing facilities with rehabilitation provide inpatient care for patients who don't require intensive care but may need medicines or other therapies.
- The Department of Veterans Affairs treats veterans with a variety of injuries and disabilities through rehabilitation that includes prosthetics and sensory aids. Leadership and acute care nurse activities are explained in **Table 13.2**.

Important Areas in Nurse Role

- Create awareness of the problem in the community.
- Reduce the consequences of the disabilities by early detection
- Assess the level of disability of an individual at community level.
- Plan and deliver early intervention.
- Organize and approach various health organizations to provide materials (prosthetic and other items).
- Organize appropriate need-based rehabilitation programs.
- Provide adequate practice in functional rehabilitation at family level.
- Provide health education to the family members to deal with disable people.
- Provide adequate recreation facilities for disables children.

TABLE 13.2: Domain 3 - Leadership and acute care nurse activities

Rehabilitation competency	Acute care nurse activities
Promote accountability for care	➢ Provides safe, ethical care ➢ Participates in quality improvement plan in healthcare agency ➢ Includes rehabilitation concepts in care
Disseminate rehabilitation nursing knowledge	➢ Promotes the inclusion of rehabilitation nursing concepts into clinical practice ➢ Seeks knowledge regarding rehabilitation concepts and clinical practice
Impact of Health Policy for People with Disability and/or Chronic Illness	➢ Advocates for all clients ➢ Includes issues that impact self-management and quality of life ➢ Supports health policy advocacy in promoting quality care
Empower client self-advocacy	➢ Respects and supports client autonomy within the acute care environment ➢ Consults interprofessional team or expert as appropriate to provide information to clients and families for informed decision-making ➢ Identifies barriers to self-advocacy

Health Teaching on ADL

- Assist the patient tolerance and nature of living at the particular environment
- Determining the nature and type rehabilitation needed
- Guiding and organizing the rehabilitation of disability.
- Providing the further complications of disability.
- Providing continuous and constant emotional support to the individual and family.
- Organizing and arranging legal, financial support to the individual and family.
- Providing health education about adjustment technique to the rehabilitation programs at community level.

Role of Rehabilitation Nurse

- Patient care plans are vital during rehabilitation and therapy. As a rehabilitation nurse, you will be required to follow your patient care and treatment plans closely.
- The nurse also be required to monitor the patients during rehabilitation and therapy to determine their progress. In some cases, such as those in which patients are making little to no progress, you may be required to help change the patients' care plans to facilitate rehabilitation.
- Basic nursing skills are used by rehabilitation nurses every day. These nursing professionals may be required to changes bandages and dressings, care for wounds, and

administer medication. Although the ultimate goal of rehabilitation is to enable patients to live as independently as possible, rehabilitation nurses may also be required to assist patients with everyday tasks, such as bathing and dressing.
- However, the main responsibility of a rehabilitation nurse is to teach patients how to deal with their disabilities. These nurses may help their patients exercise to gain strength in affected limbs, for instance, or teach them how to use adaptive devices, such as wheelchairs.
- Suffering from a disability or having a loved one who has a disability can be very confusing and frustrating at times. This is why rehabilitation nurses also act as educators and supporters in addition to their other roles. They frequently inform patients and their loved ones about their disabilities and provide support and information about treatment options.

Rehabilitation Approaches

The rehabilitation was an interdisciplinary team approach with a patient/family-centered plan of care and mutual goal setting, in which the patient is an active participant. Rehabilitation services may be providing in variety of setting such as the home, outpatient Programs, inpatient rehabilitation units or centers, acute care hospitals and skilled nursing facilities. The setting is selected on the basis of the patient's function, potential abilities and individual problems.

Major Approaches to Rehabilitation

Institution-based Rehabilitation

The rehabilitation services are delivered in an institution or home for the disabled. The services may be rendered in regional rehabilitation centers. The special rehabilitation and educational services are given to deaf and dumb and mentally retarded.

Some major institutions are:-
- National Institute for Visually handicapped, Dehradun.
- Occupation Therapy College, Mumbai
- National Institute of Mentally Handicapped, Secunderabad
- Ali Yavar Jung National Institute for the Hearing handicapped, Mumbai
- National Institute for the Orthopedically Handicapped, Kolkata.

Community-based Rehabilitation

- It a new strategy, unique concept of WHO, to provide universal coverage of rehabilitation to all segments of society. It is characterized by active role of people with disabilities, their families and the community in the rehabilitation process. There is also community involvement in the planning, decision-making and evaluation of the programs.

Objectives of community-based rehabilitation

- To involve the community to participate in the care of disabled/handicapped within the community.
- To remove physical and attitudinal behavior in the community towards disabled/handicapped.
- To provide care for the family of disabled person by community groups.
- To provide vocational and educational training for the disabled.
- To encourage the patient to perform the activity up to his maximal capacity within the framework of his disability.

Outreach Services

The professional members of rehabilitation team travel to the community and provides services to the individual, family and community.

Objectives of Outreach Services

- To reduce the consequences of the disabilities by early detection.
- To provide early intervention.
- To train family members for functional rehabilitation
- To organize special healthcare programs for disables.

The delivery of rehabilitation care is done through the following approaches:
- Homes
- Day care center
- Camps
- Outpatient clinics.

Special Nursing Approach

Rehabilitation nurses recognize the importance of integrating rehabilitation nursing principles into all levels of intervention to prevent complications or further disability and assure optimal level of independent function. Different models, concepts and approaches are essential to deal with the complexity of multiple causation, internal and external environments, psychosocial factors and variety of settings that make up nursing practice.

Rehabilitation and Disability

The term impairment, disability and handicap are closely related. According WHO estimated there are 450 million disabled in the world. In that 140 million are children with 80 percent living are given rehabilitation. The disability process is a concept describing changes in functions and social roles, due to pathological conditions.

Definition

- **Disability:** Any restriction or lack of ability to perform an activity in a manner within the range considered normal for a human being.
- **Impairment:** Any loss or abnormality psychological, physiological or anatomical structure or functions.

- **Handicap:** A handicap is a disadvantage for a given individual, resulting from impairment or a disability that limits or prevents the fulfillment of a role that is normal for that individual.

Types of Disability

- **Locomotors disability:** The disability occurs when movements in our body are affected due to diseases, injury, any absence or deformities in the joints, bones, nerves and muscles.
- **Hearing disability:** Hearing impairment means loss of 60 decibels or more in the better ear in the conversational range of frequencies. Hearing impairment or disability indicates deafness.
- **Visual disability:** Blindness is a visual activity less than 3/60 (Snellen) or its equivalent. Also blindness as an inability to account fingers in daylight at a distance of 3 meters. Blindness is a major social and economical problem in India.
- **Mental handicap:** It is otherwise called mental retardation. It is a condition of arrested or incomplete development of mind of a person, which is specially characterized by subnormal intelligence.

Causes of Disabilities

- Pregnant mother, who do not take adequate diet leads to underweight or prematurity leads to congenital anomalies or infections.
- Lack of basic health and rehabilitation services in poor communities makes disabilities more common and more severe.
- Accident is the leading cause of e disability.

Disability and rehabilitation: Rehabilitation is the optimization of the quality of life of those with established disability. This is done by the combined and coordinated use of medical, surgical, educational, physiotherapeutic, unique potentialities, skills and residual abilities.

Aims of Rehabilitation

- To make the disabled a useful, self-sufficient, and productive member of the society.
- To make life of the disabled as full and rewarding as possible.
- To allow the disabled to return to his home, work or school.

Principles of Rehabilitation

- Prevent the development of complications
- Help the disabled regain functional independence
- Help the individual develop compensatory abilities in place of disabilities and new functions in place of those lost.
- Provide the disabled person continued motivation and encouragement for participation in social activities.

International Day of Disabled Person

- The annual observance of the international day of disabled persons, 3 December, aims to promote an understanding of disability issue and mobilize support for the dignity, right and well being of persons with disability. It also seeks to increase awareness of gains to be derived from the integration of persons with disabilities in every aspects of political, social, economical and cultural life.
- A major action of the day is practical action to further implement international norms and standards concerning persons with disabilities and to further their participation in social life and development on the basis of equality.

Role and Responsibilities of Rehabilitation Nurse

Rehabilitation nurses work closely with patients with disabilities and their loved ones. As a rehabilitation nurse, you will encounter many different disabilities and have several responsibilities. For instance, you may help patients learn—or relearn—how to walk, talk, read, or write. You will also be responsible for caring for your patients' physical and emotional needs.

Job responsibilities vary greatly amongst rehab nurses depending on the place of employment. More specifically, rehabilitation nurses perform a variety of specific tasks including:

- Assisting patients to achieve and maintain maximum function and independence
- Assisting patients to adapt to a new or changed lifestyle
- Providing a therapeutic environment for patients, their families, and caregivers
- Educating patients, families, and caregivers about their disease and treatment plan
- Recording patients' medical information and vital signs
- Preparing and updating nursing care plans
- Changing wound and/or surgical dressings
- Continually assessing the patient's level of independence, injury, or disability
- Administering medications as ordered
- Performing tracheostomy care
- Administering blood products and enteral feedings via a gastrostomy tube
- Coordinating care with other healthcare professionals
- Lifting and transferring patients
- Determining if a patient is able to perform ADLs independently or with assistance.

Role of Community Health Nurse in Rehabilitation

- Assessment of the patient's physical, mental, socioeconomic and vocational status.

- Diagnosis of the therapeutic, physiotherapeutic, vocational, education, training and supportive needs of the client.
- Deciding the minimum acceptable improvement in the patient's health, capacity for independence and productivity level.
- Modification of plan of action, if necessary.
- Evaluation of the result of interventions.
- Implementing the action plan 4. Formulation of plan of action.

CONCLUSION

Rehabilitations a strategy for enhancing the quality of life of disabled people by improving service delivery, by providing more equitable opportunities and by promoting and protecting their human rights. It should deliver the service and training to people with disabilities and their family. Hence, it is necessary to mention that rehabilitation nursing is a complex task and one of the essential parts of the comprehensive nursing.

BIBLIOGRAPHY

1. Banik NDD, Nayar S, Krishna R, Bakshi S, Taskar AD. Growth pattern of Indian school children in relation to nutrition and adolescence. Indian J Pediatr. 1973;40:173–9.
2. Chaturvedi S, Kapil U, Gnanasekaran N. Nutrient intake among adolescent girls belonging to poor socioeconomic group of rural areas of Rajasthan. Indian Pediatr. 1996;33:197–201.
3. Chhabra P, Garg S, Sharma N, Bansal RD. Health and nutritional status of boys aged 6 to 12 years in a children observation home. IJPH.1996; 40(4):126–9.
4. Deb S, Dutta S, Dasgupta A, Misra R. Relationship of personal hygiene with nutrition and morbidity profile: A study among primary school children in South Kolkata. Indian J Community Medicine. 2010;35(2):280–4.
5. Dongre AR, Deshmukh PR, Garg BS. The impact of school health education program on personal hygiene and related morbidities in tribal school children of Wardha district. Indian J Comm. Med. 2006;31(1)81–2.
6. Gupta BS, Jain TP, Sharma R. Some primary schools of rural Rajasthan. Indian J Prev Soc Med. 1973;4:24–30.
7. Gutenbrunner C, Stievano A, Nugraha B, et al. Nursing–a core element of rehabilitation. Int Nurs Rev 2021. January 28.
8. Havrilla E. Rehabilitation concepts for the acute care nurse. Madridge J Nursing. 2017;2:72–75.
9. Kearney PM, Lever S. Rehabilitation nursing: invisible and underappreciated therapy. Int J Ther Rehab 2010;17:394–5.
10. Meyer T, Gutenbrunner C, Bickenbach J, et al. Towards a conceptual description of rehabilitation as a health strategy. J Rehabil Med 2011;43:765–69.
11. Spasser MA, Weismantel A. Mapping the literature of rehabilitation nursing. J Med Libr Assoc 2006; 94: E137–E42.
12. Srivastava Anurag, Srivastava Payal M, ShrotriyaVed P, et al. Nutritional status of school-age children—a scenario of urban slums in India. Archives of Public Health. 2012;70: 8.
13. Suter-Riederer S, Imhof RM, Gabriel C, et al. Consenting on principles of rehabilitation nursing care: A Delphi study. Rehabil Nurs 2018;43:E35–E41.
14. Vaughn S, Mauk KL, Jacelon CS, Larsen PD, Rye J, Wintersgill W, et al. The competency model for professional rehabilitation nursing. Rehabil Nurs 2016;41:33–44.
15. WHO expert committee. Health needs of adolescent. World Health Organisation. Report of Technical report series no: 609, 1997.
16. Who expert committee. School Health Service. World Health Organisation. Technical report series no: 30, 1950.
17. World Health Organization (WHO), the World Bank. World report on disability. Geneva: WHO; 2011.

REVIEW QUESTIONS

Long Essays

1. Define reproductive and child health. Explain evolution of maternal and child health services.
2. Describe the physiological changes in pregnancy.
3. National health mission MCH services.
4. Define school health services. Explain the objective, importance and principles of school health services.
5. Define occupational health nursing. Explain aims, objectives and occupational health services.
6. Define geriatric nursing. Describe briefly about theories of aging.
7. Describe care of differently abled physical and mental.
8. Enumerate the responsibilities for rehabilitation nurse.
9. Explain gerontological principles of rehabilitation.
10. Discuss the role of rehabilitation nurse.

Short Essays

1. Milestone in MCH care.
2. Maternal and child health development stages.
3. Mother and Child–One Unit.
4. Menstrual hygiene.
5. Phases of menstrual cycle.
6. Under five's clinic.
7. Advantages of breast milk.
8. National health mission (Rural/Urban).
9. Emergency ambulance services.
10. Government Health Insurance Schemes.
11. Employment State Insurance Scheme.
12. Health problems of school children.
13. Responsibilities of nurse school health.
14. Biological hazards and occupational health.
15. Health Acts and occupational health services.
16. Emotional care of old age.
17. Common health problems in old age.
18. National policy for persons with disabilities.

Short Answers

1. Maternity care.
2. Postpartum period.
3. Family-centered care.
4. Reproductive health.
5. Maternal child health service.
6. School health services.
7. School health program.
8. Occupational health nursing.
9. Occupational health program.
10. Ergonomics.
11. Occupational disease.
12. The lady Chelmsford League.

Chapter 13: Specialized Community Health Services and Nurse's Role

13. Complications of postnatal period.
14. Problems in breastfeeding.
15. Surakshit Matritva Aashwasan (SUMAN).
16. Pradhan Mantri Surakshit Matritva Abhiyan (PMSMA).
17. Janani Suraksha Yojana (JSY).
18. GVK EMRI (Emergency Management and Research Institute).
19. Pradhan Mantri Suraksha Bima Yojana.
20. Central Government Health Scheme (CGHS).
21. School health committee.
22. Components of school health program.
23. School health record.
24. Types of elderly abuse.
25. Legal issues in elder care.
26. Responsibilities of the home health nurse.
27. Role of community health nurse in rehabilitation.

Multiple Choice Questions

1. When India government has adopted family planning program?
   a. 1952   b. 1951
   c. 1953   d. 1949
2. In which year, the Government of India launched the Reproductive and Child Health (RCH) Program?
   a. 1994   b. 1995
   c. 1996   d. 1993
3. Which one amongst the following is not a Millennium Development Goal?
   a. Improve maternal health
   b. Combat HIV/AIDS, malaria and other diseases
   c. Ensure environmental sustainability
   d. Develop a local partnership for development
4. The MTP Act was passed in:
   a. 1949   b. 1962
   c. 1971   d. 1974
5. The family planning program started is:
   a. 1947   b. 1950
   c. 1952   d. 1960
6. The national planning program was started in:
   a. 1952   b. 1965
   c. 1955   d. 1977
7. Which of the following mentioned portals and subprograms were created under Sarva Shiksha Abhiyan (SSA)?
   a. Rashtriya Avishkar Abhiyan (RAA)
   b. Padhe Bharat Badhu Bharat
   c. Shagun Portal
   d. All of the above
8. Gujarat Chief Minister Vijay Rupani launched 'Poshan Abhiyan', a statewide mission to eradicate malnutrition among children and also launched 'PURNA' project to eliminate malnutrition among girls in the age group of 14 to 18. 'PURNA' stands for _____.
   a. Prevention of Under Nutrition and Reduction of Nutritional Anemia
   b. Prevention of Under Nutrition and Remedy of Nutritional Activities
   c. Prevention of Under Nutrition and Remedy of Nutritional Accidents
   d. None of the above
9. Janani Suraksha Yojana (JSY) is a safe motherhood intervention under the National Health Mission lanched in the year:
   a. 2004   b. 2005
   c. 2006   d. 2007
10. Janani Suraksha Yojana is a safe motherhood intervention under the
    a. National Rural Health Mission
    b. National Urban Health Mission
    c. Both a and b
    d. None of the above

ANSWERS

| 1. a | 2. b | 3. d | 4. c | 5. c | 6. a | 7. d | 8. a | 9. b | 10. a | | |

14 National Health Problems

LEARNING OBJECTIVES
1. Communicable diseases
2. Non-communicable diseases
3. Nutritional problems
4. Environmental sanitation
5. Population

COMMUNICABLE DISEASES

Malaria
- The incidence of malaria cases fluctuated between 1.3 and 1.6 million per year for the past five years (2007–2011).
- In the year 2011, there were 1.31 million reported cases of malaria in the country.
- About 95% population in the country resides in malaria endemic areas and 80% of malaria reported in the country is confined to areas consisting 20% of population residing in tribal, hilly, difficult and inaccessible areas.

Tuberculosis
- Some 1.2 million new cases annually and 0.64 million cases new smear positive of which 0.32 million cases die. Though notification rate per 1,00,000 populations at national level is much less as compared to RNTCP patient notification, there has been considerable increase in private sector notification in 2013 as compared to 2012.
- As per WHO estimations, tuberculosis prevalence in 2012 is 230 per 100,000 populations. In absolute numbers, prevalence is 28 lakhs annually and incidence per 100,000 populations is 176 in 2012.
- Morality due to TB is 2.7 lakhs annually. (Disease Specific Document for XII Plan: Tuberculosis, 2014)

Diarrheal disease: The second most common cause of death in Indian population. Diarrheal disease is responsible for one in every ten child deaths during the first five years of life worldwide, has the highest rate of incidence.

Acute respiratory infection: In India, over 4 lakh deaths annually are due to pneumonia, accounting for 13–16% of all deaths in the pediatric hospital admissions. There are some 369,000 deaths due to pneumonia among children 1–59 months.

Leprosy: India ranks first in new cases of leprosy. According to WHO, India accounted for 134,752 new cases in 2012 of a total worldwide of 232,857. India had more than 12 million people living with leprosy between 1991 and 2007. India is also one of the 16 countries ranked "worst" in 2012 with more than 1,000 new cases of leprosy.

Filariasis: Endemic in 250 districts across 20 States and Union Territories of India. About 614 million people in India are at risk of infection.

AIDS
- India has the third highest number of people living with HIV in the world with 2.1 million infected cases. This amounts to about four out of ten people infected with the deadly virus in the Asia-Pacific region. China, India, Indonesia, Myanmar, Thailand, and Vietnam account for more than 90% of the people living with HIV in the Asia-Pacific region. HIV treatment coverage is only 36% in India.
- At the end of 2013, more than 700,000 people were on antiretroviral therapy, the second largest number of people on treatment in any single country. (India has 3rd–highest number of HIV-infected people).

NON-COMMUNICABLE DISEASES

Diabetes Mellitus: India has the highest number of diabetic cases in the world. Over 77 million people in India have pre-diabetes and an estimated 40 million (**Fig. 14.1**).

Types of Non-communicable Diseases (Fig. 14.2)

Cancer
- India reports about one million new cases every year. Of the eight million cancer-related deaths in 2012, nearly

Chapter 14: National Health Problems

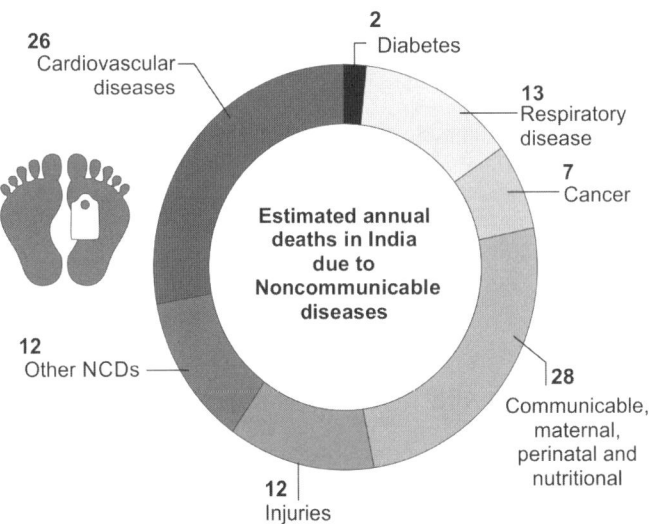

Fig. 14.1: Non-communicable death rates.

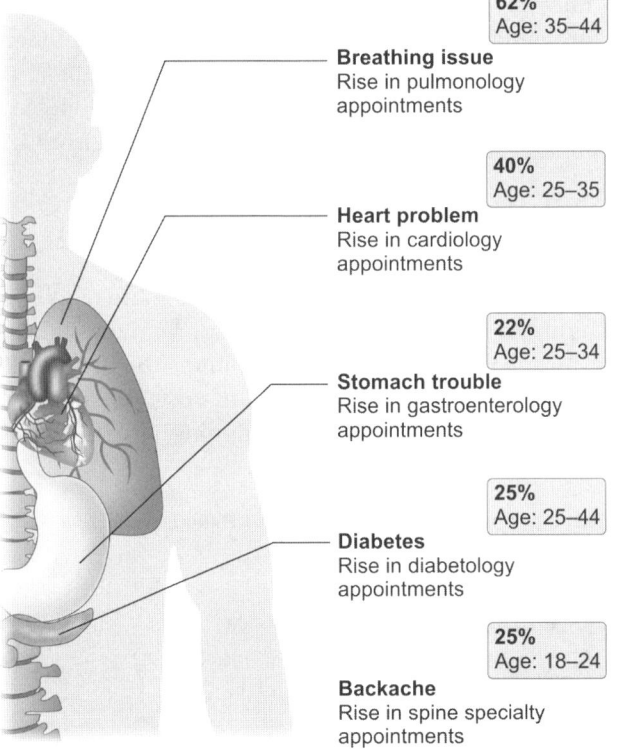

Fig. 14.2: Types of non-communicable diseases.

700,000 were in India, accounting to about 8% of the world's cancer patients.
- Again, in India, 71% deaths between 30-69 years are cancer related. As against global average of 0.5%, 15% cancers in India are in minors.
- The estimated incidence of cases of cancer in the country rose from 1,086,783 in 2013 to 1,117,269 in 2014. The estimated cancer mortality cases in the country have also risen from 478,185 in 2013 to 491,597 in 2014.
- Cancer is the second most common disease in India responsible for maximum mortality with about 0.3 million deaths per year.
- Estimated 600,000-700,000 deaths in India were caused by cancer in 2012. In age-standardized terms this figure is close to the mortality burden seen in high-income countries.
- Oral cancer ranks among the top three of all cancers in India: four in ten of all cancers in India are oral cancers. Annually, 130,000 individuals succumbs to oral cancer, approximately 14 deaths per hour.

Cardiovascular Diseases

- Prevalence of heart failure in India due to coronary heart disease, hypertension, obesity, diabetes and rheumatic heart disease ranges from anywhere between 1.3 to 4.6 million, with an annual incidence of 491,600 to 1.8 million. 2.4 million Indians die due to heart disease every year.
- Prevalence of Coronary Heart Diseases (CHDs) is between 7-13% in urban areas and 2-7% in rural areas.
- A conservative estimate indicates that there could be 30 million CHD patients in India of whom 14 million are in urban areas and 16 million in rural areas.
  - Sanitation is one of the basic determinants of quality of life and human development index
  - Earlier concept of sanitation was only limited to disposal of human excreta
  - But it also includes liquid and solid waste disposal, food hygiene and personal, domestic and environment hygiene.
- Prevalence of dyslipidemia is about 37.5% among adults of 15-64 years of age. About 25% of deaths in the age group of 25-69 years occur because of heart diseases. Heart diseases account for about 19% of all deaths across all age groups.

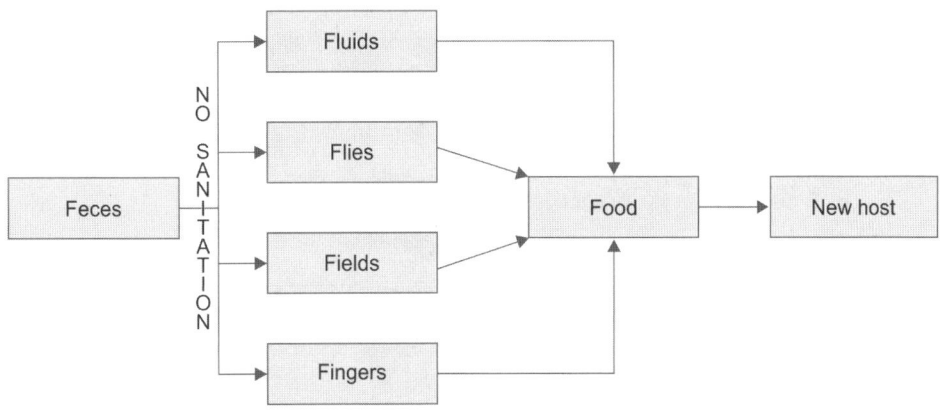

- According to the WHO, cardiovascular diseases, which affect the heart and the blood vessels resulting in heart attacks or strokes in extreme cases, account for 26% of deaths in India, or 2.5 million.
- The direct economic burden of heart disease in India could be $4.5 billion, which could increase to $18 billion if 100% of CAD patients were aware and received necessary treatment. Indirect costs would make the numbers even higher.

Blindness: Of the 37 million blind people globally, about 15 million are in India. Cataract is the most common cause of preventable blindness in India. Though about 35,000 corneas are collected annually nationwide, the annual demand is over 150,000.

ENVIRONMENTAL SANITATION PROBLEMS

- Some 400 million people defecate in open and 44% mothers dispose their children's feces in open.
- India accounts for 60% of global and 50% of its own population open defecation.
- About 48% children in India suffer from some degree of malnutrition. There is an increased female school dropout rate in the adolescent age due to lack of toilet facilities.
- Only 25% have drinking water on their premise. Sixty seven percent Indian households do not treat drinking water though it may be chemically and bacterially contaminated.
- According to Public Health Association (which year), 53%, 38% and 30% wash hands with soap after defecation, before meals and preparing food respectively.
- Nearly 80% children's feces are disposed in the open and 6% children use toilets.

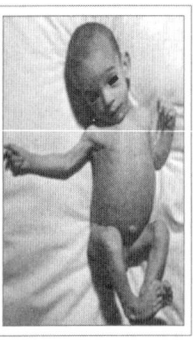

Protein-energy malnutrition
- Protein–energy malnutrition (or protein–calorie malnutrition) refers to a form of malnutrition where there is inadequate protein and calorie intake
- It is considered as the primary nutritional problem in India
- PEM is due to the 'food gap' between the intake and requirement
- Causes childhood morbidity and mortality.

MEDICAL CARE PROBLEMS

- India has a health policy, not a health service. The need-based services have primarily catered to the urban population, which houses 32% of the national population.
- The doctor population ratio stands at 1:1,700, less than the WHO prescribed 1:1,000. Reluctance by doctors to serve rural areas emerges from the feeling of professional isolation and disparity in living conditions.
- There are almost four times the medical practitioners in urban than in rural areas per 10000 population. Health problems and their causes are depicted in **Figure 14.3**.

POPULATION PROBLEM

India accounts for 17% global population and has 2.5% of the earth's land area. Overpopulation has its share of ill-effects including rising unemployment, inappropriate utilization of available manpower, inadequate infrastructure, resource scarcity, drop in production and rising costs and inequitable income distribution resulting in widening.

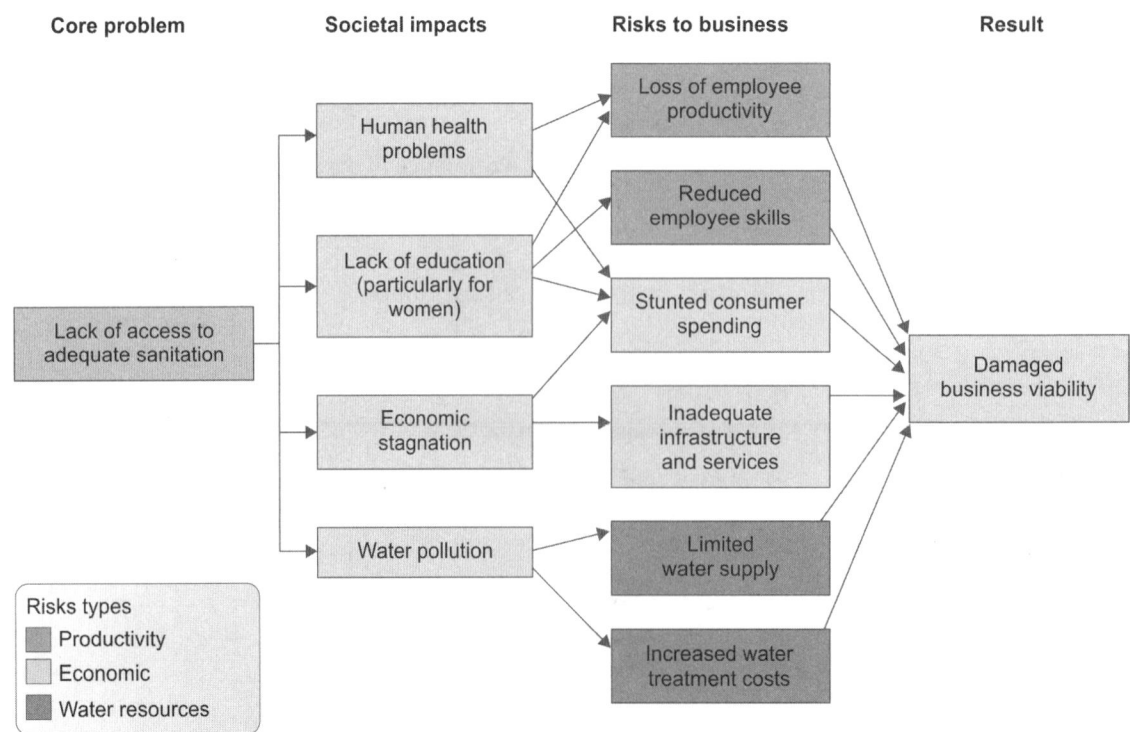

Fig. 14.3: Health problems and their causes.

Chapter 14: National Health Problems

Nutritional Problems in India

Under malnutrition makes the child susceptible to infection and results in child mortality. This accounts for 22% of the burden of disease in India and adversely affects the economic growth with an estimated adult productivity loss of 1.4% of the GDP.

Vitamin D deficiency: Vitamin D deficiency is the most under-diagnosed and under-treated deficiency in the world. Nearly 60-80% Indian population is deficient in Vitamin D. According to the WHO, the daily vitamin D requirement of 600 IU and can be obtained by a daily 15 minutes' walk in the sunlight, and yet it persists.

Calcium deficiency: Calcium deficiency and calcium deficiency-induced osteoporosis among the elderly are one of the most common causes of bone diseases and deformities. Low calcium intake predisposes to osteoporosis and hyperparathyroidism. Twenty percent girls in the age-group of 14–17 years in India suffer from calcium deficiency.

Vitamin B complex deficiencies: Nearly 80% Indians have vitamin B_{12} deficiency.

Zinc deficiency: Zinc deficiency in high among lactating women in India. Nearly 50% non-pregnant and lactating women in India have zinc.

Low birth weight: According to NFHS-3 (give year), 22% recorded were LBW (19% urban and 23% rural). On average, 28% children born in India are of LBW. Reducing LBW is an important indicator towards achieving the goal.

Protein Energy Malnutrition (PEM)

- The prevalence of stunting among under-five children is 48%, wasting 19% and underweight, 42.5%. These numbers are high in magnitude.
- Stunting is more among rural children though malnutrition is more among urban population.
- Incidence of PEM in pre-school age children is 1–2%. Prevalence of underweight children increased from 11.9% (<6 months) to 37.5% (6-11 months) to 58.5% among 12–23 months old children.

Xerophthalmia: Xerophthalmia is most common among children aged 1–3 years. An estimated 5.6% children in India suffer from eye signs of VAD. The overall prevalence of Bitot spots among children aged 1–5 years is 0.8%, which is higher than the WHO cut off point of 0.5%. The overall prevalence of night blindness is about 0.3% and of conjunctival xerosis 1.8%. (Prevalence of Vitamin A Deficiency among Preschool Children in Rural Areas, 2006).

Nutritional Anemia

- The prevalence of nutritional anemia is among the highest in the South Asian countries.
- The prevalence in India is relatively higher than that of other developing countries, affecting nearly 50% of the population. One in two women in India are anemic, including 39% having mild, 15% moderate and 2% severe anemia.
- About 55% adolescent girls suffer from anemia in India. According to the WHO, the prevalence of anemia in India is 65–75%.
- The National Nutrition Monitoring Bureau, Indian Council for Medical Research and District Level Household Survey suggest prevalence of anemia among preschool children, pregnant and lactating women and adolescent girls as high as 90%.
- NFHS-III reveals that Assam, Haryana, Jharkhand have the maximum cases of married women with anemia.
- The report further states that 84% and 92% pregnant and lactating women respectively suffered from varying degrees of anemia.
- It has been noted that women across all age groups in India have been suffering from varying degrees of anemia.

Iodine Deficiency Disorders (IDD)

- Of the 321 districts across all the states and Union Territories of India, 260 are endemic with IDD and the prevalence is more than 10%.
- In terms of numbers, an estimated 71 million people are reported to be suffering from IDD. Of the 1.5 billion populations globally at the risk of IDD, an estimated 200 Million people are in the country and 167 million living in IDD areas.
- In India, endemic belt of goiter and cretinism mainly lie along the slopes, foothills and plains adjacent to the Himalayas extending 2,400 kilometres.
- Pockets of goiter have been identified in the Aravali Hills in Rajasthan, Subvindhya hills of Madhya Pradesh, Narmada Valley in Gujarat, hilly areas of Orissa, Andhra Pradesh, tea estates of Karnataka and Kerala and the districts of Aurangabad, Pune in Maharashtra, as well.
- Inhabitants of most coastal areas, however, are relatively free of goiter. The overall prevalence of goiter among 6–11 years old children is 4%, below the cut-off to indicate endemicity of IDD.
- The proportion is higher in Maharashtra (11.9%) and West Bengal (9%) compared to elsewhere in the country. No state and/or Union Territory are free of IDD in India.
- About 54 million people are estimated to have goiter, 2.2 million cretinism and 6.6 million mild psycho-motor handicaps.

Fluorosis

- Fluorine is the abundantly available in the nature, and about 96% of fluoride in the human body is found in bones and teeth. Fluorine is often called a two-edged sword.
- Prolonged ingestion of fluoride through drinking water in excess of the daily requirement is associated with dental and skeletal fluorosis while inadequate intake of fluoride in drinking water is associated with dental caries.
- The World Health Organization has set the upper limit of fluoride concentration in drinking water at 1.5 mg/L while The Bureau of Indian Standards has laid down Indian

Standards as 1.0 mg/L as the maximum permissible limit of fluoride, with a further remark as "lesser the better."
- Fluorosis is an important public health problem in 24 countries, including India, which lies in the geographical fluoride belt that extends from Turkey to China and Japan through Iraq, Iran and Afghanistan.

SANITATION

The word "Sanitation means the science of safeguarding health. Sanitation is defined as "a way of life ". It is the quality of the living that is expressed in the clean neighborhood, and the clean community. Environmental sanitation, now being replaced by environmental health.

Definitions

- By National Sanitation Foundation of USA, "Sanitation as the quality of living which is expressed in the clean home, the clean farm, the clean, business, the clean neighborhood and the clean community. Being a way of life it must come within the people, it is nourished by knowledge and grows as an obligation and an ideal in human relations".
- WHO defines Environmental sanitation is the control of those factors in man's physical environment which exercise or may exercise a deleterious effect on his physical development, health and survival.
- Environmental health defined as an "art and science of promoting positive environmental factors and prevention and control of all the potential hazards including physical, chemical, biological and social factors which have deleterious effect in health of people".
- The environmental health has been defined as "the aspect of public health concerned with all the factors, circumstances and conditions in the environment or surrounding of humans that can exert an influence on human health and well-being".
- Environmental sanitation includes proper storage of food, collection and disposal of garbage in the proper manner, construction of rat proof buildings, godowns and warehouses and elimination of rat burrows.

Types of Environment

Since environment is a combination of physical and biological factors, it contains both living or biotic and non-living or abiotic components. On the basis of this basic structure, environment can be divided into physical or abiotic and living or biotic environment.
- **Physical or abiotic environment:** Physical environment is made up of the following states—solid, liquid, and gas. These three elements signify lithosphere, hydrosphere, and atmosphere respectively. On the basis of spatial distribution, smaller units are termed as coastal environment, plateau environment, mountain environment, Lake Environment, river environment, maritime environment, etc.
- **Living or biotic environment:** Biotic environment consists of plants (flora) and animals (fauna) including human beings as a significant factor. Thus, biotic environment can be of two types such as floral environment and faunal environment.

Apart from the above, there are social, cultural, and psychological environment.
- **Social and cultural environment:** This type of environment includes the varied aspects of socio-cultural interactions along with its outcomes such as beliefs, attitudes, stereotypes, etc. The tangible and intangible aspects of environment are included in it.
- **Psychological environment:** Psychological environment deals with the perception and experiences related to any environmental setting. Some environment may be stimulating and exciting for us, while others may be dull and boring. Psychological environment is more often used in the organizational context.

MAN–ENVIRONMENT RELATIONSHIP

Man and environment relationship is as old as the evolution of mankind. Since the evolution of man, the physical elements of the planet earth, such as terrain, soil, water, climate, flora and fauna formed man's environment. During that time man was a typically a 'physical man' because of his limited wants, requirements, and total dependence on nature.
- With the growth in social and economic activities, advancement in technologies, man expanded his own environment through design and skill to have provisions for improved and better food, shelter, access, and comfort or luxuries.
- Man's ability to survive in a variety of ecosystem and his unique ability to adapt to a great variety of external conditions make man-environment relationship quite a fascinating area of study.
- The environment in which man survives and to which he adapts himself and which he influences include physical, socio-cultural, and biological aspects.
- Man and environment has never been static and a great many factors are responsible for the shifts in man-environment relationship.

Approaches to Man–Environment Relationship

The man and environment relationship can be studied under the following approaches:

Determinism

- Friedrich Ratzel, the German geographer, was responsible for the development of the concepts of determinism, which was further expanded by Ellsworth Huntington.
- This approach is based on the concept of 'nature controls man' or 'earth made man'. According to this approach, **man is largely influenced by nature**.
- In fact, the determinism states that man is subordinate to natural environment because all aspects of human life such as physical (health and well-being), social, economic, political, ethical, aesthetic, etc. not only depend on but are dominantly controlled by the physical environment.

- World famous biologist, Charles Darwin, in 1859 laid the foundation stone of the concept of environment influences on man and other organism.

Possibilism

- Lucien Febvre, the French historian, founded the concept of Possibilism. Possibilism approach in the study of man-environment relationship is an offshoot of the criticism of environmental determinism and the impact of science and technology on such a relationship.
- Possibilism indicates that the physical environment is passive and man is the active agent at liberty to choose between wide ranges of environmental possibilities.
- According to it, the pattern of human activity is the result of the initiative and mobility of man operating within the natural framework.
- Nowadays, the role of natural elements in conditioning, though not controlling human activities, is often lost sight of.
- Possibility was largely aware of the limitations of freedom of man to dictate terms to environment.
- It was agreed upon by the possibility that man lacks the abilities to fully tame the nature and is not always victorious over it.
- As result of the above, some geographers vouched for 'cooperation with nature' or 'mutual interaction' between man and environment.

Ecological Approach

- This approach is based upon the basic principle of ecology, which is the study of mutual interaction between organisms and physical environment on the one hand, and the interaction among the organism on the other in a given ecosystem.
- This approach describes man as an integral part of nature or environment. Man, being most skilled and intelligent, has a unique role to play in maintaining a natural environment as healthy and productive as it should be.
- This approach emphasizes on wise and restrained use of natural resources, application of appropriate environmental management programs, policies and strategies keeping in view certain basic principles of ecology so that already depleted natural resources are replenished, and health and productivity of the nature is restored.

IMPORTANCE OF ENVIRONMENTAL SCIENCE

- **To realize that environmental problems are global:** Environmental science lets you recognize that environmental problems such as climate change, global warming, ozone layer depletion, acid rains, and impacts on biodiversity and marine life are not just national problems, but global problems as well. So, concerted effort from across the world is needed to tackle these problems.
- **To understand the impacts of development on environment:** It is well documented and quantified that development results in industrial growth, urbanization, expansion of telecommunication and transport systems, hi-tech agriculture and expansion of housing. Environmental science seeks to teach the general population about the need for decentralization of industries to reduce congestion in urban areas. Decentralization means many people will move out of urban centers to reduce pollution resulting from overpopulation. The goal is to achieve all this sustainably without compromising the future generation's ability to satisfy their own needs.
- **To discover sustainable ways of living:** Environmental science is more concerned with discovering ways to live more sustainably. This means utilizing present resources in a manner that conserves their supplies for the future. Environmental sustainability does not have to outlaw living luxuriously, but it advocates for creating awareness about consumption of resources and minimizing unnecessary waste. This includes minimizing household energy consumption, using disposals to dispose of waste, eating locally, recycling more, growing your own food, drinking from the tap, conserving household water, and driving your car less.
- **To utilize natural resources efficiently:** Natural resources bring a whole lot of benefits to a country. A country's natural resources may not be utilized efficiently because of low-level training and lack of management skills. Environmental science teaches us to use natural resources efficiently by:
  - Appropriately putting into practice environmental conservation methods
  - Using the right tools to explore resources
  - Adding value to our resources
  - Making sure machines are maintained appropriately
  - Thorough training of human resources
  - Provision of effective and efficient supervision
  - Using the right techniques to minimize exploitation
  - To understand behavior of organisms under natural conditions.

  Behavior is what organisms manifest to respond to, interact with, and control their environment. An animal exhibits behavior as the first line of defense in response to any change of environment. So, critical look at organism's behavior can offer insightful information about animal's needs, dislikes, preferences and internal condition providing that your evaluation of those observations firmly hinge on knowledge of species'-natural behavior.
- **To shed light on contemporary concepts such as how to conserve biodiversity:** Biodiversity is the variety of life on earth. The present rate of biodiversity loss is at an all-time high. Environmental science aims to teach people how to reverse this trend by:
  - Using sustainable wood products
  - Using organic foods
  - Embracing the 3₹—reduce, reuse, and recycle
  - Purchasing sustainable seafood
  - Supporting conservation campaigns at local levels
  - Conserving power

- Minimizing consumption of meat
- Utilizing eco-friendly cleaning products
- To understand the interrelationship between organisms in population and communities.

Organisms and humans depend on each other to get by. Environmental science is important because it enables you to understand how these relationships work. For example, humans breathe out carbon dioxide, which plants need for photosynthesis. Plants, on the other hand, produce and release oxygen to the atmosphere, which humans need for respiration. Animal droppings are sources of nutrients for plants and other microorganisms. Plants are sources of food for humans and animals. In short, organisms and humans depend on each other for survival.

- **To learn and create awareness about environmental problems at local, national and international levels:** Environmental problems at local, national and international levels mostly occur due to lack of awareness. Environmental science aims to educate and equip learners with necessary environmental skills to pass to the community in order to create awareness. Environmental awareness can be created through social media, creating a blog dedicated to creating awareness, community centered green clubs, women forums, and religious podiums.

COMPONENTS OF ENVIRONMENTAL SCIENCE

- **Ecology:** Ecology is the study of organisms and the environment interacting with one another. Ecologists, who make up a part of environmental scientists, try to find relations between the status of the environment and the population of a particular species within that environment, and if there is any correlations to be drawn between the two. For example, ecologists might take the populations of a particular type of bird with the status of the part of the Amazon rainforest that population is living in.
- **Geoscience:** Geoscience concerns the study of geology, soil science, volcanoes, and the Earth's crust as they relate to the environment. As an example, scientists may study the erosion of the Earth's surface in a particular area. Soil scientists, physicists, biologists, and geomorphologists would all take part in the study.
- **Atmospheric science:** Atmospheric science is the study of the Earth's atmosphere. It analyzes the relation of the Earth's atmosphere to the atmospheres of other systems. This encompasses a wide variety of scientific studies relating to space, astrology and the Earth's atmosphere: meteorology, pollution, gas emissions, and airborne contaminants.
- **Environmental chemistry:** Environmental chemistry is the study of the changes chemicals make in the environment, such as contamination of the soil, pollution of water, degradation of chemicals, and the transport of chemicals upon the plants and animals of the immediate environment. An example of environmental chemistry would be introduction of a chemical object into an environment, in which chemists would then study the chemical bonding to the soil or sand of the environment. Biologists would then study the now chemically induced soil to see its relationship with the plants and animals of the environment.

Natural Resources

- Natural resources are resources that exist without actions of humankind. This includes all valued characteristics such as magnetic, gravitational, electrical properties and forces, etc.
- On earth it includes sunlight, atmosphere, water, land (includes all minerals) along with all vegetation, crops and animal life that naturally subsists upon or within the previously identified characteristics and substances.
- Particular areas such as the rainforest in fatu-Hiva are often characterized by the biodiversity and geodiversity existent in their ecosystems.
- Natural resources may be further classified in different ways. Natural resources are materials and components (something that can be used) that can be found within the environment.
- Every man-made product is composed of natural resources (at its fundamental level).
- A natural resource may exist as a separate entity such as fresh water, air, and as well as any living organism such as a fish, or it may exist in an alternate form that must be processed to obtain the resource such as metal ores, rare-earth metals, petroleum, and most forms of energy.

Classifications of Natural Sources

There are various methods of categorizing natural resources, these include source of origin, stage of development, and by their renewability.

On the basis of origin, natural resources may be divided into two types:
1. **Biotic:** Biotic resources are obtained from the biosphere (living and organic material), such as forest and animals, and the materials that can be obtained from them. Fossil fuel such as coal and petroleum are also included in this category because they are formed from decayed organic matter.
2. **Abiotic:** Abiotic resources are those that come from non-living, nonorganic material. Examples of abiotic resources include land, fresh water, air, rare earth metals and heavy metals including ores, such as, gold, iron, copper, silver, etc.

Considering their stage of development, natural resources may be referred to in the following ways:
- **Potential resources:** Potential resources are those that may be used in the future for example, petroleum in sedimentary rocks that, until drilled out and put to use remains a potential resource.
- **Actual resources:** Those resources that have been surveyed, quantified and qualified and, are currently used—development, such as wood processing, depends on technology and cost.
- **Reserve resources:** The part of an actual resource that can be developed profitably in the future.

- **Stock resources:** Those that have been surveyed, but cannot be used due to lack of technology, for example, hydrogen.

RENEWABLE AND NONRENEWABLE RESOURCES

Many natural resources can be categorized as either renewable or non-renewable:

Renewable Resources

- Renewable resources can be replenished naturally. Some of these resources, like sunlight, air, wind, water, etc. are continuously available and their quantities are not noticeably affected by human consumption.
- Though many renewable resources do not have such rapid recovery rate, these resources are susceptible to depletion by over-use.
- Resources from a human use perspective are classified as renewable so long as the rate of replenishment/recovery exceeds that of the rate of consumption.
- They replenish easily compared to non-renewable resources.

Renewable	Nonrenewable
Can be replaced by natural process in a short amount of time or can be recycled	These are natural resource that either cannot be replaced or may take millions of years to replace by natural process like coal and oil
Can be reused or recycled and used multiple times	Cannot be reused or recycled
Some of the examples are: wind energy, solar power, hydroelectricity, geo thermal	Some of the examples are: Petrol, coal, natural gas, nuclear energy, fossil fuels
No harm done to the environment because of its use	Huge harm done to the environment because of the harmful emissions

Nonrenewable Resources

- Nonrenewable resources either form slowly or do not naturally form in the environment.
- Minerals are the most common resource included in this category. From the human perspective, resources are non-renewable when their rate of consumption exceeds the rate of replenishment/recovery; a good example of this are fossil fuels, which are in this category because their rate of formation is extremely slow (potentially millions of years), meaning they are considered non-renewable.
- Some resources actually naturally deplete in amount without human interference, the most notable of these being radioactive elements such as uranium, which naturally decay into heavy metals.
- The metallic minerals can be re-used by recycling them, but coal and petroleum cannot be recycled. Once they are completely used they take millions of years to replenish.

PROBLEMS ASSOCIATED WITH NATURAL RESOURCES

- **Unequal consumption of natural resources:** A major part of natural resources today are consumed in the technologically advanced or 'developed' world, usually termed 'the west'. The 'developing nations' of 'the east', including India and China, also over use many resources because of their greater human population. However, the consumption of resources per capita (per individual) of the developed countries is up to 50 times greater than in most developing countries. Advanced countries produce over 75% of global industrial waste and greenhouse gases.
- **Planning land use:** Land is a major resource, needed for not only for food production and animal husbandry, but also for industry and growing human settlements. These forms of intensive land use are frequently extended at the cost of 'wild lands', our remaining forests, grasslands, wetlands and deserts. This demands for a pragmatic policy that analyzes the land allocation for different uses.
- **Need for sustainable lifestyles**: Human standard of living and the health of the ecosystem are indicators of sustainable use of resources in any country or region. Ironically, both are not in concurrence with each other. Increasing the level of one, usually leads to degradation of other. Development policies should be formulated to strike a balance between the two.

NATURAL RESOURCES AND ASSOCIATED PROBLEMS

The effect that humanity is having on the environment is becoming ever-more important. Through our actions we are destroying habitats and endangering the lives of future generations. At this point, there is no denying the fact that our environment is changing. Hundreds of studies have been conducted to demonstrate that this is happening and it is having an effect on life around us. However, many may be unaware of the specific issues that have led to these changes. Terms like "climate change" and "genetic modification" are commonplace, but without additional information it is difficult to see why they actually matter.

Biggest Environmental Problems

- **Climate change:** The majority of the issues previously listed contributes or are linked to climate change. Statistics created by NASA state that global temperatures have risen by 1.7 degrees Fahrenheit since 1880, which is directly linked to a reduction in Arctic ice of 13.3% per decade. The effects of climate change are widespread, as it will cause issues with deforestation, water supplies, oceans and ecosystems. Each of these have widespread implications of their own, marking climate change as the major environmental issue the planet faces today.
- **Polar ice caps:** The issue of the melting of polar ice caps is a contentious one. While NASA studies have shown that the amount of ice in Antarctica is actually increasing, these rises only amount to a third of what is being lost in

the Arctic. There is strong evidence to suggest that sea levels are rising, with the Arctic ice caps melting being a major contributor. Over time, this could lead to extensive flooding, contamination of drinking water and major changes in ecosystems.

- **Transportation:** An ever-growing population needs transportation, much of which is fueled by the natural resources that emit greenhouse gases, such as petroleum. In 2014, transportation accounted for 26% of all greenhouse gas emissions. Transportation also contributes to a range of other environmental issues, such as the destruction of natural habitats and increase in air pollution.
- **Natural resource use:** Recent studies have shown that humanity uses so many natural resources that we would need almost 1,5 Earths to cover our needs. This is only set to increase as industrialization continues in nations like China and India. Increased resource use is linked to a number of environmental issues, such as air pollution and population growth. Over time, the depletion of these resources will lead to an energy crisis, plus the chemicals emitted by many natural resources are strong contributors to climate change.
- **Nitrogen cycle:** With most of the focus being placed on the carbon cycle, the effects of human use of nitrogen often slip under the radar. It is estimated that agriculture may be responsible for half of the nitrogen fixation on earth, primarily through the use and production of man-made fertilizer. Excess levels of nitrogen in water can cause issues in marine ecosystem, primarily through overstimulation of plant and algae growth. This can result in blocked intakes and less light getting to deeper waters, damaging the rest of the marine population.
- **Lowered biodiversity:** Continued human activities and expansion has led to lowered biodiversity. A lack of biodiversity means that future generations will have to deal with increasing vulnerability of plants to pests and fewer sources of fresh water. Some studies have found that lowered biodiversity has as pronounced an impact as climate change and pollution on ecosystems, particularly in areas with higher amounts of species extinction.
- **Air pollution:** Air pollution is becoming an increasingly dangerous problem, particularly in heavily-populated cities. The World Health Organization (WHO) has found that 80% of people living in urban areas are exposed to air quality levels deemed unfit by the organization. It is also directly linked to other environmental issues, such as acid rain and eutrophication. Animals and humans are also at risk of developing a number of health problems due to air pollution.
- **Ocean acidification:** Ocean acidification is the term used to describe the continued lowering of the pH levels of the Earth's oceans as a result of carbon dioxide emissions. It is estimated that ocean acidity will increase by 150% by 2100 if efforts are not made to halt it. This increase in acidification can have dire effect on calcifying species, such as shellfish. This causes issues throughout the food chain and may lead to reductions in aquatic life that would otherwise not be affected by acidification.
- **Ozone layer depletion:** Ozone depletion is caused by the release of chemicals, primarily chlorine and bromide, into the atmosphere. A single atom of either has the potential to destroy thousands of ozone molecules before leaving the stratosphere. Ozone depletion results in more UVB radiation reaching the Earth's surface. UVB has been linked to skin cancer and eye disease, plus it affects plant life and has been linked to a reduction of plankton in marine environments.
- **Acid rain:** Acid rain comes as a result of air pollution, mostly through chemicals released into the environment when fuel is burned. Its effects are most clearly seen in aquatic ecosystems, where increasing acidity in the water can lead to animal deaths. It also causes various issues for trees. Though it does not kill trees directly, acid rain does weaken them by damaging leaves, poisoning the trees and limiting their available nutrients.
- **Genetic modification of crops:** Environmental issues caused by man-made chemicals are becoming clearer. For example, there has been a 90% reduction in the Monarch butterfly population in the United States that can be linked to weed killers that contain glyphosate. There is also some speculation that genetically-modified plants may leak chemical compounds into soil through their roots, possibly affecting communities of microorganisms.
- **Waste production:** The average person produces 4.3 pounds of water per day, with the United States alone accounting for 220 million tons per year. Much of this waste ends up in landfills, which generate enormous amounts of methane. Not only does this create explosion hazards, but methane also ranks as one of the worst of the greenhouse gases because of its high global warming potential.
- **Population growth:** Many of the issues listed here result from the massive population growth that Earth has experienced in the last century. The planet's population grows by 1.13% per year, which works out to 80 million people. This results in a number of issues, such as a lack of fresh water, habitat loss for wild animals, overuse of natural resources and even species extinction. The latter is particularly damaging, as the planet is now losing 30, 000 species per day.
- **Water pollution:** Fresh water is crucial to life on Earth, yet more sources are being polluted through human activities each year. On a global scale, 2 million tons of sewage, agricultural and industrial waste enters the world's water every day. Water pollution can have harmful effects outside of contamination of the water we drink. It also distorts marine life, sometimes altering reproductive cycles and increasing mortality rates.
- **Deforestation:** The demands of an increasing population have resulted in increasing levels of deforestation. Current estimates state that the planet is losing 80,000 acres of tropical forests per day. This results in loss of habitat for many species, placing many at risk and leading to large-scale extinction. Furthermore, deforestation is estimated to produce 15% of the world's greenhouse gas emission.
- **Urban sprawl:** The continued expansion of urban areas into traditionally rural regions is not without its problems.

Urban sprawl has been linked to environmental issues like air and water pollution increases, in addition to the creation of heat-islands. Satellite images produced by NASA have also shown how urban sprawl contributes to forest fragmentation, which often leads to larger deforestation.

- **Overfishing:** It is estimated that 63% of global fish stocks are now considered overfished. This has led to many fishing fleets heading to new waters, which will only serve to deplete fish stocks further. Over fishing leads to a misbalance of ocean life, severely affecting natural ecosystems in the process. Furthermore, it also has negative effects on coastal communities that rely on fishing to support their economies.

FOREST RESOURCES

In India, forests form 23 percent of the total land area. The word 'forest' is derived from the Latin word 'foris' means 'outside' (may be the reference was to a village boundary or fence separating the village and the forest land). Forest is important renewable resources. Forest varies in composition and diversity and can contribute substantially to the economic development of any country. Plants along with trees cover large areas, produce variety of products and provide food for living organisms, and also important to save the environment.

- It is estimated that about 30% of world area is covered by forest whereas 26% by pastures.
- Among all continents, Africa has largest forested area (33%) followed by Latin America (25%), whereas in North America forest cover is only 11%. Asia and former USSR has 14% area under forest.
- European countries have only 3% area under forest cover. India's Forest Cover accounts for 20.6% of the total geographical area of the country as of 2005.

Significance of forests: Forest can provide prosperity of human being and to the nations. Important uses of forest can be classified as under:
- Commercial values
- Ecological significance
- Aesthetic values
- Life and economy of tribal

Use and Over Exploitation

A forest is a biotic community predominantly of trees, shrubs and other woody vegetation, usually with a closed canopy. This invaluable renewable natural resource is beneficial to man in many ways.

Direct Benefits from Forests

- **Fuel wood:** Wood is used as a source of energy for cooking purpose and for keeping warm.
- **Timber:** Wood is used for making furniture, tool-handles, railway sleepers, matches, ploughs, bridges, boats, etc.
- **Bamboos:** These are used for matting, flooring, baskets, ropes, rafts, cots, etc.
- **Food:** Fruits, leaves, roots and tubers of plants and meat of forest animals form the food of forest tribes.
- **Shelter:** Mosses, ferns, insects, birds, reptiles, mammals and microorganisms are provided shelter by forests.
- **Paper:** Wood and Bamboo pulp are used for manufacturing paper (Newsprint, stationery, packing paper, sanitary paper).
- **Rayon:** Bamboo and wood are used in the manufacture of rayon (yarns, artificial silk-fibres).
- **Forest products:** Tannins, gums, drugs, spices, insecticides, waxes, honey, horns, musk, ivory, hides, etc. are all provided by the flora and fauna of forests.

Indirect Benefits from Forests

- **Conservation of soil:** Forests prevent soil erosion by binding the soil with the network of roots of the different plants and reduce the velocity of wind and rain-which are the chief agents causing erosion.
- **Soil-improvement:** The fertility of the soil increases due to the humus which is formed by the decay of forest litter.
- **Reduction of atmospheric pollution:** By using up carbon dioxide and giving off oxygen during the process of photosynthesis, forests reduce pollution and purify the environment.
- **Control of climate:** Transpiration of plants increases the atmospheric humidity which affects rainfall and cools the atmosphere.
- **Control of water flow:** In the forests, the thick layer of humus acts like a big sponge and soaks rainwater preventing run-off, thereby preventing flash-floods. Humus prevents quick evaporation of water, thereby ensuring a perennial supply of water to streams, springs and wells.

Deforestation

- Forest are burned or cut for clearing of land for agriculture, harvesting for wood and timber, development and expansion of cities. These economic gains are short-term whereas long-term effects of deforestation are irreversible.
- Deforestation rate is relatively low in temperate countries than in tropics if present rate of deforestation continues we may losses 90% tropical forest in coming six decades.
- For ecological balance 33% area should be under forest cover but our nation has only 20.6% forest cover.

Causes of Deforestation

Forest area in some developed area has expanded. However in developing countries area under forest is showing declining trend particularly in tropical region. Main causes of deforestation are:

Effects of Deforestation

- Expansion of deserts
- Climate change and depletion of water table
- Loss of biodiversity, flora and fauna
- Environmental changes and disturbance in forest ecosystems.

Forest conservation and management: Forest is one of the most valuable resources and thus needs to be conserved. To conserve forest, following steps should be taken:
- Conservation of forest is a national problem, thus it should be tackled with perfect coordination between concerned government departments.
- People should be made aware of importance of forest and involved in forest conservation activities.
- The cutting of trees in the forests for timber should be stopped.
- A forestation programs should be launched.
- Grasslands should be regenerated.
- Forest Conservation Act should be strictly implemented to check deforestation.
- Awards should be instituted for the deserving.

WATER RESOURCES

The concept of water resources is multidimensional. It is not limited only to its physical measure (hydrological and hydrogeological), the 'flows and stocks', but encompasses other more qualitative, environmental and socio-economic dimensions. However, this report focuses on the physical and quantitative assessment of the resource.

Types of Water Resources
- These are defined as the average manual flow of rivers and recharge of aquifers generated from precipitation.
- It distinguishes between the natural situation (natural renewable resources), which corresponds to a situation without human influence, and the current or actual situation.
- The computation of the actual renewable water resources of a country takes account of possible reductions in flow resulting from the abstraction of water in upstream countries.

Renewable and Nonrenewable Water Resources

In computing water resources on a country basis, a distinction is to be made between renewable and non-renewable water resources.
- Renewable water resources are computed on the basis of the water cycle. In this report, they represent the long-term average annual flow of rivers (surface water) and groundwater.
- Non-renewable water resources are groundwater bodies (deep aquifers) that have a negligible rate of recharge on the human time-scale and thus can be considered non-renewable.

Natural and Actual Renewable Water Resources

Natural renewable water resources are the total amount of a country's water resources (internal and external resources), both surface water and groundwater, which is generated through the hydrological cycle. The amount is computed on a yearly basis.

- Actual resources: when taking into account the resources shared with neighboring countries (geopolitical constraints).
- Exploitable resources: according to socio-economic and environmental criteria.
- A country may have to reserve for downstream a part of its external resources (e.g., Sudan and Syria).

Surface waters include streams, rivers, lakes, reservoirs, and wetlands. In this case, the word stream represents all flowing surface water, think large rivers to small brooks and everything in between. Surface waters, because they are easily accessed, provide around 78% of the fresh water we use. The number will vary based on variables like drought. Over 1.2 billion people rely primarily on surface water in big cities around the world.

Groundwater which makes up around 22% of the water we use, is the water beneath the earth's surface filling cracks and other openings in beds of rock and sand. It exists in soils and sands that are able to retain water.

Wastewater is any water that has been affected in quality by human activities. **Wastewater** can develop from agricultural activities, urban water use, and sewer inflow and storm water runoff just to name a few. Wastewater from a municipality is also called sewage. Most of us don't want to think about it, but at times the water that swirls in the bowl ends up being treated and ends up in our taps.

Storm water: Storm water is the runoff generated when precipitation from rain and snowmelt events flows over land or impervious surfaces without percolating into the ground. This water runs over surfaces like asphalt containing pollutants like engine oil, fertilizer, and radiator fluid. Storm water not soaking into the ground ends up as surface runoff draining into rivers, lakes, streams and oceans.

WATER POLLUTION

It is a well-known fact that clean water is absolutely essential for healthy living. Adequate supply of fresh and clean drinking water is a basic need for all human beings on the earth, yet it has been observed that millions of people worldwide are deprived of this.

Sources of Pollution

The main sources of water pollution are the following:
- Discharge of untreated Raw Sewage from households and factories
- Chemicals dumped from factories
- Agricultural run-offs that make their way into our rivers and streams and groundwater sources
- Urbanization
- The rising use of synthetic organic substances
- Oil Spills
- Acid Rain caused by the burning of Fossil Fuels
- Human littering in rivers, oceans, lakes and other bodies of water. Harmful litter includes plastics, aluminum, glass and Styrofoam.

Almost everything that is a byproduct of our civilization is polluting our drinking water. Governments, through various Clean Water Acts and water resource policies have sought to regulate the discharges of pollutants in the water to minimize pollution and contamination. From 1990 to 2006, an additional 1.6 billion people had access to safe drinking water. But we are not acting fast enough and most factories still find a way to dump their toxic wastes in the sea, unseen.

Water pollution can affect us:
- **Directly:** Through consumption or bathing in a polluted stream (such as consumption of municipal water, as well as bathing in polluted lakes or beach water).
- **Indirectly:** Through the consumption of vegetables irrigated with contaminated water, as well as of fish or other animals that live in the polluted water or consume animals grown in the polluted water. This is many times more dangerous than being directly affected through consumption of water, because some pollutants bioaccumulate in fish and living organisms (their concentration in fish could be several orders of magnitude higher than their water concentration). Additionally, the toxins from the brown tide are strong and can travel via air, affecting homeowners close to the beach.

Effect of Polluted Water on Humans

Infectious diseases can be spread through contaminated water. Some of these water-borne diseases are Typhoid, Cholera, Paratyphoid Fever, Dysentery, Jaundice, Amoebiasis and Malaria.
- **Chemicals** in the water also have negative effects on our health.
- **Pesticides** can damage the nervous system and cause cancer because of the carbonates and organophosphates that they contain. Chlorides can cause reproductive and endocrine damage.
- **Nitrates** are especially dangerous to babies that drink formula milk. It restricts the amount of oxygen in the brain and cause the "blue baby" syndrome.
- **Lead** can accumulate in the body and damage the central nervous system.
- **Arsenic** causes liver damage, skin cancer and vascular diseases.
- **Fluorides** in excessive amounts can make your teeth yellow and cause damage to the spinal cord.
- **Petrochemicals** even with very low exposure, can cause cancer.

Preventive Measures
- Water-borne epidemics and health hazards in the aquatic environment are mainly due to improper management of water resources.
- Proper management of water resources has become the need of the hour as this would ultimately lead to a cleaner and healthier environment.
- In order to prevent the spread of water-borne infectious diseases, people should take adequate precautions.
- The city water supply should be properly checked and necessary steps taken to disinfect it.
- Water pipes should be regularly checked for leaks and cracks. At home, the water should be boiled, filtered, or other methods and necessary steps taken to ensure that it is free from infection.

MINERAL RESOURCES

A mineral is a pure inorganic substance that occurs naturally in the earth's crust. All of the Earth's crust, except the rather small proportion of the crust that contains organic material, is made up of minerals. Some minerals consist of a single element such as gold, silver, diamond (carbon), and sulfur. More than two-thousand minerals have been identified and most of these contain inorganic compounds formed by various combinations of the eight elements (O, Si, Al, Fe, Ca, Na, K, and Mg) that make up 98.5% of the Earth's crust. Industry depends on about 80 of the known minerals.

Definition

Minerals provide the material used to make most of the things of industrial-based society; roads, cars, computers, fertilizers, etc. Demand for minerals is increasing worldwide as the population increases and the consumption demands of individual people increase. The mining of earth's natural resources is, therefore accelerating, and it has accompanying environmental consequences.

Types of Mineral Resources

Minerals in general have been categorized into three classes' fuel, metallic and non-metallic. Fuel minerals like coal, oil and natural gas have been given prime importance as they account for nearly 87% of the value of mineral production whereas metallic and non-metallic constitutes 6 to 7% **(Fig. 14.4)**.

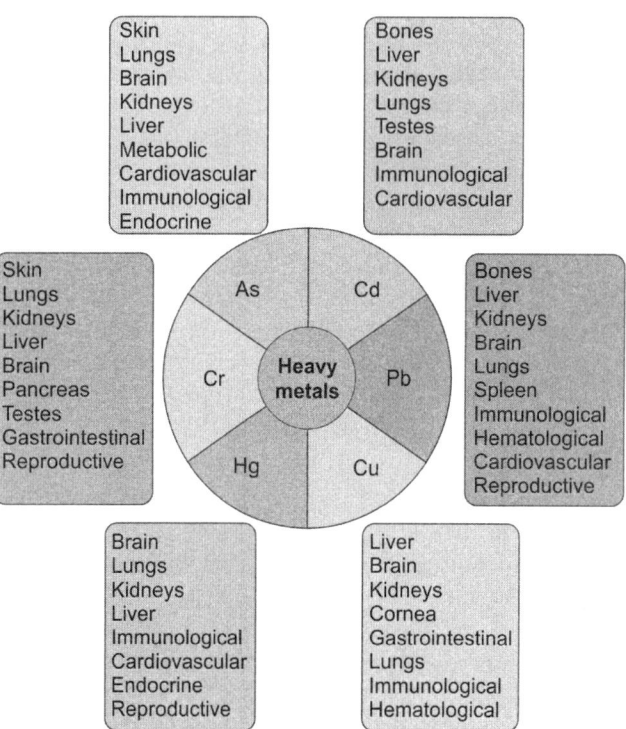

Fig. 14.4: Types of minerals used in our body by various systems.

Fuel Minerals

Coal, oil and natural gas are the basic fossil fuel. We have good reserves for coal but are very poor in more essential fuel—oils and natural gas.

- **Coal:** Proven coal reserves of the country as on January 1994 (estimated by GSI) is about 68 billion tonnes. We are mining about 250 tonnes annually and this rate is expected to go by 400-450 tonnes by 2010AD If we could maintain our mining rate of 400 tonnes per year then the coal reserves might last for about 200 years taking proven reserves as 80 billion tonnes.
- **Crude oil (petroleum):** It is believed that petroleum has been formed over a period of millions of years, through conversion of remains of microorganisms living in sea, into hydrocarbon by heat, pressure and catalytic action. The petroleum on fractional distillation and further processing provides us numerous products and by-products.
- **Natural gas:** The proven reserve for natural gas on April 1993 works out to be approx. 700 billion cubic meter (BCM). As regard to production vis a vis utilization aspect in earlier years, more than half of gas coming out of the wells remained unutilized. However, in recent years, we have achieved a utilization rate of 80–90%. Keeping in view the future demands and proven gas reserves, it is unlikely that our gas reserves might last for more than 20 years.

Mineral	Some important functions	Food sources
Boron Unknown	Important in bone retention	Fruits, leafy vegetables, nuts, legumes, beans
Calcium 1,000–1,300 mg.	Essential for growth and structural integrity of bones and teeth; nerve conduction; muscle contraction and relaxation	Yogurt, milk, cheese, tofu, fortified juices, green leafy vegetables
Chromium 50–200 µg	Participates in CHO and fat metabolism; muscle function; increases effectiveness of insulin	Whole grains, cheese, yeast
Copper 1.5–3 mg	Essential for red blood cell production, pigmentation, and bone health.	Nuts, liver, lobster, cereals, legumes, dried fruit
Iron 10–15 mg	Essential for the production of hemoglobin in red blood cells and myoglobin in skeletal muscle, and enzymes that participate in metabolism	Liver, clams, oatmeal, farina, fortified cereals, soybeans, apricot, green leafy vegetables
Magnesium 280–350 mg	Essential for nerve impulse conduction; muscle contraction and relaxation; enzyme activation	Whole grains, artichoke, beans, green leafy vegetables, fish, nuts, fruit
Manganese 2–5 mg	Essential for formation and integrity of connective tissue and bone, sex hormone production, and cell function	Nuts, legumes, whole grains
Phosphorous 800–1,200 mg	Essential for metabolism and bone development. Involved in most biochemical reactions in the body	Fish, milk, meats, poultry, legumes, nuts
Potassium 2,000 mg	Essential for nerve impulse conduction, fluid balance, and for normal heart function	Squash, potatoes, beans, fresh fruits (bananas, oranges) and vegetables (tomatoes)
Selenium 55–70 µg	Antioxidant, works with vitamin E to reduce oxidation damage to tissues	Meats, seafood, cereals
Sodium[4] 500–2,400 mg	Essential for nerve impulse conduction, muscle contraction, fluid balance, and acid	Table salt, canned and processed foods

Metallic and Nonmetallic Minerals

India is poorly endowed with mineral wealth. Except for iron ore and bauxite our share of world reserves of every other mineral is one percent or less. However, there has been a phenomenal growth in production since independence. As per estimates if the present trend of production continues, we will exhaust our reserves of all the important minerals and fuels, except coal, iron ore, limestone and bauxite, in 25 to 30 years.

Exploitation of Mineral Resources

Mining is Hazardous Occupation

- This occupation involves several health risk dust produced during mining operation are injurious to health and cause lung diseases.
- Extraction of some toxic or radioactive minerals leads to life-threatening hazards.
- Dynamite explosion during mining is very risky as fumes produced are extremely poisonous.
- Underground mining is more hazardous than surface mining as there are more chances if accidents like roof falls, flooding and inadequate ventilation, etc.

Rapid Depletion of High Grade Minerals

Increasing demand for high grade minerals has compelled miners to carry out more extraction of minerals, which require more energy sources and produce large amount of waste materials.

Wastage of Upper Soil Layer and Vegetation

Surface mining results in the complete destruction of upper soil layer and vegetation. After extraction, the wastes are dumped in an area which destroys the total surface and vegetation.

Chapter 14: National Health Problems

Mineral	Functions	Deficiency associations	Adult dose range	Food sources	Caution
Calcium	Bone and tooth formation heart and muscle function	Osteoporosis, bone spurs, muscle cramps, rheumatism	200-1500 mg	Barley, kale, unrefined grains: milk, green vegetables	Prolonged excess may cause a mineral imbalance
Magnesium	Energy processes, nerve function, enzyme activation	Stress, osteoporosis, insomnia	150-600 mg	Avocados, almonds, whole grains, grapefruit	Doses over 400 mg can cause diarrhea in some people
Potassium	pH balance, nerve function	Stress, atherosclerosis, high blood pressure	1800–5828 mg a normal	Potato peel, bananas, beans, almonds, whole grains	Do not take high supplemental doses (food sources are O.K.) when taking heart medicines without physician guidance
Sodium	pH balance, nerve function	Excess is more common and is associated with high blood pressure	Limit daily intake to 1,500 mg	Breads/rolls; pizza; sandwiches; cold cuts/cured meats; soups; burritos, tacos; savory snacks; chicken; cheese; eggs, omelets	Very few people (athletes, diarrhea/vomiting need to supplement
Phosphorus	Energy production, bones, teeth B Vit. activation	Tooth/gum disorders, impotence. equilibrium	300–600 mg	Barley, beans, fish, lentils, dark green vegetables	Prolonged, large doses can cause calcium deficiency or mineral imbalance
Iron	Red Blood cell production	Dizziness, depression, anemia	10–30 mg	Blackberries, cherries, spinach	Do NOT take iron unless told to do so by your doctor, Iron excess is associated with health problems
Zinc	Co-factor in numerous metabolic processes	Prostate enlargement, immune deficiency; atherosclerosis	15–50 mg	Wheat germ, wheat bran, pumpkin seed, avocado, sea food	Large doses (50 mg day) can cause a copper deficiency and other mineral imbalances
Copper	Red blood cell production: skeletal, heart and muscle function	Osteoporosis, digestive function, nerve disorders	2–3 mg	Green leafy vegetables, almonds, beans, sea food	Higher doses can be toxic
Manganese	Glandular function bone and ligament health	Diabetes, asthma, digestive disturbance	2–10 mg	Nuts, seeds, avocados, grapefruit, apricots	High doses may create other mineral imbalances
Chromium	Glucose metabolism; blood sugar regulation; heart function	Atherosclerosis, diabetes, hypoglycemia, high cholesterol, overweight	200–500 mcg	Whole grain cereals, molasses, meat yeast	Nontoxic at therapeutic levels
Selerium	Antioxidant, synergistic with vitamin E	Cancer prevention; aging	100–200 mcg	Brain, whole grains, onion	Prolonged excess may be toxic

Environmental Problems

Over exploitation of mineral resources resulted in many environmental problems like:

- Conversion of productive land into mining and industrial areas.
- Mining and extraction process are one of the sources of air, water and land pollution.
- Mining involves huge consumption of energy resources like coal, petroleum, natural gas, etc. which are in-turn non renewable sources of energy.
- Surface mining directly degrades the fertile soil surface thus effect ecology and climate.

Mineral Contamination and Effects on Health

Mineral contamination effects include causing disease in humans and wildlife, befouling wilderness and streams, and contributing to global warming. Although some mineral contamination is the result of natural processes, human activity is responsible for most environmental hazards.

- **Acid mine drainage:** Acid mine drainage forms when the mineral pyrite reacts with air and water to form sulfuric acid. This acidic flow dissolves heavy metals, including mercury, copper, and lead, which allows them to seep into surface or ground water.
- **Arsenic groundwater contamination:** Arsenic can contaminate groundwater when arsenic-laden minerals dissolve over time, releasing their arsenic into groundwater, but arsenic contamination is more often caused by industrial runoff waste containing arsenic. Arsenic is tasteless and odorless, making it undetectable unless ground and well water is specifically tested for arsenic. "Science Daily" reports that more than 100 million people worldwide are exposed to toxic levels of arsenic in their drinking water, which can cause diabetes and several forms of cancer even in low concentrations.
- **Asbestos contamination:** Asbestos fibers occur naturally in certain rock formations, and these fibers can easily be inhaled, causing health problems that include lung cancer, mesothelioma, and asbestosis, a condition that scars lung tissue, making it difficult for oxygen to enter the bloodstream. Plumbers, electricians, and firefighters are at increased risk of asbestos exposure compared to workers in other occupations because of asbestos's former prevalence in plumbing, electrical components, and building materials.
- **Coal burning:** The Union of Concerned Scientists reports that in one year a typical coal-burning power plant generates 500 tons of particulate matter that can exacerbate asthma and cause bronchitis, 720 tons of carbon monoxide, and 3.7 million tons of carbon dioxide, the greenhouse gas primarily responsible for global warming. Coal-burning plants also contribute to environmental hazards, including smog and acid rain.

FOOD RESOURCES

Food is essential for growth and development of living organisms. These essential materials are called nutrients and these nutrients are available from variety of animals and plants. There are thousands of edible plants and animals over the world, out of which only about three dozen types constitute major food of humans.

Food sources: The majority of people obtain food from cultivated plants and domesticated animals. Although some food is obtained from oceans and fresh waters, but the great majority of food for human population is obtained from traditional land-based agriculture of crops and livestock.

Food Crops

- It is estimated that out of about 2,50,000 species of plants, only about 3,000 have been tried as agricultural crops.
- Under different agro-climatic condition, 300 are grown for food and only 100 are used on a large scale.
- Some species of crops provide food, whereas others provide commercial products like oils, fibres, etc.
- Raw crops are sometimes converted into valuable edible products by using different techniques for value addition.
- At global level, only 20 species of crops are used for food. These, in approximate order of importance are wheat, rice, corn, potatoes; barley, sweet potatoes, cassavas, soybeans, oats, sorghum, millet, sugarcane, sugar beets, rye, peanuts, field beans, chick-peas, pigeon-peas, bananas and coconuts.
- Many of them are used directly, whereas other can be used by changing them by using different techniques for enhancing calorific value.

Livestock

- Domesticated animals are an important food source. The major domesticated animals used as food source by human beings are 'ruminants' (e.g., cattle, sheep, goats, camel, reindeer, llama, etc.).
- Ruminants convert indigestible woody tissue of plants (cellulose) which are earth's most abundant organic compound into digestible food products for human consumption.
- Milk, which is provided by milking animals, is considered to be the complete food. Other domestic animals like sheep, goat, poultry and ducker can be used as meat.

Aquaculture: Fish and seafood contributes 17 million metric tonnes of high quality protein to provide balance diet to the world. Presently aquaculture provides only small amounts for world food but its significance is increasing day by day.

World Food Problems

As per estimates of Food and Agriculture Organization (FAO), about 840 million people remain chronically hungry and out of this 800 million are living in the developing world. In last decade, it is decreasing at the rate of 2.5 million per year, but at the same time world's population is increasing.

- Target of cutting half the number of world's chronically hungry and undernourished people by 2015 will difficult to meet, if the present trend continues.
- Due to inadequate purchasing power to buy food, it is difficult to fulfil minimum calorific requirement of human body per day.
- Large number of people are in India are poor which can be attribute to equitable distribution of income.
- Food insufficiency can be divided into two categories into under-nourishment and malnourishment. Both of these insufficiencies are global problems.

Undernourishment

- The FAO estimates that the average minimum daily caloric intake over the whole world is about 2,500 calories per day.
- People who receive less than 90% of their minimum dietary intake on a long-term basis are considered undernourished.
- Those who receive less than 80% of their minimum daily caloric intake requirements are considered 'seriously' undernourished.
- Children in this category are likely to suffer from stunted growth, mental retardation, and other social and developmental disorders.

- Therefore, undernourishment means lack of sufficient calories in available food, resulting in little or no ability to move or work.

Malnourishment

- Person may have excess food but still diet suffers from due to nutritional imbalance or inability to absorb or may have problem to utilize essential nutrients.
- If we compare diet of the developed countries with developing countries people in developed countries have processed food which may be deficient in fiber, vitamins and other components whereas in the diet of developing countries, may be lack of specific nutrients because they consume less meat, fruits and vegetables due to poor purchasing power.
- Malnourishment can be defined as lack of specific components of food such as proteins, vitamins, or essential chemical elements.

The major problems of malnutrition are:
- **Marasmus:** A progressive emaciation caused by lack of protein and calories.
- **Kwashiorkor:** A lack of sufficient protein in the diet which leads to a failure of neural development and therefore learning disabilities.
- **Anemia:** It is caused by lack of iron in the diet or due to an inability to absorb iron from food.
- **Pellagra:** It occurs due to the deficiency of tryptophan and lysine, vitamins in the diet.

ENERGY RESOURCES

Energy is defined by physicists as the capacity to do work. Energy is found on our planet in a variety of forms, some of which are immediately useful to do work, while others require a process of transformation. The sun is the primary energy source in our lives. Besides, water, fossil fuels such as coal, petroleum products, water, nuclear power plants are sources of energy.

Renewable Energy Resources

Renewable energy systems use resources that are constantly replaced and are usually less polluting. Examples include hydropower, solar, wind, and geothermal (energy from the heat inside the earth). We also get renewable energy from burning trees and even garbage as fuel and processing other plants into bio-fuels.

Wind energy: The moving air or wind has huge amounts of kinetic energy, and it can be transferred into electrical energy using wind turbines. The wind moves the blades, which spins a shaft, which is further connected to a generator, which generates electricity. An average wind speed of 14 miles per hour is needed to convert wind energy into electricity. Wind-generated electricity met nearly 4% of global electricity demand in 2015, with nearly 63 GW of new wind power capacity installed.

Solar energy: Solar energy is the light and heat procured from the sun. It is harnessed using ever evolving technologies. In 2014, global solar generation was 186 terawatt-hours, slightly less than 1% of the world's total grid electricity. Italy has the largest proportion of solar electricity in the world. In the opinion of International Energy Agency, the development of affordable, inexhaustible, and clean solar energy technologies will have longer-term benefits.

Biomass energy: When a log is burned we are using biomass energy. As plants and trees depend on sunlight to grow, biomass energy is a form of stored solar energy. Although wood is the largest source of biomass energy, agricultural waste, sugarcane wastes, and other farm byproducts are also used to produce energy.

Hydropower: Energy produced from water is called hydropower. Hydroelectric power stations both big and small are set up to produce electricity in many parts of the world. Hydropower is produced in 150 countries, with the Asia-Pacific region generating 32% of global hydropower in 2010. In 2015, hydropower generated 16.6% of the world's total electricity and 70% of all renewable electricity.

Tidal and wave power: The earth's surface is 70% water. By warming the water, the sun creates ocean currents and the wind that produces waves. It is estimated that the solar energy absorbed by the tropical oceans in a week could equal the entire oil reserves of the world – 1 trillion barrels of oil.

Geothermal energy: It is the energy stored within the earth ("geo" for earth and "thermal" for heat). Geothermal energy starts with hot, molten rock (called magma) deep inside the earth which surfaces at some parts of the earth's crust. The heat rising from the magma warms the underground pools of water known as geothermal reservoirs.

LAND RESOURCES

Land area constitutes about 1/5 of the earth surface. To meet out the challenging demand of food, fiber and fuel for human population, fodder for animals and industrial raw material for agro-based industries, efficient management of land resources will play critical role. Soil, water, vegetation and climate are basic natural resources for agricultural growth and development.

Human and natural activities need space for their location and development. This space is provided by land which is put to various uses like food and energy production, waste-disposal, industrial, commercial and residential purposes.

Land houses the living species, water resources and raw material resources (minerals and ores).

Pattern of Land Use on Earth

- Arable land
- Land for pastures and meadows
- Forest land
- Urban land
- Non-agricultural land

Land-use involves economic activities leading to environmental problems like:
- Pollutant discharge
- Waste disposal
- Consumption of natural resources for economic activity
- Disturbing ecological cycles and wildlife habitats.

Desertification

Desertification is a process whereby the productive potential of arid or semiarid lands falls by ten percent or more. Desertification is characterized by devegetation and depletion of groundwater, salinization and severe soil erosion.

Causes of Desertification
- Deforestation
- Overgrazing
- Mining and quarrying

Shifting Cultivation

- Shifting cultivation is a practice of slash and burn agriculture adopted by tribal communities and is a main cause for soil degradation particularly tropical and sub-tropical regions.
- Shifting cultivation which is also popularly known as 'Jhum Cultivation' has led to destruction of forest in hilly areas.
- It is responsible for soil erosion and other problems related to land degradation in mountainous areas.

Man-induced Landslides

- Human race has exploited land resources for his own comfort by constructing roads, railway tracks, canals for irrigation, hydroelectric projects, large dams and reservoirs and mining in hilly areas.
- Moreover productive lands under crop production are decreasing because of development activities.
- These factors are affecting the stability of hill slopes and damage the protective vegetation cover. These activities are also responsible to upset the balance of nature and making such areas prone to landslides.

ROLE OF INDIVIDUALS IN CONSERVATION OF NATURAL RESOURCES

Natural resources like forests, water, soil, food, minerals and energy resources play an important role in the economy and development of a nation. Humans can play important role in conservation of natural resources. A little effort by individuals can help to conserve these resources which are a gift of nature to the mankind. Brief description of role of individual to conserve different types of natural resources is given below:

Roles to Conserve Water

- To minimize the evaporation losses irrigate the crops, the plants and the lawns in the evening, because water application during day time will lead to more loss of water due to higher rate of evapotranspiration.
- Improve water efficiency by using optimum amount of water in washing machine, dishwashers and other domestic appliances, etc.
- Install water saving toilets which use less water per flush.
- Check for water leaks in pipes and toilets and repair them promptly.
- Don't keep water taps running while they are not in use.
- Recycle water of washing of cloths for gardening.
- Installing rainwater harvesting structure to conserve water for future use.

Energy Conservation for Future Use

- Turn off all electric appliances such as lights, fans, televisions, computers, etc. when not in use.
- Clean all the lighting sources regularly because dust on lighting sources decreases lighting levels up to 20–30%.
- Try to harvest energy from natural resources to obtain heat for example drying the cloths in sun and avoid drying in washing machine.
- Save liquid petroleum gas (LPG) by using solar cookers for cooking.
- Design the house with provision for sunspace to keep the house warm and to provide more light.
- Avoid misuse of vehicles for transportation and if possible share car journey to minimize use of petrol/diesel. For small distances walk down or just use bicycles.
- Minimise the use air conditioner to save energy.

Protect Soil Health

- Use organic manure/compost to maintain soil fertility
- To avoid soil erosion does not irrigate the plants by using fast flow of water.
- Use sprinkler irrigation to conserve the soil.
- Design landscape of lawn in large area which will help to bind soil to avoid erosion.
- Provide vegetation cover by growing of ornamental plant, herbs and trees in your garden.
- Use vegetable waste to prepare compost to use in kitchen gardening.

Promote Sustainable Agriculture

- Diversify the existing cropping pattern for sustainability of agriculture
- Cultivate need based crop
- Maintain soil fertility
- Make optimum use of fertilizers, pesticides and other chemicals for production and processing of agriculture products
- Save grains in storage to minimize the losses
- Improve indigenous breeds of milch animals for sustainable dairy production systems
- Adopt post-harvest technologies for value addition.

Conservation of Energy

- Switch off light, fan and other appliances when not in use.
- Use solar heater for cooking.
- Dry the cloth in the sun light instead of driers.

- Use always pressure cookers
- Grow trees near the house to get cool breeze instead of using AC and air cooler.
- Ride bicycle or just walk instead of using scooter for a short distance.

Conservation of Water

- Use minimum water for all domestic purposes.
- Check the water leaks in pipes and repair them properly.
- Reuse the soapy water, after washing clothes for washing courtyard, carpets, etc.
- Use drip irrigation.
- Rainwater harvesting system should be installed in all the houses.
- Sewage treatment plant may be installed in all industries and institution.
- Continuous running of water taps should be avoided.
- Watering of plants should be done in the evening.

Conservation of Soil

- Grow different type plants, i.e., trees, herbs and shrubs.
- In the irrigation process, using strong flow of water should be avoided.
- Soil erosion can be prevented by sprinkling irrigation.

Conservation of Food Resources

- Cook required amount of food.
- Don't waste the food; give it to someone before spoiling.
- Don't store large amount of food grains and protect them from damaging insects.

Conservation of Forest

- Use nontimber product.
- Plant more trees.
- Grassing must be controlled.
- Minimize the use of paper and fuel.
- Avoid the construction of dam, road in the forest areas.

Equitable use of resources for sustainable lifestyle:

Sustainable development: Development of healthy environment without damaging natural resources.

Unsustainable development:
- Degradation of the environment due to over utilization of natural resources.
- Lifestyle in more developed countries
- 22% of world population, 88% of its natural resources and 85% of total global income.
- Consumption is more and pollution is more.

Lifestyle in less developed countries:
- 78% of world population, 12% of its natural resources and 15% of total global income.
- Consumption is less and pollution is less.

Causes of unsustainability: Main cause—difference between MDCs and LDCs.

Sustainable lifestyle: MDCs should have to reduce the utilization of natural resources that should have to be diverted to LDCs. This will reduce the gap between MDCs and LDCs, leads to sustainable development of the entire world.

EQUITABLE USE OF RESOURCES FOR SUSTAINABLE LIFESTYLES

In last 50 years, the consumption of resource in the society has increased many folds. There is a big gap in the consumers lifestyle between developed and developing countries.

- Urbanization has changed the lifestyle of middle class population in developing countries creating more stress on the use of natural resources.
- It has been estimated that More Developed Countries (MDC) of the world constitute only 22% of world's population but they use 88% of natural resources.
- These countries use 73% of energy resources and command 85% of income and in turn they contribute very big proportion of pollution.
- On the other hand less developed countries (LDCs) have moderate industrial growth and constitute 78% of world's population and use only 12% of natural resources, 27% of energy and have only 15% of global income.
- There is a huge gap between rich and poor. In this age of development the rich have gone richer and the poor is becoming more poorer. This has led to unsustainable growth.
- There is an increasing global concern about the management of natural resources. The solution to this problem is to have more equitable distribution of resources and income.
- Two major causes of unsustainability are over population in poor countries and over consumption of resources by rich countries.
- A global consensus has to be reached for balanced distribution of natural resources.
- For equitable use of natural resources more developed countries/rich people have to lower down their level of consumption to bare minimum so that these resources can be shared by poor people to satisfy their needs.
- Time has come to think that it is need of the hour that rich and poor should make equitable use of resources for sustainable development of mankind.

ECOSYSTEM

The interaction and interrelationship between the living community (plants, animals, and organisms) in relation to each other and the non-living community (soil, air, and water) is referred to as an **ecosystem**. Thus, an ecosystem is a structural and functional unit of biosphere. It is made up of living and non-living beings and their physical environment.

In other words, a natural ecosystem is defined as a network of interactions among the organisms and between organisms and their environment. Nutrient cycles and energy flows keep these living and non-living components connected in an ecosystem.

Functions of Ecosystems

The functions of the ecosystem are as follows:
- It regulates the essential ecological processes, supports life systems and renders the stability.
- It is also responsible for the cycling of nutrients between biotic and abiotic components.
- It maintains a balance among the various trophic levels in the ecosystem.
- It cycles the minerals through the biosphere.
- The abiotic components help in the synthesis of organic components that involves the exchange of energy.

FOREST ECOSYSTEM

An ecosystem can be as small as an oasis in a desert, or as big as an ocean, spanning thousands of miles. There are two types of ecosystem:
1. Terrestrial ecosystem
2. Aquatic ecosystem

Terrestrial Ecosystems

Terrestrial ecosystems are exclusively land-based ecosystems. There are different types of terrestrial ecosystems distributed around various geological zones. They are as follows:

Forest ecosystem: A forest ecosystem consists of several plants, animals and microorganisms that live in coordination with the abiotic factors of the environment. Forests help in maintaining the temperature of the earth and are the major carbon sink.

Grassland ecosystem: In a grassland ecosystem, the vegetation is dominated by grasses and herbs. Temperate grasslands, savanna grasslands are some of the examples of grassland ecosystems.

Tundra ecosystem: Tundra ecosystems are devoid of trees and are found in cold climate or where rainfall is scarce. These are covered with snow for most of the year. The ecosystem in the Arctic or mountain tops is tundra type.

Desert ecosystem: Deserts are found throughout the world. These are regions with very little rainfall. The days are hot and the nights are cold.

Aquatic Ecosystem

Aquatic ecosystem is ecosystems present in a body of water. These can be further divided into two types, namely:
1. **Freshwater ecosystem:** The freshwater ecosystem is an aquatic ecosystem that includes lakes, ponds, rivers, streams, and wetlands. These have no salt content in contrast with the marine ecosystem.
2. **Marine ecosystem:** The marine ecosystem includes seas and oceans. These have a larger salt content and greater biodiversity in comparison to the freshwater ecosystem.

ECOSYSTEM—SCOPE AND IMPORTANCE

Ecosystem is a part of natural environment consisting of a community of living beings and the physical environment both constantly interchanging materials and energy between them. It is the sum total of the environment or a part of nature. The environment consists of four segments as follows:

1. **Atmosphere:** The atmosphere refers to the protective blanket of gases, surrounding the earth. It sustains life on the earth. It saves the Earth from the hostile environment of the outer space. The atmosphere composed of nitrogen and oxygen in large quantity along with small percentage of other gases such as argon, carbon dioxide, and trace gases (the gases which makes up less than 1% by volume of the atmosphere).
2. **Hydrosphere:** Hydrosphere comprises all water resources such as ocean, seas, lakes, rivers, reservoirs, icecaps, glaciers, and ground water.
3. **Lithosphere:** It is the outer mantle of the solid earth. It contains minerals occurring in the earth's crust and the soil.
4. **Biosphere:** It constitutes the realm of living organisms and their interactions with the environment (atmosphere, hydrosphere, and lithosphere).

The study of ecosystem or environmental studies has been seen to be multidisciplinary in nature, hence, it is considered to be a subject with great scope. It is no more confined only to the issues of sanitation and health; rather, it is now concerned with pollution control, biodiversity conservation, waste management and conservation of natural resources.

Types of Natural Ecosystem

An ecosystem is a self-contained unit of living things and their non-living environment. Types of natural ecosystem are as follows

Biotic (living components): Biotic components in ecosystems include organisms such as plants, animals, and microorganisms. The biotic components of ecosystem comprise:
- Producers or Autotrophs
- Consumers or Heterotrophs
- Decomposers or Detritus

Abiotic (nonliving components):
- Abiotic components consist of climate or factors of climate such as temperature, light, humidity, precipitation, gases, wind, water, soil, salinity, substratum, mineral, topography, and habitat.
- The flow of energy and the cycling of water and nutrients are critical to each ecosystem on the earth. Non-living components set the stage for ecosystem operation.

Aquatic Ecosystem

- An ecosystem which is located in a body of water is known as an aquatic ecosystem.
- The nature and characteristics of the communities of living or biotic organisms and non-living or abiotic factors which interact with and interrelate to one another are determined by the aquatic surroundings of their environment they are dependent upon.
- Aquatic ecosystem can be broadly classified into Marine ecosystem and Freshwater ecosystem.

Marine Ecosystem

- These ecosystems are the biggest of all ecosystems as all oceans and their parts are included in them.
- They contain salt marshes, intertidal zones, estuaries, lagoons, mangroves, coral reefs, the deep sea, and the sea floor.
- Marine ecosystem has a unique flora and fauna, and supports a vast kingdom of species.
- These ecosystems are essential for the overall health of both marine and terrestrial environments.
- Salt marshes, seagrass meadows, and mangrove forests are among the most productive ecosystem.
- Coral reef provides food and shelter to the highest number of marine inhabitants in the world. Marine ecosystem has a large biodiversity.

Freshwater Ecosystem

- Freshwater ecosystem includes lakes, rivers, streams, and ponds. Lakes are large bodies of freshwater surrounded by land.
- Plants and algae are important to freshwater ecosystem because they provide oxygen through photosynthesis and food for animals in this ecosystem.
- Estuaries house plant life with the unique adaptation of being able to survive in fresh and salty environments. Mangroves and pickle weed are examples of estuarine plants.
- Many animals live in freshwater ecosystem. Freshwater ecosystem is very important for people as they provide them water for drinking, energy and transportation, recreation, etc.

Terrestrial Ecosystem

- Terrestrial ecosystems are those ecosystems that exist on land. Water may be present in a terrestrial ecosystem but these ecosystems are primarily situated on land.
- These ecosystems are of different types such as forest ecosystem, desert ecosystem, grassland and mountain ecosystems.
- Terrestrial ecosystems are distinguished from aquatic ecosystems by the lower availability of water and the consequent importance of water as a limiting factor.
- These are characterized by greater temperature fluctuations on both diurnal and seasonal basis, than in aquatic ecosystems in similar climates.
- Availability of light is greater in terrestrial ecosystems than in aquatic ecosystems because the atmosphere is more transparent on land than in water.
- Differences in temperature and light in terrestrial ecosystems reflect a completely different flora and fauna.

IMPORTANCE OF ECOSYSTEM

- The functional attributes of the ecosystem keep the components running together.
- Ecosystem functions are natural processes or exchange of energy that take place in various plant and animal communities of different biomes of the world.
- For instance, green leaves prepare food and roots absorb nutrients from the soil, herbivores feed on the leaves and the roots and in turn serve as food for the carnivores.
- Decomposers execute the functions of breaking down complex organic materials into simple inorganic products, which are used by the producers.
- Fundamentally, ecosystem functions are exchange of energy and nutrients in the food chain.
- These exchanges sustain plant and animal life on the planet as well as the decomposition of organic matter and the production of biomass.

All these functions of the ecosystem take place through delicately balanced and controlled processes.

ECOLOGICAL PYRAMID

Ecological pyramid refers to a graphical (pyramidal) representation to show the number of organisms, biomass, and productivity at each trophic level. It is also known as **Energy Pyramid (Fig. 14.5)**. There are three types of pyramids. They are as follows:

Pyramid of Biomass

- As the name suggests, the Biomass Pyramids shows the amount of biomass (living or organic matter present in an organism) present per unit area at each trophic level.
- It is drawn with the producers at the base and the top carnivores at the tip.
- Pyramid of biomass is generally ascertained by gathering all organisms occupying each trophic level separately and measuring their dry weight.
- Each trophic level has a certain mass of living material at a particular time called standing crop, which is measured as the mass of living organisms (biomass) or the number in a unit area.

Upright Pyramid of Biomass

- Ecosystems found on land mostly have pyramids of biomass with large base of primary producers with smaller trophic level perched on top, hence the upright pyramid of biomass.

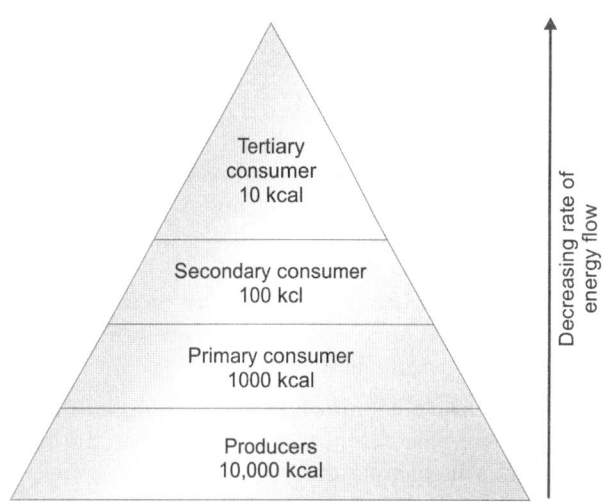

Fig. 14.5: Ecological pyramid.

- The biomass of autotrophs or producers is at the maximum. The biomass of next trophic level, i.e., primary consumers is less than the producers.
- Similarly, the other consumers such as secondary and tertiary consumers are comparatively less than its lower level respectively.
- The top of the pyramid has very less amount of biomass.

Inverted Pyramid of Biomass

- On the other hand, a reverse pyramidal structure is found in most aquatic ecosystems. Here, the pyramid of biomass may assume an inverted pattern. However, pyramid of numbers for aquatic ecosystem is upright.
- In a water body, the producers are tiny phytoplankton that grow and reproduce rapidly.
- In this condition, the pyramid of biomass has a small base, with the producer biomass at the base providing support to consumer biomass of large weight. Hence, it assumes an inverted shape.

Pyramid of Numbers

- It is the graphic representation of number of individuals per unit area of various trophic levels.
- Large number of producers tends to form the base whereas lower number of top predators or carnivores occupies the tip.
- The shape of the pyramid of numbers varies from ecosystem to ecosystem.
- For example, in an aquatic ecosystem or grassland areas, autotrophs or producers are present in large number per unit area.
- The producers support a lesser number of herbivores, which in turn supports fewer carnivores.

Upright Pyramid of Numbers

- In upright pyramid of numbers, the number of individuals decreases from the lower level to the higher level.
- This type of pyramid is usually found in the grassland ecosystem and the pond ecosystem.
- The grass in a grassland ecosystem occupies the lowest trophic level because of its abundance.
- Next comes the primary producers-the herbivores (e.g., grasshopper).
- The number of grasshoppers is quite less than that of grass. Then, there are the primary carnivores, for example, the rat whose number is far less than the grasshoppers.
- The next trophic level is the secondary consumers such as the snakes who feed on the rats.
- Then, there are the top carnivores such as the hawks who eat snakes and whose number is less than the snakes.
- The number of species decreases towards the higher levels in this pyramidal structure.

Inverted pyramid of numbers: Here, the number of individuals increases from the lower level to the higher trophic level. For example, the tree ecosystem.

Pyramid of Energy

- It is a graphical structure representing the flow of energy through each trophic level of a food chain over a fixed part of the natural environment.
- An energy pyramid represents the amount of energy at each trophic level and loss of energy at each is transferred to another trophic level.
- Energy pyramid, sometimes called trophic pyramid or ecological pyramid, is useful in quantifying the energy transfer from one organism to another along the food chain.
- Energy decreases as one moves through the trophic levels from the bottom to the top of the pyramid. Thus, the energy pyramid is always upward.

ENERGY FLOW IN ECOSYSTEM

Energy moves life. The cycle of energy is based on the flow of energy through different trophic levels in an ecosystem. Our ecosystem is maintained by the cycling energy and nutrients obtained from different external sources. At the first trophic level, primary producers use solar energy to produce organic material through photosynthesis **(Fig. 14.6)**.

- The herbivores at the second trophic level, use the plants as food which gives them energy.
- A large part of this energy is used up for the metabolic functions of these animals such as breathing, digesting food, supporting growth of tissues, maintaining blood circulation and body temperature.
- The carnivores at the next trophic level, feed on the herbivores and derive energy for their sustenance and growth.
- If large predators are present, they represent still higher trophic level and they feed on carnivores to get energy

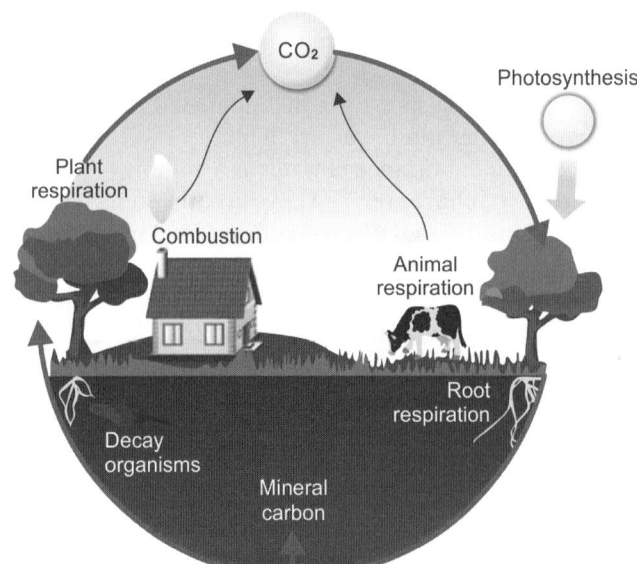

Fig. 14.6: Ecosystem-photosynthesis.

Thus, the different plants and animal species are linked to one another through food chains.
- Decomposers which include bacteria, fungi, molds, worms, and insects break down wastes and dead organisms, and return the nutrients to the soil, which is then taken up by the producers.
- Energy is not recycled during decomposition, but it is released.

Biogeochemical Cycles (Fig. 14.7)

- All elements in the earth are recycled time and again. The major elements such as oxygen, carbon, nitrogen, phosphorous, and sulfur are essential ingredients that make up organisms.
- Biogeochemical cycles refer to the flow of such chemical elements and compounds between organisms and the physical environment.
- Chemicals taken in by organisms are passed through the food chain and come back to the soil, air, and water through mechanisms such as respiration, excretion, and decomposition.
- As an element moves through this cycle, it often forms compounds with other elements as a result of metabolic processes in living tissues and of natural reactions in the atmosphere, hydrosphere, or lithosphere.
- Such cyclic exchange of material between the living organisms and their non-living environment is called Biogeochemical Cycle.

Following are some important biogeochemical cycles:
- Carbon cycle
- Nitrogen cycle
- Water cycle
- Oxygen cycle
- Phosphorus cycle
- Sulphur cycle

Carbon Cycle

- Carbon enters into the living world in the form of carbon dioxide through the process of photosynthesis as carbohydrates.
- These organic compounds (food) are then passed from the producers to the consumers (herbivores and carnivores).
- This carbon is finally returned to the surrounding medium by the process of respiration or decomposition of plants and animals by the decomposers. Carbon is also recycled during the burning of fossil fuels.

Nitrogen Cycle

- Nitrogen is present in the atmosphere in an elemental form and as such it cannot be utilized by living organisms.
- This elemental form of nitrogen is converted into combined state with elements such as H, C, O by certain bacteria, so that it can be readily used by the plants.
- Nitrogen is being continuously expelled into the air by the action of microorganisms such as denitrifying bacteria and finally returned to the cycle through the action of lightening and electrification.

Water Cycle

- The evaporation of water from ocean, rivers, lakes, and transpiring plants takes water in the form of vapors to the atmosphere **(Fig. 14.8)**.
- This vaporized water subsequently cools and condenses to form cloud and water.
- This cooled water vapor ultimately returns to the earth as rain and snow, completing the cycle.

BIODIVERSITY

Biodiversity, a shortened form of biological diversity, refers to the existence of number of different species of plants and animals in an environment.

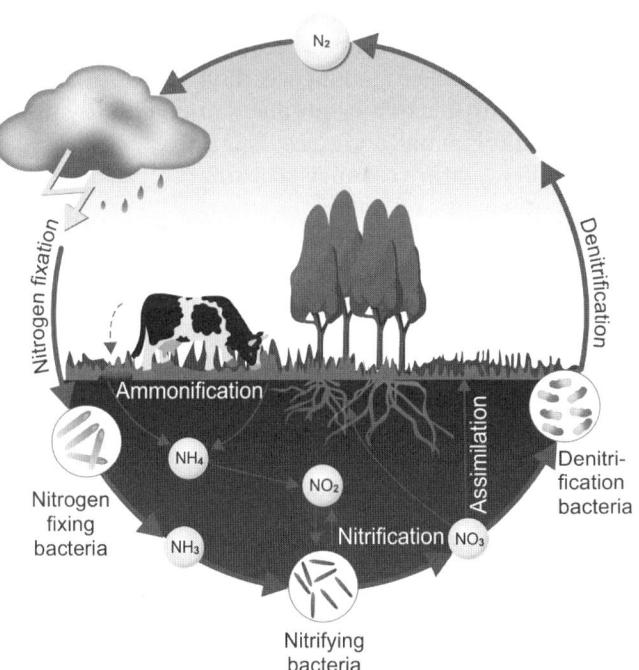

Fig. 14.7: Biogeochemical cycles.

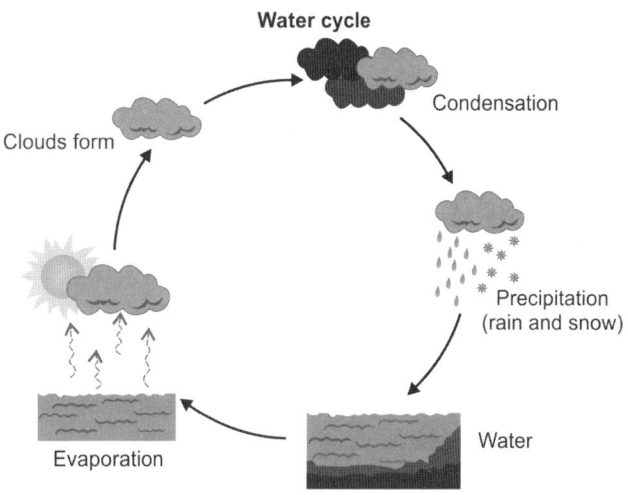

Fig. 14.8: Water cycle.

- Biological diversity means the variability among living organisms from all sources including, inter alia, terrestrial, marine, and other aquatic ecosystems and the ecological complexes of which they are part; this includes diversity within species, between species and of ecosystems.
- Biodiversity is also defined as the existence of variability among living organisms on the earth, including the variability within and between species, and within and between ecosystems.

Species Diversity

- Species diversity refers to the variety of different species of plants, animals, fungi, and organisms that are present in a region.
- It is estimated that there are above 30 million species on the earth. Species diversity is a part of diversity.
- Even within a small pond, we can notice a great variety of species. Species diversity differs from ecosystem to ecosystem.
- For example, in a tropical ecosystem more diversity is found than in temperate ecosystem.
- The most diverse group of species is invertebrates—animals without backbones.
- At present, conservation scientists have been able to identify and categorize about 1.8 million species on earth.
- Many new species are being identified. Areas that are rich in species diversity are called 'hotspots' of diversity.

Genetic Diversity

- It is the variation in genes that exists within a species. Genetic diversity corresponds to the variety of genes contained in plants, animals, fungi, and microorganisms.
- It occurs within a species as well as between species. For example, poodles, German shepherds and golden retrievers are all dogs, but they all are different in look, color, and abilities.
- Each human being is different from all others. This genetic variability is essential for a health breeding of a population of species.
- The diversity in wild species make the 'gene pool' from which crops and domestic animals have been developed over thousands of years.

Ecosystem Diversity

- It is the diversity of ecosystems, natural communities, and habitats. In other words, ecosystem diversity refers to the variety of ways that species interact with each other and their environment.
- Tropical or temperate forests, grasslands, hot and cold deserts, wetlands, rivers, mountains, and coral reefs are instances of ecosystem diversity.
- Each ecosystem corresponds to a series of complex relationships between biotic (living) and abiotic (non-living) components.

Value and Productive Use of Biodiversity

- The importance of biodiversity is second to none. It boosts the ecosystem of productivity where each species, irrespective of their size, have an important role to play.
- Greater diversity in species ensures natural sustainability for all life forms. Hence, there is a need to preserve the diversity in life on the earth.
- According to the UN sources at least 40% of the world's economy and 80% of the needs of the poor are derived from biological resources.
- In addition, the richer the diversity of life, the greater the opportunity for medical discoveries, economic development, and adaptive response to such new challenges as climate change.

SIGNIFICANCE OF BIODIVERSITY

- Environmental services from species and smooth running cycles of ecosystems are necessary at global, regional, and local levels.
- Biodiversity is essential for maintaining the water cycles, production of oxygen, reduction in carbon dioxide, protecting the soil, etc.
- It is also essential for preserving ecological processes, such as soil formation, circulation of and cleansing of air and water, global life support, fixing and recycling of nutrients, maintaining hydrological balance within ecosystems, maintaining rivers and streams throughout the year, etc.
- Biodiversity has many values such as consumptive use value, productive use value, and social values, ethical and moral values.

A healthy biodiversity offers many valuable services as follows:
- The more a region is rich in terms of biodiversity, better is the regulation of the different cycles. For example, forests regulate the amount of carbon dioxide in the air by releasing oxygen as a by-product during photosynthesis and control rainfall and soil erosion.
- Protects water resources from being depleted, contaminated, or polluted.
- Helps in soil formation and protection.
- Helps in nutrient storage and recycling.
- Helps check pollution.
- Contributes to climate stability.
- Helps an ecosystem in recovery from unpredictable events.
- Provides biological resources such as food, medicinal resources, and pharmaceutical drugs, wood products, ornamental plants, breeding stocks, etc.
- Provides recreation and tourism facilities.
- Helps in research, education, and monitoring.
- Preservation of biological resources is essential for the well-being and long-term survival of mankind.

PRODUCTIVE USE VALUE OF BIODIVERSITY

- Productive use value refers to the commercial value of products that are commercially harvested for exchange in formal markets.
- Modern civilization is invariably a gift of biodiversity. The food we eat, the medicine we take in, the furniture we use, the industries, for example, are derivatives of biological diversity.
- The agricultural crops of the present day have originated from wild varieties.
- Biotechnologists use the wild plants for developing new, high-yielding, and pest or disease resistant varieties. Biodiversity is home to original stock from which new varieties are being developed.
- Similarly, all our domesticated animals came from their wild-living ancestral species. With the help of scientific breeding techniques, animals giving better yield of milk, meat, etc. are being developed. The animal products used by modern society come from the advances made in the fields of poultry farming, pisciculture, silviculture, dairy farming, etc.
- Fossil fuels, considered to be pivotal in modern society, such as coal, petroleum, and natural gas are gifts of biodiversity from the geological past.
- Most of the pharmaceutical drugs and medicines used in the present time are extracted from different plants.
- Biodiversity provides rich storehouse for industrialists and entrepreneurs to develop new products.
- It provides agricultural scientists and biotechnologists with ample scope for developing new and better crops. New crop varieties are being developed using the genetic material found in wild relatives of crop plants though biotechnology.
- The need of the hour is the preservation of biodiversity for industrial, economic, and above all, environmental safety. This is called 'biological prospecting'.

THREATS TO BIODIVERSITY

Biodiversity is a paramount factor for the survival of the living world in general and mankind in particular. The fewer species (animals and plants) we have, the fewer people we will have on the earth. During the last few decades, loss of biodiversity is on the rise. The following are the major causes of threat to biodiversity:

Habitat Loss

- Today, major loss to biodiversity in the world has been done by man. Man has begun to overuse or misuse most of these natural ecosystems.
- Due to mindless and unsustainable resource use, once productive forest and grasslands have been turned into deserts, and wastelands have increased all over the world.
- Rapid industrialization, urbanization, and growth in population have resulted in massive deforestation and consequential habitat loss around the world.
- For instance, mangroves have been cleared for fuel-wood and prawn farming, which has led to a decrease in the habitat essential for breeding of marine fish.
- Forests all over the world, in particular tropical rainforests such as the Amazon, are under unforeseen threat largely from conversion to other land-uses.
- Scientists have estimated that human activities are likely to eliminate approximately 10 million species by the year 2050. It is also estimated that at the present rate of extinction about 25% of the world's species will undergo extinction fairly rapidly.
- Rich biodiversities such as tropical forests, wetlands, and coral reefs world over will constitute the major part of this extinction.

Poaching of Wildlife

- Poaching of wildlife for trade and commercial activities has been on the rise for the last many decades.
- It has been a significant cause of the extinction of hundreds of species and the endangerment of many more, such as whales and many African large mammal, Asian tigers, etc.
- Most extinction over the past several hundred years is mainly due to overharvesting for food, fashion, and profit.
- Illicit trade in wildlife in current times is driving many species of wild animals and plants to extinction.
- Elephants are poached for ivory; tigers and leopards for their skin; pangolins for meat and scales; and rare timber are targeted for hardwood furniture.
- The global illegal wildlife trade is estimated to be between $7 billion and $23 billion in illicit revenue annually. It is now considered the most lucrative global crime after drugs, humans, and arms.

Man-Wildlife Conflict

- Man-wildlife conflict refers to the interaction between wild animals and people and the consequential negative impact on both of them.
- Human population growth and the resultant destruction of wildlife habitat for human habitation and economic prosperity create reduction of resources or life to some people and wild animals.
- World Wide Fund for Nature (WWF) defines this conflict as "any interaction between humans and wildlife that results in a negative impact on human social, economic, or cultural life, on the conservation of wildlife population, or on the environment."
- Although man-wildlife conflict is as old as human civilization, in modern times the degree of conflict has been on the rise due to high rise in human population in the past several centuries.
- Since human populations expand into wild animal habitats, natural wildlife territory is displaced.
- Reduction in the availability of natural prey/food sources leads to wild animals seeking alternate sources.

Alternately, new resources created by humans draw wildlife resulting in conflict.
- Competition for food resources also occurs when humans attempt to harvest natural resources such as fish and grassland pasture.

There are many consequences of man versus wildlife conflicts. The major consequences are:
- Destruction of wildlife habitat
- Injury and loss of life of both humans and wildlife
- Crop damage and livestock depredation
- Damage to human property
- Decrease in wildlife population and reduction in geographic ranges
- Trophic cascades

Apart from the above, there are other causes of threat to biodiversity. Factors such as climate change, invasion of non-native species also add to biodiversity losses in some or the other.

CONVERSATION OF BIODIVERSITY

Considering the degree of threat to biodiversity around the world and the vital importance of biodiversity for living beings of which mankind is a major part, there is an urgent need to conserve biodiversity in the world. Further, we should be concerned about saving biodiversity because of the benefits it provides us—biological resources and ecosystem services, and the social and aesthetic benefits.

There are two main methods for the conservation of biodiversity:

1. **In-situ conservation:** In-situ or on-site conservation refers to the conservation of species within their natural habitats. This is the most viable way of biodiversity conservation. It is the conservation of genetic resources through their maintenance within the environment in which they occur.
   Examples—National Parks, Wildlife Sanctuaries, Biosphere Reserves, Gene Sanctuaries.
2. **Ex-situ conservation:** Ex-situ conservation means the conservation of components of biological diversity outside their natural habitats. In this method, threatened or endangered species of animals and plants are taken out of their natural habitat and placed in special settings where they can be protected and provided with natural growth. In ex-situ conservation methods, the plants and animals taken away from their habitats are taken care of in an artificially created environment.
   Examples—Captive Breeding, Gene Banks, Seed Banks, Zoos, Botanical Gardens, Aquaria, In-vitro Fertilization, Cryopreservation, Tissue Culture.

NATIONAL BIODIVERSITY ACT

National Biodiversity Act in India draws from the objectives of Convention of Biodiversity (CBD). It aims at conservation of biodiversity, sustainable use and equitable sharing of the benefits of such use.

To achieve its objectives, it has put in place a three-tier institutional structure such as:
- National Biodiversity Authority based in Chennai
- State Biodiversity Board (SBBs) in every state
- Biodiversity Management Committee (BMCs) at Panchayat/Municipality levels

The Ministry of Environment and Forestry (MoEF) is the nodal agency.

Main Provisions of the Act

- Prohibition on transfer of Indian genetic material outside the country without specific approval of the Indian Government.
- Prohibition of anyone claiming an IPR such as a patent over biodiversity or related knowledge without the permission of Indian Government.
- Regulation of collection and use of biodiversity by Indian national, while exempting local communities from such restrictions.
- Measures from sharing of benefits from the use of biodiversity including transfer of technology, monitory returns, joint research and development, joint IPR ownership, etc.
- Measures to conserve sustainable use of biological resources including habitat and species protection projects, integration of biodiversity into the plans and policies of the various departments and sectors.
- Provisions for local communities to have a say in the use of their resources and knowledge and to charge fees for this.
- Protection of indigenous or traditional laws such as registration of such knowledge.
- Regulation of the use of the genetically modified organisms.
- Setting up of national, state and local biodiversity funds to be used to support conservation and benefit sharing.
- Setting up of Biodiversity Management Committees (BMC) at local village levels.

ENVIRONMENTAL POLLUTION

Environmental pollution or simply pollution refers to undesirable changes occurring in the physical, chemical, and biological composition of natural environment consisting of air, water, and soil. Pollution also means the presence of harmful pollutants in an environment that makes this environment unhealthy to live in.

Definition

According to National Academy of Science, USA (1966), **pollution** is defined as, "An undesirable change in physical, chemical, and biological characteristics of water, air, and soil that may harmfully affect human, animal, and plant life, industrial progress, living conditions and cultural assets".

Chapter 14: National Health Problems

Meaning of Pollution

- Pollution is also viewed as 'an unfavorable alteration' in the sustaining and carrying capacity of the natural environment wholly or largely by the byproducts of human activities.
- Natural environment has an inbuilt capacity to replenish the losses or reduction in its constituents to restore it as sustainable and healthy as required.
- Ever expanding population and evolution of man into modern homo sapiens have led to rapid urbanization, industrialization and unprecedented rise in human habitations.
- All these human endeavors have, in turn, virtually perpetuated deforestation, loss of habitats for flora and fauna, depletion of natural resources at a large scale over the last couple of centuries, which have told upon the inherent resilience of the natural environment. As a result, natural environment continues to be undesirably polluted.

Pollutants

A pollutant is defined as any form of energy or matter or action that causes imbalance or disequilibrium in the required composition of natural objects such as air, water, etc. A pollutant creates damage by interfering directly or indirectly with the biogeochemical process of an organism.

Pollutants may be:

- **Natural pollutants:** Natural pollutants are caused by natural forces such as volcanic eruption and forest fire.
- **Man-made pollutants:** These refer to the release of excess amount of gases or matter by human activities. For instance, increase in the number of automobiles adds excess carbon monoxide to the atmosphere causing harmful effect on vegetation and human health.

Classification of pollution: Different types of pollution are classified based on the part of the environment which they affect or result caused by a particular pollution. Each type of pollution has its own distinctive cause and consequences.

The major types of pollution are as follows:

- Air pollution
- Water pollution
- Noise pollution
- Soil or land pollution

AIR POLLUTION

Every day, every moment, we breathe polluted air and may become a victim of air pollution. It is estimated that an average adult exchanges 15 kg of air a day, in comparison to about 1.5 kg of the food consumed and 2.5 kg of water intake. It is obvious that the quantum of pollutants that enter our body through respiration would be manifold in comparison to those taken in through polluted water or contaminated food.

Air pollution is one of the most widespread forms of pollution all over the world. Wind is the main agent of air pollution. It gathers and moves pollutants from one area to another, sometimes reducing the concentration of pollutants in one location, while increasing it in another.

Causes of Air Pollution

Apart from the natural causes of pollutants, as stated above, human interaction and resource utilization is perhaps adding more pollutants to the atmosphere.

- **Industrialization:** Industries big or small require steam to run. The steam is produced by burning fossil fuels such as coal, coke, and furnace oil. These fuels while burning release toxic gases in large amount into the atmosphere.
- **Automobiles:** To meet the demands of exploding human population, the number of automobiles is increasing at a great space. The automobile exhausts are responsible for about sixty percent of air pollution. Released carbon monoxide from the automobiles pollutes the air and harms trees and other natural vegetation. It also has ill-effects on human health.
- **Chlorofluorocarbons:** Scientists are now alarmed regarding the increased concentration of chemical substances together called chlorofluorocarbon in the atmosphere. These substances are responsible for creating holes in the ozone layer causing unwanted imbalance in the heat budget. These are produced by modern gadgets such as air conditioners, refrigerators, dyers, etc.

The adverse effects of air pollution appear in the form of poor quality of air, acidic precipitation (rain, snow and hail) and deposition, and other health hazards.

The main pollutants of air are carbon dioxide (CO_2), carbonic acid (H_2SO_2), water (H_2O), nitric acid (HNO_3O), and sulphuric acid (H_2SO_4).

Air pollution has harmful effects on natural vegetation and human health such as respiratory illnesses. Acidic precipitation is highly fatal for aquatic flora and fauna, monuments, and also for natural vegetation.

Air Pollution Control

Air pollution control is an onerous task as there is large number of pollutants involved in air pollution. Some of these are even difficult to detect. However, there can be some basic approaches to control air pollution. They are as follows:

Preventive approach: It is well said that prevention is better than cure. We can prevent pollutants of air from being produced by various ways. For instance, by changing raw materials used in industry or the ingredient of fuel from conventional to non-conventional sources of energy; by maintenance of vehicles and roads and efficient transport system; by reduction in garbage burning and shifting cultivation areas; afforestation, etc.

Dispersal approach: We can prevent air pollution by raising the heights of smokestacks in industries so as to release the pollutants high into the atmosphere.

Collection approach: Air pollution can be controlled by designing the equipment and machinery to trap pollutants before they escape into the atmosphere. To meet the standards, automobile engines have been re-designed and new cars have been equipped with devices such as the catalytic converter, which changes the pollutants into harmless substances. Because of these new devices, air pollution from car exhaust has also been reduced.

Legislation Approach

- There have been many initiatives in different countries for making laws, setting standards and norms to check air pollution and ensure quality air.
- All the highly industrialized countries of the world have certain legislations to prevent and control air pollution.
- As pollutants of air are carried by the wind from one country to another for thousands of miles, there should be global initiatives agreed upon by all countries to save the earth from the menace of air pollution.

WATER POLLUTION

Water pollution may be defined as alteration in physical, chemical, and biological characteristics of water, which may cause harmful effects on human and aquatic life.

Pollutants of Water

Following are some of the reasons for water pollution:
- Disposal of sewage and sludge into water bodies such as river, streams, and lakes.
- Inorganic compounds and minerals by mining and industrial activities.
- Use of chemical fertilizers for agricultural purposes.
- Synthetic organic compounds from industrial, agricultural, and domestic garbage.
- Oil and petroleum from tankers' accident, offshore drilling, combustion engine, etc.
- Radioactive wastes.

Water Pollution Control

- **Environmental education:** Individuals and the masses should be educated about the significance of quality of water and its impact on the economy, the society, and ecology.
- **Sewage treatment:** The household water should be treated properly to make it environmentally safe. Necessary steps should be taken to ensure that effective sewage treatment process is put in place and contaminated water does not get mixed with the fresh water bodies.
- **Accountability of industrial units:** The industrial setups should make provisions for treatment of waste materials and water, and for its safe drainage.
- **Afforestation:** Planting trees can reduce the water pollution to a large extent as they check surface soil runoff by running water.
- **Soil conservation:** Soil conservation add many inorganic substances in the surface and underground water. Soil conservation is, therefore, a useful technique to reduce water pollution.
- **Reduced use of chemical fertilizers:** Chemical fertilizers add nitrates in water bodies. Use of compost manures can help reduce the problem of eutrophication in the water bodies.
- **Financial support:** Governments should make provisions for adequate funds to the civic bodies for water pollution control.
- **Legislation and implementation of stringent environmental laws:** The need of the hour is that the government should legislate and implement strict environmental laws for the protection of water bodies, treatment of waste water, etc. The violators of such laws should be given exemplary punishment.

NOISE POLLUTION

Noise pollution refers to any unwanted and unpleasant sound that brings discomfort and restlessness to human beings. Like air and water pollution, noise pollution is harmful to human and animal life.

Noise pollution is also an important environmental hazard, which is becoming growingly injurious in many parts of the world. Noise beyond a particular level or decibel (unit of noise) tends to become a health and environmental hazard.

Sources of Noise Pollution

- Household appliances such as grinders, electric motor, washing machines
- Social gatherings such as marriages and other social parties
- Places of worship
- Commercial activities
- Construction activities
- Industrial activities
- Automobiles and transport system
- Power generators
- Agricultural equipment

Noise Pollution Control

According to the World Health Organization (WHO), of all the environmental pollution, noise is the easiest to control.

Noise pollution can be checked at home by:
- Turning off sound-making appliances when they are not in use.
- Shutting the door when noisy machines are being used.
- Lowering the volume of appliances such as television to a desirable level.
- Using earplugs while listening to music.

At mass level it can be checked by:
- Planting trees in large number to create vegetation buffer zones, which absorb noise.
- Public awareness about the need of control of noise pollution.
- Application of engineering control techniques such as alteration and modification of design to reduce noise

from equipment and machinery, and by construction of sound barriers or the use of sound absorbers in industrial and factory sites can reduce exposure to noise to a great extent.
- Construction of institutions and hospitals away from airports, railways, and highways.
- Improved building design may also reduce the impact of noise pollution.
- Stringent legislations at central and state levels to check air pollution at workplaces, urban centers, etc.

SOIL OR LAND POLLUTION

Soil pollution refers to an undesirable decrease in the quality of soil, either by man-induced sources or natural sources or by both. Soil is vital not only for the growth of plants and growing food but also cultivating raw materials for agro-based industries. Health soil is a significant prerequisite for human survival.

Definition of soil pollution: Soil pollution is defined as the reduction in productivity of soil due to presence of soil pollutants.
- Pesticides, fertilizers, organic manure, chemicals, radioactive wastes, discarded food and clothes, leather goods, plastic, paper, bottles, tin cans and carcasses contribute towards soil pollution.
- Industrial wastes contain chemicals like iron, lead, mercury, copper, zinc, cadmium, aluminum, cyanides, acids, alkalies, etc that reach soil either directly through water or indirectly through air (acid rain).
- Improper and continuous use of herbicides, fungicides and pesticides to protect crops from pests and fungi alter the basic composition of soils and make it toxic for plant growth.
- Organic insecticides like DDT, Aldrin, Benzene-hexachloride, etc used against soil borne pests accumulate in the soil due to slow degradation by soil and water bacteria. They result in stunted growth of plants and reduced size of fruit. Their bye-products of degradation reach animals including man through food chain.
- Radioactive wastes from mining and nuclear processes may reach soil via water or as 'fall-out'. From soil they reach plants and live stock from where they enter human beings through milk and meat. This causes retarded and abnormal growth in human beings.
- Human and animal excreta used as organic manure to increase crop yield, pollute soil by contaminating soil and vegetable crops with pathogens that may be present in excreta.
- Intensification of agricultural production by excessive irrigation, excessive fertilizers, pesticides, insecticides, etc. causes soil pollution.

Classification of Solid Wastes

- Municipal waste
- Hospital waste
- Hazardous waste

Effective solid waste management can be carried out in the following ways:
- Sanitary landfills
- Composting
- Landfills
- Incineration and pyrolysis (a process of combustion in the absence of oxygen)
- Vermiculture or earthworm farming
- Bioremediation or the use of micro-organism (bacteria and fungi)
- Reuse, reduce, and recycle.

Causes of Soil Erosion

- Deforestation at large scale
- Over-grazing
- Mining
- Decrease in soil microorganisms
- Excessive use of chemical fertilizers
- Excessive use of irrigation
- Lack of humus content
- Improper and unscientific rotation of crops

Soil pollution leads to many harmful consequences such as decrease in agricultural production; reduced nitrogen fixation; reduction in biodiversity; silting of tanks, lakes and reservoirs; diseases and deaths of consumers in the food chain due to use of chemical fertilizers and pesticides, etc.

Soil Pollution Control

- Adoption of soil-friendly agricultural practices.
- Use of compost manures in place of chemical fertilizers; Use of bio-fertilizers and natural pesticides help in minimizing the usage of chemical fertilizers and pesticides
- Scientific rotation of crop to increase soil fertility.
- Proper disposal of industrial and urban solid and liquid wastes.
- Planting of trees to check soil erosion in slopes and mountainous regions.
- Controlled grazing.
- Reduction in the heaps of garbage and refuse.
- The principles of three R.s: **Recycle, Reuse**, and **Reduce:** help in minimizing generation of solid waste.
- Formulation and effective implementation of stringent pollution control legislation.
- Improved sewage and sanitation system in urban areas.

Solid Waste Management

- It refers to the collecting, treating, and disposing of solid material that is discarded or is no longer useful.
- Solid waste management is an important aspect of urban area management.
- Improper disposal of municipal solid waste can create unsanitary conditions, which can lead to environmental pollution and the outbreak of vector-borne disease.
- The task of solid waste management presents complex technical challenges. They also pose various economic, administrative, and social problems which need urgent attention.

- The major sources of solid waste are households; agricultural fields; industries and mining, hotels and catering; roads and railways; hospitals and educational institutions; cultural centers and places of recreation and tourism, etc. Plastic waste is also a solid waste.

MARINE POLLUTION

Marine pollution is the introduction of substances or energy from humans into the marine environment resulting in such deleterious effects as harm to living resources, hazards to human health, hindrance to marine activities including fishing, impairment of quality for use of seawater, and reduction of amenities

There can be several causes of ocean pollution, but the leading causes include sewage, toxic chemicals from industries, nuclear waste, thermal pollution, plastics, acid rain, and oil spillage.

Sewage: Sewage is defined as the wastewater and its component excrements that are transported in the sewer system. Sewage is mostly comprised of the human waste from toilet flushing, dirty water from bathing and even animal waste. Most of the wastes find their way into the ocean waters through the sewer systems.

Industrial chemicals: Another major pollutant is the chemicals from industries and from the fertilizers and other farm products that are carried by run-off water into the ocean waters. Many industries dump their waste materials and chemicals into the ocean waters. These chemicals pollute the ocean by altering the pH level of the waters. Most aquatic plants and animals cannot survive in adverse pH levels.

Nuclear waste: Another major ocean pollutant is the nuclear waste, which is mostly produced from industrial, medical, and also scientific procedures that use radioactive material. The common industries that produce nuclear waste include power stations, the military, and the reprocessing plants. This radiation enters the food chain through kelp and plankton, and once the marine animals consume these plants they become contaminated.

Thermal pollution: Thermal pollution is the lowering of water quality by any method that tends to change the water temperature. Thermal pollution occurs when power plants and manufacturing companies release hot water into the water streams and oceans and thus causing a change in temperature by raising the temperatures higher. The sudden change in temperature causes reduction in the oxygen supply and this greatly affects the ecosystem composition. Aquatic plants and other organisms that are adapted to a certain temperature range get killed abruptly by the sudden change in temperature by a process known as thermal shock.

Plastics: Plastic pollution mainly involves the accumulation plastic in the ocean waters and thus causing adverse effects on marine organisms. Marine organisms are affected by the plastics through direct ingestion of the plastic wastes and also through exposure to chemicals that are within the plastics.

Acid rain: Acid rain is not a major cause of ocean pollution, but it also contributes to water pollution. Erupting volcanoes, fossil fuels, rotting vegetation, and nitrogen oxides when released into the atmosphere react with water and other substances in the air to form sulphuric and nitric acid. The wind blows these chemicals across the atmosphere, and when it rains, these chemicals find their way into the marine waters. Acid rain makes water acidic and thus destroys the marine life as most aquatic organisms cannot survive in acidic conditions.

Oil spills: Oil spillage is another primary cause of ocean pollution in that the oil forms a layer on the water preventing oxygen circulation. Lack of oxygen in the ocean waters results in the destruction of marine life over a long period. Therefore, it is necessary to prevent these pollutants from entering the oceans to protect the marine animals and plants.

Effects of Marine Pollution

- The contamination of water by excessive nutrients is known as nutrient pollution, a type of water pollution that affects the life under water. When excess nutrients like nitrates or phosphates get dissolved with the water it causes the eutrophication of surface waters, as it stimulates the growth of algae due to excess nutrients.
- Most of Benthic animals and plankton are either filter feeders or deposit feeders take up the tiny particles that adhere to potentially toxic chemicals. In the ocean food chains, such toxins get concentrated upward.
- This makes estuaries anoxic as many particles combine chemically depletive of oxygen.
- When the marine ecosystem absorbs the pesticides, they are incorporated into the food webs of the marine ecosystem. After getting dissolved in the marine food webs, these harmful pesticides causes' mutations, and also results in diseases, which can damage the entire food web and cause harm to the humans.
- When toxic metals are dumped or flown into the oceans through drains, it engulfs within the marine food webs.
- It affects the biochemistry, reproduction process, can affect the tissue matter. These can cause a change to tissue matter, biochemistry, behavior, reproduction, and suppress and alter the marine life's growth.
- Marine toxins can be transferred to several animals feeding on the fish or fish hydrolysate as a meal; toxins are then transferred to dairy products and meat of these affected land animals.

Steps to Prevent Marine Pollution

- Stop using plastic and littering garbage as they not only choke up the drains but also releases into the oceans.
- Ensure that chemicals mentioned above are not used anywhere near the streams of water and try cutting down on the usage of such chemicals.

- For farmers, they need to switch from chemical fertilizers and pesticides and move towards the usage of organic farming methods.
- Use public transport and reduce the carbon footprint by taking small and substantial measures that will not help in reducing the pollution from the environment but will ensure a safe and healthy future for the upcoming generations.
- Prevent from any oil or chemical spill in the oceans and if in case there is an oil or chemical spill near you volunteer and help in cleaning out the ocean water.
- Volunteer or initiate beach cleanup activities and spread awareness about the same in the nearby vicinity.

THERMAL POLLUTION

Thermal pollution is the degradation of water quality by any process that changes ambient water temperature. A common cause of thermal pollution is the use of water as a coolant by power plants and industrial manufacturers.

Definition

The term thermal pollution has been used to indicate the detrimental effects of heated effluent discharge by various power plants. It denotes the impairment of quality and deterioration of aquatic and terrestrial environment by various industrial plants like thermal, atomic, nuclear, coal-fired plants, oil field generators, factories, and mills.

Sources of Thermal Pollution

- Nuclear power plant
- Coal-fired power plant
- Industrial effluents
- Domestic sewage
- Hydroelectric power
- Thermal power plant

The discharged effluents of these sources have a higher temperature than the intake water that reduces the concentration of oxygen from the water which causes the deleterious effects on the marine ecosystem.

Harmful Effects of the Thermal Pollution

The harmful effects of the thermal pollution are discussed below:

- **Reduction in dissolved oxygen:** The pollutant from various industrial plants are heated decreases the concentration of oxygen with an increase in the temperature of water.
- **Change in water properties:** The decrease in density, viscosity and solubility of gases in water increases the setting speed of suspended particles which seriously affect the food supplies of aquatic organism.
- **Increase in toxicity:** The concentrated pollutant causes the rise in the temperature of water which increases the toxicity of the poison present in water. The toxicity in water will increase the death rate in marine life.
- **Disruption of biological activities:** Temperature changes disrupt the entire marine ecosystem because changes in temperature causes change in physiology, metabolism and biological process like respiration rate, digestion, excretion and development of an aquatic organism.
- **Damage of biotic organism:** Aquatic organisms like juvenile fish, plankton, fish, eggs, larva, algae and protozoa which pass through screens and condenser cooling system are extremely sensitive to abrupt temperature changes. They are habitual of warmer water may suddenly face increase or decrease in temperature of water bodies and thus die because of sudden changes in the temperature of water.

Thermal Pollution is Prevented

The following measures can be taken to prevent or control high temperature caused by thermal pollution:

- Heated water from the industries can treated before discharging directly to the water bodies.
- Heated water from the industries can be treated by the installation of cooling ponds and cooling towers.
- Industrial treated water can be recycled for domestic use or industrial heating.
- Through artificial lakes: In this lake industries can discharge their used or heated water at one end and water for cooling purposes may be withdrawn from the other end. The heat is eventually dissipated through evaporation.

Hence, we can say any kind of pollution may directly or indirectly affect humans because the loss of biodiversity causes changes that affect all the aspects of the environment.

NUCLEAR HAZARDS AND THEIR IMPACT ON HEALTH

Radionuclides are elements (uranium 235, uranium 283, thorium 232, potassium 40, radium 226, carbon 14 etc.) with unstable atomic nuclei and on decomposition release ionizing radiations in the form of alpha, beta and gamma rays. Out of the known 450 radioisotopes only some are of environmental concern like strontium 90, tritium, plutonium 239, argon 41, cobalt 60, cesium 137, iodine 131, krypton 85, etc. These can be both beneficial and harmful, depending on the way in which they are used.

- Radioactive substances when released into the environment are either dispersed or become concentrated in living organisms through the food chain.
- Other than naturally occurring radioisotopes, significant amounts are generated by human activity, including the operation of nuclear power plants, the manufacture of nuclear weapons, and atomic bomb testing.
- For example, strontium 90 behaves like calcium and is easily deposited and replaces calcium in the bone tissues.
- It could be passed to human beings through ingestion of strontium-contaminated milk. Again another example is tritium, which is radioactive hydrogen.

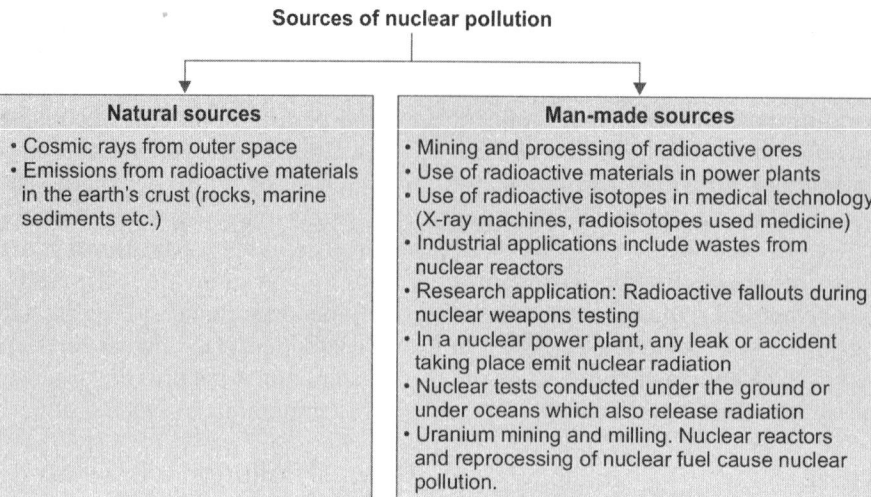

Fig. 14.9: Sources of nuclear pollution.

Sources of Nuclear Pollution (Fig. 14.9)

The sources of radioactivity include both natural and man-made.

Effects of Nuclear Pollution

- **Somatic effects:** Somatic effects the function of cells and organs. It causes damages to cell membranes, mitochondria and cell nuclei resulting in abnormal cell functions, cell division, growth and death.
- **Genetic effects:** Genetic effects are for the future generations. Radiations can cause mutations, which are changes in genetic makeup of cells. These effects are mainly due to the damages to DNA molecules. People suffer from blood cancer and bone cancer if exposed to doses around 100 to 1,000 roentgens.

Management of Radioactive Waste

- The radioactive waste which comes out from industry, nuclear reactors should be stored and allowed to decay either naturally in closed drums or in very large underground air tight cemented tanks (Delay and Decay).
- The intermediate radioactive waste should be disposed off into the environment after diluting it with some inert materials (Dilute and Disperse).
- Now-a-days small quantities of high activity wastes are converted into solids such as concrete and then it is buried underground or sea (Concentrate and contain).

Control Measures

- Laboratory generated nuclear wastes should be disposed off safely and scientifically.
- Nuclear power plants should be located in areas after careful study of the geology of the area, tectonic activity and meeting other established conditions.
- Appropriate protection against occupational exposure.
- Leakage of radioactive elements from nuclear reactors, careless use of radioactive elements as fuel and careless handling of radioactive isotopes must be prevented.
- Safety measure against accidental release of radioactive elements must be ensured in nuclear plants.
- Unless absolutely necessary, one should not frequently go for diagnosis by X-rays.
- Regular monitoring of the presence of radioactive substance in high risk area should be ensured.

Among the many options for waste disposal, the scientists prefer to bury the waste in hundreds of meters deep in the earth's crust is considered to be the best safety long-term option.

GLOBAL ENVIRONMENTAL PROBLEMS

Climate refers to the usual weather of a place. Climate differs from season to season, from region to region. A combination of all the climates of the world is termed as the Earth's climate.

Climate Change

Climate change is real, and the evidence is all around us. While the changes to the earth's climate are nothing new, it is apparent recent effects are having a devastating impact on countless people, places, and wildlife. If you want to know what climate change really is and why it matters, then keep reading to learn more about its causes, effects, and practical solutions to stopping it.

Concept of Climate Change

- Climate change refers to a change or changes in the usual weather condition found in a place or region.
- Changes could be experienced in the rainfall or snowfall pattern, temperature, etc. Climate change is also a change in Earth's climate.
- Climate change is now a much-discussed concept around the globe.
- It is because it is now experienced that the world temperature is increasing during these years.
- The global average surface temperature is believed to have increased by 0.6 + 0.2°C over the last century. Globally, 1998 was the warmest year and the 1990s was the warmest decade on record.

- Many countries have experienced increases in rainfall, particularly in the countries situated in the mid to high latitudes.
- In some regions, such as parts of Asia and Africa, the frequency and intensity of droughts have been observed to increase in recent decades.
- Episodes of El Nino, which creates great storms, have been more frequent, persistent, and intense since mid-1970s compared with the previous 100 years.
- All these signs show that the earth's climate is changing, making it more difficult for mankind to survive.

Causes of Climate Change

- Climate changes on its own in nature. Earth's distance from the sun, volcanic eruption at large scale, heavy rainfall for longer period, are the instances of natural phenomena that influence the Earth's climate.
- These are natural and have nothing to do with our present concern about climate change.
- What concerns us today is the rise in global temperature, especially. Most scientists say that human activities have caused certain changes in the natural climate of the earth.
- Most scientists agree that the main cause of current global warming is human expansion of the 'greenhouse effect'.
- Greenhouse effect is the increase in the number of certain gases that include carbon dioxide (CO_2), methane, nitrous oxide (N_2O), water vapor, chlorofluorocarbons (CFCs), etc.
- Greenhouse gases are produced naturally and trap heat in the Earth's atmosphere like a blanket.
- When there is increased concentration of such gases in the atmosphere mostly by burning fossil fuels, there is a proportionate increase in the temperature of the Earth's atmosphere. It is called global warming.

Significant human-led factors responsible for climate change are:
- Exponential growth in human population.
- Massive and unplanned urbanization and industrialization over the last century.
- Burning of fossil fuels such as coal, petroleum, and natural gas at huge scale to meet the growing energy needs of the bulging world population.
- Change in lifestyle and massive increase in the number of machinery, gadgets, etc.

Impact of Climate Change on Human Environment

- It is now clear that climate change causes unwanted alterations in the natural systems.
- The environmental consequences of climate change are extreme heat waves, rising sea levels, changes in precipitation resulting in flooding and droughts, intense hurricanes, and degraded air quality.
- The above phenomenal changes directly and indirectly affect the physical, social, and psychological health of human beings.

Frequency in Weather-related Disasters

- Changes in precipitation create changes in the availability and quantity of water and also results in extreme weather events, such as intense storms, flooding and droughts.
- Frequency in all these weather phenomena sometimes lead to human causality in great proportion apart from huge loss of property, mostly in developing and underdeveloped countries.

Human Health

- Climate change affects the prerequisites of human health such as clean air and water, sufficient and healthy food, natural constraints to infectious disease agents and the adequacy and security of shelter.
- The report of the WHO Commission on Social Determinants of Health points out that disadvantaged communities are likely to shoulder a disproportionate share of the burden of climate change because of their increased exposure and vulnerability to health threats.

Large Scale Displacement of People

- Climate change affects such as desertification, rising sea levels and severity of weather related disasters along with the spread of epidemics can destroy or affect human habitation causing people to seek shelter elsewhere.
- Deteriorating environment and depleting resources can result in human conflicts at all levels.
- The Intergovernmental Panel on Climate Change (IPCC) has estimated that there will be over 150 million environmental migrants by 2050 and the number will be perplexing due to complexity of the issue and lack of data.

Apart from the above, following are some other consequences of climate change:
- Change in hydrological cycle and water supply
- The Inter-Tropical Convergence Zone (ITCZ) may move northward in the northern hemisphere causing rapid changes in rainfall pattern.
- Increase in tropical and temperate cyclones, cloud cover, tornadoes and storms.
- Changes in pressure belts and atmospheric circulation
- Warming of ocean water may endanger the corals worldwide
- Expansion of deserts and more desertification within deserts.
- Effect on food supply and international trade of grains.
- National parks, sanctuaries and biosphere reserves may be altered.
- Countries such as Maldives and greater parts of Netherlands etc. may submerge under water.
- Climate change is making food crops less nutritious. Rising carbon dioxide emissions lead to iron and zinc deficiencies in food crops.

GLOBAL WARMING

Global warming occurs when carbon dioxide (CO_2) and other air pollutants and greenhouse gases collect in the atmosphere and absorb sunlight and solar radiation that have bounced off the earth's surface. Normally, this radiation would escape into space—but these pollutants, which can last for years to centuries in the atmosphere, trap the heat and cause the planet to get hotter. That's what's known as the greenhouse effect.

Global Warming Causes

Global warming is a serious issue and is not a single issue but a number of environmental issues. Global warming is a rise in the surface temperature of the earth that has changed various life forms on the earth. The issues that cause global warming are divided into two categories include "natural" and "human influences" of global warming.

Global warming is primarily a problem of too much carbon dioxide (CO_2) in the atmosphere—which acts as a blanket, trapping heat and warming the planet. As we burn fossil fuels like coal, oil and natural gas for energy or cut down and burn forests to create pastures and plantations, carbon accumulates and overloads our atmosphere. Certain waste management and agricultural practices aggravate the problem by releasing other potent global warming gases, such as methane and nitrous oxide.

Natural Causes of Global Warming

- The climate has continuously changing for centuries. The global warming happens because the natural rotation of the sun that changes the intensity of sunlight and moving closer to the earth.
- Another cause of global warming is greenhouse gases. Greenhouse gases are carbon monoxide and sulphur dioxide it trap the solar heats rays and prevent it from escaping from the surface of the earth. This has caused the temperature of the earth increase.
- Volcanic eruptions are another issue that causes global warming. For instance, a single volcanic eruption will release amount of carbon dioxide and ash to the atmosphere. Once carbon dioxide increase, the temperature of earth increase and greenhouse trap the solar radiations in the earth.
- Finally, methane is another issue that causes global warming. Methane is also a greenhouse gas. Methane is more effective in trapping heat in the atmosphere that carbon dioxide by 20 times.

Human Influences on Global Warming: Human influence has been a very serious issue now because human do not take care the earth. Human that cause global warming are more than natural causes global warming. The earth has been changing for many years until now it is still changing because of modern lifestyle of human. Human activities include industrial production, burning fossil fuel, mining, cattle rearing or deforestation.

Effect of Global Warming

- The greenhouse gases will stay in the atmosphere for many years since hundreds years ago. However, the effect that global warming will cause on earth are extremely serious.
- There are many effects that will happen in the future if global warming continues. That includes polar ice caps melting, economic consequences, warmer waters and more hurricanes, spread of diseases and earthquake.
- First effect is polar ice caps melting. As the temperature increase, the ice at the North Pole will melt. Once the ice melt the first effect will be raise on sea levels because the melting glaciers become oceans.
- Another effect is the species loss of habitat. Species that include polar bears and tropical frogs will be extinct due to climate change. Besides, various birds will migrate to other places because animals are not like humans. They cannot adapt the habitat that changes their living or temperature.
- Next effect is more hurricanes will occur and economic consequences still affect as well. Hurricane causes damage to houses and government need to spend billions of dollars in damage and people need places to stay or have been killed. Once a disaster happens many people have died and diseases happen.
- Diseases are more serious because it can spread to other people very fast and more people will get the disease and the disease maybe come more serious because of different weather.

Solution to Stop Global Warming

- Now there are solutions that we can stop global warming. However, we human and governments need to move forward to implement the global warming solutions.
- To reduce global warming we can do to reduce the contribution of greenhouse gases to the atmosphere. Therefore, the solutions that we can reduce global warming are reducing gasoline, electricity and our activities that cause global warming.
- To reduce gasoline mean we have a choice to choose a hybrid car that reduce using gasoline. Besides, petrol price are increasing. If a person everyday drives to work they need to pump petrol after 3 days and causes carbon dioxide.
- Another way to reduce gasoline is taken public transport or carpool to work. It can help reduce carbon dioxide and save cost.
- Another way to reduce global warming is recycle. Recycle can reduce garbage by reusing plastic bags, bottles, papers or glass. For instance, when we buy foods, we can use our own containers instead of plastic bags.
- Another example is after finish drinking the water from the bottle; we can reuse it or use our own bottle. If all this is being reuse, human can reduce deforestation and help save environment. Besides, turn off electricity if unused.
- It can save thousands of carbon dioxide and buy product that have energy saving because it saves cost and save environment.
- Finally, human should stop open burning such as burning dry leafs or burning garbage. It will release carbon

dioxide and toxic if burning garbage with plastic. Besides, government should reduce deforestation because the earth temperatures are increasing. Trees will help to improve the temperature on earth.

HAZARDOUS WASTE MANAGEMENT

Hazardous waste (HW) is defined as any substance, in solid, liquid or gaseous form, which has no use in future and which causes danger or is likely to cause danger to health and environment.

The hazardous waste requires to be disposed of in a secured manner in view of their characteristic properties. When HWs are not used efficiently by the waste generators, they cause severe pollution of land, surface, and ground water.

Components of Hazardous Waste Management

- Identification of hazardous waste generation by industries and other sources.
- Characterization of hazardous waste pertaining to physical, chemical, and general characteristics and properties pertaining to ignitability, corrosiveness, reactivity and toxicity.
- Quantification of hazardous waste in order to facilitate safe disposal.
- Identification of sites for disposal.
- Environmental impact assessment should be conducted and public acceptance should be accepted for the sites.
- Hazardous waste management rules are notified to ensure safe handling, generation, processing, treatment, package, storage, transportation, use reprocessing, collection, conversion, and offering for sale, destruction, and disposal of hazardous waste.

Proper treatment, storage prior to treatment or disposal of hazardous waste is the need of the hour. Governments should make provisions for and prepare guidelines for the industries and other hazardous waste generating sources for safe disposal or treatment of hazardous waste.

WASTEWATER MANAGEMENT

Wastewater refers to any water that is not clean or is adversely affected in quality by human-induced activities. Wastewater originates from a combination of domestic, industrial, commercial, or agricultural activities.

Wastewater treatment or **management** refers to the processes used to convert wastewater into an effluent that can be either returned to the water cycle with negligible environmental impact or can be reused.

The major objective of wastewater treatment is generally to allow human and industrial effluents to be disposed of without danger to human health or unacceptable damage to the natural environment.

Wastewater Treatment Process

Phase separation: It transfers impurities into a non-aqueous phase.

Sedimentation: Sedimentation is a physical water treatment process using gravity to remove suspended solids from water. Solid particles entrained by the turbulence of moving water may be removed naturally by sedimentation in the still water of lakes and oceans.

Filtration: Suspension of fine solids may be removed by filtration through physical barriers such as coarser screens or sieves.

Oxidation: This process diminishes the biochemical oxygen demand of wastewater and may reduce the toxicity of some impurities. Advanced oxidation processes (AOPs) are a set of chemical treatment of wastewater purported to remove organic and also inorganic materials in waste water by oxidation through reaction with hydroxyl radicals.

Chemical oxidation may remove some persistent organic pollutants and concentrations remaining after biochemical oxidation.

Wastewater treatment plants are set up for effective treatment of wastewater. They may be distinguished by the type of wastewater to be treated. They are as follows:
- Sewage treatment plants
- Industrial wastewater treatment plants
- Agricultural wastewater treatment plants.

POPULATION EXPLOSION AND ITS PRESSURE ON ENVIRONMENT

Finite Resources

- Most resources being finite since the very beginning and natural limit to resource generation being slow, constant rise in the number of people on the earth exerts undue pressure on world resources.
- Population growth and the resultant increase in human habitations in the last couple of centuries has taken away a considerable portion of natural vegetation, cultivable lands, and above all the natural habitats of wild animals.
- There has been loss of biodiversity and resultant ecological imbalance in severity in the current times.

More People, More Demand, More Waste

- With the advent of science and technology man's need for comfort and luxury has multiplied many times.
- This has necessitated the production of a great number of goods and services in the world.
- Not only the huge population (7.4 billion in 2016), but also the lifestyle, consumption patterns in modern time directly affect the environment.
- More people demand more resources and generate more waste.
- Clearly one of the challenges of a growing population is that the mere presence of so many people sharing a limited number of resources strains the environment.

Rapid Urbanization and Industrialization

- Rapid urbanization and industrialization during the last century in most part of the world has not only destroyed

a substantial part of natural vegetation but also forced many wild animals on the verge of extinction.
- Apart from the pressure on the resources due to high growth in population, technological and scientific innovations, rapid rise in automobile population, electronic gadgets, machinery and equipment have added a great number of pollutants to the environment. As a result, environmental degradation has risen to an irrecoverable level.
- Developed countries where the levels of consumption are high add more to pollution than other countries.
- A child born in a country, where the levels of material and energy use are high, places a greater burden on the earth's resources than a child born in a poorer country.
- Nonetheless, sustainable development can be pursued more easily when population size is stabilized at a level consistent with the productive capacity of the ecosystem.

Crazy Consumerism

- Consumption, although necessary for the economy, can be hazardous to the environment.
- Consumerism is a social and economic order that supports and encourages the acquisition of goods and services in ever increasing amounts.
- Man has developed an unprecedented craze for a mushrooming number of products and services available in the world market.
- This has been aggravated by improved marketing strategies, alluring advertisements, and consumer-friendly services offered by companies and outlets.
- Approximately 2 billion people belonging to the "consumer class" are characterized by desire for processed food, desire for bigger houses, cars, durables, etc. to maintain their desired lifestyles.
- Consumerism has become more acute in developing countries such as India and China than that in developed countries due to the rise in population in the former.

Reasons for Crazy Consumerism

- Growing materialistic tendencies among the modern man.
- Easy access to markets due to faster development in transport and communication.
- Effective marketing and advertising strategies.
- Rising income levels in most part of the world.
- Globalization and liberalization.
- Rapid rise in income generation ways.
- Greed to possess more and more.

Impact of Crazy Consumerism

- Increasing consumerism has led to excessive production of goods and services, which in turn has led to enormous pressure on natural environment and natural resources.
- Resource depletion, environmental degradation, and pollution have become the order of the day.
- Mankind has reached the height of environmental pollution from where it seems very difficult to return.
- Race for comfort and luxury has vitiated the environment disproportionately.
- Excessive demand for consumer products has created most of the current environmental imbalances and these imbalances have already caused ecological disaster in different places all over the world.
- Consumerism has resulted in heaps of waste in urban and also in rural areas which lead to a pollution of environment.
- Mounting e-waste in the world, especially in developed countries, is causing more harm to the environment.
- Popularity of plastic for various purposes is adding severely to air, water, and land pollution.

OZONE DEPLETION

Ozone is a form of oxygen in which three atoms of oxygen combine to form a single molecule of ozone. It is normally not found in the lower atmosphere. It exists in the stratosphere between 20 and 50 kilometers above the surface.

- The presence of ozone is of singular importance because it filters out the incoming ultraviolet (UV) radiation and thus acts as a screen against ultraviolent radiation that can increase the occurrence of skin cancer, cataracts, and other diseases of eyes.
- It also affects the body defense mechanism, which increases the vulnerability of infectious diseases.
- Increased ultraviolet radiation can seriously affect plant and fish production.

Ozone depletion refers to the wearing out or reduction of the amount of ozone in the stratosphere. It was first identified in 1970s due to the advent of supersonic aircraft, which fly in the lower stratosphere and emit nitrogen oxides.

Ozone Depleting Substances

- Ozone depleting substances are those substances which deplete the ozone layer.
- It is found that the major cause of ozone depletions is the CFC (Chlorofluorocarbons) gases.
- CFCs are used for a wide range of applications including refrigerant, foaming agents, plastic manufacturing, fire extinguishing agents, solvents for freezing food, cleaners for electronic components fine retardant, solvents, aerosol, propellants, and the production of foamed plastics.

Other ozone depleting substances controlled by Montreal Protocol (discussed in a subsequent chapter) are:
- Halon
- Carbon tetrachloride (CCl_4), methyl chloroform (CH_3CCl_3)
- Hydrobromofluorocarbons (HBFCs)
- Hydrochlorofluorocarbons (HCFCs)
- Methyl bromide (CH_3Br)
- Bromochloromethane (CH_2BrCl)

There are serious consequences of ozone depletion. The following are some of the significant consequences of ozone depletion:

- Plants and animals vary in their tolerance of ultraviolet rays. The ultraviolet rays damage DNA (the genetic code in every living being). Crops such as soybean are the worst affected.
- Animals and humans also have adapted to UVB radiation. In case of depletion of the ozone layer, there is danger of melanoma—a type of skin cancer. The disease is now almost epidemic in the United States.

POLICY AND LEGISLATION

In the previous chapters, we have learnt about the environment, ecosystem, natural resources, biodiversity and its importance for the living world, especially for mankind. We have also learnt how environmental problems such as pollution and climate change affect and threaten our survival. There is a need for knowing the legal and constitutional provisions for protecting and nurturing the nature. In this chapter, we will learn about such provisions and acts.

Need for Policy and Legislation

- It has always been the desire of man to have clean air, clean water and environment free of toxins and pollutants. In the first half of the last century, there were few legal and constitutional mechanisms in place to protect the environment and the natural resources found in a country.
- Increasing pollution and mounting pressure on air, water and land quality led to environmental legislations being designed to protect the environment from harmful actions.
- Due to the current state of the environment, policy makers in every country need to place a top priority on environmental policy.
- Natural resources, both renewable and non-renewable and wildlife are continuously being under threat.
- It is estimated that considering the present rate of exploitation of such resources we are going to be devoid of many important resources in near future.
- Unless we take care of them and resort to a sustainable use, we will make our posterity live without resources. Hence, there is a need for environmental policies and legislations.

Environmental Policy

- Policy refers to a set of principles or plans agreed upon by a government or an organization to be carried out in a particular situation.
- Environmental policy is defined as "any action deliberately taken to manage human activities with a view to prevent, reduce, or mitigate harmful effects on nature and natural resources, and to ensure that man-made changes to the environment do not have harmful effects on human or the environment".
- Environmental policy usually covers air and water pollution, waste management, ecosystem management, biodiversity protection, and the protection of natural resources, wildlife and endangered species.
- Proper policies and legislations at the national and the international levels can reduce the venomous pollution and help protect biodiversity and natural resources.

Environmental Legislation

- Environmental legislation is a set of laws and regulations which aim at protecting the environment from harmful actions.
- Legislation may take many forms, including regulation of emissions that may lead to environmental pollution, taxation of environment- and health-damaging activities, and establishing the legal framework for trading schemes, for example, carbon emissions.
- Other actions may rely on voluntary agreements. Among major current legislative frameworks are those relating to environmental permitting, and those mandating environment and health impact assessments?

Environmental Protection Act

- Most of the countries in the world have enacted Environmental Protection Acts considering the need for the protection of our environment.
- In the US, the National Environmental Policy Act (NEPA) of 1970 promotes the enhancement of the environment and established the President's Council on Environmental Quality (CEQ).
- It is referred to as the 'Environmental Magna Carta' in the USA because it was an early step towards the development of US' environmental policy. Other environmental acts in the USA are as follows:
  - Clean Air Act of 1970 and 1990
  - Clean Water Act of 1972
  - Endangered Species Act of 1973
  - Resource Conservation and Recovery Act of 1976
  - National Forest Management Act of 1976
  - Surface Mining Control and Reclamation Act of 1977
  - Comprehensive Environmental Response, Compensation and Liability Act of 1980.

Environmental Protection Acts in India

In the Constitution of India, it is clearly stated that it is the duty of the state to 'protect and improve the environment and to safeguard the forests and wildlife of the country'. It imposes a duty on every citizen 'to protect and improve the natural environment including forests, lakes, rivers, and wildlife'. There are a number of environmental acts enacted in India. Some of the important legislations in this respect are:

- Wildlife Protection Act, 1972
- Forest (Conservation) Act, 1980
- Water (Prevention and Control of Pollution) Act, 1974
- The Air (Prevention and Control of Pollution) Act, 1981
- Environmental Protection Act, 1986
- Handling and Management of Hazardous Waste Rules, 1989

- The National Environmental Tribunal Act, 1995
- The Biological Diversity Act, 2002.

Environmental Protection Act, 1986

- Environmental Protection Act, 1986, was a statutory response that came into effect a year after the tragic Bhopal Gas Tragedy and is considered an umbrella legislation as it addresses many loopholes in the existing environmental laws.
- It was enacted as per the spirit of the Stockholm Conference held in June 1972 to take suitable measures for the protection and reinvigoration of environment and related matters.
- The Environment (Protection) Act is applicable to whole of India including Jammu and Kashmir. It came into force on November 19, 1986. EPA 1986 was enacted largely to implement the decisions made at the UN Conference on Human Environment held at Stockholm in June, 1972.
- It was to coordinate the activities of the various regulatory agencies under the existing laws.
- It also seeks collection and dissemination of information on environmental pollution.
- A lot have been done to protect and improve the environment world over. However much remains to be done for building a sustainable society.
- New mechanisms are being put in place to expedite the process of protecting and improving the environment.
- For example, new institutions—the National Environment Management Authority (NEMA) and the State Environment Management Authorities (SEMA)—in India have been proposed as full-time technical organizations with the capacity to process all environmental clearance applications in a time-bound manner.

Acts Related to Air Pollution

- **The Factories Act and Amendment, 1948** was the first to express concern for the working environment of the workers. The amendment of 1987 has sharpened its environmental focus and expanded its application to hazardous processes.
- **The Air (Prevention and Control of Pollution) Act, 1981** provides for the control and abatement of air pollution. It entrusts the power of enforcing this act to the Central Pollution Control Board (CPCB).
- **The Air (Prevention and Control of Pollution) Rules, 1982** defines the procedures of the meetings of the Boards and the powers entrusted to them.
- **The Atomic Energy Act, 1982** deals with radioactive waste.
- **The Air (Prevention and Control of Pollution) Amendment Act, 1987** empowers the central and state pollution control boards to meet with grave emergencies of air pollution.
- **The Motor Vehicles Act, 1988** states that all hazardous waste is to be properly packaged, labeled, and transported.

Acts Related to Water Pollution

- **The Indian Fisheries Act, 1897**—establishes two sets of penal offences whereby the government can sue any person who uses dynamite or other explosive substance in any way (whether coastal or inland) with the intent to catch or destroy any fish, or poisonous fish in order to kill.
- **The River Boards Act, 1956**—enables the states to enroll the central government in setting up an Advisory River Board to resolve issues in inter-state cooperation.
- **The Merchant Shipping Act, 1970**—aims to deal with waste arising from ships along the coastal areas within a specified radius.
- **The Water (Prevention and Control of Pollution) Act, 1974**—establishes an institutional structure for preventing and abating water pollution. It establishes standards for water quality and effluent. Polluting industries must seek permission to discharge waste into effluent bodies. The CPCB (Central Pollution Control Board) was constituted under this Act.
- **The Water (Prevention and Control of Pollution) Cess Act, 1977**—provides for the levy and collection of cess or fees on water consuming industries and local authorities.
- **The Water (Prevention and Control of Pollution) Cess Rules, 1978**—contains the standard definitions and indicates the kind of and location of meters that every consumer of water is required to affix.
- **The Coastal Regulation Zone, 1991**—notification puts regulations on various activities, including construction. It gives some protection to the backwaters and estuaries.

Acts Related to Forests

- **The Indian Forest Act and Amendment, 1984**—is one of the many surviving colonial statutes. It was enacted to 'consolidate the law related to forest, the transit of forest produce, and the duty to be levied on timber and other forest produce'.
- **The Wildlife Protection Act and Rules, 1973**—and Amendment 1991 provides for the protection of birds and animals and for all matters that are connected to it, whether it be their habitat or the waterhole or the forests that sustain them.
- **The Forest (Conservation) Act and Rules, 1981**, provides for the protection of and the conservation of the forests.
- **The Biological Diversity Act, 2002** is an act to provide for the conservation of biological diversity, sustainable use of its components, and fair and equitable sharing of the benefits arising out of the use of biological resources and knowledge associated with it.

TOWARDS SUSTAINABLE FUTURE

According to the United Nations, "Sustainable development is the development that meets the needs of the present without compromising the ability of future generations to meet their own needs." Sustainable development requires meeting the basic needs of all and aims to provide all the opportunity to meet their aspirations to lead a better and healthy life.

Concept of Sustainable Development

Our living standards should be in tune with the limit of the world's ecological means. However, many of us live beyond it and have scant regard for long-term sustainability. Economic growth and development is required to be in commensurate with the limits of the ecology and environment. It is required largely by the sustainable development.

- Sustainable development requires setting limits in terms of population or resource use beyond which lies ecological disaster.
- It warns every one of us against surpassing the ultimate limits of the natural system, or else face dire consequences.
- It also requires that long before mankind crosses these limits, the world must ensure equitable access to the constrained resource and use technology towards it.
- Economic growth and development obviously involve changes in the physical ecosystem. However, it should not cross the limits of regeneration and natural growth.
- For instance, renewable resources such as forests and fish stocks need not be depleted provided the rate of use is within the limits of regeneration and natural growth.
- Sustainable development requires that the rate of depletion of non-renewable resources should foreclose as few future options as possible.
- It requires flourishing biodiversity and, hence, it vouches for the conservation of plant and animal species.
- It also vouches for a type of development where the adverse impacts on the quality of air, water, and other natural elements are minimized so as to sustain the ecosystem's overall integrity.
- Sustainable development is a wholesome process of change in which the use of resources, investment, the orientation of technological development and institutional changes are all in harmony with and enhance both the current and future potential to meet human needs and aspirations.

17 NEW UNDEVELOPMENT GOALS FOR 2030

1. End poverty in all its forms everywhere.
2. End hunger, achieve food security and improved nutrition, and promote sustainable agriculture.
3. Ensure healthy lives and promote well-being for all at all ages.
4. Ensure inclusive and equitable quality education and promote lifelong learning opportunities for all.
5. Achieve gender equality and empower all women and girls.
6. Ensure availability and sustainable management of water and sanitation for all.
7. Ensure access to affordable, reliable, sustainable and modern energy for all.
8. Promote inclusive and sustainable economic growth, full and productive employment, and decent work for all.
9. Build resilient infrastructure, promote inclusive and sustainable industrialization, and foster innovation.
10. Reduce inequality within and among countries.
11. Make cities and human settlements inclusive, safe, resilient, and sustainable.
12. Ensure sustainable consumption and production patterns.
13. Take urgent action to combat climate change and its impact.
14. Conserve and sustainably use the oceans, seas, and marine resources for sustainable development.
15. Protect, restore, and promote sustainable use of terrestrial ecosystems, sustainably manage forests, combat desertification, halt and reverse land degradation, and halt biodiversity loss.
16. Promote peaceful and inclusive societies for sustainable development, provide access to justice for all and build effective, accountable, and inclusive institutions at all levels.
17. Strengthen the means of implementation and revitalize the global partnership for sustainable development.

The new goals replace the eight Millennium Development Goals adopted at a Summit in 2000, which expired at the end of 2015.

ENVIRONMENTAL EDUCATION

- Environmental education is a multi-disciplinary field integrating disciplines such as biology, chemistry, physics, ecology, earth science, atmospheric science, mathematics, and geography.
- Environmental education (EE) aims at increasing the consciousness and knowledge about the various aspects of environment and also about the major environmental problems facing the world today.
- It also spreads awareness among the masses with special emphasis on educators, voluntary works, youth and women with a view to promote conservation of nature and its resources.
- It develops and makes room for implementation of innovative, region-specific educational programs and materials for conservation education and sensitizes children on environment.
- It includes all efforts to make general public aware of the knowledge of the environmental challenges through media and print materials.
- UNESCO (United Nation Educational, Scientific, and Cultural Organization) emphasizes the role of EE in safeguarding future global developments of societal quality of life (QOL), through the protection of the environment, eradication of poverty, minimization of inequalities, and insurance of sustainable development.
- Today, environmental education has become one of the most popular academic study world-over. There are special institutions coming up in the world to impart higher degrees on environmental education.

Environmental Health and Sanitation (Fig. 14.10)

- Concept of environment health and sanitation.
- Concept of safe water, sources of water, waterborne diseases, water purification processes, household purification of water.

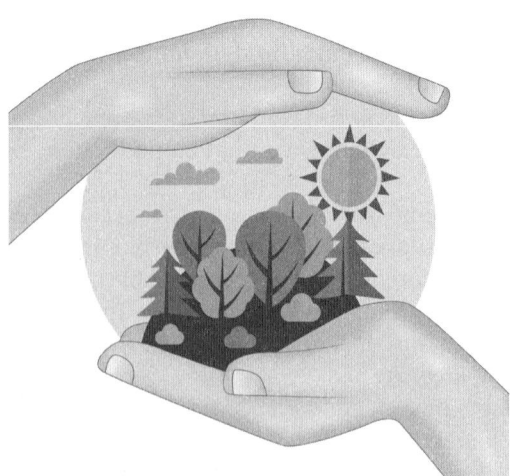

Fig. 14.10: Environmental heath.

- Physical and chemical standards of drinking water quality and tests for assessing bacteriological quality of water.
- Concepts of water conservation—rainwater harvesting and water shed management.
- Concept of pollution prevention—air and noise pollution, Role of nurse in prevention of pollution.
- Solid waste management, human excreta disposal and management and sewage disposal and management.
- Commonly used insecticides and pesticides.

CONCEPT OF ENVIRONMENTAL HEALTH AND SANITATION

Environmental health is broader than hygiene and sanitation; it encompasses hygiene, sanitation and many other aspects of the environment that are not included in this module such as global warming, climate change, radiation, gene technology, flooding and natural disasters. It also involves studying the environmental factors that affect health.

Definitions

The World Health Organization's definition is as follows:
- Environmental health addresses all the physical, chemical, and biological factors external to a person, and all the related factors impacting behaviors. It encompasses the assessment and control of those environmental factors that can potentially affect health.
- Hygiene generally refers to the set of practices associated with the preservation of health and healthy living. The focus is mainly on personal hygiene that looks at cleanliness of the hair, body, hands, fingers, feet and clothing, and menstrual hygiene.
- Sanitation means the prevention of human contact with wastes, for hygienic purposes. It also means promoting health through the prevention of human contact with the hazards associated with the lack of healthy food, clean water and healthful housing, the control of **vectors** (living organisms that transmit diseases), and a clean environment.

Factors Affecting Environmental Health

- **Population explosion:** The rapid increase in our population is having harmful and unfavorable effect on our environment. It is creating problems due to overcrowding, depletion of natural resources and development of man made resources by industrialization, green revolution etc. Increasing population is also creating slum partially due to its natural growth and partially due to its migration from rural areas to urban areas in search employment.
- **Industrialization:** The industries have multiplied not only in magnitude but also in variety. All the industries generate loss of waste product such as gases, effluents, solid matters thermal waste, etc. these wastes often are released directly into the air, rivers, streams, and drain on the land which deteriorate our environment and cause harmful effects on human health.
- **Urbanization:** People from village migrate to town and cities for employment, education, etc., resulting in overcrowding and slums most of the time on unauthorized land. This situation not only creates administrative problems but also adverse effects on environment and results in many physical, mental and social health problems.
- **Modern agricultural practices:** Chemical fertilizers are used to increase agricultural production for meeting agricultural demands of ever increasing population, in addition insecticides are added and sprayed to destroy pests and micro organisms it also causes harmful effects of living organisms.
- **Deforestation;** Deforestation refers to reducing, removing of forest. Deforestation is there because of fire wood required by human being, demand on wood construction of houses, building, industries, dams, roads and highways and expansion of land for cultivation. Deforestation also reduced the amount of cultivation. Deforestation also reduces the amount of water being transferred from the ground to the air because of reduced trees. This phenomenon is causing change in the climate. All these situations have adverse effect on the environment health.
- **Radioactive substances:** The radioactive substances are used in the laboratories, hospitals and power plants, where nuclear bombs are manufactured. Some of the radioactive wastes from nuclear power plants are discharged directly into the air and water and pollute these.
- **Natural calamities:** Natural calamities are grave disasters of misfortune of great magnitude which occur by nature cause, disruption of the environment. These calamities include floods, earthquakes, droughts, cyclones, volcanoes, landslides, avalanches and tidal waves in the seas.

Chapter 14: National Health Problems

Dimensions of Environmental Sanitation

Environmental sanitation is (a) the promotion of hygiene and, (b) the prevention of disease and other consequences of ill-health, relating to environmental factors. Environmental sanitation cover two basic dimensions:

Environmental factors: These are environmental factors which impact on the infectious agents and transmission of disease. These include:
- Disposal of human excreta
- Sewage
- Household waste and other waste likely to contain infectious agents
- Water drainage
- Domestic water supply
- Housing

Sanitation Practices

These are various hygienic practices of the communities, basic knowledge, skills and human behaviors as well as social and cultural factors concerning health, life-styles and environmental awareness. These include:
- Personal hygiene (washing, dressing, eating, etc.)
- Household cleanliness (kitchen, bathroom cleanliness, etc.)
- Community cleanliness (waste collection, common places, etc.)

Environmental sanitation strongly depends on social and cultural practices and beliefs and these have to be considered when planning interventions.

Components of Hygiene and Environmental Health

Description	Concerns
Personal hygiene	Hygiene of body and clothing
Water supply	Adequacy, safety (chemical, bacteriological, physical) of water for domestic, drinking and recreational use
Human waste disposal	Proper excreta disposal and liquid waste management
Solid waste management	Proper application of storage, collection, disposal of waste. Waste production and recycling
Vector control	Control of mammals (such as rats) and arthropods (insects such as flies and other creatures such as mites) that transmit disease
Food hygiene	Food safety and wholesomeness in its production, storage, preparation, distribution and sale, until consumption
Healthful housing	Physiological needs, protection against disease and accidents, psychological and social comforts in residential and recreational areas
Institutional hygiene	Communal hygiene in schools, prisons, health facilities, refugee camps, detention homes and settlement areas
Water pollution	Sources, characteristics, impact and mitigation
Occupational hygiene	Hygiene and safety in the workplace

Types of Sanitation

Sanitation means the prevention of human contact with wastes, for hygienic purposes. It also means promoting health through the prevention of human contact with the hazards associated with the lack of healthy food, clean water and healthful housing, the control of **vectors** (living organisms that transmit diseases), and a clean environment. It focuses on management of waste produced by human activities. There are different types of sanitation relating to particular situations, such as:

- **Basic sanitation:** It refers to the management of human feces at the household level. It means access to a toilet or latrine.
- **Onsite sanitation:** The collection and treatment of waste at the place where it is deposited.
- **Food sanitation:** It refers to the hygienic measures for ensuring food safety. Food hygiene is similar to food sanitation.
- **Housing sanitation:** It refers to safeguarding the home environment (the dwelling and its immediate environment).
- **Environmental sanitation:** The control of environmental factors that form links in disease transmission. This category includes solid waste management, water and wastewater treatment, industrial waste treatment and noise and pollution control.
- **Ecological sanitation:** The concept of recycling the nutrients from human and animal wastes to the environment.

Health Hazards of Environment

- **Danger of ozone depletion:** Atmospheric ozone absorbs ultraviolet range (260–320 nm) and plants and animals from its damaging effects, loss of ozone from the earth's outer atmosphere can bring ozone from the earth's outer atmosphere can bring about serious consequences for human health. Potential direct health effects are erythema (sunburn), Keratitis (acute), skin cancer and cataracts (chronic). Potential indirect health effects are increased susceptibility to cutaneous infection and carcinogenesis.
- **Effects of dust on health:** Dust contains particles of the size ranging from 1 to 200 microns. Dust particles less than 5 microns can get through nose and throat and are carried down to lungs, while some dusts are not harmful, fibrous dust particles causes' ill health.
- **Disease caused due to water pollution:** The diseases caused by direct transmission are cholera, typhoid fever, salmonella infections, hepatitis, diarrhea, schistosomiasis, amoebic dysentery, typhoid fever, etc. are some of the directly transmitted human diseases due to water pollution. Indirectly transmitted diseases are malaria, yellow fever, dengue, encephalitis, filariasis, onchocerciasis, schistosomiasis, etc.
- **Noise pollution and health effects:** Noise can disturb people's work, rest sleep and communication. It can damage hearing and produce psychological, physiological and at times pathological reactions. Noise can induce

stress in the form of high blood pressure, fatigue and irritability.
- **Radiation and health effects:** The diseases that is likely due to radioactive pollution are lung cancer, secondary cancer leukemia, etc. Bones, lung thyroid, lens of the eye skin, etc. are some of the human organs which are affected by the radiation.
- **Pesticide pollution and health effects:** Today people all over the world are facing the health hazards caused by extensive and persistent use of pesticides. Besides widespread poisoning of wildlife and livestock, pesticides take a heavy toll on human lives. It is feared that the death rate from pesticides poisoning is more than the death rate of infectious diseases like polio, diphtheria, tetanus, etc.

Strategies to Improve Environmental Sanitation

- Sanitation needs to be addressed as a whole, including improvement of facilities, environmental conditions and behavioral change;
- Sanitation programs should be demand-based and the community should be fully involved in the process;
- High risk group should be identified for better targeting of funds and efforts;
- Sanitation should be a component of other health-promoting or disease control programs;
- Awareness needs to be raised and sanitation set as a priority in national and local governments, and also in the population at large;
- Systems have to be sustainable; cost-sharing and cost-recovery need to be addressed carefully.

WHO's Role

- Assess health impacts of various elements of environmental sanitation;
- Assess effectiveness of existing environmental sanitation programs;
- Assess the health and socioeconomic benefits of environmental sanitation interventions on the basis of preventable burden of disease and their cost-effectiveness;
- Identify efficient interventions;
- Identify research and development needs;
- Identify high risk groups;
- Direct interventions to groups most in need.

Role of Environmental Health in Public Health

Environmental health is a part of public health where the primary goal is preventing disease and promoting people's health. Environmental health is associated with recognizing, assessing, understanding and controlling the impacts of people on their environment and the impacts of the environment on the public. The role of the environmental health worker, therefore, includes the following functions of public health:

- Improving human health and protecting it from environmental hazards.
- Developing liaison between the community and the local authority, and between the local and higher levels of administration.
- Acting independently to provide advice on environmental health matters; designing and developing plans of action for environmental health.
- Initiating and implementing health/hygiene, sanitation and environmental programs to promote understanding of environmental health principles.
- Enforcing environmental legislation.
- Monitoring and evaluating environmental health activities, programs and projects.

CONCEPT OF SAFE WATER

Man's life in the universe or on the moon will be impossible without water that is prime necessity of life. The 34th World Health Assembly in a resolution emphasized that safe drinking water is a basic element of "Primary healthcare" which is the key to the attainment of "health for all" by the year 2000 AD. Water is also integrated with other PHC components because it is an essential part of health education, food and nutrition and also MCH.

Safe and wholesome water defined as:
- Free from pathogenic agents
- Free from harmful chemical substances
- Pleasant to the taste, i.e., free from color and odor
- Usable for domestic purposes.

Purposes of Water

- **Domestic use:** On domestic front, water is required for drinking, cooking, washing and bathing, flushing of toilets, gardening, etc.
- **Public purposes:** Cleaning streets, recreational purposes like swimming pools, public fountains, fire production and public parks.
- **Industrial purposes:** Water is important for industries too, not only for their processing and washing but also for producing captive power (electricity) using steam tubing.
- **Agriculture purpose:** Water is used for irrigation to the plants.
- **Power production:** Water is used for power (electricity) production from hydropower and steam power.
- **Trade and business:** Hospitals, hostels, restaurants, diaries, and places of worship where large number of people gather, dhobi (washman's unit) require water for both drinking, bathing and washing.

Sources of Water

Water is primarily derived from the ocean. In tropical regions like India the evaporation of water into the air is great and it has been estimated that about 700 gallons are evaporated every minute from each square mile of ocean surface. There are three sources:

- **Rain water:** Rain is the purest in nature and prime source of water. A part of the rain water sinks into the ground to form ground water, part of it evaporates back into the atmosphere, and some returns off to form streams and rivers which flow ultimately into the sea. It is purest in nature; physically it is clear, bright and sparking.

- **Surface water:** The origin of this is again rainwater. Many of the Indian cities and towns depend upon the surface water. Examples of surface water include rivers, tanks, lakes, wades (water source which are dry, expect in rainy season), non-mad reservoirs depend upon surface water source, which are 1. Impounding reservoirs 2. Rivers and streams and 3. Tanks, ponds and lakes.
  - *Impounding resources:* There are artificial lakes constructed usually of earthwork or masomy in which large quantities of surface water is stored. Dams built across rivers and mountain streams also provide large reserves of surface water. The area drinking into the reservoir is called "catchments area". Impounding reservoirs usually furnish a fairly good quality of water.
  - *Rivers:* River water is turbid during rainy season it may be clear in other seasons. Clarity of water is no guarantee that the river water is safe for drinking. River water contains dissolved and suspended impurities of all kinds. The bacterial count, including the human intestinal organisms may be very high. The chief drawback of river water is that it is always grossly polluted and is quite unfit for drinking without treatment.
  - *Tank:* In some of Indian villages tanks are important sources of water supply, perhaps the only source. Tanks are large excavations in which surface water is stored. Tank water is always subject to contamination. In our country cattle and other domestic animals are washed in the tanks, sometimes vehicles like Lorries are brought near the tanks and washed, clothes are also washed in tanks. If the tank water is drunk without being boiled, disinfected or having undergone treatment of any kind which is responsible for an incalculable number of cases of sickness and death, particularly of children.
- **Ground water:** Ground water is the cheapest and the most practical way of providing water to small communities. Ground water is safer the surface water, as the ground itself acts as successful filtering medium. It is likely to be free from pathogenic agents. It is cool and colorless. It requires no treatment and even during dry season the supply of water may be assured. The usual ground water sources are well and spring. Well have been classified into shallow and deep wells dug and tube wells.
  - *Wells:* Wells are the common and main source of water supply in Indian villages and towns.
    Shallow wells: Shallow wells tap subsoil layers in the ground. They yield limited quantities of water and the water is notoriously liable to pollution unless care is taken in well construction.
    Deep wells: A deep well is one which taps water from the water-bearing stratum below the first impervious layer in the ground. Deep wells are usually machine dug and may be several hundred meters deep. Deep wells furnish the safest water and are often the most satisfactory sources of water supply.
    Sanitary wells: which is properly located well-constructed and protected against contamination with a view to yield a supply of safe water? It should be tapped in good soil and located at least 150 ft away from any sewage farm. A parapet wall around the well up to height of at least 2.5. Feet (70-75 cm) should be provided above the ground.
    Tubewells: Tubewell water is bacteriologically safe, and are also cheap in comparison to other sources of supply. Shallow tubewells or driven wells have become largest individual source of water supply to the rural community.
  - *Springs:* Springs are found when ground water is made to overflow upon the surface. Springs are considered as natural wells cropping out at places whether geological conditions are favorable. There are four varieties of springs 1. Main springs, 2. Intermittent springs, 3. Surface or shallow land springs and 4. Hot or thermal springs.

WATER-BORNE DISEASES

- **Water-borne diseases:** It classified as viral, bacteria, protozoal, helminthic, leptospira. Viral diseases include hepatitis A and E and poliomyelitis, bacterial diseases are cholera, typhoid, dysentery, and protozoal disease are amebiasis and giardiasis, helminthic disease are roundworm and thread worm.
- **Water-associated disease:** High nitrogen content in the water causes methemoglobinemia, cretinism and endemic goiter are associated with consumption of water which is deficient in iodine. Dental caries caused by the consumption of water deficient in fluorine and dental and skeletal fluorosis due to excess of fluorine.

WATER PURIFICATION PROCESSES

Water available in nature from surface or underground sources is described as "raw" water. It requires to purity before it can be supplied to the community. The aim of purification is to protect the water supply by removing organic matter, suspended and dissolved matter in water. The nature of purification is determined by the quality of raw water and impurities present.

Purification on Large Scale

Large scale purification method is suitable when supply is to be made for large communities as in urban town or city. The purpose of water treatment is to produce water that is safe and wholesome.

Storage: Storage provides a reserve of water from which further pollution is excluded. As a result of storage, a very considerable amount of purification takes place. In natural purification physical, chemical and biological process are taken place.

Physical process: Physical action of stored water helps to settle the impurities down in 24 hours time due to gravity. Thus water becomes clear. This allows sunlight to penetrate and thereby reduces the work of filters.

Chemical process: Chemical process of stored water in aerobic bacteria oxidizes the organic matter in water with the aid of dissolved oxygen. It reduces the content of free ammonia and increases nitrates.

Biological process: Biological process of storage helps in reducing the amount of bacteria present in water, the pathogens die in 5–7 days of storage. The optimum period of storage is about 10–14 days.

Filtration

Large scale water purifications second stage is filtration, 98-99% of the bacteria are removed by filtration. Two types of filters are in use biological or slow sound filters and the rapid sand or mechanical filters.

- **Slow and filter:** Slow sand system or biological system was introduced in England for the first time in 1804. These filter beds consist of water tight rectangular basins usually made of masonry. Each unit has to be at least 50" × 40" × 15" and the bottom, an acre or more.

  Advantages of slow sand filter:
  - Equipment needed is simple
  - Supervision is simple
  - Quality of filtered water is high
  - Simple to construct and operate.

  Elements:
  - **Supernatant water:** The supernatant water above the sand bed, whose depth varies from 1 to 1.5 meter, serves two important purposes 1. It promotes downward flow of water through sand beds. 2. It provides waiting period of some hours (3 to 12 hours).
  - **Sand bed:** A coarse gravel layer of bricks or broken stone at the bottom of the bed for a thickness of 6"–12" above this another layer of gravel 12 inches deep is placed. Above this 3–5 feet fine sand is placed. Above the sand 4–5 feet water is allowed to stand for filtering. There is a perforated tubular drain at the bottom of the bed to collect the filtered water.
  - **Under drainage system:** It consists of porous or perforated pipes which serve the dual purpose of providing an outlet for filtered water, and supporting the medium above filter box consists of 3 elements—supernated water, sand bed and under drainage system.
  - **Filter control:** The purpose of these devise is to maintain a constant rate of filtration. Venturi meter used to measures the bed resistance or loss of head. Filters may run for weeks or even months without cleaning. When the bed resistance increases to such an extent that regulating valve has to be kept fully open. It is the time to clean the filter bed.

  Disadvantages
  - Filtration is open, possibility of contamination is more.
  - Sedimentation takes place before filtration.
  - Large area is required.
  - Less feasibility in operation.
- **Rapid sand filter:** Rapid sand filtration of water first installed in 1885 at USA. Rapid sand filters are of two types—the gravity type (Paterson's filter) and the pressure type (Candy's filter).

  Advantage of Rapid Sand Filter:
  - It deals with raw water directly
  - Filter best occupy less space
  - Filtration more than 40–50% of slow sand filter
  - Washing of the filter is easy.
  - More flexibility in operation.

  Steps of Rapid Sand Filtration:
  - **Coagulation:** Chemical coagulant such as alum or aluminum sulphate at dosage of 1 to 4 gravis per gallon of water or 5–40 milligram per liter. This process gallon the chemical to get well mixed with water.
  - **Flocculation:** Treated water is gently and slowly stirring to 'flocculation hydroxide is formed.
  - **Sedimentation:** Coagulated water is led into sedimentation tank for a period of 2 to 6 hours. Before the water is admitted into rapid sand filters 95% of flocculent precipitate is removed.

Disinfection

Chemical or an agent used be potentially useful as a disinfectant in water supplies. The chemical used should be capable of destroying the pathogenic organisms in the water. It should be ready and dependable availability at reasonable cost permitting convenient, safe and accurate application to water.

Chlorination

Chlorine is an oxidizing agent and when added to water leads to the formation of hydrochloric acids. This disinfecting action is mainly due to the hypochlorous acid and to a small extent due to the hypochlorite ions. Chlorine kills pathogenic bacteria, apart from its germicidal effect; it removes turbidity, color and odor.

Principles of Chlorination

- Water should be clear and free from turbidity.
- Estimate the chlorine demand.
- Residual chlorine needs to kill bacteria and viruses
- Recommended free chlorine concentration should be 0.5 mg/L for one hour.

Methods of Chlorination

- **Chlorine gas**: It most convenient, cheap quick in action and easy to apply. "Paterson's chloronome" measures regulate and administer gaseous chlorine.
- **Chloramines:** Are the compounds of chlorine and ammonia. They are slower action, so it is not usually used.

- **Perchloron:** Perchloron or high test hypochlorite (H.T.H) is a calcium compound which carries 60–70% available chlorine.

Measurements

- **Orthotolidine (07) test:** It enables both free combined chlorine in water to be determined with speed and accuracy. The test is carried out be adding 0.1 mL of reagent to 1 mL of water. The yellow color produced in matched against suitable standards or color discs.
- **Orthotolidine-Arsenite (OTA) Test:** is a modification of the OT test to determine the free and combined chlorine residuals separately.

HOUSEHOLD PURIFICATION OF WATER

Physical Method

- **Boiling:** Boiling for 5–10 minutes helps in killing bacteria. Boiling removes temporary hardness of the water.
- **Distillation:** Water is subjected to chemical purification; this process is done in chemical laboratories. It is not economical.
- **Ozone:** Ozonized air brought into contact with water in quantities 1–3 mg into purifies 1 litre of water.
- **Ultraviolet ray:** Ultraviolet rays can disinfect water.

Chemical Method

- **Katadyn process:** When water is allowed to pass through a filter consisting of this Katadyn sand minute particles in the form of silver ions enter the solution that in turn attracts oxygen from the air dissolved in water and this action kills bacteria.
- **Potassium permanganate:** It is a powerful oxidizing agent but not a satisfactory agent for disinfecting water as it has a few drawbacks like causing decolourization, smell and taste.
- **Chlorinated lime or bleaching powder:** Bleaching powder contains 35% of available chlorine. But on exposure to air, light and moisture, it loses its chlorine content, when mixed with fresh lime, it retains its strength.
- **Iodine:** It is used in the forms of NESFIELD'S Tables. A 2 gain tablet of sodium iodine and equal quantity of citric acid will kill typhoid and cholera in a few minutes.

PHYSICAL AND CHEMICAL STANDARDS OF DRINKING WATER

The evolution of standards for the quality control of public water supplies has to take into account the limitations imposed by local factors in the several regions of the country. The Environment Hygiene Committee (1949) recommended that the objective of a public water supply should be to supply water "that is absolutely free from risks of transmitting diseases, is pleasing to the senses and is suitable for culinary and laundering purpose" and added that "freedom from risks is comparatively more important than physical appearance or hardness" and that safety is an obligatory standard and physical and chemical qualities are optional within a range.

Physical and chemical quality of drinking water: The physical and chemical quality of drinking water should be in accordance with the recommended guidelines presented **(Table 14.1)**.

TABLE 14.1: Recommended guidelines for physical and chemical parameters.

S. No.	Characteristics	*Acceptable	**Cause for rejection
1.	Turbidity (NTU)	1	10
2.	Color (Units on platinum cobalt scale)	5	25
3.	Taste and odor	Unobjectionable	Objectionable
4.	pH	7.0 to 8.5	<6.5 or >9.2
5.	Total dissolved solids (mg/L)	500	2000
6.	Total hardness (as $CaCO_3$) (mg/L)	200	600
7.	Chlorides (as Cl) (mg/L)	200	1000
8.	Sulphates (as SO_4) (mg/L)	200	400
9.	Fluorides (as F) (mg/L)	1.0	1.5
10.	Nitrates (as NO_3) (mg/L)	45	45
11.	Calcium (as Ca) (mg/L)	75	200
12.	Magnesium (as Mg) (mg/L)	=30	150
13.	Iron (as Fe) (mg/L)	0.1	1.0
14.	Manganese (as Mn) (mg/L)	0.05	0.5
15.	Copper (as Cu) (mg/L)	0.05	1.5
16.	Aluminum (as Al) (mg/L)	0.03	0.2
17.	Alkalinity (mg/L)	200	600
18.	Residual chlorine (mg/L)	0.2	>1.0
19.	Zinc (as Zn) (mg/L)	5.0	15.0
20.	Phenolic compounds (as Phenol) (mg/L)	0.001	0.002
21.	Anionic detergents (mg/L) (as MBAS)	0.2	1.0
22.	Mineral oil (mg/L)	0.01	0.03

Contd...

Contd...

S. No	Characteristics	*Acceptable	**Cause for rejection
Toxic minerals			
23.	Arsenic (as As) (mg/L)	0.01	0.05
24.	Cadmium (as Cd) (mg/L)	0.01	0.01
25.	Chromium (as hexavalent Cr) (mg/L)	0.05	0.05
26.	Cyanides (as CN) (mg/L)	0.05	0.05
27.	Lead (as Pb) (mg/L)	0.05	0.05
28.	Selenium (as Se) (mg/L)	0.01	0.01
29.	Mercury (total as Hg) (mg/L)	0.001	0.001
30.	Polynuclear aromatic hydrocarbons (PAH) (mg/L)	0.2	0.2
31.	Pesticides (total, mg/L)	Absent	Refer to WHO guidelines for drinking water quality Vol.I.-1993
Radio Activity+			
32.	Gross Alpha activity) Bq/l	0.1	0.1
33.	Gross Beta activity (ßq/l)	1.0	1.0

Notes:
* The figures indicated under the column 'Acceptable' are the limits up to which water is generally acceptable to the consumers.
** Figures in excess of those mentioned under 'Acceptable' render the water not acceptable, but still may be tolerated in the absence of an alternative and better source but up to the limits indicated under column "Cause for Rejection" above which the sources will have to be rejected.

BACTERIOLOGICAL QUALITY OF WATER

Organisms	Guidelines
All water intended for drinking E.coli or thermotolerant coliform bacteria b,c	Must not be detectable in any 100-mL sample
Treated water entering the distribution system	
E coli or thermotolerant coliform Bacteria b	Must not be detectable in any 100-mL sample
Total coliform bacteria	Must not be detectable in any 100 mL sample

Contd...

Treated water in the distribution system	
E. coli or thermotolerant coliform Bacteria	Must not be detectable in any 100 mL sample
Total coliform bacteria	Must not be detectable in any 100 mL sample. In the case of large supplies, where sufficient samples are examined, must not be present in 95% of samples taken throughout any 12-month period

Source: WHO guidelines for Drinking Water Quality Vol.1—1993.

- Immediate investigative action must be taken if either *E. coli* or total coliform bacteria are detected. The minimum action in the case of total coliform bacteria is repeat sampling; if these bacteria are detected in the repeat sample, the cause must be determined by immediate further investigation.
- Although *E. coli* is the more precise indicator of fecal pollution, the count of thermotolerant coliform bacteria is an acceptable alternative. If necessary, proper confirmatory test must be carried out. Total coliform bacteria are not acceptable indicators of the sanitary quality of rural water supplies, particularly in tropical areas where many bacteria of no sanitary significance occur in almost all untreated supplies.
- It is recognized that, in the great majority of rural water supplies in developing countries, fecal contamination is widespread. Under these conditions, the national surveillance agency should set medium term targets for progressive improvement of water supplies, as recommended in volume 3 of WHO guidelines for drinking water supply 1993.

Recommended Treatment for Different Water Sources to Produce Water with Negligible Virus Risk

Type of source	Recommended treatment
Ground Water Protected, deep wells; essentially free of fecal contamination	Disinfection
Unprotected, shallow wells; fecally contaminated	Filtration and disinfection
Surface Water Protected, impounded upland water; essentially free of fecal contamination	Disinfection
Unprotected, impounded upland water or upland river; fecal contamination	Filtration and disinfection
Unprotected lowland rivers; fecal contamination	Predisinfection or storage, filtration, disinfection
Unprotected water shed; heavy fecal contamination	Predisinfection or storage, filtration, additional treatment and disinfection
Unprotected water shed; gross fecal contamination	Not recommended for water supply

CONCEPTS OF WATER CONSERVATION

- Water conservation encompasses the policies, strategies and activities made to manage fresh water as a sustainable resource, to protect the water environment, and to meet current and future human demand.
- The goals of water conservation efforts include: ensuring availability of water, energy conservation, habitat conservation.

Conservation Planning

- These plans serve as guidelines for overall water resource management and set targets for smaller, local utilities to provide adequate water supplies.
- Comprehensive plans are increasingly popular as a method of combining supply and conservation projects.

Benefits

- Conservation benefits to the customer include reduced water bills and greater water supplies that help in better economic development.
- Environmental benefits include ecosystem and habitat protection.
- Decreased water demand also has positive implications for tourism, especially for the recreational use of waterways.
- Water conservation can be achieved through stronger plumbing codes, promotion of conservation devices, pricing levels, and public education.

Common characteristics: Each state program is distinctive with regards to particular geographic, hydrologic, and political characteristics; each contains features common to all. The major characteristics include:
- Needs to simplify and coordinate resource planning efforts;
- Efforts to extend limited supplies prior to initiating new source development projects;
- Reductions in residential, industrial, and agricultural demand; and
- Improvements in the efficiency of older supply infrastructure.

Irrigation hours ordinance: Communities may enact a minimum rule that limits lawn and garden **irrigation** to restricted hours, generally during early morning or late evening when less sunlight and winds minimize water evaporation.

Xeriscape landscape: Xeriscape, or "dry gardening," is defined as a method of improving the character of land that maximizes water conservation by the use of site-appropriate plants and an efficient watering system.

The principles of Xeriscape include:
- Developing plans and designs that consider exposure, slope, view, and soils;
- Creating practical turf areas with type and location determined by landscape purpose and function;
- Evaluating and improving soils, and when appropriate, adding peat moss or compost to improve root development, water penetration, and water retention;
- Using appropriate plant selection according to water needs so minimum usage will allow maximum conservation;
- Watering efficiently with properly designed irrigation systems and with well managed plant groupings of similar watering needs; and
- Using organic mulch that minimizes evapotranspiration, reduces weed growth, slows erosion, and helps reduce soil temperature fluctuations.

Ultra-Low-Volume Fixtures

The installation of ultra-low-volume (ULV) plumbing fixtures in new construction is often required to save water while still providing desired services. Permit regulations usually specify that fixtures possess a maximum flow volume when pressure is (for instance) 80 pounds per square inch. In this case, the maximum flow volume is normally 1.6 gallons per flush for toilets; 2.0 gallons per minute for faucets; and 2.5 gallons per minute for showerheads. The goal is to attain ongoing savings without behavioral changes.

Rain Sensor Device

This measure requires that any person purchasing or installing an automatic sprinkler system must install and operate a rain sensor device or an automatic switch. This equipment will override the irrigation cycle of the sprinkler system when adequate rainfall has occurred.

Water Conservation-based Rate Structure

A conservation rate structure is a pricing system used by utilities that provides financial incentives for users to reduce their water demands. Rates generally entail one of the following:
- Increasing block rates, where the marginal cost to users increases in two or more steps as use increases; or
- Seasonal pricing, in which water consumed in the peak demand season is charged a higher rate than in the off-peak season.

Leak Detection and Repair Program

Public water supply systems desire to attain a 10% or less unaccounted-for water loss. When actual loss is greater, then the implementation of leak detection programs is required. The program must include auditing procedures, and in-field leak detection and repair efforts.

Public education program: Public information will inform citizens of opportunities to reduce water use, give reasons why they should choose to practice conservation, and publicize the conservation options being promoted. Nearly all users can be affected by public information efforts, although they are typically targeted at the uses with the broadest participation.

Commercial and Industrial Users

All individual commercial and industrial users submit a conservation plan that generally includes audits of water use; implementation of cost-effective conservation measures; employee conservation awareness programs; and feasibility studies of using reclaimed water.

Social Acceptability

- Water conservation is not an isolated activity and its social acceptability is related to many factors such as the characteristics of the utility market; the pricing system; and economic, political, technological, and willingness to conserve.
- By the time that water conservation is necessary, the public has already developed established use patterns and may be resistant to changing these patterns.
- To change social consciousness about water resources, an understanding of all the issues is critical.
- Public perception often is influenced by an effective campaign to highlight the positives of these new decisions.
- Drought situations often highlight the need for conservation measures and increase social acceptability.

RAINWATER HARVESTING

Rainwater harvesting is a type of harvest in which the rain drops are collected and stored for the future use, rather than allowing it to run off. Rainwater can be collected from rivers or roofs and redirected to a deep pit (well, shaft, or borehole), aquifer, a reservoir with percolation, or collected from dew or fog with nets or other tools. Its uses include water for gardens, livestock, irrigation, domestic use with proper treatment, indoor heating for houses, etc. The harvested water can also be used as drinking water, longer-term storage, and for other purposes such as ground water recharge.

Importance of Rainwater Harvesting

- Rainwater harvesting or the collection of rainwater in a proper way, can be a permanent solution to the problem of water crisis in different parts of the world.
- Although the earth is three-fourths water; very little of it is suitable for human consumption or agriculture. Rainfall is unpredictable and there is a constant shortage of water in countries which are agriculture dependent or generally drought prone.
- A bad monsoon means low crop yield and shortage of food. Even animals suffer from scarcity of water. Africa and the Indian subcontinent face acute water crisis during the summer months. The farmers are the most affected because they do not get sufficient water for their fields. Rainwater harvesting therefore is an ideal solution for farmers who depend on monsoon for consistent water supply.
- Unavailability of clean water compels the consumption of polluted water, giving rise to water-borne diseases and high rate of infant mortality. In recent studies, it has been observed that in Lima (Peru) nearly 2 million people do not have access to any water supply and those who do have access get water supply which has a high possibility of being contaminated.
- If rainwater, which comes for free, can be collected and stored, instead of letting it run off, it could be an alternative to back up the main water supply especially during dry spells. Its importance will not be limited to an individual family but can be used by a community as well.
- The importance of rainwater harvesting lies in the fact that it can be stored for future use. Just as it can be used directly so also the stored water can be utilized to revitalize the ground level water and improve its quality. This also helps to raise the level of ground water which then can be easily accessible.
- In areas having sparse and irregular rainfall, scarcity of water is a persistent problem. It cannot be completely resolved but can be mitigated through rainwater harvesting. Rainwater harvesting is an ideal solution to water problems in regions which receive inconsistent rainfall throughout the year.

Methods of Rainwater Harvesting

The most common methods for rainwater harvesting are:

- **Surface run off harvesting:** Surface run off harvesting is most suitable in urban areas. Here rain water flows away as surface run off and can be stored for future use. Surface runoff rainwater in ponds, tanks and reservoirs built for this purpose. This can provide water for farming, for cattle and also for general domestic use.
- **Roof top rainwater harvesting:** Roof top water harvesting can be done in individual homes or in schools. For this the first requirement is to intercept the rainwater to flow towards a definite direction. The water should reach a bucket or a tank through pipes made from wood or bamboo. In urban areas PVC pipes can be used. Roof top rainwater can be harvested through existing tube wells. In areas where the aquifer that holds the ground water has dried up, tubewells source deeper into the soil for water. Roof top rainwater harvesting can be done through these dried up tube wells to rehydrate the dried subsoil water level.

WATERSHED MANAGEMENT

The word "watershed" introduced in 1920 was used for the "water parting boundaries". Watershed is that land area which drains or contributes runoff to a common outlet. Watershed is defined as a geohydrological unit draining to a common point by a system of drains. All lands on earth are part of one watershed or other. Watershed is thus the land and water area, which contributes runoff to a common point.

Types of Watershed Management

Watershed is classified depending upon the size, drainage, shape and land use pattern.

- Macro watershed: 1,000–10,000 ha
- Micro watershed: 100–1,000 ha

- Mini watershed: 10–100 ha
- Mille watershed: 1–10 ha

Objectives of Watershed Management
- Production of food, fodder, fuel
- Pollution control
- Over exploitation of resources should be minimized
- Water storage, flood control, checking sedimentation
- Wildlife preservation
- Erosion control and prevention of soil, degradation and conservation of soil and water
- Employment generation through industrial development dairy fishery production.
- Recharging of ground water to provide regular water supply for consumption and industry as well as irrigation.
- Recreational facility.

Main Components of Watershed
- Soil and water conservation,
- Water harvesting and water management,
- Alternate land use system.

Irrigation Projects
- Major—Covered >10,000 ha of catchments command area (CCA)
- Medium—2,000 to 10,000 ha of CCA
- Minor—<2,000 ha of CCA.

Steps in Watershed Management
Watershed management involves determination of alternative land treatment measures for, which information about problems of land, soil, water and vegetation in the watershed is essential. In order to have a practical solution to above problem it is necessary to go through four phases for a full scale watershed management.

Program
- Recognition phase
- Restoration phase
- Protection phase
- Improvement phase

Recognition Phase
It involves following steps:
- Recognition of the problem
- Improvement phase
- Analysis of the cause of the problem and its effect
- Development of alternative solutions of problem.

Restoration Phase
It includes two main steps:
1. Selection of best solution to problems identified
2. Application of the solution to the problems of the land

Protection Phase
This phase takes care of the general health of the watershed and ensures normal functioning. The protection is against all factors which may cause determined in watershed condition.

Improvement Phase
This phase deals with overall improvement in the watershed and all land is covered. Attention is paid to agriculture and forest management and production, forage production and pasture management, socioeconomic conditions to achieve the objectives of watershed management.

Water Resources Development Plan
Water resource management plays a vital role in sustainable development of watershed which is possible only through the implementation of various water harvesting technique. The efficient way for sub-surface water storage, soil moisture conservation or ground water recharge technologies should be adopted properly under water resource development plan.

Various Measures Adopted Under Soil and Water Harvesting
- Vegetative barriers
- Building of contour bunds along contours for erosion
- Furrow/Ridges and Furrow ridge method of cultivation across the slope.
- Irrigation water management through drip and sprinkler methods.
- Planting of horticultural contour species on bunds.

Watershed Management Programs
- **Drought Prone Area Program (DPAP):** Year of start: 1970–71
  Objectives: Area development program through restoration of ecological balance and optimum utilization of land, water, livestock and human resources to mitigate the effect of drought.
- **Desert Development Program (DDP):** Year of start: 1977–78
  Objectives: Mitigate the effect of drought in the desert area and restore ecological balance.
- **National Watershed Development Program for Rainfed Agriculture (NWDPRA):** Year of start: 1986–87
  Objectives: To conserve and utilize rainwater from both arable and nonarable lands on watershed basis. To increase the productivity of crops and to increase the fuel, fodder and fruit resources through appropriate alternate land use system.
- **Control of Shifting Cultivation:** Year of start: 1986–87
  Objectives: Restoring ecological balance in hilly areas and improving socioeconomic conditions.
- **World Bank Assisted Integrated Watershed Development Project:** Year of start: 1990
  Objectives: To arrest the problems of environmental degradation and promote sustainable increase in agriculture production and to enhance vegetative

technology of soil and water conservation for rainwater conservation and for increasing crop, forage, fuel wood and timber yield of the area.

Watershed Management Practices

In Terms of Purpose
- To increase infiltration
- To increase water holding capacity
- To prevent soil erosion.

Method and Accomplishment

Vegetative Measures/Agronomical Measures
- Strip cropping
- Pasture cropping
- Grass land farming
- Woodlands

Engineering Measures/Structural Practices
- Contour bunding
- Terracing
- Construction of earthen embankment
- Construction of check dams
- Construction of farm ponds
- Construction of diversion
- Gully controlling structure
- Rock dam
- Establishment of permanent grass and vegetation
- Providing vegetative and stone barriers

Rainwater Harvesting

Rainwater harvesting means collection and storage of rainwater by some mechanism to make water available for future use. An appreciable amount of precipitation, which is generally lost as surface flow, can be harvested and stored for useful purposes like drinking and providing supplemental irrigation to the crops.

CONCEPT OF POLLUTION PREVENTION: AIR AND NOISE POLLUTION, ROLE OF NURSE IN PREVENTION OF POLLUTION

Air

The immediate environment of man comprises of air on which depends all forms of life. Apart from supplying the life giving oxygen, air and atmospheric conditions severe functions. Every living creature on the earth depends upon air for its survival. For the maintenance of healthy life, pure and clean atmospheric air is necessary.

Functions of Air
- Human body is cooled by the air contact.
- The special senses of hearing and smell function through air transmitted stimuli.
- Air purifies the blood by interchange of oxygen with carbon dioxide in the lung.
- Atmospheric air regulates body temperature.
- Air acts as a channel for carrying bacteria.
- Recent development of man's adventure into outer space has breaded the concept of air movements.

Composition of Air

Air is a mechanical mixture of gases. The normal composition of external air by volume is approximately as follows:

Nitrogen—78.1%
Oxygen—20.93%
Carbon dioxide—0.03%

The balance is made up of other gases which occur in traces, e.g., argon, neon, krypton, xenon, and helium. Air also contains water vapor, traces of ammonia and suspended matter such as dust, bacteria, vegetable fibers, offensive odors from sewers industries and offensive trades, etc.

Air is a need of the body: Air is essential for maintenance of life. Air supplies oxygen to human body, which is essential for life. Air supplies oxygen to human body, which is essential for life. Clean air is necessary for our health and longevity. An average person breathes 35 lbs of air each day, which is about 6 times of his food and water intake the oxygen in the air is the force in each cell of the body.

Air has two important functions, i.e., interchanges of gases during respiration and regulation of body temperature. An adult at rest breathes at the rate of eighteen times a minute. During respiration, 500 cubic centimeters or 22 cubic inches of air passes in and out of the individual's lungs, each time he respires.

Respiration is a process of inspiration and expiration, air in the lungs loses 4% of oxygen that is absorbed by the blood in the pulmonary capillaries, and gains carbonic acid from the venous blood to the extent of 3.5 to 4%. The expired air is warm and the carbonic acid is given off by an adult at rest is 0.7 cubic foot I one hour. This might reach up to nearly 2 cubic feet during physical activity.

Feeling of suffocation or discomfort is experienced by the occupants in sufficiently ventilated rooms and also complaints of headache, drowsiness and inability to concentrate. There is also the risk of droplet infection and lowered resistance to disease. Discomfort is a subjective sensation which people experience an ill-ventilated and over-crowded room.

Temperature, humidity, air movement and heat radiation are the factors determine the "cooling power" of the air with respect to the human body.

Indices of Thermal

Thermal comfort is a complex entity. Much work was done in the past to determine what constitute "thermal comfort". Several indices have been put forward from time to time to express thermal comfort and heat stress. These are as follows:
- Air temperature
- Air temperature and humidity
- Cooling power

- Effective temperature
- Corrected effective temperature

An instrument designed by Hill called "KATA THERMOMETER" is used to determine cooling power in a room. This instrument measures the rate of the heat loss from the surface at approximate body temperature. Of 98.4°F, fresh comfortable room has a dry kata reading of 6 of and above wet indices for thermal comfort. and above. These used as indices for thermal comfort.

Comfort zones: Comfort is quite a complex subjective experience which depends not only on physical, physiological factors but also on psychological factors which are difficult to determine. Considering only the environmental factors, "Comfortable thermal conditions are those under which a person can maintain normal balance between production and loss of heat, at normal body temperature and without sweating. Comfort zones evaluated in India as below.

Human feeling	Temperature
Pleasant and cool	69°F or 21°C
Comfortable and cool	69–76°F or 21–24°C
Comfortable	77–80°F or 24°C–27°C
Hot and uncomfortable	81°F + or 28°C
Intolerably hot	86°F + or 30°C

Global warming: It is the build up in the atmosphere of carbon dioxide and other gases such as methane, chlorofluorocarbons, nitrous oxide, ozone and others.

Causes of Global Warming

- **Population growth:** The world population which is just over 5 billion expected to double in the next 60 years. Population increase automatically results in more energy usage, driving more miles, producing more garbage.
- **Emission of gases:** Emission of gases in the course of day to day human activities in another cause for global warming. Gases like carbon dioxide, methane.

Health Effects due to Global Warming

People especially those who are elderly, very young or sick are not good at dealing with extremes of temperature. Mortality from coronary heart disease and stroke increases when the average temperature exceeds the normal. A further increase in temperature causes cardiovascular and respiratory diseases. Other diseases like mosquito-borne malaria, dengue fever, encephalitis, yellow fever, etc. can also prevent due to the changes in temperature and humidity.

Air Pollution

Air pollution may be defined as any atmospheric condition in which certain substances are present in such concentrations that they can produce undesirable effects on man and his environment. Air pollution refers to the presences of foreign materials such as smoke, harmful gases dust, vapours and fine particles in the atmospheric which are harmful for human being, animals, vegetations, buildings, monuments, etc.

Sources of Air Pollution

- **Natural pollution:** Natural pollution of the atmosphere occurs due to dust storms, eruption of volcanoes, results of lightening and floods, etc.
- **Industries:** Industrial enterprises emit various gases and particulate matter such as sulfur dioxide, nitrogen oxide, cement dust, carbon monoxide, etc.
- **Automobilism:** Automobiles are the major sources of air pollution because of the number of vehicles are increasing. The major pollutant emitted by the automobiles is nitrogen oxide, hydrocarbons, carbon-monoxide, lead and benzene.
- **Chemical fertilizers:** They are used to increase agriculture production, it produces pollutants like nitrogen oxide, sulfur dioxide, ammonia and urea dust which pollute the air in the community.
- **Tobacco smoke:** Smoking in the house and public places pollute the air. The tobacco smoke emits nicotine which is very injurious to health.

Air Pollution and Health

Air pollution affects human health directly as well as indirectly, direct effects of air pollution occur at individual level and the indirect effect appears at global level. The chemical contaminants enter human system mainly through three avenues.

- Inhalation (breathing) the air—borne contaminants find their way into the lungs.
- Absorption—many gaseous and liquid materials are absorbed to a limited extend through the skin. Phenol, creosol, aniline, etc. are examples of skin absorption.
- Ingestion—ingestion of toxic materials may result from sources such as food, drinks, etc.

Disease caused by prolonged exposure to dust

Dust and illnesses

Dust	Dust diseases
1. Silica	Silicosis
2. Coal	Pneumoconiosis
3. Asbestos	Asbestosis
4. Cotton	Byssinosis
5. Bagasse	Bagassosis

Chemical and Illness

Sulphur dioxide emissions cause suffocation, irritation of throat and eyes and respiratory diseases. The principal effect of carbon monoxide on human being and animals is its interference with transfer of oxygen in the body. Health hazards of nitrogen oxides are bronchitis and edema of lungs. The major problem with hydrocarbons is their ability to react with nitrogen oxide through photo-chemical reaction in sunlight to produce "smog" smog can result in serious sight and respiration problems. Thus, hydrocarbons may be cancer producing. Lead, mercury, cadmium, etc. affect kidney, blood vessels, liver and central nervous system.

Systemic Illness and Air Pollution

- **Respiratory system:** Bronchitis, asthma, emphysema
- **Central venous system:** Heart attack by carbon monoxide
- **Central nervous system:** Reduced ability to concentrate, irritation, hyperactivity in children below five years. Lead can cause permanent brain damage.
- **Eye problems:** Irritation, conjunctivitis and even blindness.
- **Cancer:** Inhalation of diseases and petrol exhaust can cause lung cancer. Some of the hydrocarbons can cause anemia and blood cancer.

Prevention and Control of Air Pollution

Air pollution can cause many health disorders in man related to respiratory system, cardiovascular system, nervous system and eye. These problems can be prevented and controlled by taking appropriate measures of prevention and control of pollution.

- **Contaminated method:** This is done by various mechanical devices, e.g., in factories exhaust fans, suction apparatus, air cleaning device, etc. are installed to effect ventilation and cleaning of air before discharge into the atmosphere.
- **Replacement method:** Pollution producing substances and processes are replaced with non-polluting substances and process. Replacement of coal based electricity production plants by hydroelectric power and wind powered generators are used.
- **Dilution:** It refers to reducing of pollutants in the air which can be done by extensive planting of trees and vegetation around industrial and residential area.
- **Disinfection of air:** This method includes mechanical ventilation which helps in reducing vitiated air and bacterial density, ultraviolet radiation for disinfecting operation theater and infectious wards.
- **Legislative method:** Government law, which can set some norms for precautionary measures to be implemented by the factories, automobiles, etc.
- **International action:** WHO established regional centers at various places in worldwide. These laboratories are set up to study the air pollution level.
- **Dust control:** It can be done frequent wet dusting and wet cleaning of floors of health centers, hospitals wards, houses and roads, etc.

LIGHTING

Lighting is essential for efficient vision. If the lighting conditions are not ideal the visual apparatus is put to strain which may lead to general fatigue and loss of efficiency. Imperfect light is one of the causes of ill health and accidents. Good lighting in houses, schools, factories, offices or any work area is essential for efficient vision. Inadequate light may cause damage to eye and produce physical and mental discomfort.

Factors Essential for Good Lighting

- **Sufficiency:** The light should be sufficient, 15 to 20 footcandles are the minimum required for satisfactory vision.
- **Distribution:** Distribution of light in any place should be uniform.
- **Absence of glare:** Glare creates acute discomfort and reduces the critical vision.
- **Absence sharp shadows:** Slight shadow is inevitable but sharp and contrasting shadows are disturbing.
- **Steadiness:** The light should be constant, flickering cause's eye strain and may lead to accidents.
- **Color of light:** Very bright flashing colors may harm our eyes and would cause discomfort.
- **Surroundings:** Ceilings and roof should have a reflection factor of 80% contrasting colors are often used to prevent accidents.

Types of Lighting

- **Natural lighting:** Natural lighting is derived partly from the visible sky and partly from reflection. Natural lighting also depends upon the time of the day, season, weather and atmospheric pollution. This can be obtained effectively with suitable planning of location and orientation of building.
- **Artificial lighting:** Artificial lighting should be as close as possible to daylight in composition. Artificial light needs consistency, uniformity and adequacy. Some common methods of proving artificial lights and candles, oil lamps or lanterns, gas light and electric lighting.

Requirements of Good Lighting

- Lighting is natural or artificial has to be good.
- Good lighting promotes good vision to works.
- Very bright flashing colors should be avoided, it may harm our eyes.
- Glare should be prevented since glare creates acute discomfort.
- Distribution of light in any place should be uniform.
- Light should be constant, flickering cause eye strain.
- Good lighting needs consistency, uniformity and adequacy.

Measurements of Lighting

Light is measured for the amount and for intensity by the standard candle. Candle power is the standard measurement of artificial lighting. Light is a narrow wavelength band of electromagnetic radiation from about 380 to 780 nm (nanometer). Light containing all visible waves is perceived as white.

- **Luminous intensity:** Which is the 'power' of a light source considered as a point radiating in all directions: this is measure as candelus or candle power.
- **Luminous flux:** Which is the flow of light related to a unit of solid angle measured in lumens?

- **Illumination or luminance:** Which is the amount of light reaching a surface measured in lux, per unit area?
- **Brightness or luminance:** Which is the amount of light reflected from a surface measured in lamberts?

Effects of Light on Health

Good light promotes good vision to the workers. The eyes of the workers need to be protected by means of goggles to avoid excess of light in welding process. Translucent shading is good for street lighting and also for lighting of hospital wards to prevent accidents. The observation that daylight could cause the in vitro degradation of bilirubin is now being used as a therapeutic measure in premature infants with hyperbilirubinemia other biologic effects of light include activity, the stimulation of melanin synthesis, the activation of precursors of vitamin D, adrenocortical secretion and food consumption.

VENTILATION

Ventilation is the modern concept implies not only the removal of vitiated air and replacement of fresh air but also control of the quality of incoming air in relation to its temperature, humidity and purity with a view to provide a thermal environment this is comfortable.

Definition

Ventilation also defined as "the science of maintaining atmospheric conditions which are comfortable and helpful to the human body". Ventilation should be adequate. Most of the ill effects attribute to bad air are due to overcrowding.

Types of Ventilation

Natural Ventilation

It is the simplest system of ventilating small dwellings, schools and offices, etc. There are three factors operate this process of natural ventilation- diffusion of gases, wind, and difference of temperature.

- **Diffusion:** Air passes through the smallest openings or spaces by diffusion. This is a slow process and therefore is not relied upon as the sole means of ventilation.
- **Inequality of temperature:** Air flows from high pressure point to low pressure point. When air is heated or when the heats of the expired air reaches atmosphere, air tend to expand, rise up and escape through opening provided high up in a room.
- **Wind:** The wind is an active force in ventilation. When it blows through a room, it is called perflation. Doors and windows facing each other provide **"cross ventilation"**.

Mechanical Ventilation

Mechanical ventilation may be of the following types: exhaust ventilation, plenum ventilation, balanced ventilation and air conditioning.

- **Exhaust ventilation:** In this system, air is extracted or exhausted to the outside by exhaust fans widely used in industries to remove dusts, fumes and other concentrated contaminants at their source.
- **Plenum ventilation:** Fresh air is blown into the room be centrifugal fans so as to create a positive pressure and displaced the vitiated air. Plenum or propulsion system is used for supplying air to air-conditioned buildings and factories.
- **Balanced ventilation:** This combination of the exhaust and plenum system of ventilation. When this system is employed, natural system of ventilation is entirely dispensed.
- **Air conditioning:** Air conditioning is defined as "The simultaneous control of all, or at least the first three of those factors affecting both the physical and chemical conditions of the atmosphere within any confined space or room. Air conditioning is popular in large institutions, hospitals, industries and dwellings".

Standards of Ventilation

- **Cubic space:** Different workers have advocated standards for the minimal fresh air supply ranging from 300 to 3000 cft per hour per person.
- **Air change:** Air change is more important than the cubic space requirement. It is recommended that in the living rooms, there should be 2 or 3 air change in one hour, in work rooms and assemblies 4 to 6 air changes.
- **Floor space:** It is more important that cubic space. The optimum floor space requirements per person vary 50 to 100 sq.ft heights in excess of 10 to 12 feet are ineffective from the point of view of ventilation.

Minimum Air Space Requirement Per Head

- Residence—1,000 cft per adult
    - 500 cft per child
    - 50 cft minimum per worker
- General hospital—1,200 cft per patient
- Infectious disease hospital—1,440 cft per patient
- Lodging house—400 cft per person
- Shop—300 cft person
- Soldier—600 cft per soldier

Effects and Prevention of Ventilation

- Ventilation defined as the science of maintaining atmospheric conditions which are comfortable and helpful to the human body.
- A sick person requires 2,000 cu.ft air per hour for the physical physiological and psychological recovery.
- Inadequate floor space creates the problem of overcrowding, excessive humidity, overheating and final results in stagnation of air. Secondly, the limited floor space favors droplet infection.
- Infectious disease hospital floor space should be 144 sq.ft for general hospital 100 sq.ft. It is important for nurses to bear these aspects in mind in order to provide good therapeutic environment for patients in the wards as well for the individuals in the community in order to maintain optimum health.

- Vacuum or extraction system should be used in large halls, auditoriums and are popular in industries to remove dust, fumes, etc.
- Air conditioning system become essential particularly operation theaters, recovery rooms, intensive care units, blood banks, premature units in the hospitals to regulate the body temperature.

RADIATION

Radiation is a process of energy transfer from one body to another. Ionizing radiations are emitted when atoms decay or disintegrate by natural or artificial means, and release energy, subatomic particles and electromagnetic waves. The electromagnetic waves produced by ionizing radiations are X-rays and gamma rays.

- **Radioactive substances:** The substances which emit invisible ionizing radiations due to nuclear disintegration are called as radioactive substances. For example, uranium, radium, thorium and polonium.
- **Radioactivity:** The emission of invisible ionizing radiations from radioactive substances is known as radio activity.
- **Radioactive pollution:** The presence of invisible ionizing radiations produced from radioactive substances in atmosphere, water, food, etc. which are harmful refers to radioactive pollution.

Types of Radiations

The important subatomic particles which emit ionizing radiation are alpha particles, beta particles, neutrons and protons. All the form of ionizing radiation produces identical biological effects by causing ionization of atoms within cells.

- **Alpha particles:** They are positively charged very harmful (10 times more powerful than X-ray, gamma or beta rays) Alpha particles have little penetrating powers in the body.
- **Beta particles:** They are negatively charged they can penetrate the skin but generally do not reach deep. These beta particles can damage the skin affect eyes.
- **Gamma rays:** They are electromagnetic radiations they are short wave length, high penetrating power and more dangerous than alpha and beta rays.
- **X-rays:** They are manmade electromagnetic radiations and are great use in medical field. These are also highly hazardous when used frequently.

Sources of Radioactive Pollutions

- **Natural sources:** Natural sources of radioactive pollution are cosmic as well as terrestrial in origin. Terrestrial radiation enters the human body directly through irradiated water, vegetables, cereals and fruits and also indirectly through fish obtained from irradiated water, milk, and meat of animals fed on irradiated sources.
- **Nuclear sources:** Nuclear explosions release fission products in high atmosphere which fall out on earth or are washed down by rain. The radiation eventually reaches man directly or indirectly via respiratory, alimentary and mucocutaneous routes. A reactor accident, when it occurs, releases radioactive gases and particles in the environment exposing the reactor staff as well as adjacent inhabitants or radiation hazards.
- **Medical sources:** The demand for medical applications of radiation in diagnostic and therapeutic fields is on the increase. The use of ultrasonography, computerized axial tomography, magnetic resonance imaging is used to achieve diagnostic precision and improved quality of medical care. Medical radiation is the largest man-made source of radioactive pollution and a potential hazard for hospital personnel.
- **Industrial sources:** Currently radioisotopes are being used in monitoring soil fertility nitrogen fixation and plant breeding. Other industries that use radiation material are those dealing with chemicals, petroleum, food products and rocks and ores. Milling and refining of uranium carries a risk of exposure for miners.

Radioactive Pollution and Health

Radioactive substances have been responsible for advancement in medicine, informatics, communication, agriculture, industries, space technology, etc. But have many harmful effects on human health.

- **Acute radiation syndrome:** The initial phase or the period of prodromal symptoms, the intermediate phase or the period of progressive disease.
- **Abnormal pregnancy outcome:** Exposure to ionizing radiation in the implementation phase of an embryo, i.e., 9 to 10 days after conception leads to death of the fetus which obviously escapes notice at that stage 2–6 weeks of gestation, carries a high risk of malformation. During 8–15 weeks gestation carries a high risk of microcephaly and mental retardation.
- **Temporary sterility:** A temporary period of sterility, lasting up to 3 years, may develop after exposure to high dose of ionizing radiation.
- **Shortening of life-span:** Exposure to massive doses of radiation has been implicated in fast aging and shortening of life span.
- **Predisposition to cataract:** Lens of the eye which is particularly sensitive to radiation can develop opacities or frank cataract.
- **Chronic exposure to low level radiation:** Can cause many somatic and genetic problems. In early stages, it can cause depigmentation of skin and loss of hair. In long run of the body like blood cancer, various parts of the body like thyroid, lungs, bones, etc.

Prevention and Control of Radiation

- Use radiation therapy within safe limits and when absolutely required.
- Safe disposal of radioactive waste substances
- Initial efforts to stop nuclear explosion
- Avoidance of unnecessary X-ray examination especially children and pregnant women.
- Underground testing of nuclear explosion

- Through monitoring and surveillance of X-ray plants and workers.
- Application of protective measures while carrying any diagnostic or therapeutic procedure involving use of the radioactive substances.
- Monitoring of level of concentration in the industries labs and nuclear medicine departments.
- Creating awareness among people regarding radioactive radiations.

METEOROLOGICAL ENVIRONMENT

Meteorology is the science that deals with the atmosphere and its phenomena including weather and climate.

Meteorological environment: Meteorological environment includes temperature, humidity, wind and rainfall. These factors keep on changing between different places at the same time or at the same place at different times. The behavior of meteorological factors at a particular time of a place denotes the weather of the place. Climate has a profound influence on all aspects of life patterns of populations. Climate shapes the physical, biological and social environment of places. Climate affects the health and nutritional status of populations and also the spectrum of diseases to which they are exposed.

Types of Climate

- **Tropical type of climate:** In the tropical region, the sun is always shining vertically overhead and the temperature is uniformly high all round the year.
- **Desert type of climate:** Desert climate is very dry, the temperature is very high during the day and the evaporation is excessive. The afternoons are characterized by dust storms, but nights are cold and become very chilly during winter season.
- **Mediterranean type:** This climate is usually characterized by short, wet and mild winters, and long warm and dry summers. Mediterranean region area situated near deserts has hot summers and areas near sea coasts have cool summers.
- **European type of climates:** Proximity to the ocean keeps the summers cold and the warm currents that wash the shores make the winter's warm and mild rainfalls through the year.
- **Monsoon type of climates:** Monsoon lands have typically winter, summer and rainy seasons. The winter is relatively cold and dry; the summer is hot and dry.

Elements of Climate

The meteorological factors like temperature, humidity, wind and rainfall keep on changing between different places at the same time or at the same place at different times.

- **Atmospheric pressure:** The atmospheric pressure at the surface of earth, close to sea level, averages 760 mm Hg per square inch of earth's surface. The greater the humidity of a place in a particular day, the lower the weight of the air column as indicated by the reading of the atmospheric pressure. A depression in atmospheric pressure is obviously an indicator of ensuring rainfall.
- **Air temperature:** Several geographical factors such as altitude, latitude, direction of wind and proximity to sea influence the air temperature of a place. Air temperature does not remain the same even at the same places; it undergoes seasonal as well as diurnal variations in response to various meteorological factors.
- **Air humidity:** Moisture content in the air is expressed in terms of absolute or relative humidity. Absolute humidity is the weight of water vapour per unit volume of air and relative humidity is the percentage of moisture present in the air, complete saturation being taken as 100% humidity.
- **Air movement:** Air movement is initiated by disturbance in the atmospheric equilibrium. Constant changes occurring in the temperature and humidity of air produce variations in the density of air columns.
- **Climate influences** the indoor and outdoor life activities and determines food, shelter and clothing of people. Climate affects the health and nutritional status of populations and also the spectrum of diseases to which they are exposed.

Measurements of Climate

- **Atmospheric pressure:** The instruments used for measuring atmospheric pressure are of two kinds: mercurial barometers and android barometers. The mercurial barometer generally used in meteorological laboratories is Fortin's barometer. It is always fixed at one place in a room and duly protected from sun, rain, wind, and source of heat. Aneroid barometer is portable and handy, it is useful in situations where accurate measurements are not necessary such as for ascertaining heights while climbing mountains or ascending through airplanes.
- **Air temperature:** Several kinds of thermometers are used for measuring temperature of air, the commonly used ones are ordinary thermometer, maximum thermometer, minimum thermometer, Six's thermometer, globe thermometer and wet globe thermometer.
- **Air humidity:** Relative humidity is a better indicator of thermal comfort than absolute humidity. Several types of instruments are available for measuring air humidity, some of are dry and wet bulb thermometers, sling psychometer and Assmann psychometer.
- **Air movement:** Air movement is initiated by disturbance in the atmospheric equilibrium. High velocity in the outdoor air is conventionally measured by an anemometer and the very low density in the indoor air is estimated by using Kata thermometer.
- **Rainfall:** The instrument used for measuring rainfall is a rain gauge. It consists of copper funnel with a sharp rim usually 5 in diameter, an outer case which holds the funnel in place and an inner container located at the bottom for collecting the rainwater.

HOUSING

A WHO Expert Group (1961) on public health aspects of housing prefers to use the term "residential environment" which is defined as the physical structure that man uses and the environs of the structure including all necessary services, facilities, equipment and devices needed or desired for the physical and mental health and the social well-being of the family and the individual. Good housing essential for good health, security, shelter and comfort and for good working conditions. The type of housing will depend upon many different factors such as climate, races, community's socio – cultural standards and economic standards, etc.

Principles and Objectives of Healthful Housing

- **Shelter:** A good housing provides shelter to inhabitants against wind and weather. The shelter should be spacious enough to provide room for sitting, sleeping, cooking, and socializing needs of the family members.
- **Safety:** A house should provide a safe environment characterized by clean air, pure water, safe food and hygienic living. Safety also demands that the house should be accident proof, fire proof and quake proof.
- **Security:** It must serve as an insurance against loss of life and loss of property and valuables.
- **Privacy:** It must provide privacy of a bathroom, privacy of a change room and privacy of a bedroom.

Criteria for Healthful House

An expert committee of the WHO recommended the following criteria of healthful housing:
- Healthful housing provides physical protection and shelter.
- Provides adequately for cooking, eating, washing and excretory functions.
- It is designed, constructed, maintained and used in a manner such as to prevent the spread of communicable diseases.
- Provides for protection from hazards of exposure to noise and pollution.
- It is unsafe physical arrangements due to construction or maintenance and from toxic or harmful materials.
- Encourage personal and community development, promotes social relationships, reflects a regard for ecological principles and by these means promotes mental health.

Housing Standards

The standards are no longer confined to narrow health criteria. Social and economic characteristics such as family income, family size and composition, standards of living, life style, stage in life cycle, education, cultural factors must be taken into consideration in determining housing standards.
- **Site:** The soil selected for the house should be dry and safe. Housing site should be away from fields, marshy area, trenching ground traffic, etc. Soil should be suitable for laying sound foundation.
- **Set back:** Proper lighting and ventilation, there should be an open space all round house—this called set back. Set back should be such that there is no obstruction to lighting and ventilation.
- **Floor:** The floor should be smooth, usually made up of cement, red brick or stone chips. It should be free from cracks and crevices to prevent any insect breeding.
- **Walls:** Walls should be strongly built of burnt brick and plastered both inside and outside and then white washed. It should admit no dampness if exposed to rain.
- **Roof:** The number of living rooms should not be less than ten feet in the absence of air conditioning for comfort. The roof should have a low heat transmittance coefficient.
- **Rooms:** The number of living rooms should not be less than two, at least one of which can be closed for security. The number of area of rooms should be increased according to size of the family.
- **Floor area:** Floor area of a living room should be at least 120 sq.ft. For one person at least 100 sq.ft of floor space should be allowed. Room should not be overcrowded.
- **Windows:** Every room should be provided with at least 2 windows, at least one of them should open directly on to an open space.
- **Lighting:** The daylight factor should exceed 1% over half the floor area.
- **Kitchen:** The kitchen must be protected against dust and smoke, adequately lighted, provided with arrangements for storing food, fuel and provisions, provided with water supply and drainage.
- **Privy:** A sanitary privy is a must in every house, belonging exclusively to it and readily accessible.
- **Bathing and washing:** The house should have facilities for bathing and washing belongings exclusively to it and providing proper privacy.

Effects of Poor Housing

Housing is an important part of man's total environment in promoting health. It is difficult, however, to demonstrate the specific cause and affect relationships because housing embraces so many facts of environment. By deductive reasoning, a strong relationship can be established between poor housing and following conditions:
- **Respiratory infections:** Common cold, tuberculosis, influenza, diphtheria, bronchitis, measles, whooping cough etc.
- **Skin infections:** Scabies, ringworm, impetigo, leprosy.
- **Rat infestation:** Plague
- **Arthropods:** House flies, mosquitoes, Fleas and bugs
- **Accidents:** A substantial proportion of house accidents are caused by some defect in the home and its environment.
- **Morbidity and mortality:** High morbidity and mortality rates are observed where housing conditions are sub-standard.
- **Psychosocial effects:** These effects must not be overloaded. These sense of isolation felt by the persons living in the upper floors of high buildings is now well known to have harmful effects.

- **Overcrowding:** It refers to the situation in which more people are living within a single dwelling than there is space for so that movement is restricted privacy scheduled, hygiene impossible rest and sleep difficult.
- **Physical health:** It is clear though infectious disease spread rapidly under conditions of overcrowding.
- **Overcrowding** is a health problem; it may promote spread of respiratory infections such as tuberculosis, influenza and diphtheria.

TOWN PLANNING

Town planning provides the key to organized growth and development to town. Its objective is to promote physical, mental social and psychosocial well-being of the town population by ensuring healthful residential environment.

Objectives of Town Planning
- Uniform distribution of population
- Undisturbed ecosystem
- Pollution-free environment
- Organized traffic
- Communication system healthy
- Healthy peaceful and productive living conditions.

Importance of Town Planning
- Elimination of hazardous and congested housing units
- To prevent unsanitary surroundings
- Infiltrating slums and industrial establishments
- To prevent traffic hazards.

Elements of Town Planning

Zonalization

Zonalization aims at scientific and organized placement and distribution of various activity areas of town life in manner that obviates encroachments and healthily interactions. Zonalization safeguards the peace and tranquility or residential families without restricting their access to other areas for satisfying their basic needs.

Types of Zonalization
- **Residential zone:** It may comprise a series of sub-zones, each suiting the socioeconomic level of a particular population segment. Accordingly, the plan may have provision for developing separate sub-zones having detached, semi detached or attached layouts.
- **Silent zone:** It should be developed for hospitals, schools, offices and libraries which need special protection from noise pollution.
- **Market zone:** It should have a central location for the convenience of the residing families the consume the market products.
- **Traffic zone:** Traffic zone should be placed a reasonable distance from the residential area. The main traffic roads should not pass through the residential zone or the silent zone.
- **Industrial zone:** It should not be allowed to grow in the vicinity of the township. Industries which do not contribute to environmental pollution may be placed in the industrial zone on the side nearer to the residential area.
- **Intervening zones:** Which separate the residential area from traffic and industrial zones should be developed into green belt areas bearing flower beds, shrubs and trees.

Supportive Services

A town planning is incomplete without adequate provision of supportive services like road transport system, municipal services, public amenities, communication facilities and the like:
- **Road transport:** Regulation of traffic can be ensured by diverting the main traffic roads away from the residential and silent zones.
- **Municipal services:** It includes piped water supply, sewage and drainage systems and solid waste disposal services.
- **Public amenities:** It includes school hospitals, libraries, marriage halls cinema halls, community centers, post-office, police station, fire brigade, telephone booths, etc.

DISPOSAL OF SOLID WASTE

The term **"Solid wastes"** includes garbage (food wastes) rubbish (paper, plastic, wood, throw away containers, glass) demolition products (bricks, masonry, pipes), sewage treatment residue (sludge and solids form the coarse screening of domestic sewage) dead animals, manure and other discarded materials.

Refuse may be defined as solid or semi-solid waste matter produced in the normal course of human activities. The nature, composition and volume of refuse produced vary between different countries, different seasons, different life styles and life activities of population.

Composition of Refuse
- **Decomposable refuse:** This generally includes organic material of human or animal origin excluding excreta. It includes discarded food items, vegetable peelings, dung of cattle, excreta of dogs and hags, droppings of birds and bodies of dead animals, etc.
- **Non-decomposable component:** It includes combustible items like leaves, twigs, paper, packing materials, rags, etc. non-combustible items like grit, pieces, pottery pieces, tins, bottles, etc. The non-decomposable refuse items have a tendency to get scattered and thereby spread filthiness all around.

Health Hazards of Accumulated Solid Waste

There is a correlation between improper disposal of solid wastes and incidence of vector-borne diseases. Therefore in all civilized countries, there is an efficient system for its periodic collection, removal and final disposal without risk to health.

- It decomposes and favors fly breeding.
- It attracts rodents and vermin.
- The pathogens which may be present in the solid waste may be conveyed back to man's food through flies and dust.
- There is a possibility of water and solid pollution.
- Heaps of refuse present an unsightly appearance and nuisance from bad odour.

Sources of Refuse

- **Domestic refuse:** It includes kitchen garbage arising during preparation, distribution and consumption of food items, it comprises vegetable peelings, discarded fruits and various food remnants. Domestic refuse also includes rubbish or non-decomposable and combustible waste items.
- **Street refuse:** It includes decomposable and non-decomposable, combustible and non-combustible waste items issuing from markets, hotels, offices, etc. It also includes street sweeping consisting of rubbish and organic waste matter.
- **Industrial refuse:** It includes metal shavings metal cuttings, metal scrapping, grit, dust, cinder and various type of discarded items.
- **Constructional refuse:** It includes and, grit, gravel, stone pieces, brickbats, wood shaving and variety of discarded items.
- **Hospital refuses:** It contains both organic and inorganic waste items such as laboratory waste, dressing, human tissues, needles and syringes.
- **Stable refuse:** It is composed of horse dung, cow dung, strew, hey and discarded animal feeds, etc.

Storage and Collection of Refuses

- **Storage:** Before the refuse is taken for disposal it has to be collected in proper receptacles or containers. The galvanized steel dust bin with close fitting cover is a suitable receptable for storing refuse. The capacity of a bin will depend upon the number of user and frequency of collection. Refuse is stored in the paper sack and the sack is substituted. Public bin cater for a longer number of people. They are usually without cover in India because people do not like to touch them. They are kept on a concrete platform raised 2 to 3 inches above ground level to prevent flood water entering the bin. In bigger municipalities, the bins are handled and emptied mechanically by lorries fitted with cranes.
- **Collection:** The method of collection depends upon the funds available. House to house collection is by far the best method of collecting refuse. In India, there is no house to house collection system. People are expected to dump the refuse in the nearest public bin. The refuse is then transported in refuse collection vehicles to the place of ultimate disposal. The environmental hygiene committee (1949) recommended that municipalities and other local bodies should arrange for collection of refuse not only form the public bins but also from individual houses. There is a wide variety of refuse collection vehicles of all shapes and size. The largest arrival in the western countries is the "Dustless Refuse Collector" which has a totally enclosed body.

Methods of Disposal

Unsanitary Methods

- **Hog feeding:** It continues to be a traditional way of refuse disposal in certain areas and certain cultures of the world. It provides cheap method of raising pig stock and a cheap means of refuse disposal for habitations that indulge in this practice for economic reasons.
- **Stacking:** Stacking or piling-up of refuse and cow dung usually observed in rural India, is a traditional practice. Stacks attract flies, birds and rats and also lead to soil and water pollution.
- **Salvaging:** It is an unhealthy practice of screening refuse dumps to recover objects that can be reclaimed and reused. Salvaging is a reverse process whereby some of the filth is a reverse process whereby some of he filth is returned to the area wherefrom it was removed for disposal.
- **Pumping:** Pumping of refuse openly in an unsanitary manner in peri-urban areas by municipalities and corporations is a hazardous practice that threatens the health population living in adjoining areas.

Sanitary Methods of Refuse Disposal

- **Composting:** It is an integrated method of refuse disposal, has been in practice in many parts of the world, since ancient times, albeit with regional differences. Basically there are two methods of composting in vogue, the anaerobic and aerobic methods. In Indian situation, the aerobic method as Indoor method.
- **Aerobic method (Indoor method):** In this method a pit of 30 ft × 14 ft × 2 ft with a slope is dug refuse, cow dung or horse dung, urine are mixed and piled, layer by layer up to 2 inches thick. Watering is done and the whole pit is filled in 6 days or less. The whole process goes on for 90 days and then the product is removed.
- **Anaerobic method (Bangalore method):** In this method, trenches are dug 15 to 30 feet deep, These 8 feet broad and not more than 3 feet deep. These trenches should be located at ½ mile from city or town limits. The procedure of composting in this method is first a thickness of 6" refuse is spread at the bottom of the trench as the first layer. Over this a layer of night soil is spread alternately till the heap rises to one foot above the ground level till the point reaches where the top layer ends up with refuse with 9 inches thickness.
- **Sanitary landfill:** Sanitary landfill or controlled tipping is the most hygienic process of refuse disposal, suitable for land filling. Sanitary landfill consists in lying of dry and condensed refuse in layers with intervening earth partitions or covering to prevent nuisance due to fly breeding.

- **Incineration:** Incineration or burning is suitable method of refuse disposal in congested areas where place is not available for sanitary landfill. It is the method of choice for hospital refuse which include infected organic waste, burning kills bacterial flora and ova of insects and converts the infected material into an innocuous mass.
- **Disposal of excreta:** Human excreta are a source of infection. It is an important cause of environmental pollution. Every society has a responsibility for its safe removal and disposal so that it does not constitute a threat to public health.

Health Hazards of Improper Excreta Disposal

- Soil pollution
- Water pollution
- Contamination of food
- Propagation of flies
- **Disease caused:** Typhoid and paratyphoid fever, dysenteries, diarrheas, cholera, hook worm disease, ascariasis, viral hepatitis, and similar other intestinal infections and parasitic infestations.
- **Transmission of fecal-borne disease:** Human excreta of a sick person or a carrier of disease is the main focus of infection. It contains the disease agent which is transmitted to a new host through various channels.
  1. Water, 2. Finger, 3. Flies, 4. Soil, 5. Food
- **Sanitation barrier:** Sanitation barrier is the barrier can be provided by a 'Sanitary latrine' and a disposal pit.

Hygienic Requirement of Sanitary Latrines

- A water seal arrangements for receiving excreta
- Plenty of water for flushing and ablution
- Adequate ventilation for letting off offensive gases.
- Hygienic system for disposal of excreta.
- Health education of the community on hygienic living can facilitate the use of sanitary latrines in rural areas.

Types of Latrines

Service Latrines

- **Bucket latrine:** It consists of a collection chambers made of brick or cement with an opening at rear for manual service. The collection chamber provides space for accommodating a bucket or pail of impervious material.
- **Commode toilet:** Commode toilet is very simple in structure, consisting of porcelain or enameled pan or pot supported by a wooden or iron stand, the top of which forms the seat. The seat is covered with a tight closing or self-closing lid to ward off fly nuisance.
- **Chemical closet:** It consists of a corrosion resistant metal tank usually of 500 L capacity. The tank has a seat at the top provided with a seat cover. It is also connected to a ventilating pipe that passes through the house roof. The tank is filled with an alkaline solution. Caustic soda and phenol, and a tap covering of crude oil.
- **Biogas plant supplement:** A biogas plant provides a scientific way of disposing of excreta from bucket latrines or commode toilets without polluting the environment.

Nonservice Latrines

Nonservice latrines are sanitary because they do not require any manual handling of excreta, nor do they cause any soil or water pollution. Nonservice latrines have provision for in-situ treatment of excreta by the action of soil bacteria, aerobic as well as anaerobic.

- **Shallow trench latrine:** A row of seats provided across a shallow trench. A temporary screening arrangement for privacy. Direct disposal into the trench. At the end of defecation, the user cover the excreta with excavated earth, useful in temporary habitations.
- **Deep trench latrine:** A row of seats provided across a deep trench. Wooden planks put across the trench for squatting purpose. Partition walls raised in between the seats for privacy. Direct disposal of excreta into the trench, used for semi-permanent habitations.
- **Direct pit latrine:** A concrete squatting plate fixed on the top of a circular pit. There is no water seal system. The excreta fall directly into the pit through a drop hole. A suitable enclosure with provision for ventilation is created for privacy and shelter. It intended to serve a family of 4–5 members for several years.
- **VIP latrine:** A concrete squatting plate fixed on top of a pit. The excreta fall directly into the pit through a drop hole. There is no provision for a water seal. When the pit contents rise up to one meter below ground level, its squatting plate is removed and it is topped with earth cover to allow anaerobic putrefaction of excreta.
  Intended to serve a family of 4–5 members for several years.
- **Septic tank latrine:** A water closet complete with pan, trap, flushing cistern and ventilation pipe assembly is connected to an underground septic tank and seepage pit system. The seating arrangements may be squatting type or sitting type. Usually placed in a bathroom that provides privacy and comfort.

  The sewage that collects in the septic tank undergoes anaerobic putrefaction. It is an ideal water seal latrine which is designed to meet the requirements of families in towns and cities having water supply but no sewage system.
- **Aqua privy:** One or more squatting plates each having a central drop hole with foot rests on either side. The drop hole is connected to drop pipe which remains submerged in water contained in a water tight masonry tank. An outlet pipe connects the tank with a seepage pit or subsurface irrigation system. Superstructure is built on the top of the tank for providing privacy and shelter. The fecal matter that collects in the tank undergoes anaerobic putrefaction. It is a feasible alternative to septic latrine in areas where there is no sewage system.

COMMONLY USED INSECTICIDES AND PESTICIDES

Pesticides are chemical substances that are meant to kill pests. In general, a pesticide is a chemical or a biological agent such as a virus, bacterium, antimicrobial, or disinfectant that deters, incapacitates, kills, pests.

This use of pesticides is so common that the term pesticide is often treated as synonymous with plant protection product. It is commonly used to eliminate or control a variety of agricultural pests that can damage crops and livestock and reduce farm productivity. The most commonly applied pesticides are insecticides to kill insects, herbicides to kill weeds, rodenticides to kill rodents, and fungicides to control fungi, mold, and mildew.

Definition of Pesticides

The Food and Agriculture Organization (FAO) has defined pesticide as: any substance or mixture of substances intended for preventing, destroying, or controlling any pest, including vectors of human or animal disease, unwanted species of plants or animals, causing harm during or otherwise interfering with the production, processing, storage, transport, or marketing of food, agricultural commodities, wood and wood products or animal feedstuffs, or substances that may be administered to animals for the control of insects, arachnids, or other pests in or on their bodies.

Types of Pesticides

These are grouped according to the types of pests which they kill.
1. Insecticides—insects
2. Herbicides—plants
3. Rodenticides—rodents (rats and mice)
4. Bactericides—bacteria
5. Fungicides—fungi
6. Larvicides—larvae

- **Biodegradable:** The biodegradable kind is those which can be broken down by microbes and other living beings into harmless compounds.
- **Persistent:** While the persistent ones are those which may take months or years to break down.

Another way to classify these is to consider those that are chemical forms or are derived from a common source or production method.

Chemically-related Pesticides

- **Organophosphate:** Most organophosphates are insecticides, they affect the nervous system by disrupting the enzyme that regulates a neurotransmitter.
- **Carbamate:** Similar to the organophosphorus pesticides, the carbamate pesticides also affect the nervous system by disrupting an enzyme that regulates the neurotransmitter. However, the enzyme effects are usually reversible.
- **Organochlorine insecticides:** They were commonly used earlier, but now many countries have been removed Organochlorine insecticides from their market due to their health and environmental effects and their persistence (e.g., DDT, chlordane, and toxaphene).
- **Pyrethroid:** These are a synthetic version of pyrethrin, a naturally occurring pesticide, found in chrysanthemums (Flower). They were developed in such a way as to maximize their stability in the environment.
- **Sulfonylurea herbicides:** The sulfonylureas herbicides have been commercialized for weed control such as pyrithiobac-sodium, cyclosulfamuron, bispyribac-sodium, terbacil, sulfometuron-methyl Sulfosulfuron, rimsulfuron, pyrazosulfuron-ethyl, imazosulfuron, nicosulfuron, oxasulfuron, nicosulfuron, flazasulfuron, primisulfuron-methyl, halosulfuron-methyl, flupyrsulfuron-methyl-sodium, ethoxysulfuron, chlorimuron-ethyl, bensulfuron-methyl, azimsulfuron, and amidosulfuron.
- **Biopesticides:** The biopesticides are certain types of pesticides derived from such natural materials as animals, plants, bacteria, and certain minerals.

Examples of Pesticides

Examples of pesticides are fungicides, herbicides, and insecticides. Examples of specific synthetic chemical pesticides are glyphosate, Acephate, Deet, Propoxur, Metaldehyde, Boric Acid, Diazinon, Dursban, DDT, Malathion, etc.

Benefits of Pesticides

The major advantage of pesticides is that they can save farmers. By protecting crops from insects and other pests. However, below are some other primary benefits of it.
- Controlling pests and plant disease vectors.
- Controlling human/livestock disease vectors and nuisance organisms.
- Controlling organisms that harm other human activities and structures.

Effects of Pesticides

- The toxic chemicals in these are designed to deliberately released into the environment. Though each pesticide is meant to kill a certain pest, a very large percentage of pesticides reach a destination other than their target. Instead, they enter the air, water, sediments, and even end up in our food.
- Pesticides have been linked with human health hazards, from short-term impacts such as headaches and nausea to chronic impacts like cancer, reproductive harm.
- The use of these also decreases the general biodiversity in the soil. If there are no chemicals in the soil there is a higher soil quality, and this allows for higher water retention, which is necessary or plants to grow.

CONCLUSION

Environmental science is the study of the effects of natural and unnatural processes, and of interactions of the physical components of the planet on the environment. Environmental science involves different fields of study. Most often, the study of environmental science includes the study of climate change, natural resources, energy, pollution, and environmental issues. In environmental sciences, ecologists study how plants and animals interact with each other, chemists study the living and non-living components of the environment, geologists study the formation, structure and history of earth, biologists study the biodiversity, Physicists are involved in thermodynamics, computer scientists are involved in technical innovations and computer modeling and biomedical experts study the impact of environmental issues on our health and social lives.

BIBLIOGRAPHY

1. Alrumman SA, El-kott AF, Kehsk MA. Water pollution: Source and treatment. Ame j Environ Eng. 2016;6(3):88–98.
2. Bibi S, Khan RL, Nazir R, et al. Heavy metals in drinking water of Lakki Marwat District, KPK, Pakistan. World App Sci j. 2016; 34(1):15–19.
3. Briggs D. Environmental pollution and the global burden of disease. British Med. Bull. 2003;68:1–24.
4. Gibbons, Whit. "Whither Our Air and Water?" The World and I vol. 14, issue 6 (June 01, 1999):184.
5. Gleick, Peter H. "Safeguarding Our Water: Making Every Drop Count." Scientific American vol. 284, no. 2 (February 01, 2001):38.
6. Juneja T, Chauhdary A. Assessment of water quality and its effect on the health of residents of Jhunjhunu district, Rajasthan: A cross sectional study. Public health and epidem. 2013;5(4):186–91.
7. Khan MA, Ghouri AM. Environmental Pollution: Its effects on life and its remedies. Arts, Science and Comm. 2011;2(2):276–85.
8. Khan N, Hussain ST, Saboor A, et al. Physiochemical investigation of the drinking water sources from Mardan, Khyber Pakhtunkhwa, Pakistan. Int. Phy Sci. 2013;8(33): 1661–71.
9. McEvoy, T. J. Positive Impact Forestry: A Sustainable Approach to Managing Woodlands. Washington, DC: Island Press, 2004.
10. Pawari MJ, Gawande S. Ground water pollution and its consequence. Int. Eng Res and Gen Sci. 2015;3(4):773–76.
11. Smith, W. Brad, Patrick D. Miles, John S. et al. Forest Resources of the United States. Washington, DC: U.S. Department of Agriculture Forest Service, 2002.
12. Vickers, Amy. Water Use and Conservation: Homes, Landscapes, Industries, Businesses, Farms. Amherst, MA: Water Plow Press, 2001.

REVIEW QUESTIONS

Long Essays

1. Define non-communicable diseases. Briefly explain the types of non-communicable diseases.
2. Define sanitation. Explain the types of environment.
3. Define natural sources. Discuss the classifications of natural sources.
4. Discuss and compare the renewable and nonrenewable resources.
5. Define forest resources. Enumerate the direct and indirect benefits of forest resources.
6. Define deforestation. Explain the causes and effects of deforestation.
7. Define water pollution. Explain the sources and effects of polluted water on humans.
8. Define energy source. Explain the renewable energy resources.
9. Enumerate role of individuals in conservation of natural resources.
10. Define ecosystem. Explain the types of natural ecosystem.
11. Define environmental pollution. Explain in detail about air pollution.
12. Explain the effects of marine pollution. Enumerate steps to prevent marine pollution.
13. Describe 17 new undevelopment goals for 2030.
14. Explain the concept of pollution prevention: air and noise pollution, role of nurse in prevention of pollution.

Short Essays

1. Environmental sanitation problems.
2. Nutritional problems in India.
3. Nutritional anemia.
4. Iodine Deficiency Disorders (IDD).
5. Approaches to man–environment relationship.
6. Importance of environmental science.
7. Components of environmental science.
8. Natural resources and associated problems.
9. Renewable and nonrenewable water resources.
10. Types of mineral resources.
11. Exploitation of mineral resources.
12. Mineral contamination and effects on health.
13. Define food sources, explain the world food problems.
14. Equitable use of resources for sustainable lifestyles.
15. Ecosystem—scope and importance.
16. Ecological pyramid.
17. National Biodiversity Act.
18. Importance of ecosystem.
19. Energy flow in ecosystem.
20. Significance of biodiversity.
21. Productive use value of biodiversity.
22. Threats to biodiversity.
23. Man-Wildlife conflict.
24. Conversation of biodiversity.
25. Soil or land pollution.
26. Harmful effects of the thermal pollution.
27. Nuclear hazards and their impact on health.
28. Impact of climate change on human environment.
29. Components of hazardous waste management.
30. Population explosion and its pressure on environment.
31. Ozone depleting substances.
32. Environmental Protection Act.
33. Global environmental problems.
34. Environmental education.
35. Components of hygiene and environmental health.
36. Household purification of water.
37. Methods of rainwater harvesting.
38. Commonly used insecticides and pesticides.

Short Answers

1. Communicable diseases.
2. Malaria.
3. Tuberculosis.
4. Population problem.
5. Medical care problems

6. Protein energy malnutrition.
7. Vitamin D deficiency.
8. Low birth weight.
9. Fluorosis.
10. Ecological approach.
11. Types of water resources.
12. Metallic and nonmetallic minerals.
13. Aquaculture.
14. Undernourishment.
15. Land resources.
16. Man-induced landslides.
17. Conservation of water.
18. Aquatic ecosystem.
19. Pyramid of biomass.
20. Pyramid of energy.
21. Biogeochemical cycles.
22. Carbon cycle.
23. Ecosystem diversity.
24. Water pollution control.
25. Sources of noise pollution.
26. Effects of nuclear pollution.
27. Causes of climate change.
28. Global warming causes.
29. Factors affecting environmental health.
30. Dimensions of environmental sanitation.
31. Water-borne diseases.
32. Principles of chlorination.
33. Bacteriological quality of water.
34. Meteorological environment.
35. Principles and objectives of healthful housing.
36. Criteria for healthful house.
37. Effects of poor housing.

Multiple Choice Questions

1. Which of the following non-infectious diseases is the most lethal?
   a. Cancer   b. Diabetes
   c. AIDS   d. Obesity
2. Which of the following is not a pathogenic biological agent?
   a. Fungi   b. Radiations
   c. Virus   d. Mycoplasma
3. Sanitation is defined as "a way of life". It is the quality of the living that is expressed in the clean:
   a. Neighborhood   b. Clean community
   c. Both a and b   d. None of the above
4. Which of the following is the main reason for producing the atmospheric greenhouse effect?
   a. Absorption and re-emission of ultraviolet radiations by the atmosphere
   b. Absorption and re-emission of infrared radiations by the atmosphere
   c. Absorption and re-emission of visible light by the atmosphere
   d. None of the above
5. The year declared as the "water year" by the Indian Government is
   a. 2010   b. 2005
   c. 2006   d. 2007
6. Which of the following energy is stored in the earth?
   a. Mechanical energy
   b. Solar energy
   c. Chemical energy
   d. Geothermal energy
7. The forest cover in our country has recently increased due to:
   a. Increase in natural forest growth
   b. Increase in net sown area
   c. Plantation by different agencies
   d. None of the above
8. Which one of the following is not a direct outcome of environmental destruction?
   a. Biological loss
   b. Loss of cultural diversity
   c. Severe droughts
   d. River Valley Projects
9. What is the process of removal of forest cover of an area called?
   a. Afforestation
   b. Deforestation
   c. Pollution
   d. Greenhouse effect
10. Which of the following are the primary causes of water pollution?
    a. Plants
    b. Animals
    c. Human activities
    d. None of these
11. Which of the following is a waterborne disease?
    a. Typhoid   b. Cholera
    c. Diarrhea   d. All of the above
12. Which of the following is not a waterborne disease?
    a. Measles   b. Typhoid
    c. Cholera   d. Hepatitis

ANSWERS

| 1. a | 2. b | 3. b | 4. b | 5. d | 6. d | 7. c | 8. c | 9. b | 10. c | 11. d | 12. a |

National Health Programs

LEARNING OBJECTIVES

1. National ARI Control Programme
2. Revised national tuberculosis control programme (RNTCP)
3. National antimalaria programme
4. National Filarial Control Programme
5. National Guinea Worm Eradication Programme
6. National Leprosy Eradication Programme
7. National AIDS Control Programme
8. STD Control Programme
9. National Program for Control of Blindness
10. Iodine Deficiency Control Programme
11. Expanded Program of Immunization
12. National Family Welfare Programme
13. National Water Supply and Sanitation Programme
14. Minimum Needs programme
15. National Diabetes Control Programme
16. Polio Eradication: Pulse Programme
17. NPSP
18. National Cancer Control Programme
19. Yaws Eradication Programme
20. National Nutritional Anemia Prophylaxis Programme
21. 20 Points Programme
22. ICDS Programme
23. Mid-day Meal Programme
24. National Mental Health Programme
25. Adolescent Health Programme
26. Role of Nurse in the National Health Programme

TERMINOLOGY

- **Basic needs:** Besides minimum needs, they cover the aspects of equity, social justice and human rights also.
- **Distributive justice:** It refers to equal opportunities for employment and sources to income and access to social services by all.
- **Environment:** Natural ecosystem or balance between land, water, flora and fauna.
- **Food security:** To ensure availability of food for all at affordable costs.
- **Human development:** Improvement in the quality of life.
- **ILO:** International Labor Organization, a sister organization of United Nations.
- **Needs:** Facilities/services like housing, health and nutrition, elementary education, safe drinking water and sanitation, which are necessary for improving living standards.
- **Promotive health:** It refers to nutrition, hygiene and sanitation.

NATIONAL ARI CONTROL PROGRAMME

The National ARI Control Programme was launched in 1989 in order to reduce the mortality attributed to pneumonia, and rationalize the use of drugs in the management of patients with ARI. WHO's standard ARI case management guidelines were adopted to achieve these objectives. **Figure 15.1** explained the factors causes for acute respiratory infections.

ARI Control

- Improving the primary medical care services and developing better methods for early detection, treatment and prevention of acute respiratory infection is the best way to control ARI.
- Mortality rate due to pneumonia is reduced if treated correctly.
- Education of mothers about pneumonia because compliance with treatment and seeking proper care when child suffers determine outcome of the disease.

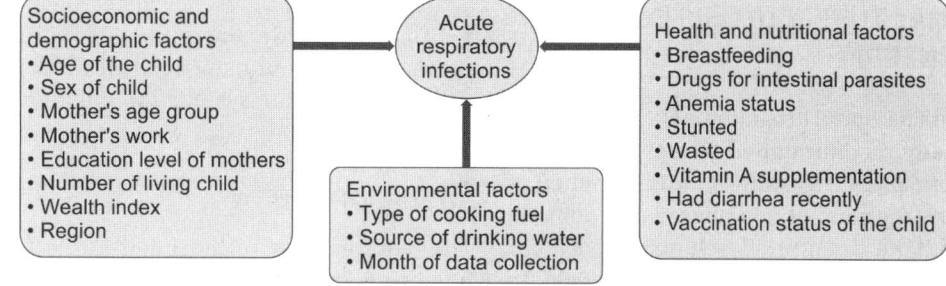

Fig. 15.1: Factors causes acute respiratory infections.

ARI Control Programs

Crux of the program is to identify children with ARI at the community level by training the field workers to recognize easily and reliably identifiable clinical signs of ARI and early reference WHO protocol comprises three steps:
1. Case finding and assessment
2. Case classification
3. Institution of appropriate therapy

Step 1: Case finding and assessment
- Cough and difficult breathing in children < 5 years age
- Fever is not an efficient criterion

Step 2: Case classification: Children grouped into 2:
- Infants <2 months and older children
- Signs to be looked: In younger children like feeding difficulty, lethargy, hypothermia, convulsions.

In Infants <2 months
- Pneumonia is diagnosed if RR 60/min with other clinical signs
- All should be hospitalized
- All should receive IV medications
- Minimum duration of 10 days
- Combination of Ampicillin and Gentamicin

Step 3: Institution of appropriate therapy: Antibiotics

Prevention of ARI

- Breastfeeding infants exclusively (no other food or drinks, not even water) for the first six months breast milk have excellent nutritional value and it contains the mother's antibodies which help to protect the infant from infection.
- Avoiding irritation of the respiratory tract by indoor air pollution, such as smoke from cooking fires; avoid the use of dried cow dung as fuel for indoor fires.
- Immunization of all children with the routine Expanded Program on Immunization
- Feeding children with adequate amounts of varied and nutritious food to keep their immune system strong.
- Control the spread of respiratory bacteria by educating parents to avoid contact as much as possible between their children and patients who have ARIs.
- People with ARIs should cough or sneeze away from others, hold a cloth to the nose and mouth to catch the airborne droplets when coughing or sneezing
- Immunization also increases control, by reducing the reservoir of infection in the community and increasing the level of herd immunity.

REVISED NATIONAL TUBERCULOSIS CONTROL PROGRAMME (RNTCP)

The Revised National TB Control Programme (RNTCP), based on the internationally recommended Directly Observed Treatment Short-course (DOTS) strategy, was launched in 1997 expanded across the country in a phased manner with support from World Bank and other development partners. Full nationwide coverage was achieved in March 2006. In terms of treatment of patients, RNTCP has been recognized as the largest and the fastest expanding TB Control Program in the world. RNTCP is presently being implemented throughout the country.

- Under the program, diagnosis and treatment facilities are provided free of cost to all TB patients. For quality diagnosis, designated microscopy centers have been established for every one lac population in the general areas and for every 50,000 population in the tribal, hilly and difficult areas.
- More than 13,000 microscopy centers have been established in the country. Free treatment services are available for TB at all Government hospitals, Community Health Centers (CHC), Primary Health Centers (PHCs).
- DOT centers have been established near to residence of patients to the extent possible. All public health faculties, subcenters, Community Volunteers, ASHA, and Women Self-Groups, etc. also function as DOT Providers/DOT Centers.

Estimated TB Burden in India (as per Global TB Report 2015)

- **Incidence:** 2.2 million new TB cases annually—167 cases per 100,000 populations
- **Prevalence:** 2.5 million cases—195 cases per 1,00,000 population
- **Deaths:** About 220,000 deaths each year—17 deaths per 1,00,000 population
- Approximately 5% of TB patients estimated to be HIV +ve
- DR-TB (Drug resistant-TB)
- 2.2% in new cases and 15% in previously treated cases.

India is highest TB burden country in the world, accounting for nearly 23% of the global incidence. In 2014, out of the estimated global annual incidence of 9.6 million TB cases; 2.2 million were estimated to have occurred in India.

Goal of the Program

The goal of TB Control Program is to decrease mortality and morbidity due to TB and cut transmission of infection until TB ceases to be a major public health problem in India.

Objectives of the Program

- To reduce the incidence of and mortality due to TB
- To prevent further emergence of drug resistance and effectively manage drug-resistant TB cases
- To improve outcomes among HIV-infected TB patients
- To involve private sector on a scale commensurate with their dominant presence in healthcare services
- To further decentralize and align basic RNTCP management units with NRHM block level units within general health system for effective supervision and monitoring.

Strategic Pillars

The requirements for moving towards TB elimination have been integrated into the four strategic pillars of "Detect-Treat-Prevent-Build" (DTPB).

- **Detect:** Find all DS-TB and DR-TB cases with an emphasis on reaching TB patients seeking care from private providers and undiagnosed TB in high-risk populations.
- **Treat:** Initiate and sustain all patients on appropriate anti-TB treatment wherever they seek care, with patient-friendly systems and social support.
- **Prevent** the emergence of TB in susceptible populations
- **Build** and strengthen enabling policies, empowered institutions and human resources with enhanced capacities.

Action List

For achieving the goals of the NSP 2017–2025, the following critical components of the program will be addressed on priority. The next set of actions includes:
- Ministry of Health and Family Welfare (MoHFW) will evolve a scheme to address the patients seeking care in private sector. The scheme will have suitable incentives for the private doctors and patients to report TB cases coupled with another scheme to provide free of cost medicines to TB patients going to a private doctor/institute.
- A robust, modern MIS system will be developed to monitor the newly diagnosed as well as existing cases of TB on delivery of the drug kit to the patient, compliance to treatment regimen etc. The MIS system will have suitable linkages with the private pharmacy on sale of anti-TB drugs thereby integrating those patients into the MIS.
- The availability of rapid molecular tests will be suitably augmented so that these diagnostic facilities are also made available for patients referred by any private doctor or institute.
- To improve the compliance of the TB patients to the treatment regimen, MoHFW will start customized SMS services to the individual patients on regular basis reminding them about the time to consume the drugs.
- The MoHFW will establish mechanisms for facilitating nutritional support to the TB patients, including financial support through DBT mode.
- The MoHFW will work on a scheme to provide suitable incentives to the States doing well in RNTCP. The incentives will also be linked with performance in "Swachh Bharat Mission".
- **TB Corpus Fund:** To improve financial sustainability in the TB sector the program will mobilize additional resources to accelerate TB control efforts, for which the 'Bharat Kshay Niyantran Pratishthan' (India TB Control Foundation) is proposed. Activities like nutrition support for TB patients, active case finding in prisons, slums, tribal area, sputum collection and transport in difficult areas will be carried out.

Tracking the Progress

A national level annual review of the program will be undertaken by the TB elimination board chaired by the Prime Minister's Office (PMO). Apart from the SDG related indicators the review will also track program performance and provide directives to enhance the ease of Program implementation at all levels.

NATIONAL ANTIMALARIA PROGRAMME

Malaria is one of the major communicable diseases affecting mankind, caused by Plasmodium parasite, transmitted by the bite of infective female Anopheles mosquito. There are four plasmodium species, *P. vivax* (Pv), *P. falciparum* (Pf), *P. malaria* (Pm) and *P. ovale* (Po).

Malaria is one of the serious public health problems in India. At the time of independence malaria was contributing 75 million cases with 0.8 million deaths every year prior to the launching of National Malaria Control Program in 1953. A countrywide comprehensive Program to control malaria was recommended in 1946 by the Bhore committee report that was endorsed by the Planning Commission in 1951. The National Program against Malaria has a long history since that time. In April 1953, Government of India launched a National Malaria Control Program (NMCP) with the following objectives:
- To bring down malaria transmission to a level at which it would cease to be a major public health problem; and
- Thereafter an achievement was to be maintained by each state to hold down the malaria transmission at low level indefinitely.

Strategies under NMCP

- Principal operational activities under the control program comprised of residual insecticide spray of human dwelling and cattle sheds;
- Malaria control teams were organized and directed by the state antimalaria organization to carry out surveys and to monitor the malaria incidence in the control areas; and
- Antimalarial drugs were made available for patients reporting to an Institution.

Modified Plan of Operation

In 1977, attempts at malaria eradication were given up and under the review policy, a modified plan of operation (MPO) was adopted.

Objectives

- To reduce period of sickness and to prevent deaths due to Malaria
- To maintain industrial and agricultural progress
- To retain the achievements gained so far.

Activities

- Establishing District Malaria Control Societies
- Fever Treatment Depot
- Malaria Voluntary Link Worker Scheme
- PADA Worker Scheme
- Insecticide spraying (selective)
- Early case detection and prompt treatment (EDPT)
- Identification of high-risk areas
- Biological measures—Guppy fishes

- Insecticide impregnated mosquito nets
- Chemoprophylaxis—preventive treatment for pregnant mothers
- Antimalaria campaign

World Bank assisted Enhanced Malaria Control Project.
In the State, 14 tribal districts and Navi Mumbai Corporation is identified for implementation of the project. District Malaria Control Societies have been established.

Components

- Early Detection and Prompt Treatment (EDPT).
- Selective Vector Control.
  - Insecticide spray in selected villages.
  - Antilarval measures.
  - Personal protection methods.

Under the scheme 1, 77,646 mosquito nets impregnated with insecticide have been distributed in 28 villages.

The pregnant mothers are given prophylactic treatment for Malaria in the high risk area.
  - Training to Health Personnel.
  - Inputs ego vehicles, equipment and diagnostic kits.

Antimalaria Campaign

Since last five years, the month of June is celebrated for Antimalaria campaign. This is to involve the community in the Antimalaria measures. Following messages are given:
- Examination of blood in every case of fever is necessary.
- In case of malaria, radical treatment is must.
- Clean environment will prevent mosquito-breeding places.
- Use of mosquito net for personal protection.
- Cooperate health workers in the spraying activity.
- Malaria with headache, vomiting, unconsciousness indicates serious symptoms, contact hospital immediately.

Urban Malaria Scheme

The proposal of Urban Malaria Scheme (UMS) was sanctioned in 1971 when it was realized that urban malaria was a significant problem and if effective antilarval measures were not undertaken in urban areas, the proliferation of malaria cases from urban to rural might occur in a bigger way. In this scheme all the towns having more than 40,000 populations and showing more than 2 API in last 3 years are to be covered. At present 131 towns and cities in 19 states and union territories are under the UMS.

Enhanced Malaria Control Project

Enhanced Malaria Control Project (EMCP) was launched in April 1997 with the assistance of the World Bank. This is directly benefiting the six crore Tribal Population of the eight peninsular states covering 100 districts and 19 urban areas. However, the population living in other malaria endemic areas is also benefited, as the strengthening of the components of IEC, Training and Management Information System has covered the entire country.

Selection of PHCs is based on:

- Annual Parasitic Incidence (API) is more than 2 for last 3 years;
- Plasmodium falciparum cases are more than 30% of the malaria cases;
- 25% population of the PHC is tribal; and
- The area has been reporting deaths due to malaria and also has the flexibility to direct resources to any needy areas in case of outbreak of malaria.

Objectives of EMCP

- Effective control of malaria to bring reduction in malaria morbidity;
- Prevention of death due to malaria;
- Consolidation of the gain achieved so far.

Strategies

- Early case detection and prompt treatment;
- Vector control by indoor residual insecticide spray in rural areas with API of 2 per 100 and above in the preceding three years with appropriate insecticide and by recurrent antimalaria in urban areas;
- Health Education and community participation.

Components of EMCP

- Early case detection and prompt treatment
- Selective vector control
- Legislative measures
- Personal protective measures
- Epidemic planning and Rapid Response and Intersectoral Coordination
- Institutional and Management Capacities Strengthening
- Operation Research
- Community Participation.

Antimalaria Drug Policy

The National Antimalaria Drug Policy was drafted in 1982 to combat the increasing level of resistance to chloroquine detected in Pf. However, there was large scale malaria epidemics reported in recent times that has generated great concerns. An expert committee was formulated under the chairmanship of DGHS to revise the drug treatment policy and the committee submitted its recommendations.

NATIONAL FILARIA CONTROL PROGRAMME

After pilot project in Orissa from 1949 to 1954, the National Filaria Control Programme (NFCP) was launched in the country in 1955 with the objective of delimiting the problem, to undertake control measures in endemic areas and to train personnel to man the program. The main control measures were mass DEC administration, antilarval measures in urban areas and indoor residual spray in rural areas.

NFCP Strategy

- Recurrent antilarval measures at weekly intervals.
- Environmental methods include source reduction by filling ditches, pits, low lying areas, deweeding, desilting, etc.
- Biological control of mosquito breeding through larvivorous fish.
- Anti-parasitic measures through 'detection' and 'treatment' of microfilaria carriers and disease person with DEC by Filaria Clinics in towns covered under the Program.

Concept of the Program

- The National Filarial Control Programme was launched in 1955.
- The activities are mainly confined to urban area.
- However, the program has been extended to rural area since 1994.
- The population covered under National Filarial Control Programme is 53.68 lakhs.

Objectives

- To train professional and ancillary personnel required for the program.
- To carry out survey in different part of the state.
- Reduction of problem in unsurveyed area.
- Control in urban area through recurrent anti-parasitic measure.

Activities of NFCP

- Recurrent weekly antiviral operations and biological control of vector through larvivorous fish.
- Source reduction through environmental and water management.
- Diagnosis and treatment of microfilaria carriers and management of cases.
- Information, education and communication for community awareness.

Detection of Carriers

- Through the immuno-chromatographic card test is used to detect the infection in human and mosquitoes.
- It is done with night blood smear examination.
- It is costlier.

Mass Drug Administration

Chemotherapy: EX-Diethylcarbamazine.
1. Bancroftian filariasis: Dose: 6 mg/kg/body-weight/day/orally
2. Brugian filariasis: Dose: 3–6 mg/kg/body-weight/day

Strategy

- Revised control strategy for lymphatic filariasis was adopted in 1996.
- The components of the revised strategy were:
- Single dose mass diethylcarbamazine therapy at dose of 6 mg/kg body weight once a year.
- Management of acute and chronic filariasis through referral services at selected centers.
- Continuation of antivector measures in all the National Filarial Control Programme towns as complimentary to antiparasitic measures.

Role of Nurse

The functions of a community health nurse have been classified as follows:

- **Administration:** She provides direction and leadership to those whom she supervises. She is responsible for planning, implementation, and evaluation of a practical plan of nursing administration in the primary health centers and its associated subcenters.
- **Communication:** She should maintain good working relationship with members of health team. She is a link between the patient, the family and the doctor. She participates in staff and community meetings.
- **Nursing:** She provides comprehensive nursing care to individuals and families. She should support to the patient and family. Provides proper health education and proper administration of drug.
- **Teaching:** Nurse should teach to the patient and family regarding: Disease condition, Risk factors, Treatment, Prevention, Home care.
- **Researcher:** The nurse should have knowledge regarding current updates.

Responsibilities of Nurse

- To go for home visit in community.
- To find out the cases of filariasis in the community.
- To provide proper nursing care to the patients.
- To provides health education to the patients and family members.
- Advise to the patients for follow-up.
- Advise to patient and family for proper sanitation.

NATIONAL GUINEA WORM ERADICATION PROGRAMME

- Dracunculosis or Guinea Worm (GW) disease is caused by the nematode Dracunculus medinensis. The adult female guinea worm, measuring 60–100 cm in length, emerges through the skin, usually lower limbs, causing swelling, ulceration and discomfort to the patients.
- The GW infection is transmitted to a person when an active GW patient with the ulcer enters into unsafe drinking water—source the anterior end of the emerging guinea worm is ruptured.
- The contact with water bursts a loop of the uterus discharges its thousand of embryos into water. Cyclops present in the water ingests these embryos.
- When a person drinks water containing infected Cyclops, the gastric juice of man kills the Cyclops and activates the larvae which then penetrate the gut wall and migrate,

usually to the retroperitoneal connective tissues, when they mature into male and female adult worms in about 6 months after entering into human body.
- The male worm is smaller in size, dies immediately after copulation and gets absorbed in the body. The female then, migrate to that part of the body which are likely to come in contact with water.

Important Strategy Adopted to Eradicate the GW
- GW case detection and continuous surveillance through active case search operations and regular monthly reporting
- GW case management
- Vector Control by the application of Tempos in unsafe water sources eight times a year and use of fine nylon mesh/double layered cloth strainers by the community to filter Cyclops in all the affected villages
- Health education
- Trained manpower development
- Provision and maintenance of safe drinking water supply on priority in GW endemic villages
- Concurrent evaluation and operational research.

Implementation
- The endemic State Health Directorate through Primary Healthcare system implemented the program.
- The Ministry of Rural Development, Government of India and State Public Health Engineering Departments (Rural Water Supply) assist the program in provision and maintenance of safe drinking water supplies and conversion of unsafe drinking water sources, like step wells, and ponds on priority in the guinea worm affected areas.
- District Medical Officer and PHC medical officer were responsible for planning, implementation, monitoring and supervision of the GWEP.
- Annually the Task Force Group under the chairmanship of Director General of Health Services, Government of India, reviewed the GWEP in depth.
- This task Force Group was constituted by:
    - Director and Deputy Director (Helminthology) of NICD Delhi as convener and coordinator of the work
    - Directors of Health and Medical Services, GWEP-officers, chief engineers (Rural Water Supply) of GW endemic states.
    - Director/Advisor of National Water Mission as members
    - Experts from WHO, UNICEF, Center Health Education Bureau (CHEB), Planning Commission and related organizations.

Achievement
- At the beginning of the Program, i.e., in 1984, there were around 40,000 GW cases in 12,840 villages in 89 districts of 7 endemic states.
- During 1996, only 9 guinea worm cases have been recorded in three villages from Jodhpur (Rajasthan), rest of the country continued to remain free from GW.
- Banwari Lal 25 years old from Jodhpur in Rajasthan was the last case in India in 1996 (Lancet 2000).

"Guinea Worm Disease Free"
- "Zero" incidence has been maintained since August 1996 through active surveillance and intensified field monitoring in the endemic areas.
- In the Meeting of WHO in February 2,000 the India has been certified for the elimination of Guinea Worm Disease and on 15th February 2001 declared India as "Guinea Worm Disease Free".

NATIONAL LEPROSY ERADICATION PROGRAMME

The National Leprosy Eradication Programme is a centrally sponsored Health Scheme under the National Health Mission of the Ministry of Health and Family Welfare, Government of India. The program is headed by the Deputy Director of Health Services (Leprosy) under the administrative control of the Directorate General Health Services, Government of India. While the NLEP strategies and plans are formulated centrally, the program is implemented by the States/UTs. The major concern of the program is to detect cases of leprosy at an early stage and provide complete treatment, free of cost, in order to prevent occurrence of Grade II Disability (G2D) in affected persons. Under NLEP, it is aimed to reduce G2D per million populations to less than 1 per million populations and to have zero G2D among new child cases aligned with the target given by Global Leprosy Strategy 2016–20.

Vision: "Leprosy-free India" is the vision of the NLEP.

Objectives
- To reduce Prevalence rate less than 1/10,000 population at subnational and district level.
- To reduce Grade II disability % <1 among new cases at National level
- To reduce Grade II disability cases <1 case per million populations at National level.
- Zero disabilities among new Child cases.
- Zero stigma and discrimination against persons affected by leprosy.

Strategies for Leprosy Elimination in India
- Integrated anti-leprosy services through General Health Care system.
- Early detection and complete treatment of new leprosy cases.
- Carrying out household contact survey for early detection of cases.
- Involvement of Accredited Social Health Activist (ASHA) in the detection and completion of treatment of Leprosy cases on time.
- Strengthening of Disability Prevention and Medical Rehabilitation (DPMR) services.
- Information, Education and Communication (IEC) activities in the community to improve self-reporting to Primary Health Center (PHC) and reduction of stigma.
- Intensive monitoring and supervision at Health and Wellness Centers and Block Primary Health Center/Community Health Center.

Milestones in NLEP

1955: National Leprosy Control Programme (NLCP) launched
1983: National Leprosy Eradication Programme launched
1983: Introduction of Multidrug therapy (MDT) in Phases
2005: Elimination of Leprosy at National Level
2012: Special action plan for 209 high endemic districts in 16 States/UTs
2014: Upgraded Simplified Information System Implementation
2016: Rights of Persons with Disabilities Act, 2016.

2017–2019 New Initiatives

- Active Case Detections Campaigns (14 days) in high endemic districts
- Focused Leprosy Campaign (FLC) in low endemic districts
- ASHA Based Surveillance for Leprosy Suspects (ABSULS)
- Grade II Disability Epidemiological Investigation
- Implementation of Postexposure Prophylaxis (administration of Single Dose of Rifampicin)
- Sparsh Leprosy Awareness Campaigns
- Introduction of NIKUSTH—A real time leprosy reporting software across India.

2019

- External Evaluation of NLEP by World Health Organization.
- Convergence of leprosy screening with Comprehensive Primary Health Care Program of Ayushman Bharat, to screen 30+ years population at HWCs.
- Convergence of leprosy screening with Rashtriya Bal Swasthya Karyakram (RBSK) to screen children (0–18 years) at Anganwadi Centers and Government schools.

2020

- Active Case Detection and Regular Surveillance (ACD and RS) guidelines rolled out.
- Convergence of NLEP with Rashtriya Kishore Swasthya Karyakram (RKSK) for counseling the children of teen age group (13–19 years) about leprosy at Adolescent Friendly Clinics.

Healthcare Interventions for Leprosy Patient

Leprosy is a chronic infectious disease caused by the acid fast bacillus *Mycobacterium leprae*. Some important health interventions for leprosy patient are pointed out in the below:

- Diagnose the impaired tissue integrity and monitor the characteristics of the lesion such as size, color, odor and drainage.
- Clean the wounds with saline or nontoxic substances as indicated.
- Apply sterile bandage to cover the wounds and maintain aseptic technique.
- Examine the wound damage daily during each dressing changes.
- Compare the changes of ulcer daily and record regularly.
- Routinely monitor temperature and color of skin.
- Encourage the affected people to maintain regular medical care with multidrug therapy (MTD).
- Keep continue follow-up the affected leprosy patient to identify relapse of leprosy disease.
- Monitor any signs of adverse effects regarding medications and take proper action.
- Protect hands and feet to avoid inadvertent injury and prevent chronic disability.
- Keep skin moist to prevent dryness and fissuring and avoid ulceration or infection of skin.
- Educate the patient to avoid plastic footwear or gloves which trap moisture and cause ulceration.
- Ensure adequate intake of fluid to maintain optimal skin hydration.
- Ensure proper rest and nutrition of the affected leprosy patient.
- Ensure proper treatment nursing of eye inflammation to preserve vision.
- Ensure moisture of nasal mucosa with 0.9% saline and essential fatty acids.
- Educate the patient and family member about the consequence of leprosy.
- Nurses should educate the leprosy patient about the signs and symptoms of relapse and disease exacerbation.
- Closely monitor the family and community people for development of leprosy signs and symptoms.
- Provide knowledge and increase awareness about advance signs of neuropathy.
- Nurses should educate the community people about signs and symptoms and mode of transmission of leprosy.
- Educate the patient and family members about importance of continuing treatment with Multidrug therapy (MDT) and evaluate the efficacy of Multidrug therapy (MDT).
- Identify patients who are not collecting drug on time and identify the reasons and take effective actions.
- Nurses should arrange health campaigns for early detection of leprosy and start early treatment.
- Public awareness and education campaigns are necessary to eliminate social stigma and isolation associated with the disease.
- Increase awareness among family members and community people to reduce discrimination to leprosy patient.
- Provide information to community people that leprosy is an infectious disease but curable with treatment.
- Inform the community people that leprosy treatment is available and free of cost.
- Also informed the community people, treated persons are no longer infectious.
- Nurses can increase awareness among people by arranging quizzes, essay competitions with prizes, public talks, game, puppet shows, posters and leaflets, religious leaders, local public representative and the mass media.
- Give psychological support to leprosy patient that they can able to live a normal life after proper treatment.

National AIDS Control Programme

The National AIDS Control Programme (NACP), launched in 1992, is being implemented as a Comprehensive Program for Prevention and Control of HIV/AIDS in India. Over time, the focus has shifted from raising awareness to behavior change, from a national response to a more decentralized response and to increasing involvement of NGOs and networks of People living with HIV (PLHIV).

The NACP I started in 1992 was implemented with an objective of slowing down the spread of HIV infections so as to reduce morbidity, mortality and impact of AIDS in the country.

In November 1999, the second National AIDS Control Project (NACP II) was launched (i) to reduce the spread of HIV infection in India, and (ii) to increase India's capacity to respond to HIV/AIDS on a long-term basis.

NACP III was launched in July 2007 with the goal of Halting and Reversing the Epidemic over its five-year period.

NACP IV, launched in 2012, aims to accelerate the process of reversal and further strengthen the epidemic response in India through a cautious and well defined integration process over the next five years.

NACP-IV—Objectives

- Reduce new infections by 50% (2007 Baseline of NACP III)
- Provide comprehensive care and support to all persons living with HIV/AIDS and treatment services for all those who require it.

Key Strategies

- Intensifying and consolidating prevention services, with a focus on high risk groups (HRGs) and vulnerable population.
- Increasing access and promoting comprehensive care, support and treatment.
- Expanding IEC services for (a) general population and (b) high risk groups with a focus on behavior change and demand generation.
- Building capacities at national, state, district and facility levels.
- Strengthening strategic information management system.

Key Priorities under NACP IV

- Preventing new infections by sustaining the reach of current interventions and effectively addressing emerging epidemics.
- Prevention of parent to child transmission.
- Focusing on IEC strategies for behavior change in HRG, awareness among general population and demand generation for HIV services.
- Providing comprehensive care, support and treatment to eligible PLHIV.
- Reducing stigma and discrimination through Greater involvement of PLHA (GIPA).
- De-centralizing rollout of services including technical support.
- Ensuring effective use of strategic information at all levels of program.
- Building capacities of NGO and civil society partners especially in states with emerging epidemics.
- Integrating HIV services with health systems in a phased manner.
- Mainstreaming of HIV/AIDS activities with all key central/state level Ministries/ departments will be given a high priority and resources of the respective departments will be leveraged. Social protection and insurance mechanisms for PLHIV will be strengthened.

Package of Services Provided under NACP IV

Prevention Services

- Targeted Interventions for High Risk Groups and Bridge Population (Female Sex Workers (FSW), Men who have Sex with Men (MSM), Transgenders/Hijras, Injecting Drug Users (IDU), Truckers and Migrants).
- Needle-Syringe Exchange Program (NSEP) and Opioids Substitution Therapy (OST) for IDUs.
- Prevention Interventions for Migrant population at source, transit and destination.
- Link Worker Scheme (LWS) for HRGs and vulnerable population in rural areas.
- Prevention and Control of Sexually Transmitted Infections/Reproductive Tract Infections (STI/RTI).
- Blood Safety.
- HIV Counseling and Testing Services.
- Prevention of Parent to Child Transmission.
- Condom promotion.
- Information, Education and Communication (IEC) and Behavior Change Communication (BCC).
- Social Mobilization, Youth Interventions and Adolescent Education Program.
- Mainstreaming HIV/AIDS response.
- Work Place Interventions.

Care, Support and Treatment Services

- Laboratory services for CD4 Testing and other investigations.
- Free First line and second line Anti-Retroviral Treatment (ART) through ART centers and Link ART Centers (LACs), Centers of Excellence (COE) and ART plus Centers.
- Pediatric ART for children.
- Early Infant Diagnosis for HIV exposed infants and children below 18 months.
- HIV-TB Coordination (Cross-referral, detection and treatment of co-infections).
- Treatment of Opportunistic Infections.
- Drop-in Centers for PLHIV networks.

New Initiatives Under NACP IV

- Differential strategies for districts based on data triangulation with due weightage to vulnerabilities.
- Scale up of Programs to target key vulnerabilities.

- Scale up of Opioids Substitution Therapy (OST) for IDUs.
- Scale up and strengthening of Migrant Interventions at Source, Transit and Destinations including roll out of Migrant Tracking System for effective outreach.
- Establishment and scale up of interventions for Transgenders (TGs) by bringing in community participation and focused strategies to address their vulnerabilities.
- Employer-Led Model for addressing vulnerabilities among migrant labor
- Female Condom Program.
- Scale up of multi-drug regimen for prevention of parent to child transmission (PPTCT) in keeping with international protocols.
- Social protection for marginalized populations through mainstreaming and earmarking budgets for HIV among concerned government departments.
- Establishment of Metro Blood Banks and Plasma Fractionation Center.
- Launch of Third Line ART and scale up of first and second Line ART.
- Demand promotion strategies specially using mid-media, e.g., National Folk Media Campaign and Red Ribbon Express and buses (in convergence with the National Health Mission).

STD CONTROL PROGRAM

Sexually transmitted diseases (STD) are major health problems all over the world including India, although available data on the magnitude of STDs in India is of questionable quality. The annual incidence of STD in India as reported to the Central Bureau of Health Intelligence during 1989 was approximately 14 million. Community-based studies and other limited studies suggest that HIV rates are high in both rural and urban areas.

- A National STD Control Programme has been in operation since the mid-1950s. The program is clinic-based, however, and covers only 5% of all STD patients in the country, with the majority of patients attending private healthcare providers, the informal sector, or resorting to self medication.
- In acknowledgement of the need to strengthen the STD control program, especially in the context of the recently launched AIDS control program, efforts are being made to extend the existing program at the community level through existing private healthcare services in the country.
- A phased approach to implementing the STD Control Program in the 32 states and union territories has been adopted.
- This programmatic extension from the clinic to the community has become a necessity as the vast majority of patients are being treated without laboratory investigation by private practitioners.
- Efforts to control STDs should focus upon increasing the availability and acceptance of curative and preventive measures by individual patients and the community.
- Sustained support from national and international agencies will be needed in order for this new strategy to be successful.

Objectives of STD
- Explain the epidemiological impact of sexually transmitted disease
- Discuss ways to reduce risk for STDs
- Examine how condoms can reduce risk for STDs
- Describe the clinical presentation of STD
- Outline the management, complication and prevention of STD

Strategies
- Case detection case is on essential part of any control Program.
    - Screening screenings the testing of apparently healthy volunteers from the general population for the early detection of disease.
    - High priority is given to screening of special groups, pregnant women, blood donors, industrial workers, army, police, refugees, convicts restaurant and hotel staff, etc.
    - Contact tracing: it is the term used for technique by which the sexual partners of diagnosed patients are identified, located, investigated and treated.
    - Cluster testing here the patients are asked to name other persons of eighth sex who more in the same socio-sexual environment there persons are then screened (e.g., blood testing) this technique has been shown almost to double the number of case found.
- **Case holding and treatment:** there is a tendency on a part of patients suffering from STDs to disappear or drop out before treatment is complete.
- **Epidemiological treatment:** It consists of the administration of full therapeutic dose of treatment to persons recently exposed to STD while awaiting the results of lab test.
- **Personal prophylaxis:** i. Contraceptives: mechanical barriers can be reamended for personal prophylaxis against STDs ii. Vaccines: the development of a vaccine for hepatitis B has raised hope that vaccine will be found for other STDs.
- Health education is an integral part of STD control Program. It is help the individual alter behavior in an effort to avoid STDs that is minimize disease acquisition and transmission.

Control of STDs: The aim of the control Program for STDs is the prevention of ill health resulting from the above conditions through various intervention 1. primary prevention (prevention of infection). 2. secondary prevention (minimize the adverse effects of infection).

National Sexually Transmitted Disease Control Programme
- STD Control Programme has been in operation in India since 1949.

- The program is based on in the specialized facilities offering clinical service for diagnosis and treatment of SDT.
- Government of India has established 62 surveillance centers for screening persons practicing high risk behavior, 29 zonal blood testing centers in 4 metropolitan cities and additional 89 blood testing centers in 83 large cities for screening all pooled plasma for HIV infection.
- 62 surveillance centers functioning in 33 cities have also been identified as zonal blood testing centers for screening blood samples received from the blood bank.
- With this testing facilities have now become available at 110 cities of country.
- The facilities currently providing STD control are: 5 regional STD a. Delhi b. Chennai c. Hyderabad d. Nagpur e. Calcutta
- Skin-leprosy—STD clinics in medical colleges and in some district and taluka hospitals.
- STD Control Program has been merged with AIDS Control Program.
- The National Venereal Diseases Control Programme was established in 1949 as per the advice of Bhore Committee which recommended the following:
  - To introduce compulsory notification
  - Free treatment to all patients seeking treatment
  - Facilities to be provided free for personal prophylaxis.
  - Adequate diagnostic facilities
  - Follow-up to be maintained
  - Mass education of public regarding cause and prevention of venereal disease
  - Measure to reduce prostitution to be considered essential.

Nurse's Responsibility of a Community Health Nurse in STDs

- Case finding:
  - Interviewing the patient
  - Assist doctor with examination and diagnosis
  - Recognition of symptoms
  - Taking history skillfully
  - Education
- Managing clinics and follow-up
  - Home visits to care for patients and families
  - Follow up the contacts
- All pregnant mothers who are having sexually transmitted disease must be visit as frequently as possible and made to attend the clinic for treatment
- Prevention:
  - Visits to newborn infants
  - Helping babies with congenital syphilis to have hospital care
  - Teaching care under supervision
- The nurse's job in providing the care and treatment to the family when diagnosed will be a difficult task, especially in India, where people are still not aware of the seriousness of this disease. Community health nurse has to spend considerable amount of time in getting the patient to complete the course of the treatment.

NATIONAL PROGRAMME FOR CONTROL OF BLINDNESS

National Programme for Control of Blindness was launched in the year 1976 as a 100% Centrally Sponsored Scheme with the goal to reduce the prevalence of blindness from 1.4% to 0.3%. As per survey in 2001–02, prevalence of blindness is estimated to be 1.1%. Rapid Survey on Avoidable Blindness conducted under NPCB during 2006–07 showed reduction in the prevalence of blindness from 1.1% (2001–02) to 1% (2006–07). Various activities/initiatives undertaken during the Five Year Plans under NPCB are targeted towards achieving the goal of reducing the prevalence of blindness to 0.3% by the year 2020.

Goals and Objectives of NPCB in the XII Plan

Goals

- To reduce the prevalence of blindness (1.49% in 1986–89) to less than 0.3%.
- To establish an infrastructure and efficiency levels in the Program to be able to cater new cases of blindness each year to prevent future backlog.

Objectives

- To reduce the backlog of blindness through identification and treatment of blind at primary, secondary and tertiary levels based on assessment of the overall burden of visual impairment in the country.
- Develop and strengthen the strategy of NPCB for "Eye Health" and prevention of visual impairment; through provision of comprehensive eye care services and quality service delivery.
- Strengthening and upgradation of RIOS to become center of excellence in various sub-specialties of ophthalmology.
- Strengthening the existing and developing additional human resources and infrastructure facilities for providing high quality comprehensive Eye Care in all Districts of the country.
- To enhance community awareness on eye care and lay stress on preventive measures.
- Increase and expand research for prevention of blindness and visual impairment.
- To secure participation of Voluntary Organizations/Private Practitioners in eye care.

Strategies to Achieve the Objectives

- Decentralized implementation of the scheme through District Health Societies (NPCB).
- Reduction in the backlog of blind persons by active screening of population above 50 years, organizing screening eye camps and transporting operable cases to eye care facilities.
- Development of eye care services and improvement in quality of eye care by training of personnel, supply of high-tech ophthalmic equipment, strengthening follow up services and regular monitoring of services;

- Screening of school age group (Primary and Secondary) children for identification and treatment of Refractive Errors, with special attention in under-served areas;
- Public awareness about prevention and timely treatment of eye ailments;
- Special focus on illiterate women in rural areas. For this purpose, there should be convergence with various ongoing schemes for development of women and children;
- To make eye care comprehensive, besides cataract surgery, provision of assistance for other eye diseases like Diabetic Retinopathy, Glaucoma Management, Laser Techniques, Corneal Transplantation, Vitreoretinal Surgery, Treatment of Childhood Blindness, etc.
- Construction of dedicated Eye Wards and Eye OTs in District Hospitals in NE States and few other States as per need;
- Development of Mobile Ophthalmic Units [renamed as Multipurpose District Mobile Ophthalmic Units (MDMOU)] in the district level for patient screening and transportation of patients;
- Continuing emphasis on Primary Healthcare (eye care) by establishing Vision centers in all PHCs with a PMOA in position.
- Participation of community and Panchayat Raj institutions in organizing services in rural areas;
- Involvement of Private Practitioners in the Program.

Main Causes of Blindness

- Cataract (62.6%)
- Refractive error (19.70%)
- Corneal blindness (0.90%)
- Glaucoma (5.80%)
- Surgical complication (1.20%)
- Posterior capsular opacification (0.90%)
- Posterior segment disorder (4.70%)
- Others (4.19%)
- Estimated National Prevalence of Childhood Blindness/ Low vision is 0.80 per thousand.

IODINE DEFICIENCY CONTROL PROGRAM

Realizing the magnitude of the problem, the Government of India launched a 100% centrally assisted National Goiter Control Programme (NGCP) in 1962. In August 1992, the National Goiter Control Programme was renamed as National Iodine Deficiency Disorders Control Programme (NIDDCP) with a view of wide spectrum of Iodine Deficiency Disorders like mental and physical retardation, deaf-mutism, cretinism, stillbirths, abortions, etc. The program is being implemented in all the States/UTs for entire population.

Goals

- To bring the prevalence of IDD to below 5% in the country
- To ensure 100% consumption of adequately iodized salt (15 ppm) at the household level.

Objectives

- Surveys to assess the magnitude of Iodine Deficiency Disorders in the districts.
- Supply of iodized salt in place of common salt.
- Resurveys to assess iodine deficiency disorders and the impact of iodated salt after every 5 years in the districts.
- Laboratory monitoring of iodized salt and urinary iodine excretion.
- Health education and publicity.

Policy

On the recommendations of Central Council of Health in 1984, the Government took a policy decision to Iodate the entire edible salt in the country by 1992. The program started in April, 1986 in a phased manner. To date, the annual production of iodated salt in our country is 65 lakh metric tones per annum.

Nodal Ministry: Ministry of Health and Family Welfare is the nodal Ministry for implementation of National Iodine Deficiency Disorders Control Programme.

Financial assistance to all states/UTs for the following:
- Human resource of State IDD Cell, i.e., Technical Officer, Statistical Assistant and LDC and State IDD monitoring laboratory, i.e., Lab Technician and Lab Assistant.
- Health education and publicity activities including global IDD Day activities.
- Conducting district IDD survey/resurvey to assess magnitude of IDD.
- Procurement of salt testing kits by State/UTs for IDD endemic districts for creating awareness at the community level about consumption of iodized salt and monitoring of salt for presence of adequate iodine at household level (since 2013–14).
- Performance based incentive to ASHA @ ₹ 25/- per month for conducting 50 salt samples testing by STK at household/community level (since 2013–14).

Under NIDDCP financial assistance is also being provided to Salt Commissioner's Office, Jaipur, (M/o Industries) which is responsible for promoting production of iodized salt, monitoring, distribution and quality control of iodized salt at the production level through nine quality control laboratories.

Achievements: Over the years the Total Goiter Rate (TGR) in the entire country is reduced significantly. Production of iodized salt in the country reached to 65.00 lakh MT which is adequate to meet the requirement of population.
- The consumption of adequately iodized salt at household level has been increased from 51.1% (as per NFHS III report 2005–06) to 71.1% (as per CES report, 2009).
- Regulation 2.3.12 of Food Safety and Standards (Prohibition and Restriction on Sales), Regulation, 2011 restricts the sale of common salt for direct human consumption unless the same is iodized.

- National Reference Laboratory for monitoring of IDD has been set up at NCDC, Delhi. Four Regional laboratories one each at NIN, Hyderabad, AIIH and PH, Kolkata, AIIMS and NCDC, Delhi have been set up to conduct training, monitoring, quality control of salt and urine testing.
- For effective implementation of NIDDCP 35 States/UTs have established IDD Control Cells in their State Health Directorate. 35 States/UTs have set up State IDD monitoring laboratories in their respective States/UTs.
- Extensive IEC activities have been carried out to create awareness about the regular consumption of iodated salt in prevention and control of IDD through Doordarshan, All India Radio, Directorate of Field Publicity, Song and Drama, Directorate of Advertising and Visual Publicity.

EXPANDED PROGRAMME OF IMMUNIZATION

The Expanded Programme on Immunization (EPI) was initiated in India in 1978 with the objective to reduce morbidity and mortality from diphtheria, pertussis, tetanus, poliomyelitis and childhood tuberculosis by providing immunization services to all eligible children and pregnant women by 1990.

EPI covers vaccination services implemented in order to ensure the immunization of all vulnerable age groups by preventively reaching out to them before they contract and develop infectious diseases: pertussis, diphtheria, tetanus, measles, rubella, mumps, tuberculosis, polio, chickenpox, hepatitis A, hepatitis B, invasive *Streptococcus pneumoniae* and invasive *Haemophilus influenzae* type B.

- This program aims to control, and eventually, eradicate these infections with a special focus on decreasing the incidence of these infectious diseases and associated deaths.
- The EPI was established in 1976 to ensure that infants/children and mothers have access to routinely recommended infant/childhood vaccines.
- Six vaccine-preventable diseases were initially included in the EPI: tuberculosis, poliomyelitis, diphtheria, tetanus, pertussis and measles.
- In 1986, 21.3% "fully immunized" children less than fourteen months of age based on the EPI Comprehensive Program review.

The basic vaccines provided through the EPI have included:
- *Haemophilus influenzae* Type B (Hib) preventing meningitis and pneumonia;
- Hepatitis B, protecting against liver viral infections and their consequences;
- Measles, preventing a viral disease that can result in high fever and rash and possibly lead to encephalitis or death;
- Mumps, preventing a contagious viral infection that can cause painful swelling of the parotid gland, fever, headache, muscle aches and might lead to meningitis;
- Rubella, preventing a viral disease that can cause fetal death or congenital rubella syndrome leading to defects of the brain, heart, eyes and ears during early pregnancy;
- Poliomyelitis, preventing a viral disease that can cause irreversible paralysis;
- Diphtheria, preventing a serious disease caused by a toxin that can cause a thick coating in the back of the nose or throat that makes it hard to breathe or swallow;
- Tetanus, preventing an infection by a bacterium growing in contaminated wounds or unclean umbilical cord leading to death;
- Pertussis, preventing whooping coughs, a highly contagious respiratory tract infection.

Global Situation

Burden: In 2002, WHO estimated that 1.4 million of deaths among children under 5 years due to diseases that could have been prevented by routine vaccination. This represents 14% of global total mortality in children under 5 years of age.

Burden of diseases: The immunization coverage of all individual vaccines has improved. (Demographic Health Survey 2003 and 2008). Fully Immunized Child (FIC) coverage improved by 10% and the Child Protected at Birth (CPAB) against Tetanus improved by 13% compared to any prior period.

Interventions/Strategies

Program Objectives/Goals

Over-all goal: To reduce the morbidity and mortality among children against the most common vaccine-preventable diseases.

Specific Goals

- To immunize all infants/children against the most common vaccine-preventable diseases.
- To sustain the polio-free status of the Philippines.
- To eliminate measles infection.
- To eliminate maternal and neonatal tetanus.
- To control diphtheria, pertussis, hepatitis b and German measles.
- To prevent extrapulmonary tuberculosis among children.

NATIONAL FAMILY WELFARE PROGRAMME

Family welfare includes not only planning of birth, but they welfare of wholes family by means of total family healthcare. The Family Welfare Program has high priority in India because its success depends upon the quality of life of all citizens.

- It was started in the year 1951.
- In 1977, the government of India redesignated the National Family Planning Programme as the National Family Welfare Programme also changed the name of the ministry of health and family planning to ministry of health and family welfare.
- It is a reflection of the government anxiety to promote family planning through the total welfare of the family.
- It is aimed at achieving a higher end, i.e., to improve the quality of life of the people.

- India is the first country in the world that implemented the Family Welfare Program at government level.
- Health is a part of concurrent list but centers provides 100% assistance to states for this program.

Concept of Family Welfare Program

- The concept of welfare is basically related to quality of life.
- As such it includes education, nutrition, health employment, women's welfare and right, shelter, soft drinking water all vital factors associated with the concept of welfare.
- It is centrally sponsored Program. For this, the states receive 100% assistance from central government.
- The emphasis is on child family.
- Also, emphasis is on spacing methods along with terminal methods.
- The current policy is to promote family planning on the basis of voluntary and informed acceptance with full community participation.
- The services are taken to every doorstep in order to motivate families to accept the small family norm.

Aims and Objectives of Family Welfare Program

The Government of India in the Ministry of Health and Family Welfare has started the operational aims and objective of Family Welfare Program as follows:

- To promote the adoption of small family size norm, on the basis of voluntary acceptance.
- To promote the use of spacing method.
- To arrange for clinical and surgical service so as to achieve the set target.
- To ensure adequate supply of contraceptive to all eligible couple within easy reach.
- Participation of voluntary organization/local leaders/local self government, in Family Welfare Program at various level.
- Using the means of mass communication and interpersonal communication to overcome the social and cultural hindrance in adopting the program or extensive use of public health education for family planning.

Goals of the Family Welfare Program

- Reduction of death rate from 10 (in 1992) to 9 per 1000.
- Raising couple protection rate from 43.3 (in 1990) to 60%.
- Reduction in average family size from 4.2 (in 1990) to 2.3
- Decrease in infant mortality rate from 79 (in 1992) to less than 60 per 1000 live birth.

Impact of Family Welfare Activities

- Nearly 98% of women and 99% men in the age group 15 and 49 have a good knowledge about one or more methods of contraception. Adolescents seem to be well aware of the modern method of contraception.
- Over 97% of women and 95% of men are knowledgeable about female sterilization, which is the most popular modern parmanent method of family planning. While only 79% of women and 80% of men have heard about male sterilization.
- 93% of men have awareness about the usage of condom while only 74% of women are aware of the same.
- Around 80% of men and women have a fair knowledge about contraception pills.

Importance of Family Welfare Program

- The year 2010–2011 ended with 34.9 million family planning acceptor at national level comprising of 5.0 million sterilization, 5.6 million IUD insertion, 16 million condom user and 8.3 million oral pills users. As against 35.6 million families planning acceptors in 2009–2010.
- Over the decades, there has been a substantial increase in contraception use in India.

Strategies of Family Welfare Programme

- **Integration with health service:** Family Welfare Programme has been integrated with other health service instead of being a separate service.
- **Integration with maternity and child health:** Family Welfare Programme has been integrated with maternity and child health. Public are motivated for post delivery sterilization, abortion and use of contraception.
- **Concentration in rural area:** Family Welfare Programme are concentrated more in rural areas at the level of subentries and primary health center. This is in addition to hospitals at district, state and central levels.
- **Literacy:** There is a direct correlation between illiteracy and fertility. So stress and priority is given for girl's education, fertility rate among educated female are low.
- **Breastfeeding:** Breastfeeding is encouraged. It is estimated that about 5 million birth per annum can be prevented through breastfeeding.
- **Rising the age for marriage:** Under the child marriage bills (1978), the age of marriage has been raised to 21 years for male and 18 years for female. This has some impact on fertility.
- **Minimum need program:** It was launched in 5th year plan with an aim to raise the economical standards. Fertility is low in higher income groups. so fertility rate can be lowered by increasing economical standard.
- **Incentive:** Monetary incentive has been given in Family Planning Programme, especially for poor classes. But these incentives have not been very effective. So the Program must be on voluntary basis.
- **Mass media:** Motivation through radio, television, cinema, news paper, puppet shows and folk dance is an important aspect of this Program.

ROLE OF COMMUNITY HEALTH NURSE IN FAMILY WELFARE SERVICES

Community health nurse has a vast role in family welfare service.

Survey Work

- Collecting demographic facts.
- Making list of homes and finding out housing location.

- Collecting information about pregnant mother, eligible couples, and infants.

Educational Function and Motivation

Explaining the importance and necessity of family planning to masses:
- Using various techniques of teaching and communication to propagate the message of family planning to common man.
- Motivating the eligible couple to use contraceptive and educating them about its uses.
- Motivating people for family planning operation or permanent contraception.

Managerial Function

- Conducting clinics.
- Deciding the date and place of clinics.
- Arranging equipment and other resources at clinics.
- Arrangement and distribution of contraceptives.
- Insertion and removal of IUD.
- Organizing family planning camps.
- Arranging family planning operation (sterilization) of male and female through special camps.
- Making arrangements at the camps and follow aseptic techniques for the operation.
- Motivating eligible couple and preparing them for the operation.
- Assisting the doctor in operation.
- Maintaining the records.
- Keeping the eligible couple register update.
- Maintaining the register of sterilization cases, contraceptives user, and pregnant mothers.
- Maintaining other records related to family planning.
- Liaison work
- Soliciting the cooperation of NGOs/voluntary organization.

NATIONAL WATER SUPPLY AND SANITATION PROGRAMME

Drinking water and sanitation facilities are very important and crucial for achieving the goal of "HEALTH FOR ALL". Safe drinking water supply and basic sanitation are so intrinsically linked to human and ecosystem health that they, along with proper hygiene form the most essential components of a safe and healthy life.

Approximately 80–90 % of untreated sewage is discharged directly into rivers and streams, the main source water supply in cities. Human feces remains one of the World's most dangerous pollutants, spreading microbes that cause Typhoid, Cholera, Diarrheal illness, Amoebic Dysentery, and other virulent disease (WHO 1999).

The Union Government of India appointed the Environmental Hygiene Committee (1948-49), which recommended a comprehensive plan for providing safe water supply and sanitation to the population. Thereafter the National Water Supply and Sanitation Programme was launched in 1954. The United Nations declared 1981-1990 as the "International Drinking Water Supply and Sanitation Decade". The following targets were fixed by the Indian Government for the decade:
- 100% Urban and Rural Water Supply
- 50% Urban Sanitation
- 25% Rural Sanitation

The Guinea Worm Eradication Programme was linked up with this decade. In 1986, the National Drinking Water Mission (NDWM) also known as the Rajiv Gandhi Drinking Water Mission (RGDWM) was launched in order to provide scientific and cost effective content to the Centrally Sponsored Accelerated Rural Water Supply Programme.

In 1990, United National General Assembly accepted the following guidelines given in the New Delhi Declaration for Water Supply and Sanitation:
- Protection of environment and safeguard of health through the integrated management of water resources and solid waste.
- Organizational reforms, changing attitudes and behavior and full participation of women.
- Community management of services, and strengthening local Institutions.
- Sound financial practices, and application of appropriate technology.

Rural Sanitation Program

Under this program, the following activities were considered:
- Demand driven low cost sanitation approach
- Involvement of private bodies, NGOs to provide sanitation facilities
- Entrusting Panchayati Raj Institutions and local administration the responsibility of operation and maintenance of water supply and sanitation.
- Achieving zero incidences of Guinea worm disease by 1993 and total eradication by 1995 by improving water quality.
- Improving sanitation in rural areas through IEC Programs, and introducing the concept of total environmental Sanitation.
- Converting all existing dry latrines to low cost sanitary latrines.

Urban Sanitation Programme

Under this programme, the following activities were considered:
- Providing reasonable level of sanitation facility to a large population.
- Total elimination of dry latrines and manual scavenging.
- Low cost on-site sanitation in unsewered parts of cities parts of cities, small and medium towns.
- Technological innovations to improve the re-usability of the recycled waste.
- Polluter paying principle should be applied to finance waste disposal programs.
- Involvement of NGOs, private sector and community.
- Converting all existing dry latrines to low cost sanitary latrines.

- Recycling the treated effluents for horticulture, irrigation, water harvesting and transport system for solid waste disposal.

MINIMUM NEEDS PROGRAM

The Minimum Needs Program (MNP) was introduced in the first year of the Fifth Five Year Plan (1974–78), to provide certain basic minimum needs and improve the living standards of people. It aims at "social and economic development of the community, particularly the underprivileged and underserved population". It also promoted equality as from now poor will be able to get basic needs.

Components

The main components of the MNP are:
- Provision of facilities for universal elementary education for children up to the age of 14 at the nearest possible places to their homes.
- Adult education to improve literacy among the persons above the age of 15 years.
- Development of rural public health facilities. These would include preventive medicine, family planning, and nutrition, early detection of morbidity and referral services.
- Supply of drinking water to problem villages suffering from chronic scarcity of safe sources of water.
- Provision of all-weather roads to all villages having a population of 1,500 persons or more.
- Provision of housing or developed home sites for the houseless in rural areas.
- Environmental improvement in slums.
- Rural electrification.

Principles

Two basic principles are observed during the implementation of minimum needs program:
1. The facilities under MNP are to be first provided in those areas which are at present underserved so as to remove disparities among different areas.
2. The facilities under MNP should be provided as a package to an area through intersectoral area projects to have a greater impact.

Objectives

Rural Health

The objectives to be achieved by the end of the Eighth Five Year Plan are:
- One peripheral health center for 30,000 population in plains and 20,000 population in tribal and hilly areas.
- One subcenter for a population of 5000 people in the plains and for 3,000 in tribal and hilly areas.
- One community health center for a population of 100,000.
- The establishments of peripheral health centers, their up gradation also come under MNP.

Nutrition
- To extend support of nutrition to 11 million eligible persons.
- To consolidate mid-day meal program and link it to health, potable water and sanitation.

NATIONAL DIABETES CONTROL PROGRAMME

Diabetes is one of the major causes of premature illness and death worldwide. Diabetes prevalence is increasing in every country in the world, and the toll is climbing in terms of human lives as well as the costs to society. Diabetes is a metabolic disease which is characterized by high blood sugar levels. It can be caused either due to the lack of insulin (type 1 diabetes) or because the body's cells fail to respond to the insulin produced (type 2 diabetes). Some of the common symptoms of diabetes are hunger, frequent urination and increased thirst. While type 1 diabetes is usually genetic, type 2 diabetes is caused more by lifestyle factors. It is one of the common 'lifestyle diseases' which is plaguing people in the developed countries and often has a causal link to heart diseases, hypertension and obesity.

Objectives
- Prevention of diabetes through identification of high risk subjects and early intervention in the form of health education.
- Early diagnosis of disease and appropriate treatment morbidity and mortality with reference to high risk group.
- Prevention of acute and chronic metabolic, cardiovascular, renal and ocular complication of the disease.
- Provision of equal opportunity for physical attainment and scholastic achievement for the diabetic patients.
- Rehabilitation of those partially or totally handicapped diabetes people.

POLIO ERADICATION: PULSE PROGRAMME

With the global initiative of eradication of polio in 1988 following World Health Assembly resolution in 1988, Pulse Polio Immunization Programme was launched in India in 1995. Children in the age group of 0–5 years administered polio drops during National and Sub-national immunization rounds (in high risk areas) every year. Around 17.4 crore children of less than five years across the country are given polio drops as part of the drive of Government of India to sustain polio eradication from the country.

The last polio case in the country was reported from Howrah district of West Bengal with date of onset 13th January 2011. Thereafter no polio case has been reported in the country. WHO on 24th February 2012 removed India from the list of countries with active endemic wild polio virus transmission.

Objective

The Pulse Polio Initiative was started with an objective of achieving hundred percent coverage under Oral Polio

Vaccine. It aimed to immunize children through improved social mobilization, plan mop-up operations in areas where polio virus has almost disappeared and maintain high level of morale among the public.

Steps Taken by the Government to Maintain Polio Free Status in India

- Maintaining community immunity through high quality National and Sub-National polio rounds each year.
- An extremely high level of vigilance through surveillance across the country for any importation or circulation of poliovirus and VDPV is being maintained. Environmental surveillance (sewage sampling) have been established to detect poliovirus transmission and as a surrogate indicator of the progress as well for any programmatic interventions strategically in Mumbai, Delhi, Patna, Kolkata Punjab and Gujarat.
- All States and Union Territories in the country have developed a Rapid Response Team (RRT) to respond to any polio outbreak in the country. An Emergency Preparedness and Response Plan (EPRP) has also been developed by all States indicating steps to be undertaken in case of detection of a polio case.
- To reduce risk of importation from neighboring countries, international border vaccination is being provided through continuous vaccination teams (CVT) to all eligible children round the clock. These are provided through special booths set up at the international borders that India shares with Pakistan, Bangladesh, Bhutan Nepal and Myanmar.
- Government of India has issued guidelines for mandatory requirement of polio vaccination to all international travelers before their departure from India to polio affected countries namely: Afghanistan, Nigeria, Pakistan, Ethiopia, Kenya, Somalia, Syria and Cameroon. The mandatory requirement is effective for travelers from 1st March 2014.
- A rolling emergency stock of OPV is being maintained to respond to detection/importation of wild poliovirus (WPV) or emergence of circulating vaccine derived poliovirus (cVDPV).
- National Technical Advisory Group on Immunization (NTAGI) has recommended Injectable Polio Vaccine (IPV) introduction as an additional dose along with 3rd dose of DPT in the entire country in the last quarter of 2015 as a part of polio endgame strategy.

Progress

- South-East Asia Region of WHO has been certified polio free. The Regional Certification Commission (RCC) on 27th March 2014 issued certificate which states that "The Commission concludes, from the evidence provided by the National Certificate Committees of the 11 Member States, that the transmission of indigenous wild poliovirus has been interrupted in all countries of the Region."
- India has achieved the goal of polio eradication as no polio case has been reported for more than 3 years after last case reported on 13th January, 2011.
- WHO on 24th February 2012 removed India from the list of countries with active endemic wild poliovirus transmission?
- There are 24 lakh vaccinators and 1.5 lakh supervisors involved in the successful implementation of the Pulse Polio Program.

NATIONAL CANCER CONTROL PROGRAMME

In India, it is estimated that there are 2 to 2.5 million cancer patients at any given point of time with about 0.7 million new cases coming every year and nearly half die every year. Two-third of the new cancers are presented in advance and incurable stage at the time of diagnosis. More than 60% of these affected patients are in the prime of their life between the ages of 35 and 65 years. With increasing life expectancy and changing lifestyles concomitant with development, the number of cancer cases will be almost three times the current number.

- It has long been realized that cancers of the head and neck in both sexes and of the uterine cervix in women are the most common malignancies seen in the country.
- The age adjusted incidence rate per 100,000 for all types in India in urban areas range from 106-130 for men and 100-140 for women but still lower than USA, UK and Japan rates. Fifty percent of all male cancers are tobacco related and 25% in female (total 34% of all cancers are tobacco related).
- There are predictions of incidence of 7 fold increase in tobacco related cancer morbidity in between 1995-2025.
- To control this problem the Government of India has launched a National Cancer Control Programme in 1975 and revised its strategies in 1984-85 stressing on primary prevention and early detection of cancer.

Goals

- The primary prevention of tobacco related cancers;
- Secondary prevention of cancer of the uterine cervix, mouth, breast etc.; and
- Tertiary prevention includes extension and strengthening of therapeutic services including pain relief on a national scale through regional cancer centers and medical colleges (including dental colleges).

IX Plan focuses on:
- Identification of IEC activities so that people seek care at the onset of symptoms.
- Provision of diagnostic facilities in primary and secondary care level so that cancers are detected at early stages when curative therapy can be administered.
- Filling up of the existing gaps in radiotherapy units in a phased manner so that all diagnosed cases do receive therapy without any delay as near to their residence as feasible.
- IEC to reduce tobacco consumption and avoid lifestyle which lead to increasing risk of cancers.

Organizational Structure

- It would be at two levels—Central Government and State Government—with linkage through the Central Council of Health.
- It is suggested that respective executive committee should be assisted by a newly constituted National Cancer Control Board at the central and stage levels by the corresponding Cancer Control Boards.
- The full time officer-in-charge of cancer control is an oncologist who heads the Cancer Control Cell at the Directorate General of Health Services.

Regional Cancer Research and Treatment Centers

- There are 17 regional cancer research centers in India at present. Their main functions are: Cancer Detection and Diagnosis, Provision of Therapy, after care and rehabilitation, Education and Training, Cancer Registration and Research.
- Coordination with the medical colleges and the general health infrastructure is the essential feature.
- The core requirements of a Regional Cancer Center are divisions of surgical oncology, radiation oncology, and medical oncology with support from department of anesthesiology, pathology, cytopathology, hematology, biochemistry and radiodiagnosis with appropriate equipment and staff.

District Cancer Control Program

This program was launched in 1990–91 and under this program each state and union territory has advised to prepare their projects on health education, early detection, and pain relief measures. For this they can get up to ₹ 15 lakh one time assistance and ₹ 10 lakh for four years recurring assistance. The district program has five elements:

1. Health education
2. Early detection
3. Training of medical and paramedical personnels
4. Palliative treatment and pain relief
5. Coordination and monitoring.

The District Programs are linked with Regional Cancer Centers/Government Hospitals/Medical Colleges. For effective functioning each district where Program is started have one District Cancer Society that is chaired by local Collector/Chief Medical Office. Other members are Dean of medical college, Zila Parishad representative, NGO representative, etc.

Comprehensive Antitobacco Program

Consumption

- It is estimated that 80–85% of tobacco is consumed for smoking either as bidis/cigarette. Almost 13% chew tobacco either with pan or lime. Almost 15% are addicted to both habit of chewing and smoking.
- Only 1–3% use tobacco either in the form of stuff or oral use. Smoke contain more than 40 substance which cause cancer, heart disease, respiratory illness, visual impairment, etc. 29% of males age 15 and above smoke and 28% chew masala or tobacco.
- While 3% only the women smoke and more than 10% chew pan masala or tobacco (NHFS-II). Most common form is bidi which is 34% of the total tobacco consumption.

Impact

- In India, more than 2,000 persons die every day and about 8 lakh people die every year due to tobacco-related diseases.
- Tobacco use can cause spontaneous abortion, premature delivery, and intrauterine growth retardation.
- Even passive smoking can cause lung cancer, respiratory illness, heart diseases, nasal sinus cancer, premature aging and intrauterine effects.

National Cancer Registry Programme

National Cancer Registry Programme was launched in 1982 by Indian Council of Medical Research (ICMR) to provide true information on cancer prevalence and incidence.

Objectives

- To generate authentic data on the magnitude of cancer problem in India;
- To undertake epidemiological investigations and advice control measures; and
- Promote human resource development in cancer epidemiology.

Tobacco Free Initiatives

WHO established the Tobacco Free Initiatives (TFI) in 1998. Long-term mission of TFI of WHO is to reduce smoking prevalence and tobacco consumption in all countries and among all groups, and thereby reduce the burden of disease caused by tobacco.

The Goals of the TFI are:

- Galvanize global support for evidence based tobacco control policies and actions;
- Build new partnerships for action and strengthen existing ones;
- Heighten awareness of the need to address tobacco issues at all levels of society;
- Accelerate the implementation of national, regional and global strategies;
- Commission policy research to support rapid, sustained and innovative actions; and
- Mobilize resources to support required action.

WHO has developed partnership with UNICEF, World Bank, CDC, Environment Protection Agency, US National Institute of Health, International NGOs, private sector, and Academic Centers for tobacco prevention work. In 53rd and 54th World Health Assembly all member states reaffirmed for the actions required to control tobacco.

YAWS ERADICATION PROGRAM

Yaws is a disfiguring and debilitating non-venereal disease. It is a highly infectious disease transmitted by direct (person-to-person) contact. Skin shows early lesions, which on healing show little scarring. Disease can be progressive involving bone and cartilage and causing disability.

- Yaw does not have extra human reservoir of infection and can be cured by single injection of long acting penicillin (Benzathine Benzyl).
- Yaws occur in remote, hilly and forest areas that have limited acceptability to healthcare services. Cases of Yaws have been reported from 27 districts in 9 states (Andhra Pradesh, Assam, Bihar, Gujarat, Madhya Pradesh, Maharashtra, Orissa, Tamil Nadu, and Uttar Pradesh).

Clinical Features

- **Primary/early stage:** Primary sore (mother yes) appears as a large papule, about 6 cm in diameter, or as a vesicle on the knee or near the mouth. The scabs become macule and later a papilloma. Infective serous fluid exudes from the lesion.
- **Secondary stage:** After 6–8 weeks rashes resemble a raspberry "framboesia" develop. They fall off without pain. Periosteum and bone may be involved.
- **Tertiary or later stage:** It occurs after about 5 years or more and is characterized by gummatous lesion near bones and joints. Gondou, a swelling by the side of nasal bridge and gandosa ulcerative lesion on palate are two special form of the stage.

Treatment

Benzathine penicillin G is the drug of choice in a dose of 1.2 million units for all cases and contacts, and half that dose (0.6 million units) for children under 10 years of age. In penicillin sensitive cases, erythromycin or tetracycline is used in recommended doses for a period of 15 days.

The WHO recommended three modes of treatments:
1. **Total mass treatment:** In areas where yaws is hyperendemic (>10% prevalence of clinically active yaws) treatment is given to all irrespective of disease status of person.
2. **Juvenile mass treatment:** In mesoendemic communities 6–10% prevalence), treatment is given to all cases and to all children under 15 years of age and other obvious contacts of infectious cases.
3. **Selective mass treatment:** In hypoendemic (<5% prevalence), treatment is confined to cases, their household and other obvious contacts of infectious cases.

National Health Policy: "Eradication of Yaws by 2005"

Yaws Eradication Program

The program was started in 1996–97 in Koraput districts of Orissa then extended to endemic states as a centrally sponsored health scheme with the objectives of:
- Interrupting the transmission of yaws infection (no case) in the country; and
- Eradication of Yaws, (i.e. no seroreactivity to RPR/VDRL in children below 5 years of age) from the country.

The Government of Andhra Pradesh, Gujarat, Madhya Pradesh, Orissa have taken several initiatives for interruption of infection by mass administration of single dose of penicillin in the affected areas. "Yaws Cells" have been established in Division of Epidemiology to coordinate all activities.

Program Strategy
- Manpower development
- Detection of cases
- Treatment of cases and contacts
- IEC involving multi-sectors approach

Operation Component

The case detection is carried out by active surveillance, i.e., house-to-house visit by trained paramedical workers and treatment of cases and contacts simultaneously and immediately after detection. In such cases, a colored recognition cards are given to patient.

Program Management

The National Institute of Communicable Diseases (NICD) has been identified as the nodal agency for Planning, guidance, coordination, monitoring and evaluation of the Program. The program is implemented by the State Health Directorate of yaws endemic states utilizing existing health care delivery system with the coordination and collaboration of Department of Tribal Welfare and other related institutions, Director General of Health Services, Ministry of Health forms the task force to coordinate and review program.

NATIONAL NUTRITIONAL ANEMIA PROPHYLAXIS PROGRAMME

Nutritional anemia is a major public health problem in India. The NNAPP was started in 1970. It is a centrally sponsored scheme. Anemia especially affects women in the reproductive age group and young children. It is estimated that over 50% of pregnant women suffer from anemia. Nutritional anemia, due to iron and folic acid deficiency, is directly or indirectly responsible for about 20% of maternal deaths. Anemia is also a major contributor cause of high incidence of premature births, low birth weight and perinatal mortality. Presently, 22 million adult and 30 million child beneficiaries are being covered under the Program (Guidelines for National Nutritional Anemia Prophylaxis Program, Ministry of Health and Family Welfare, Government of India, 1990).

Objectives

The program aims at significantly decreasing the prevalence and incidence of anemia in women in reproductive age group, especially pregnant and lactating women, and preschool children.

Specific Objectives of the Program

- To assess the baseline prevalence of nutritional anemia in mothers and young children through estimation of hemoglobin (Hb) levels.

- To put the mothers and children with low Hb levels (less than 10 g and less than 8 g respectively) on anti-anemia treatment.
- To put the mother with Hb level more than 10 g/dL and children with Hb more than 8 g/dL on the prophylaxis program.
- To monitor continuously the quality of the tablets, distribution and consumption of the supplements.
- To assess periodically the Hb levels of the beneficiaries.
- To motivate the mothers to consume the tablets through relevant nutrition education (and to give to their children also).

Beneficiaries

The scheme beneficiaries are children in 1–5 years of age, pregnant and nursing mothers, female acceptor of terminal methods of family planning and IUDs.

The target beneficiaries of the scheme are 50% of total pregnant and nursing mothers and 25% of total women acceptors of terminal methods and IUDs. The target child population is 50% of total population in the age group of 1–5 years.

Activities

The program focuses on the following activities:
- Promotion of regular consumption of foods rich in iron.
- Supply of iron and folate supplements in the form of tablets (folifer tablets) to the target group.

Identification and treatment of severely anemic cases. The recommended daily dosages of iron and folic acid (IFA) tablets are as follows:
- Adult women: 60 mg elemental iron + 0.5 mg folic acid
- Children (1–5 years): 20 mg elemental iron + 0.1 mg folic acid.

For young children, who cannot swallow, liquid syrup containing the same amount of IFA was given (2 mL at a time). This has been discontinued since 1991.

Organization: The program is implemented through the Primary Health Centers and its subcenters. The multipurpose worker female and other para-medics in the PHCs are responsible for the distribution of IFA tablets (adult and pediatric doses) to beneficiaries. The functionaries of ICDS scheme assist in implementation of Program.

20 POINT PROGRAM

The Twenty Point Program was initially launched by Prime Minister Indira Gandhi in 1975 and was subsequently restructured in 1982 and again on 1986. With the introduction of new policies and Programs it has been **finally restructured in 2006** and it has been in operation at present. The Programs and Schemes under TPP—2006 are in harmony with the priorities contained in the National Common Minimum Program, the Millennium Development Goals of the United Nations and SAARC Social Charter. The restructured Program, called Twenty Point Program-2006 (TPP-2006), was approved by the Cabinet on 5th October, 2006.

Objective of Twenty Point Program

The basic objective of the 20-Point Program is to eradicate poverty and to improve the quality of life of the poor and the under privileged population of the country. The program covers various socioeconomic aspects like poverty, employment, education, housing, health, agriculture and land reforms, irrigation, drinking water, protection and empowerment of weaker sections, consumer protection, environment, etc.

20 Points

The 20 points of the program and its 66 items have been carefully designed and selected to achieve the above objectives. The 20-Point Program consisted following:
1. Attack on rural poverty
2. Strategy for rained agriculture
3. Better use of irrigation water
4. Bigger harvest
5. Enforcement of land reforms
6. Special programs for rural labor
7. Clean drinking water
8. Health for all
9. Two child norm
10. Expansion of education
11. Justice for SC/ST
12. Equality for women
13. New opportunities for women
14. Housing for the people
15. Improvement for slums
16. New strategy for forestry
17. Protection of environment
18. Concern for the consumer
19. Energy for the villages
20. A responsive administration

20 Points as defined in 2006

The TPP further restructured in 2006 had following points:
1. Poverty eradication
2. Power to people
3. Support to farmers
4. Labor welfare
5. Food security
6. Clean drinking water
7. Housing for all
8. Health for all
9. Education for all
10. Welfare of SC/ST/OBC and minorities
11. Women welfare
12. Child welfare
13. Youth development
14. Improvement of slums
15. Environment protection and afforestation
16. Social security

17. Rural Roads
18. Energizing of rural areas
19. Development of backward areas
20. IT enabled and e-governance

The monitoring of the program at the center has been assigned to the Ministry of Statistics and Programme Implementation, Government of India. The management information system relating to Twenty Point developed by the Ministry consists of a monthly Progress Report (MPR) and yearly Review of the Program, Point-wise, Item-wise and State-wise. The monthly report covers progress on the implementation of the program for 20 crucial points for which there is pre-set physical targets and the Yearly Review presents an analytical review of the performance of all the items under the program.

ICDS PROGRAM

The Integrated Child Development Service (ICDS) Scheme providing for supplementary nutrition, immunization and pre-school education to the children is a popular flagship Program of the government. Launched in 1975, it is one of the world's largest programs providing for an integrated package of services for the holistic development of the child. ICDS is a centrally sponsored scheme implemented by state governments and union territories. The scheme is universal covering all the districts of the country.

The scheme has been renamed as Anganwadi Services.

Objectives

- To improve the nutritional and health status of children in the age-group 0–6 years;
- To lay the foundation for proper psychological, physical and social development of the child;
- To reduce the incidence of mortality, morbidity, malnutrition and school dropout;
- To achieve effective coordination of policy and implementation amongst the various departments to promote child development; and
- To enhance the capability of the mother to look after the normal health and nutritional needs of the child through proper nutrition and health education.

Beneficiaries

- Children in the age group of 0–6 years
- Pregnant women and
- Lactating mothers.

Services under ICDS

The ICDS Scheme offers a package of six services, viz.
- Supplementary nutrition
- Pre-school nonformal education
- Nutrition and health education
- Immunization
- Health check-up and
- Referral services

Three of the six services viz. immunization, health check-up and referral services are related to health and are provided through National Health Mission and Public Health Infrastructure. The services are offered at Anganwadi Centers through Anganwadi Workers (AWWs) and Anganwadi Helpers (AWHS) at grassroots level.

Guidelines for Performance Incentives under POSHAN Abhiyaan

Population Norms for Setting up of AWCs/Mini-AWCs:
- There will be 1 Anganwadi center (AWC) for population of 400-800; 2 AWCs for 800-1600; 3 AWCs for 1600-2400 and thereafter in multiples of 800-1 AWC.
- The norms for one AWC for Tribal/Riverine/Desert, Hilly and other difficult areas will be 300-800.
- Norms for one Mini AWC will be 150-400.
- Norms for Anganwadi on Demand (AOD)—Where a settlement has at least 40 children under 6 years of age but no AWC

ICDS Systems Strengthening and Nutrition Improvement Project (ISSNIP)

The overall goal of the project is to improve nutritional and early childhood development outcomes of children in India. Key objectives of Phase 1 are to support the GoI and the selected States to:
- Strengthen the ICDS policy framework, systems and capacities, and facilitate community engagement, to ensure greater focus on children under three years of age in the project districts; and
- Strengthen convergent actions for improved nutrition outcomes in the stipulated districts.

MID-DAY MEAL PROGRAM

Mid-Day Meal Scheme was started in India from 15th August 1995 under the name of 'National Program of Nutritional Support to Primary Education (NP-NSPE)'. In October 2007, NP-NSPE was renamed as 'National Program of Mid-Day Meal in Schools,' which is popularly known as Mid-Day Meal Scheme. Recently, the Vice President of India has proposed the inclusion of milk in mid-day meals of children. Hence, it is important to know the importance of the scheme for the IAS Exam.

Mid-day Meal Scheme Latest News

In September 2021, the Mid-Day Meal Scheme was renamed 'PM POSHAN' or Pradhan Mantri Poshan Shakti Nirman. PM POSHAN will extend the hot cooked meals to students studying in pre-primary levels or Bal Vatikas of government and government-aided primary schools, in addition to those already covered under the mid-day scheme.

PM POSHAN

The revamped scheme has been launched for 5 years, from 2021–22 to 2025–26, with a budget of ₹ 1,30,794.90 crore. The government hopes it will benefit 11.80 crore children studying in 11.20 lakh schools across India. The scheme is different from the mid-day meal scheme in the following ways:

- Apart from providing nutritional meals to schoolchildren, the revamped scheme will also focus on monitoring the nutritional levels of schoolchildren.
- A nutritional expert will be appointed in each school to ensure that the BMI, weight levels and hemoglobin levels of the students are monitored.
- In districts with a high prevalence of anemia, special provisions for nutritional items would be made.
- The government is also considering developing nutrition gardens on school campuses with active participation by students.
- There could also be cooking competitions held under the scheme to promote ethnic cuisine and innovative menus based on local ingredients.

Aspirants can read similar articles from the links mentioned below:

Mid-day meal scheme aims to:
- Avoid classroom hunger
- Increase school enrolment
- Increase school attendance
- Improve socialization among castes
- Address malnutrition.

Empower Women through Employment

The main objectives of the MDM scheme are:
- To increase the enrolment of the children belonging to disadvantaged sections in the schools.
- Leading enrolment to increased attendance in the schools.
- To retain children studying in classes 1–8.
- To provide nutritional support to the children of the elementary stage in drought-affected areas.

Salient Features of Mid-day Meal Scheme

- It is the world's largest school meal program aimed to attain the goal of universalization of primary education.
- The Ministry of Education (earlier known as the Ministry of Human Resources and Development) is the authorized body to implement the scheme.
- It is a centrally sponsored scheme hence cost is shared between the center and the states. (Center's share–60%).
- Tamil Nadu is the first state to implement the mid-day meal scheme.

NATIONAL MENTAL HEALTH PROGRAMME

The Government of India has launched the National Mental Health Programme (NMHP) in 1982, keeping in view the heavy burden of mental illness in the community, and the absolute inadequacy of mental healthcare infrastructure in the country to deal with it.

NMHP has three components:
1. Treatment of mentally ill
2. Rehabilitation
3. Prevention and promotion of positive mental health.

Aims
- Prevention and treatment of mental and neurological disorders and their associated disabilities.
- Use of mental health technology to improve general health services.
- Application of mental health principles in total national development to improve quality of life.

Objectives
- To ensure availability and accessibility of minimum mental healthcare for all in the foreseeable future, particularly to the most vulnerable and underprivileged sections of population.
- To encourage application of mental health knowledge in general healthcare and in social development.
- To promote community participation in the mental health services development and to stimulate efforts towards self-help in the community.

Strategies
- Integration mental health with primary health care through the NMHP.
- Provision of tertiary care institutions for treatment of mental disorders.
- Eradicating stigmatization of mentally ill patients and protecting their rights through regulatory institutions like the Central Mental Health Authority, and State Mental Health Authority.

Mental Healthcare
- The mental morbidity requires priority in mental health treatment
- Primary healthcare at village and subcenter level
- At Primary Health Center level
- At the District Hospital level
- Mental Hospital and teaching Psychiatric Units.

District Mental Health Program

Components
- Training programs of all workers in the mental health team at the identified Nodal Institute in the State.
- Public education in the mental health to increase awareness and reduce stigma.
- For early detection and treatment, the OPD and indoor services are provided.
- Providing valuable data and experience at the level of community to the state and Center for future planning, improvement in service and research.

Agencies like World Bank and WHO have been contacted to support various components of the Program. Funds are provided by the Government of India to the state governments and the nodal institutes to meet the expenditure on staff, equipment, vehicles, medicine, stationary, contingencies, training, etc. for initial 5 years and thereafter they should manage themselves. Government of India has constituted central Mental Health Authority to oversee the implementation of the Mental Health Act 1986. It provides for creation of state Mental Health Authority also to carry out the said functions. The National Human Rights Commission also monitors the conditions in the mental hospitals along with the government of India and the states are currently acting on the recommendation of the joint studies conducted to ensure quality in delivery of mental care.

ADOLESCENT HEALTH PROGRAM

Adolescents are individuals aged between 10 and 19 years. Adolescence is important phase in the life span of an individual, with long-term influence on his/her overall health. In order to promote Adolescent Health in a holistic manner, a multi-component intervention targeting both determinants of health problems and their consequences is imperative. Ministry of Health and Family Welfare -National Health Mission, along with Government of Kerala has put in place a comprehensive health Program for adolescents, i.e., Rashtriya Kishor Swasthya Karyakram (RKSK)/Adolescent Health Programme.

Vision

The Adolescent Health Programme envisions that all adolescents in Kerala are enabled to realize their full potential by:
- Making informed and responsible decisions related to their health and well-being
- Accessing the existing services and support systems for resolving issues.

Mission

- To increase the availability and access to information about health to all adolescents.
- To increase accessibility and utilization of quality adolescents health service.
- To develop multi-sectorial partnerships to create safe and supportive environments for adolescents.
- To institute special strategies to target adolescents residing in geographic pockets or negative socio-economic environments, which make them vulnerable to health and nutrition risks.

Guiding Principles

The adolescent health strategy adheres to the following key principles:
- Adolescent participation and leadership
- Equity, Gender Equity, inclusion
- Strategic partnerships.

Objectives

The specific objectives of the program are:
- Improve nutrition
- Enable/enhance sexual, reproductive and maternal health
- Enhance mental health
- Prevent/reduce injuries and violence
- Prevent substance misuse
- Address noncommunicable diseases prevention.

Strategies

Nutrition
- To reduce the prevalence of malnutrition among adolescents
- To reduce prevalence of Iron Deficiency Anemia among adolescents.

Sexual and Reproductive Health

- To improve knowledge, attitude and behavior in relation to SRH
- To promote healthy menstrual hygiene practices among adolescent girls
- To reduce teenage pregnancies by giving knowledge about risks of early conception.

Mental health: To address mental health concern of adolescents.

Injuries and violence: To promote favorable attitudes against injuries and violence, including GBV among adolescents

Substance misuse: To raise awareness on adverse effects and consequences of substance misuse.

Noncommunicable diseases: To promote behavior change for prevention of NCDs, hypertension, stroke, cardiovascular diseases, cancer and diabetes through healthy lifestyles and promotion of physical activity.

ROLE OF NURSE IN THE NATIONAL HEALTH PROGRAMME

Patient treatment is the primary responsibility of community health nurses staff. In addition, community health nurses provide community members with information about their well-being in order to decrease disease and death occurrence. They plan educational assemblies, conduct health screenings, hand-out fliers, administer immunizations, and dispense medications.
- Nurse must know government department and their activities noting where and whom advice can be obtained.
- Nurse should study the various government and other forms for reports that are required weekly, monthly/quarterly/yearly from CH department.
- Find out and discuss about different social activities and self-help project in the community, their value and effect upon the community.
- In addition the responsibility includes: Case finding, case Holding, Follow-up, referrals, records and education.
- This role or approach in community can be implemented by suing nursing process. Nurse must be active participant in each and every National Health Programme. As he/she is the key person for health team he/she needs to be alert, attentive and supporter.

Chapter 15: National Health Programs

CONCLUSION

National Health Programme globally accepted to see change in health status of community people. To achieve goals towards health such programs are helpful to achieve or know about health and disease. Various international agencies like WHO, UNICEF, UNFPA as also number of foreign agencies like SIDA, DANIDA, NORAD and USAID have been providing technical and material assistance in the implementation of these programs.

BIBLIOGRAPHY

1. Basavanthappa BT. Community Health Nursing, 1st Edition. New Delhi: Jaypee Brothers; 1998. pp. 319–21.
2. Chalkey AM. A Textbook for the Health Worker, 1st Edition. New Delhi: N.A.I. Limited, Publisher;1985. pp. 330–40.
3. Kumari Neelam. Essentials of Community Health Nursing, 1st Edition. Jalandhar: PV Books: Jalandhar; 2011. pp. 225–26.
4. Park K. Essentials of Community Health Nursing, 4th Edition. Jabalpur: Banarasidas Bhanot Publisher: 2004. pp. 225–26.
5. Swarnkar K. Community Health Nursing, 2nd Edition. Indore: N.R. Brother; 2008. pp. 639–42.

REVIEW QUESTIONS

Long Essays

1. Revised National Tuberculosis Control Programme (RNTCP).
2. National AIDS Control Programme.
3. National programme for control of blindness.
4. Role of Community Health Nurse in Family Welfare Services.
5. Minimum Needs Program.
6. National Diabetes Control Programme.
7. Role of nurse in the national health programme.

Short Essays

1. National ARI Control Programme.
2. National Antimalaria Programme.
3. Enhanced Malaria Control Project.
4. National Filarial Control Programme.
5. National Guinea Worm Eradication Programme.
6. National Leprosy Eradication Programme.
7. Strategies for Leprosy Elimination in India.
8. STD Control Program.
9. Iodine Deficiency Control Program.
10. National Family Welfare Programme.
11. National Water Supply and Sanitation Programme.
12. Polio Eradication: Pulse Programme.
13. National Cancer Control Programme.
14. Yaws Eradication Program.
15. National Nutritional Anemia Prophylaxis Programme.
16. ICDS Program.
17. National Mental Health Programme.
18. Adolescent Health Program.

Short Answers

1. ARI Control.
2. Urban Malaria Scheme.
3. Healthcare Interventions for Leprosy Patient.
4. Causes of Blindness.
5. Expanded Programme of Immunization.
6. Aims and Objectives of Family Welfare Program.
7. Impact of Family Welfare Activities.
8. Rural Sanitation Program.
9. Urban Sanitation Programme.
10. District Cancer Control Program.
11. Objective of Twenty Point Program.
12. Mid-day meal program.
13. PM Poshan.
14. Salient Features of Mid-day Meal Scheme.
15. District Mental Health Program.

Multiple Choice Questions

1. Which one of the following is the main target of family welfare programs?
    a. Couples in the fertile age
    b. Male after fertile age
    c. Children below 12 years
    d. Women after fertile age
2. What is the main aim of Janani Suraksha Yojana which is the programme by the Family Welfare programme?
    a. Reducing maternal and neonatal mortality
    b. To encourage people to use safe sexual methods
    c. To provide pensions to widow women
    d. To provide shelters to poor people
3. Which of the following mentioned portals and sub-programmes were created under Sarva Shiksha Abhiyan (SSA)?
    a. Rashtriya Avishkar Abhiyan (RAA)
    b. Padhe Bharat Badhu Bharat
    c. Shagun Portal
    d. All of the above
4. The causative of tuberculosis is:
    a. Virus
    b. Bacterium
    c. Malnutrition
    d. Protozoan
5. The BCG vaccine is administered for immunity against:
    a. Malaria
    b. Tuberculosis
    c. Jaundice
    d. Hepatitis
6. The community development programme is means:
    a. To bring about a special and economic change in village life through the effort of the villagers themselves
    b. To arrange welfare programmes for women and children
    c. To improve agriculture product through better manure and seeds
    d. To plan development programme in a village high population of 60 and 80 thousand
7. Under NMEP, the function of fever depot treatment is:
    a. Diagnosis of cases + spraying
    b. Collection of slides + treatment of fever
    c. Treatment fever cases only
    d. Treatment + slide collection + spraying
8. All of the following statements about National Malaria Control Programme are true except:
    a. Number of slides examined should amount to at least 10% of the population under surveillance in a year
    b. Annual parasite incidence based on active and passive surveillance and cases confirmed by blood examination

Chapter 15: National Health Programs

    c. Annual blood examination rate is calculated from the number of slides examined per 100 cases of fever
    d. The slide positivity rate provides information on the trend of malaria transmission

9. National aids control programme launched in the year _____.
    a. 1990
    b. 1991
    c. 1988
    d. 1987

10. RNTCP test was introduced in _____.
    a. 1993
    b. 1904
    c. 1980
    d. 1990

11. Which one of the following is the activity of the Family Welfare Programme?
    a. Malnutrition programme
    b. Child marriage
    c. IUD programme
    d. One child one nation policy

12. What is the main aim of Janani Suraksha Yojana which is the programme by the Family Welfare Programme?
    a. To provide pensions to widow women
    b. To provide shelters to poor people
    c. To encourage people to use safe sexual methods
    d. Reducing maternal and neonatal mortality.

ANSWERS

1. a	2. a	3. d	4. b	5. b	6. a	7. b	8. c	9. d	10. a	11. c	12. d

16 CHAPTER

Demography and Family Welfare

LEARNING OBJECTIVES

Demography
1. Concept
2. Trends in the world and in India
3. Concept of fertility and infertility
4. Small family norm

Family Welfare
5. Concept, importance, aims and objectives
6. Family planning methods
7. Family planning counseling
8. National Family Welfare Policy
9. National Family Welfare Programme
10. Role of a nurse in the family planning programme

INTRODUCTION

The word 'Demography' is a combination of two Greek words, 'Demos' meaning people and 'Graphy' meaning science. Thus, demography is the science of people. In the middle of the nineteenth century in 1855, the word 'Demography' was first used by a French writer Achille Guillard. Demography is the branch of social size, structure, which deals with the study of size, structure and distribution of populations, along with the spatial and temporal changes in them in response to birth, migration, aging and death. Demography is the study of human populations—their size, composition and distribution across space—and the process through which populations change. Births, deaths and migration are the 'big three' of demography, jointly producing population stability or change.

DEFINITIONS

- Demography is the "study of human populations in relation to the changes brought about by the interplay of births, deaths, and migration".
- "Demography is the statistical description and analysis of human population".—Wrong
- Demography is the "statistical and mathematical study of the size, composition and spatial distribution of human populations, and of the changes over time, in these aspects through the operation of the five processes of fertility, mortality, marriage, migration and social mobility"—Bogue
- Demography is the "scientific study of human population in which includes study of changes in population size, composition and its distribution".

CONCEPT OF DEMOGRAPHY

A population's composition may be described in terms of basic demographic features—age, sex, family and household status–and by features of the population's social and economic context—language, education, occupation, ethnicity, religion, income and wealth. The distribution of populations can be defined at multiple levels (local, regional, national, global) and with different types of boundaries (political, economic, and geographic). Demography is a central component of societal contexts and social change **(Fig. 16.1)**.

Uses of Demography

- Demography is very useful for understanding social and economic problems and identifying potential solutions.
- Demographers are engaged in social planning, market research, insurance forecasting, labor market analysis, economic development and so on.
- They work for private firms and public agencies at local, regional, national and international levels.

Demographic Factors (Fig. 16.2)

- **Age:** Under 12, 12 to 17, 18 to 24, 25 to 34... (these typically go on at 10-year increments)
- **Sex (gender):** Male, female, other nonbinary identities
- **Income level:** Under $15,000, $15,000 to $24,999, $25,000 to $34,999... (distribution brackets will vary based on who is being sampled)
- **Race:** Caucasian, African American, American Indian, Latino, Asian, Pacific islander
- **Ethnicity:** Jewish, Arab, Irish, Dutch, Russian, Swedish
- **Employment status:** Employed, unemployed, self-employed, retired, disabled
- **Education level:** High school, some college, undergraduate degree, graduate degree
- **Number of children:** None, 1 to 2, 3 to 5, 5 or more...
- **Living status:** Own, rent, lease, other

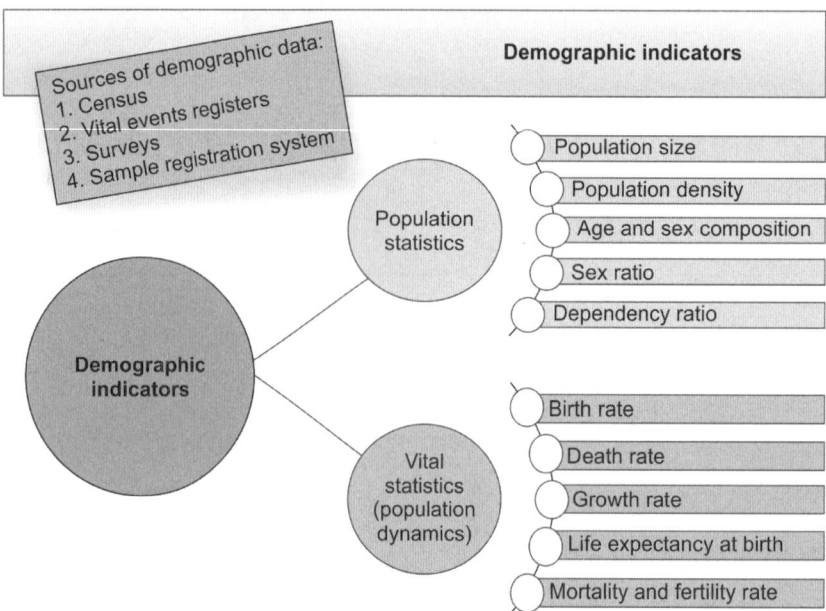

Fig. 16.1: Demographic indicators.

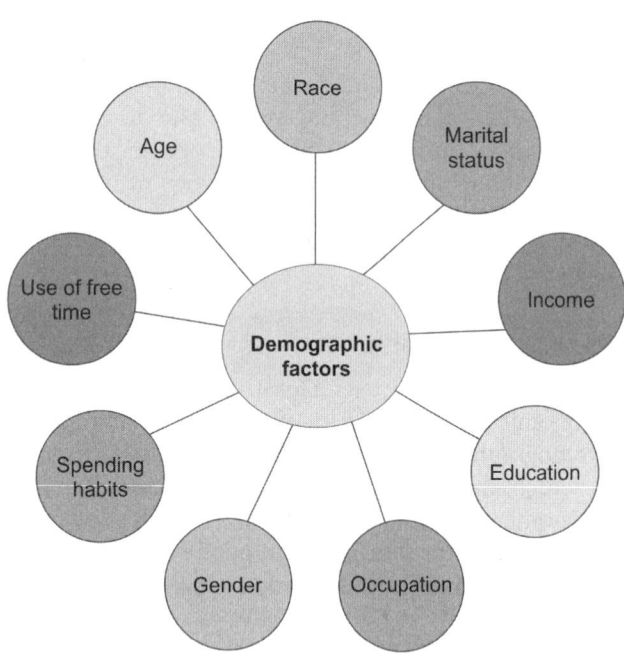

Fig. 16.2: Demographic factors.

- **Location (geographical data):** Zip code, city, county, state, country
- **Political affiliation:** Republican, Democrat, independent
- **Marital status:** Single, married, separated, widowed
- **Religious affiliation:** Muslim, Buddhist, Hindi, Catholic, Jewish
- **Social class:** Lower class, middle class, upper class
- **Nationality:** American, Mexican, German, Swiss, Finnish, French.

IMPORTANCE OF DEMOGRAPHY

With the majority of developing countries facing population explosion, the study of population and its problems has become very important in every sphere of an economy.

For the Economy

- The study of demography is of immense importance to an economy.
- Population studies help us to know how far the growth rate of the economy is keeping pace with the growth rate of population.
- If population is increasing at a faster rate, the pace of development of the economy will be slow.
- The government can undertake appropriate measures to control the growth of population and to accelerate the development of the economy.

For Society

- Population studies have much importance for the society. When population is increasing rapidly, the society is faced with innumerable problems.
- Shortages of basic services like water, electricity, transport and communications, public health, education, etc. arise.
- Along with these, problems of migration and urbanization are associated with the growing population which further led to the law and order problem.

For Economic Planning

- Data relating to the present trend in population growth help the planners in formulating policies for the economic plan of the country.
- They are kept in view while fixing targets of agricultural and industrial products, of social and basic services like schools and other educational institutions, hospitals, houses, electricity, transport, etc.
- Population data are also used by the planners to project future trends in fertility and to formulate policy measures to control the birth rate.

For Administrators

- Population studies are also useful for administrators who run the government. In under-developed countries, almost all social and economic problems are associated with the growth of population.
- The administrator has to tackle and find solutions to the problems arising from the growth of population. They are migration and urbanization which lead to the coming up of shanty towns, pollution, drainage, water, electricity, transport, etc.
- These require improvement of environmental sanitation, removal of stagnant and polluted water, slum clearance; better housing, efficient transport system, clean water supply, better sewerage facilities, control of communicable diseases, provision of medical and health services, especially in maternal and child welfare by opening health centers, opening of schools, etc.

For Political System

- The knowledge of demography is of immense importance for a democratic political system. It is on the basis of the census figures pertaining to different areas that the demarcation of constituencies is done by the election commission of a country.
- The addition to the number of voters after each election helps to find out how many have migrated from other places and regions of the country.
- Political parties are able to find out from the census data the number of male and female voters, their level of education, their age structure, their level of earning, etc.
- On this basis, political parties can raise issues and promise solutions in their election manifestos at the time of elections.

Scope of Demography

- Demography is the science of population. In its most general meaning, a population is a set of people who live in a specific land area: a commune, a district, a country or a continent, etc.
- A formal demography is concerned with the size, distribution, structure and changes of population.

Size: Size is the number of units (inhabitants) in the population.

Distribution: Distribution is the arrangement of the population at a given time, geographically or among various types of residential areas.

Structure

- Is the distribution of characteristics such as age, gender groups, etc. among the population.
- Additional characteristics of the units such as marital status, occupation educational level, ethnic characteristics, socioeconomic status, etc.

Change: It is the increase or decrease of the total population or of the one of its structural units.

Narrow Scope

- Population is constantly changing over time.
- The components of change in a population are births, deaths and migration.
- Thus, one generation will be replaced by another younger generation by birth and death process.
- This is a natural change or demographic reproduction.

Broader Scope

- The broader scope of demographic reproduction includes migration. It means the movement of people from place to place.
- Migration has great influence on population change.
- Within a country or an area, this movement does not affect the total size of the population.
- It changes the structure of the population and area as well as the living conditions of immigrants and out-migrants.
- This process may also influence the behavior of the inhabitants, especially out-migrants.
- Migrations have great influence on population change.

Demographic Indicators

- Measurement of mortality
- Measurement of morbidity
- Measurement of disability
- Measurement of natality
- Measurement of the presence, absence or distribution of the characteristics or attributes of the disease.
- Measurement of medical needs, healthcare facilities, utilization of health services and other health related events.
- Measurement of the presence, absence or distribution of the environmental and other factors suspected of causing the disease.
- Measurement of demographic variables.

Examples of Demographic Indicators

- Crude birth rate (CBR)
- General fertility rate (GFR)
- Crude death rate (CDR)
- Infant mortality rate (IMR)
- Life expectancy (LE)
- Total fertility rate (TFR)
- Gross reproduction rate (GRR)
- Net-reproduction rate (NRR)

DEMOGRAPHIC CYCLE

The demographic cycle, or population cycle, refers to the evolution over time of the population profile of a country, region or other defined geographical area. A population cycle theory has been postulated in terms of the socioeconomic history of industrialized countries (**Fig. 16.3**). Four stages of population change have been identified in the demographic cycle:

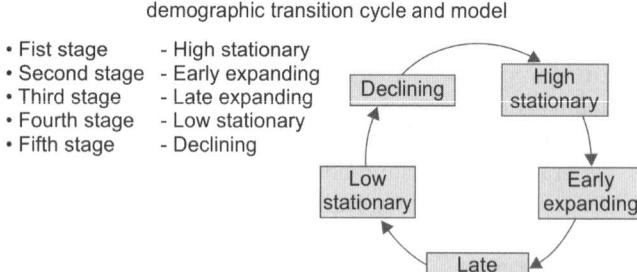

Fig. 16.3: Demographic transition cycle.

- The first high stationary phase marked by high birth and high death rates and relatively low population;
- The second phase with uneven population density due to increased urbanization and industrialization;
- The third phase where the birth and death rates are much lower resulting in a relatively steady population growth; and
- The fourth phase of population cycle which is characterized by stagnation or an actual decline in the total population of a country due to an excess of deaths over births.

Stages

First stage (High stationary): It is characterized by both high birth rate and high death rate it is found when the country is economically most backward. So the population remains stationary. India was in this stage till 1920.

Second stage (Early expanding): It begins with the declining of death rate while the birth rate remains unchanged. So this stage experiences the beginning of large increase of population. Because of improvements in food supply and sanitation, our life span increases. These changes have brought due to improvements in basic healthcare, farming techniques, education and access to technology. At present many developing countries of Asia and Africa are in this stage.

Third stage (Late expanding): Death rate declines further and birth rate begins to fall. Yet there is large increase of population since birth exceeds deaths. Due to access to contraceptives, increased wages, urbanization, a reduction in subsistence agriculture, an increase in the status and education of women, an increase in parental investment in the education of children and other social changes. India appears to be this stage.

Fourth stage (Low stationary): It is characterized with low birth rate and low death rate. So the population becomes stationary. Due to changing lifestyle and stationary working condition, high obesity and many diseases are caused in this stage aging population is predominant. Japan, Sweden, Belgium, Denmark and Switzerland are in this stage.

Fifth stage (Declining): Population begins to decline as birth rate is lower than death rate. East European countries like Germany and Hungary and north European countries like Sweden, Norway are now in this stage.

WORLD POPULATION TRENDS

Population growth is the increase in the number of individuals in a population. Global human population growth amounts to around 83 million annually, or 1.1% per year. The global population has grown from 1 billion in 1800 to 7.774 billion in 2020. It is expected to keep growing, and estimates have put the total population at 8.6 billion by mid-2030, 9.8 billion by mid-2050 and 11.2 billion by 2100. Many nations with rapid population growth have low standards of living, whereas many nations with low rates of population growth have high standards of living.

Demographic Trends (Fig. 16.4)

Global level: The population of the world is not uniformly distributed over the globe. It is mainly concentrated in the developing countries. Demographic profile of this countries and their health status is greatly influenced by their levels of socioeconomic development. UNICEF has grouped the countries of the world into three categories—industrialized, developing and least developed.

The world population stood at 6 billion by year 2000 and the population growth was 6 billion in 2000. The statistical indices used to assess the health profile of the countries of the world are both crude and specific. The difference between crude birth rate and crude death rate for comparing the health status of countries are infant mortality rate (IMR), under five mortality rate (UFMR) and maternal mortality rate (MMR).

Indian level: India is the second populous country in the world. The population size is about 1027 million in 2001. The population size is about 1,000 million between 1991 and 2001. According to 2001 census the child population, the total number of children of 0–6 years 15.78 crores out of which male children are 8.19 crores and female children are 7.59 crores. The sex ratio in India has been generally adverse to women, i.e., 1 number of women per 1,000 men has generally been less than 1000. Kerala has a sex ratio of 1,058 females per 1,000 males in 2001.

In the Indian census, density is defined as the number of persons, living per square kilometer. The family size refers

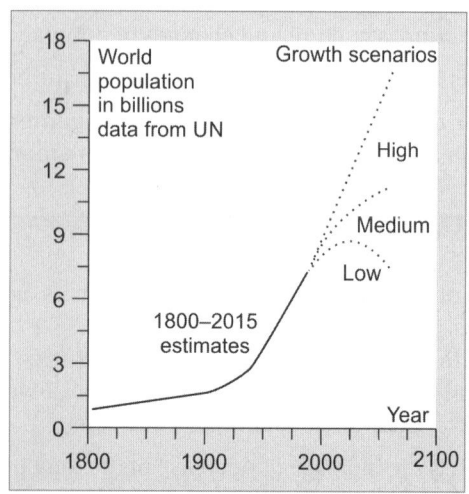

Fig. 16.4: Demographic trends.

to the total number of persons in the family. The family size depends upon numerous factors viz, duration of marriage, education of the couple, the number of live births and living children, preference of male children, desired family size, etc.

Urbanization is a recent phenomenon in the developing countries. The proportion of the urban population in India has increased from 10.84% in 1901 to 25.72% in 1991 and was 27.8 in the year 2001. The factor is expectancy at birth has continued to increase globally over the living longer and they have a right to a long life in good health rather than one of pain and disability.

World Population Prospects 2019

- Confirms that the world's population continues to grow, albeit at a slowing rate;
- Points to the challenges facing some countries and regions related to rapid population growth driven by high fertility;
- Notes that population size is decreasing in some countries due to sustained low fertility or emigration;
- Underscores the opportunities available to countries where a recent decline in fertility is creating demographic conditions favorable for accelerated economic growth;
- Highlights the unprecedented aging of the world's population;
- Confirms the ongoing global increase in longevity and the narrowing gap between rich and poor countries, while also pointing to significant disparities in survival that persist across countries and regions;
- Describes how international migration has become an important determinant of population growth and change in some parts of the world.

CONCEPT OF FERTILITY AND INFERTILITY

Infertility

- Infertility is a disease of the male or female reproductive system defined by the failure to achieve a pregnancy after 12 months or more of regular unprotected sexual intercourse.
- Infertility affects millions of people of reproductive age worldwide—and has an impact on their families and communities. Estimates suggest that between 48 million couples and 186 million individuals live with infertility globally.
- n the male reproductive system, infertility is most commonly caused by problems in the ejection of semen (1), absence or low levels of sperm, or abnormal shape (morphology) and movement (motility) of the sperm.
- In the female reproductive system, infertility may be caused by a range of abnormalities of the ovaries, uterus, fallopian tubes, and the endocrine system, among others.
- Infertility can be primary or secondary. Primary infertility is when a pregnancy has never been achieved by a person, and secondary infertility is when at least one prior pregnancy has been achieved.
- Fertility care encompasses the prevention, diagnosis and treatment of infertility. Equal and equitable access to fertility care remains a challenge in most countries; particularly in low and middle-income countries. Fertility care is rarely prioritized in national universal health coverage benefit packages.

Causes of Infertility

Infertility may be caused by a number of different factors, in either the male or female reproductive systems. However, it is sometimes not possible to explain the causes of infertility.

In the female reproductive system, infertility may be caused by:
- Tubal disorders such as blocked fallopian tubes, which are in turn caused by untreated sexually transmitted infections (STIs) or complications of unsafe abortion, postpartum sepsis or abdominal/pelvic surgery;
- Uterine disorders which could be inflammatory in nature (such as such endometriosis), congenital in nature (such as septate uterus), or benign in nature (such as fibroids);
- Disorders of the ovaries, such as polycystic ovarian syndrome and other follicular disorders;
- Disorders of the endocrine system causing imbalances of reproductive hormones. The endocrine system includes hypothalamus and the pituitary glands. Examples of common disorders affecting this system include pituitary cancers and hypopituitarism.

Male reproductive system, infertility may be caused by:
- Obstruction of the reproductive tract causing dysfunctionalities in the ejection of semen. This blockage can occur in the tubes that carry semen (such as ejaculatory ducts and seminal vesicles). Blockages are commonly due to injuries or infections of the genital tract.
- Hormonal disorders leading to abnormalities in hormones produced by the pituitary gland, hypothalamus and testicles. Hormones such as testosterone regulate sperm production. Examples of disorders that result in hormonal imbalance include pituitary or testicular cancers.
- Testicular failure to produce sperm, for example due to varicoceles or medical treatments that impair sperm-producing cells (such as chemotherapy).
- Abnormal sperm function and quality. Conditions or situations that cause abnormal shape (morphology) and movement (motility) of the sperm negatively affect fertility. For example, the use of anabolic steroids can cause abnormal semen parameters such sperm count and shape.

Environmental and lifestyle factors such as smoking, excessive alcohol intake and obesity can affect fertility. In addition, exposure to environmental pollutants and toxins can be directly toxic to gametes (eggs and sperm), resulting in their decreased numbers and poor quality, leading to infertility.

Female Infertility Treatment

Treatments for infertility include:
- **Medications:** Fertility drugs change hormone levels to stimulate ovulation.

- **Surgery:** Surgery can open blocked fallopian tubes and remove uterine fibroids and polyps. Surgical treatment of endometriosis doubles a woman's chances of pregnancy.

Male Infertility Treated

Treatments for male infertility include:
- **Medications:** Medications can raise testosterone or other hormone levels. There are also drugs for erectile dysfunction.
- **Surgery:** Some men need surgery to open blockages in the tubes that store and carry sperm. Varicocele surgery can make sperm healthier and can improve the odds of conception.

Fertility Treatment Options for all Genders

Some couples need more help conceiving. To increase pregnancy odds, a woman may first take medications to stimulate ovulation before trying one of these options:
- **Intrauterine insemination (IUI):** A healthcare provider uses a long, thin tube to place sperm directly into the uterus.
- **In vitro fertilization (IVF):** IVF is a type of assisted reproductive technology (ART). It involves harvesting the eggs at the end of the stimulation and placing sperm and eggs together in a lab dish. The sperm fertilize the eggs. A provider transfers one of the fertilized eggs (embryo) into the uterus.
- **Intracytoplasmic sperm injection (ICSI):** This procedure is similar to IVF. An embryologist (highly specialized lab technician) directly injects a single sperm into each of the harvested eggs and then a provider transfers an embryo into the uterus.
- **Third-party ART:** Couples may use donor eggs, donor sperm or donor embryos. Some couples need a gestational carrier or surrogate. This person agrees to carry and give birth to your baby.

SMALL FAMILY NORM

India is the first country in 1952 to implement established population policies, in a series of Five Year Plans starting from 1951. In the First Five Year plan, from 1951 to 1956, it has been recognized by the Planning Commission that a population policy is necessary and family planning is identified as an important component of the legislation, hence family planning received 100% funding from the central government. In the next five years, from 1956 to 1961, the method of sterilization is emphasized, and by the next 5 years, family planning programs are placed as national priority **(Fig. 16.5)**.
- Fertility rates for literate women are 2.2 while for non-literate people it is 4.
- While knowledge of family planning is universal, only 36% of married women aged 13 to 49 currently use modern contraceptives.
- Place of residence, education and religion are strongly related to both fertility and contraceptive use.
- Government programs push female sterilization at a young age 97%.

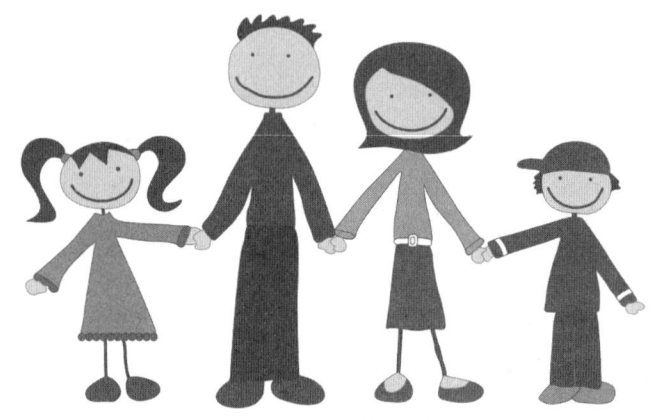

Fig. 16.5: Small family.

Aims and Objectives

The following are the aims and objectives:
- To determine the views about family size and ideal spacing.
- To determine the degree of knowledge about various contraceptive methods.
- To know the family size amongst population not adopting small family norm.
- To know the reason for nonacceptance of family planning methods.

Effects of Family Size

- **Basic human needs:** Food clothing, shelter, basic education and primary health are basic needs of human. If the family size is small, the perception share will be more.
- **Economical needs:** Income, savings and resources may not be sufficient to meet if the family size is large. Low savings income and large family size will not help in further development.
- **Food and nutrition:** The larger the family size will not be able to meet the nutritive requirements of the members of family.
- **Socioeconomic:** Large family size result in migration of rural people to urban areas in search for employment resulting in urban slums and associated socioeconomic problems.
- **Larger family size:** has shown higher morbidity and mortality among mothers and children.
- **Education:** It is hard for the large family to give proper education to their children.

Factors Involve Small Family

- Sociocultural background of the society.
- Socioeconomic aspects of the family.
- Health center and health workers involvement and participation.
- Family health services or programs effectiveness.
- Education background of the individual and family members.
- Effective contraceptive delivery services.
- Health education and mass media participation.

- Legal issues by governmental sectors by maintaining proper records and reports.
- Statistical system of particular area.
- Periodical evaluation and revision of policies and procedures.

Benefits

There are some very clear benefits to having a small family:
- Each child receives more parental attention and educational advantages, which generally raise her self-esteem **(Fig. 16.6)**.
- Children in small families, especially first and only children, tend to have higher school and personal achievement levels than do children of larger families.
- The financial costs of maintaining a household are lower.
- It is easier for both parents to combine careers with family life.
- The general stress level is lower because there often are fewer conflicts and less rivalry.

Challenge

A small family promises well-nourished and healthy family affiliates. Furthermore, children in a small family will get more love and concentration from their parents. Generally, a family is a group, which is made up of two parents and their kids living jointly as a unit. It also consists of all the successors of a common precursor. In general, a family is a social unit of two or more individuals, related by marriage, blood, or adoption and having a common pledge to the mutual relationship.
- Population explosion
- Poverty
- Lack of health, education and livelihood opportunity
- Migration
- Environment pollution Scheduled Caste and Other Backward Communities are affected and the solution of problems through this project intervention will benefit the target SC and OBC community.

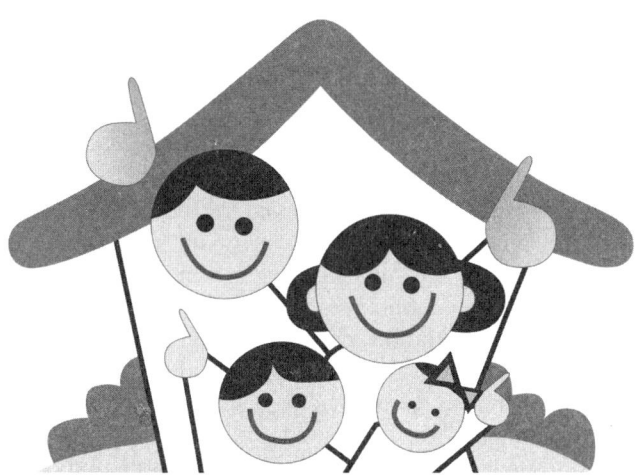

Fig. 16.6: Advantages of small family.

Hazards of Large and Unplanned Family

- Too early marriages leads to hazards and pregnancy and child birth, i.e. abortion, stillbirth, premature birth and increase chances to develop cancer of cervix, also discontinuation of job and education.
- Too early pregnancy leads to increase risk from pregnancy and child birth, LBW, sickness and ill health mother, increasing mortality and morbidity rate.
- Too frequent pregnancies lead to LBW, cancer and also economic hardships, parents attention is divided among children.
- Too many pregnancies also lead to un happiness and disharmony in the family and difficulty in providing proper education to children.
- The late pregnancies lead to lose social status and also congenital abnormalities.

Advantages of Adopting Small Family Norm

Dominant civilizing norms habitually influence couples in their option of family size. Depending on the background, this option can be traced to cultural, religious, or socioeconomic reasons, like the necessity for support in old age. However, it is established that a family with two or fewer kids provides several benefits to both the children and the parents. Here are the top 10 benefits of a small family.

1. **Better life quality for children:** Kids of smaller families get more attention to higher quality from their parents, causing higher achievements. Kids with one or no siblings can perform better in edification, as parents hold a restricted amount of emotional and economic resources these happen to be diluted, meaning their quality diminishes as the number of kid increases.
2. **Amplified economic success:** Children with fewer siblings are capable of attaining amplified economic success and communal positions. Furthermore, the decision to limit the size of a family can be understood as a strategic option to perk up the socioeconomic success of kids and grandkids in modern societies.
3. **Better life quality for parents:** Parents are greatly benefitted by a small family. The expenditure, such as of supporting a kid from cradle to university, such as schoolbooks, uniforms, trips, provisions, university fees, etc., is greatly reduced. Moreover, fewer kids create a more controllable impact on family finances, thus relieving strain and emotional pressure levels.
4. **Less pressure on family budgets:** Parents of a small family experience less pressure on family budgets, making them to make both ends meet easily, and to make them doing essential shopping without any difficulty by buying quality products.
5. **Maximum level of happiness:** The levels of happiness are maximized when the number of kids is limited to two for each family. Those who turn into a parent at their young age, which is habitually related to having a bigger family, reported descending happiness trajectories, whereas happiness levels were maximized when parents

were older and had previously acquired financial and educational resources.

6. **Less strain for mothers in small family:** Mothers with one or two children experience less strain when compared to those having two or more children. This allows mothers to pay more attention to the welfare of their children.
7. **A small family is an ecologically sustainable option:** The size of a family plays a vital role in preventing and highlighting climate change. Actually, it may be the solitary campaign for ecologically friendly lifestyles, which really counts. Considering further influences impacts of climate change, such as the loss of certain species, a small family makes even more ecological sense.
8. **Smaller families are inclined to have optimistic effects on the life of a woman:** Women are usually responsible for child-rearing activities. A smaller number of kids would offer women additional time to develop individually and professionally. Smaller families could boost the empowerment of women, together with men, assuming more responsibility. Moreover, women who bear their first kid at their 30s tend to have fewer kids are better off professionally and economically, as well as in terms of welfare.
9. **Condensed health risk in small family:** Parents are much benefitted with a small family, which include abridged expenses on food, additional time to devote to leisure or work, increased caring attention per kid, and condensed health risk.
10. **Higher levels of education in small family:** Young individuals are more probable to attain higher levels of education if their family is restricted to one or two kids. While socioeconomic factors are pertinent, family size has a considerable impact on the encouragement and attention children get at home.

Advantages for Mother

- Maintain her health
- Loss of fear about unwanted pregnancy
- Less strain and worry due to less children
- More time and energy for children
- Have more time for education, vocational
- Better job opportunities
- Can save child's health.

Advantages to Child

Child will have conducive atmosphere for his proper physical and psychological growth and development. Child gets proper nutrition, education, prenatal care and love.

Advantages to Father

- Father can provide children with better education, comfort, food clothing, and recreation.
- He will be more relaxed and enjoy good health.
- He will improve living standards, better health.

Advantages for Community

- Small family leads to conservation of natural resources and savings.
- Small family norm helps the nation to have enough schools, hospitals, and other basic services.
- Small family yields more employments.
- Happiness, peace, harmony and prosperity.

Practices for Small Family Norm

Small family norm has to become a way of life, for this population should be educated.

Goals of Health Worker

- Supply necessary information, for education and motivation.
- Assist client to evaluate contraceptive information and services.
- To encourage them for continuous use of contraception
- The health personnel should be properly trained with proper knowledge to motivate people.
- The service agency should be properly geared for effective implementation, monitoring and evaluation of contraceptive services.
- Effective delivery of contraceptive services at the door step of people is effective.
- For promoting acceptance of FP the IMR has to be brought down.

Barriers

- Religious point: desiring a son
- Children considered social security at old age.
- Ethical uneasiness about MTP
- Death rate of infant is high
- Lack of recreation.

In order to Remove Barriers

Government should take certain measures:
- Provide recreation facilities.
- Educate poor and illiterate regarding small family norm.
- Voluntary maternity of women should have a proper place of information.
- Make FP program a peoples program.
- Role of voluntarily organizations.

FAMILY PLANNING

Family planning may involve consideration of the number of children a woman wishes to have, including the choice to have no children, as well as the age at which she wishes to have them. These matters are influenced by external factors such as marital situation, career considerations, financial position, and any disabilities that may affect their ability to have children and raise them. If sexually active, family planning may involve the use of contraception and other techniques to control the timing of reproduction.

Definition

Family planning is the planning of when to have children and the use of birth control and other techniques to implement such plans. Other techniques commonly used include sexuality education prevention and management of sexually transmitted infection preconception counseling and management, and infertility management.

Key Facts

- 214 million Women of reproductive age in developing countries who want to avoid pregnancy are not using a modern contraceptive method.
- Some family planning methods, such as condoms, help prevent the transmission of HIV and other sexually transmitted infections.
- Family planning/contraception reduces the need for abortion, especially unsafe abortion.
- Family planning reinforces people's rights to determine the number and spacing of their children.
- By preventing unintended pregnancy, family planning/contraception prevents deaths of mothers and children.

Objectives

- To avoid unwanted births
- To bring about wanted births
- To regulate the intervals between pregnancies
- To control the time at which births occur in relation to the ages of the parent
- To determine the number of children in the family.

Importance of Family Planning in India

- Increased population has adverse effect on our per capita income. More than 40% India's population live below the "poverty line" Poverty leads to sickness and sickness to poverty. People suffer from serious illness and they can't get adequate medications due to poverty.
- Population explosion has created; various social problems like unemployment, overcrowding, illiteracy, low standard of living urban deterioration, inadequate housing poor/inadequate nutrition.
- As the family size increases, parents will not able to cope up with the increased family demands because family income is not increased comparing to family size. This leads to family disturbances, unhappiness and insecurity, etc.
- Mother's general health gets impaired with increased number of pregnancies. The adverse effects of repeated pregnancies lead to problems of anemia in a mother and that she becomes susceptible to any infection.
- As there is no spacing of children, the child gets very little attention. This causes malnutrition negligence and other problems in the child.
- To avoid all the problems family planning is necessary because of health and happiness of family depends on the size of the number of children the family has.

Scope of Family Planning Services

- The proper spacing and limitation of births
- Advice on sterility
- Education for parenthood
- Sex education
- Screening for pathological conditions related reproductive system
- Genetic counseling
- Premarital consultation and examination
- Carrying out pregnancy tests
- Marriage counseling
- The preparation of couples for the arrival of their child
- Providing services for unmarried mothers
- Teaching home economics and nutrition
- Providing adoption services.

Benefits of Family Planning/Contraception

Promotion of family planning—and ensuring access to preferred contraceptive methods for women and couples—is essential to securing the well-being and autonomy of women, while supporting the health and development of communities (**Fig. 16.7**).

Types of Family Planning Methods

Hormonal

These methods contain hormones called estrogen and progestin that are similar to the estrogen and progesterone a woman makes in her own body. They include pills, injections, and implants. Hormonal methods work by preventing eggs from being released from the ovaries, thickening cervical mucus to prevent sperm from entering the uterus, and thinning the lining of the uterus to prevent implantation of fertilized egg.

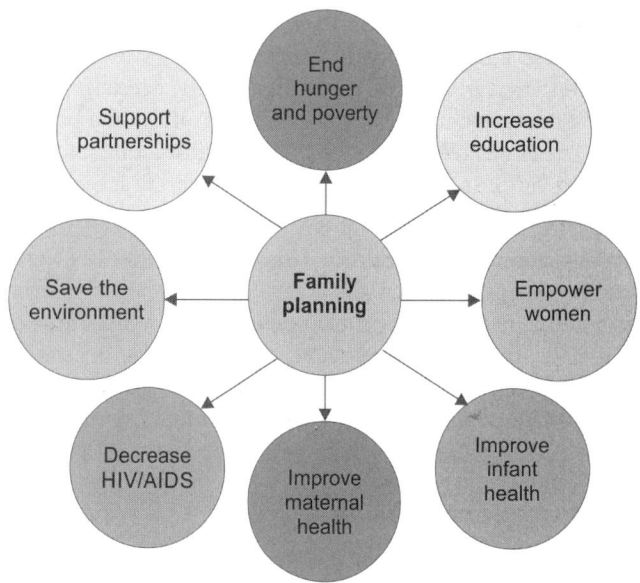

Fig. 16.7: Benefits of family planning/contraception.

Barrier

These are devices that attempt to prevent pregnancy by physically preventing sperm from entering the uterus. The sperm is thus blocked from reaching the egg. They include male condoms, female condoms, cervical caps, diaphragms and contraceptive sponges with spermicides. They do not change the way the woman's or man's body works and cause very few side effects.

Intrauterine Devices

The IUD is a small plastic or copper device inserted into the uterus by a trained health worker. It works by creating a hostile environment for the sperm. They can last for 5–12 years.

Sterilization

- There are operations that make it almost impossible for a man or a woman to have any children. Since these operations are permanent, they are only good for those women or men who are certain that they do not want any more children.
- The surgery for the man is known as Vasectomy in which the tubes that carry the sperm from the testicles to the penis are cut. The operation does not change a man's ability to have sex or to feel sexual pleasure.
- The surgery for the woman is known as tubal ligation and as the name implies the tubes that carry the eggs to the uterus are cut or tied.
- It does not change a woman's monthly bleeding or her ability to have sex and sexual pleasure.

Natural Methods

These are methods to avoid pregnancy that does not require the use of any devices or chemicals or medicines. The methods are breastfeeding for the first 6 months also known as lactational amenorrhea and the fertility awareness method.

Lactational amenorrhea: This method involves the use of a woman's natural postpartum infertility which occurs after delivery and may be extended by breastfeeding. Breastfeeding exclusively for the first six months can prevent the ovaries from releasing an egg. This method does not cost anything but it is most effective for only the first 6 months after childbirth.

Fertility awareness method: This method requires that a woman is aware of when she is fertile during her menstrual cycle and to avoid having unprotected sexual intercourse on those days. To follow this method, women need to accurately and precisely chart their fertility, either through basal body temperature changes or changes in cervical mucus, or by following the calendar.

Emergency Contraception

Emergency methods are ways for women to avoid pregnancy after having unprotected sex. They are only effective if used soon after having sex. They work primarily by preventing ovulation or fertilization. They include pills and intrauterine devices.

Advantages of Family Planning

- **Preventing pregnancy-related health risks in women:** Family planning allows spacing of pregnancies and can delay pregnancies in young women at increased risk of health problems and death from early childbearing. It prevents unintended pregnancies, including those of older women who face increased risks related to pregnancy. Family planning enables women who wish to limit the size of their families to do so. Evidence suggests that women who have more than 4 children are at increased risk of maternal mortality. By reducing rates of unintended pregnancies, family planning also reduces the need for unsafe abortion.
- **Reducing infant mortality:** Family planning can prevent closely spaced and ill-timed pregnancies and births, which contribute to some of the world's highest infant mortality rates. Infants of mothers who die as a result of giving birth also have a greater risk of death and poor health.
- **Helping to prevent HIV/AIDS:** Family planning reduces the risk of unintended pregnancies among women living with HIV, resulting in fewer infected babies and orphans. In addition, male and female condoms provide dual protection against unintended pregnancies and against STIs including HIV.
- **Empowering people and enhancing education:** Family planning enables people to make informed choices about their sexual and reproductive health. Family planning represents an opportunity for women to pursue additional education and participate in public life, including paid employment in non-family organizations. Additionally, having smaller families allows parents to invest more in each child. Children with fewer siblings tend to stay in school longer than those with many siblings.
- **Reducing adolescent pregnancies:** Pregnant adolescents are more likely to have preterm or low birth-weight babies. Babies born to adolescents have higher rates of neonatal mortality. Many adolescent girls who become pregnant have to leave school. This has long-term implications for them as individuals, their families and communities.
- **Slowing population growth:** Family planning is key to slowing unsustainable population growth and the resulting negative impacts on the economy, environment, and national and regional development efforts.

Health Aspects of Family Planning

- **Women's health:** Maternal mortality, morbidity of women of child bearing age, nutritional status (weight changes, hemoglobin level, etc.) preventable complications of pregnancy and abortion.
- **Fetal health:** Fetal mortality (early and late fetal death); abnormal development.
- **Infant and child health:** Neonatal, infant and pre-school mortality, Health of the infant at birth (birth weight), Vulnerability to diseases.

Welfare Concept

- Family planning is associated with numerous misconceptions—one of them is its strong association in minds of people with sterilization.
- The recognition of its welfare concept came only a decade and half after its inception, when it was named Family Welfare Program.
- The concept of welfare is very comprehensive and basically related to quality of life.

FAMILY PLANNING PROGRAMME

Family planning services are defined as "educational, comprehensive medical or social activities which enable individuals, including minors, to determine freely the number and spacing of their children and to select the means by which this may be achieved".

History of Family Planning in India

- Population growth has been a cause of worry for the Government of India since a very long time. Just after independence, the Family Planning Association of India was formed in 1949.
- The country launched a nationwide Family Planning Program in 1952, a first of its kind in the developing countries.
- This covered initially birth control programs and later included under its wing, mother and child health, nutrition and family welfare.
- In 1966, the ministry of health created a separate department of family planning.
- The then ruling Janata Government in 1977 developed a new population policy, which was to be accepted not by compulsion but voluntarily.
- It also changed the name of Family Planning Department to Family Welfare Program.

Goal: Improve pregnancy planning and spacing, and prevent unintended pregnancy.

Objectives of Family Planning Programme

- Reduce infant mortality rate
- Encourage late marriages
- Improve women's health
- Control of communal diseases.

Centrally Sponsored Program

This is a centrally sponsored program, for which 100% help is provided by the Central to all the states of the country. The main strategies for the successful implementation of the FWP program are:

- FWP is integrated with other health services
- Emphasis is in the rural areas
- child family norm to be practiced
- Adopting terminal methods to create a gap between the birth of 2 children
- Door-to-door campaigns to encourage families to accept the small family norm
- Encouraging education for both boys and girls
- Encouragement of breastfeeding
- Proper marriageable adopted (21 years for men and 18 years for women)
- Minimum Needs Program launched to raise the standard of living of the people.
- Monetary incentives given to poor people to adopt family planning measures.
- Creating widespread awareness of family planning through television, radio, news papers, puppet shows, etc.

Family planning services include:

- Contraceptive services
- Pregnancy testing and counseling
- Pregnancy–achieving services including preconception health services
- Basic infertility services
- Sexually transmitted disease services
- Broader reproductive health services, including patient education and counseling
- Breast and pelvic examinations
- Breast and cervical cancer screening
- Sexually transmitted infection (STI) and human immunodeficiency virus (HIV) prevention education, counseling, testing, and referral.

Barriers to people's use of family planning services include:

- Cost of services
- Limited access to publicly funded services
- Limited access to insurance coverage
- Family planning clinic locations and hours that are not convenient for clients
- Lack of awareness of family planning services among hard-to-reach populations
- No or limited transportation
- Inadequate services for men
- Lack of youth-friendly services.

Benefits of Using Family Planning

Family planning provides many benefits to mother, children, father, and the family.

Mother

- Enables her to regain her health after delivery.
- Gives enough time and opportunity to love and provide attention to her husband and children.
- Gives more time for her family and own personal advancement.
- When suffering from an illness, gives enough time for treatment and recovery.

Children

- Healthy mothers produce healthy children.
- Will get all the attention, security, love, and care they deserve.

Father

- Lightens the burden and responsibility in supporting his family.
- Enables him to give his children their basic needs (food, shelter, education, and better future).
- Gives him time for his family and own personal advancement.
- When suffering from an illness, gives enough time for treatment and recovery.

Importance of Family Planning in India

- Family planning is not confined to only birth control or contraception. It is important as whole for the improvement of the family's economic condition and for better health of the mother and her children.
- First of all, family planning highlights the importance of spacing births, at least 2 years apart from one another.
- According to medical science, giving birth within a gap of more than 5 years or less than 2 years has a seriously affect the health of both the mother and the child.
- Giving birth involves costs and with an increase in the number of children in a family, more medical costs of pregnancy and birth are involved, along with incurring high costs of bringing up and rearing the children.
- It is the duty of the parents to provide food, clothing, shelter, education to their children. Family planning, if adopted, has an effective impact on stabilizing the financial condition of any family.

Impact of Family Planning Programme in India

The initiatives taken by the Government in implementing the Family Planning Programme have significant impact on the country as a whole. India was the first country in the world to establish a government family planning program way back in 1952. According to 2011 Family Welfare Program, some major achievements are as follows:

- Awareness of one or more methods of contraception.
- Increase in contraceptives use over the years.
- Knowledge of female sterilization, which is considered to the most safest and popular method of modern family planning.
- Increase in the use of condoms.
- Increased knowledge about contraceptive pills.
- Fertility rate low among educated women.
- Fertility rate low among higher income groups.

Suggestions for the Family Welfare Programme

Following are some of the important suggestions that can be normally advanced are achieving further success in the implementation of family planning programme:

- The family welfare program be completely integrated and coordinated along with the public health measures.
- Enrolment of more sincere, experienced and sympathetic personnel for the implementation of the programme.
- Increasing production and free distribution of contraceptives among the poor people.
- Raising the age of marriage for both sex through both legal and social sanction.
- Offering higher incentives for sterilization.
- Liberalizing abortion for married women.
- Withdrawing maternity benefits to those women violating two-child norm.
- Adoption of Chinese system of incentives in respect of job, salary hike, promotion, housing, ration, etc. to those who have been following small family norm.
- Introduction of disincentive schemes in the form of increased taxation and withdrawal of other facilities, etc. for those people who refuse to accept the small family norm.
- Making adequate provision for substantial reduction in the infant mortality rate and also to enhance the child survival rate for the successful adoption of small family norm.
- To strengthen the monitoring of the entire program so as to reduce leakages and misutilization to the minimum.
- Adoption of a strong political will by all the political parties for the universal implementation of family planning program and also for adoption of incentive and disincentive package in connection with small family norm.
- **Publicity:** In order to send the message of family planning, its importance and method to the general masses, wide publicity must be made. Misconceptions about the harmful effect of birth control devices should be removed from the mind of the people through publicity. With the help of mass media like T.V., Radio, Cinema, Newspapers, Journals or by pamphlets the task of publicity can be made successfully.
- **Spread of education and motivation:** By raising the rate of literacy and to make the people more conscious about health and family welfare along with adoption of small family norm, the Government can popularize family welfare programs among the people.
- Spread of education among women and participation of women in various job opportunities and other social activities can raise their social status which can indirectly contribute towards containing the birth rate of population of the country. Moreover, the family planning program staff should try to motivate people in general to adopt the family planning or birth control devices so as to accept the idea of small family norm.

BIRTH CONTROL PILLS

Birth control pills are oral contraceptives that must be taken daily. The method is often recommended for both women who are religious in remembering daily doses and those who desire to restore fertility quickly.

Advantages

- Aside from its birth control properties, the pill also has health benefits. Both progestin-only and combination pills lighten periods, reduce the intensity of menstrual cramps, and lessen the possibility of ectopic pregnancies.

- The combination pill specifically helps prevent bone thinning, acne, ovarian cysts and cancers, breast cysts, endometrial cancers, infections in the uterus, fallopian tubes, and ovaries, anemia, PMS, and iron deficiency.
- Women on the pill can get pregnant immediately after stopping it—one of the reasons why most women prefer the method. Also, taking the pill is made easier to remember with easy to bring small pill packs.

Disadvantages

- The most popular thing that women don't like about birth control pills is the daily routine of taking it. The use of alarms and reminder apps or pill pack just next to you may help in remembering, but not a complete assurance. Also, like other medications, pills have their own set of side effects.
- While they usually go away after a couple of months, most women on pills experience changes in sexual desire, bleeding between periods, nausea, and sore breasts.

BARRIER METHODS

Diaphragms, female and male condoms, as well as cervical caps all belong to the barrier family planning methods. Basically, they work in preventing the sperm from getting close or in contact to the egg **(Fig. 16.8)**.

For the methods to be effective, these must be anchored before the actual copulation takes place. While thousands do not like the methods because somehow it inhibits spontaneity, barriers prevent the spread of diseases as well as promote sharing of birth control responsibilities.

Advantages

- Barrier methods are simple to use, widely available and must be used before intercourse only.
- They protect both parties from possible spread of sexually transmitted diseases and, often, are not contraindicated against most allergies.
- Female condoms, specifically, are unlikely to tear even during the roughest sexual techniques and can be inserted many hours before the sexual intercourse.

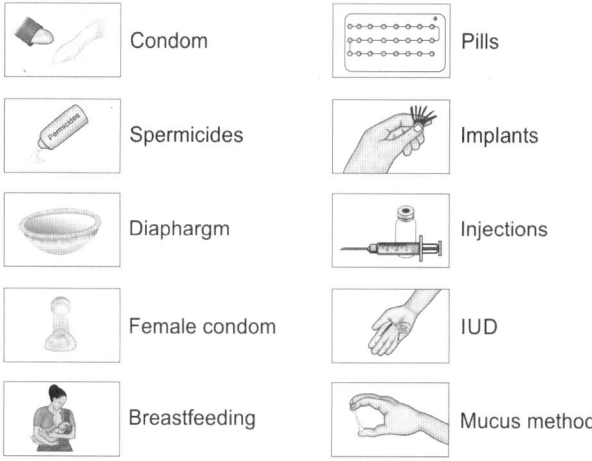

Fig. 16.8: Barrier method.

Disadvantages

- It is extremely rare to use the male condoms perfectly as they are easily torn apart. Also, frequent users report reduced arousal during sexual intercourse with the use of it.
- Female condoms, on the other hand, is easily dislodged and may result to the penis inserting between the vaginal wall and the condom instead.
- There were circumstances where women report a "noisy" method experience during the intercourse.

LONG-TERM CONTRACEPTIVE METHODS

For individuals who would want to get pregnant in the future, but are not into regularly prepping up against contraception, long-term methods are the best tools to use.

The methods include vaginal ring, contraceptive shots, intrauterine device or IUD, and implantable rod. All these are not easily reversible and non-hormonal. However, fertility immediately returns when the woman decides to discontinue its use.

Advantages

- The long-term effect of not having to remember daily routines is the biggest advantage of using these methods.
- It is extremely effective in preventing pregnancy although a few methods halt menstrual periods.

Disadvantages

- The long-term contraceptive methods do not protect either of the parties from contacting sexually transmitted infections. Also, most of these methods require surgeries for both the insertion procedure and the removal of it.
- While there are rare instances of infections in areas of tool implantation, the most common side effects include weight gain, nervousness, irregular menstrual periods, hair loss, and episodes of depression.
- Most importantly, it is not for use of all women. Those with maintenance medications are discouraged from using any of the long-term contraceptive methods.

NATURAL FAMILY PLANNING (NFP)

NFP is the sole option that produces no negative health impact and is completely free. The American College of Obstetricians and Gynecologists explained that NFP only necessitates full awareness of a woman's body's cycles especially when she is the most fertile **(Table 16.1)**.

When the main goal of copulation is to produce pregnancy, intercourse during the fertile times is the way to do it. However, if it is for avoiding pregnancy, the practice of abstinence during periods of fertility should be done.

Advantages

- The healthiest fertility regulation method, natural family planning neither interferes with the menstrual cycle nor

TABLE 16.1: Natural family planning methods.	
Method	Description
Basal body temperature charting	Identifies the luteal phase of the menstrual cycle by postovulatory increase in basal body temperature; all other days are considered fertile
Calendar calculation	Predicts the fertile period by menstrual dating
Cervical mucus monitoring	Identifies beginning and end of the fertile period from cervical secretions
Lactational amenorrhea	Maximizes suppression of ovulation during breastfeeding; effectiveness limited to six months postpartum
Symptothermal method	Based on cervical mucus monitoring; calendar calculations or basal body temperature charting monitoring provides redundancy

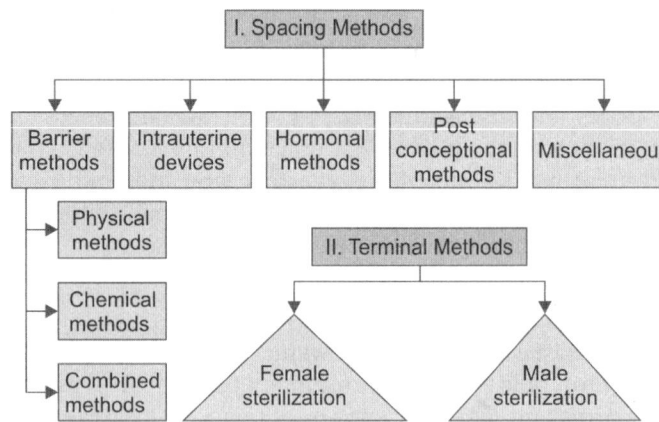

Fig. 16.9: Spacing and terminal family planning methods.

make use of chemicals and hormones that pollute the environment.
- NFP is also easy to use and familiarize and is highly effective amongst women regardless of a woman's stage of reproductive life.
- Both culture and religion permit the use of natural family planning because of its moral principles, while constantly promoting better couple communication.

Disadvantages

- The primary disadvantage is abstinence when a woman's biology is the most interested in being intimate. For most couples, it requires a huge lifestyle change.
- Also, the practice of NFP needs training from a healthcare professional to establish the unique physiology of a woman's cycle.
- Maternal health is one of the biggest factors why effective family planning campaign is being pushed worldwide. It revolves around the holistic condition of a woman from pregnancy through recovering after giving birth.
- While it is true that motherhood is a fulfilling and positive journey, millions of women associate the experience with medical complications, emotional suffering, and death.
- When women are given the chance to space their pregnancies and limit it through their personal choice of contraceptive method, they are also given the right to a healthy well-being and pleasant motherhood.

NATURAL METHODS OF SPACE METHODS

Natural family planning (NFP) is the method that uses the body's natural physiological changes and symptoms to identify the fertile and infertile phases of the menstrual cycle. Such methods are also known as fertility-based awareness methods **(Fig. 16.9)**.

Advantages

Natural family planning methods are generally the preferred contraceptive method for women who do not wish to use artificial methods of contraception for reasons of religion, or who, due to rumors and myths, fear other methods.

Disadvantages

Natural family planning methods are unreliable in preventing unwanted pregnancy. It takes time to practice and use them properly, which adds to their unreliability. Additionally, natural family planning methods do not protect against sexually transmitted infections (STIs), including the human immunodeficiency virus (HIV). You should advise couples to use condoms to protect against STIs.

Effectiveness: The effectiveness of any method of natural family planning can vary from couple to couple, and all these methods are less effective for couples who do not follow the method carefully.

Types of Natural Family Planning Methods

In order to understand the ways that natural family planning methods can prevent pregnancy, it is important for you to know each type and its techniques of use. There are three major classifications of natural family planning methods:
- Periodic abstinence (fertility awareness) method
- Use of breastfeeding or lactational amenorrhea method (LAM)
- Coitus interruptus (withdrawal or pulling out) method.

Periodic Abstinence (Fertility Awareness) Methods

During the menstrual cycle, the female hormones estrogen and progesterone cause some observable effects and symptoms:
- Estrogen produces alterations in the cervical mucus, which changes from thick, opaque and sticky to thin, clear and slippery as ovulation approaches.
- Progesterone produces a slight rise in basal body temperature (temperature at rest) after ovulation. Otherwise, the function of progesterone on the cervical mucus is just the opposite effect of estrogen—it makes the cervical mucus thick, opaque and sticky.

Observation of these changes provides a basis for periodic abstinence methods. There are three common techniques used in periodic abstinence methods, namely:

- Rhythm (calendar) method
- Basal body temperature (BBT) method
- Cervical mucus (ovulation) method.

CALENDAR OR RHYTHM METHOD

- This method is the most widely used of the periodic abstinence techniques.
- The calendar method is a calculation-based approach where previous menstrual cycles are used to predict the first and the last fertile day in future menstrual cycles.
- This method requires a good understanding of the fertile and infertile phases of the woman's menstrual cycle.
- It is based on the regularity of the menstrual cycle and the fact that an ovum (egg) can only be fertilized within 24 hours of ovulation.

Advantages: This method does not require daily monitoring of fertility indicators.

Disadvantages: It is associated with a high failure rate and can be difficult to use in the case of irregular menstrual cycles. It also takes a long time to learn and use it properly. Challenges in family planning is discussed in **Figure 16.10**.

BASAL BODY TEMPERATURE (BBT) METHOD

- The basal body temperature method is based on the slight increase in the body temperature of women at rest by about 0.3–0.5°C during and after ovulation, due to the action of an increased level of progesterone secreted by the corpus luteum.
- The rise in body temperature sustained for three consecutive days indicates that ovulation has occurred, and it remains at this increased level until the start of the next menstrual cycle.
- In this section, you will learn about when the rise in body temperature occurs, and what women need to know in order to use this method properly.

- This natural family planning method may be selected if the woman is not willing to touch her genitalia to check her cervical secretions (as in the cervical mucus method), but is willing to abstain from sexual intercourse with her spouse for long periods of time.
- It is difficult for a woman to use natural family planning methods if her menstrual cycle is irregular, as it may disturb the subtle changes in body temperature and cervical secretions, as a result of hormonal effects.

Advantages

- No side-effects for this method.
- Encourages discussion about family planning between couples.
- High failure rate if the couple do not clearly understand the method.

Disadvantages

- Requires several days of abstinence.
- Needs a longer duration to practice, understand and use properly.
- False interpretation or indications in the case of fever, as this may mislead the result of BBT.
- A special thermometer may be required.

CERVICAL MUCUS METHOD (CMM)

The cervical mucus method (or Billings method) is based on the recognition and interpretation of changes in cervical mucus and sensations in the vagina, due to the effect of changes in estrogen levels during the menstrual cycle. This method is also an ovulation method used by women trying to get pregnant and have a child **(Fig. 16.11)**.

Mechanism of Action of CMM

You may remember from the description of natural family planning methods, that the rise in the level of estrogen during the menstrual cycle influences the cervical gland to

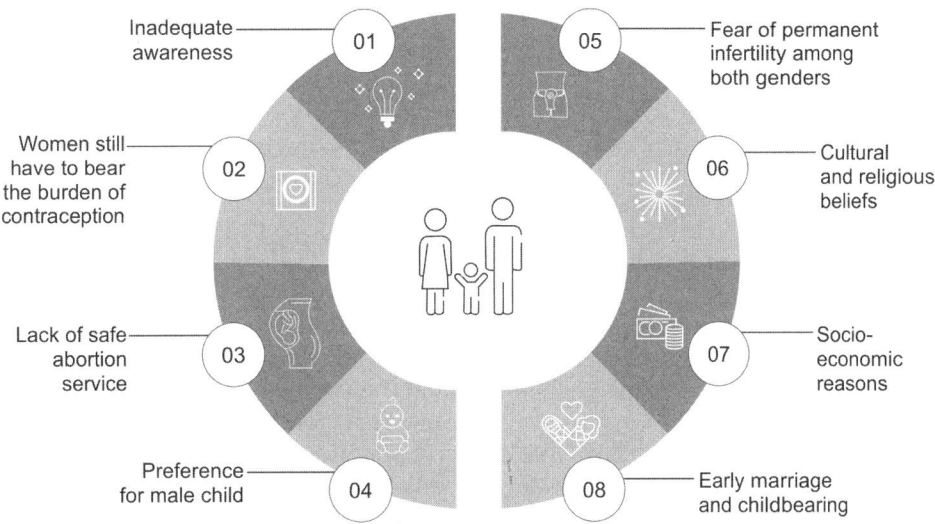

Fig. 16.10: Challenges in family planning.

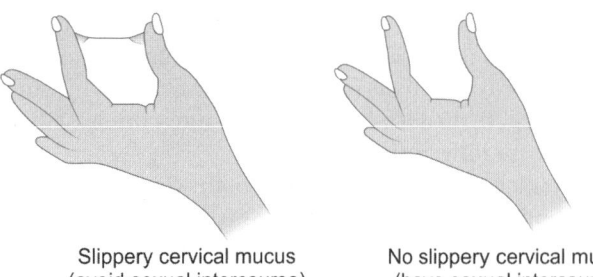

Fig. 16.11: Cervical mucus method.

secrete mucus that changes from a sensation of dryness in the vagina (characterized by thick, viscous and sticky mucus), to a sensation of wetness in the vulva (characterized by thin, white, slippery and stretchy thread-like, transparent strands-similar to uncooked egg white), during ovulation.

Using this method, these are the times when it is safe to have sexual intercourse:

- After menstruation ends the dry days (absence of cervical secretions) will start, and during these days it is safe to have sexual intercourse every other night until a woman starts to feel wet in her vagina. Every other night is suggested, as it will help women from confusing semen with cervical mucus.
- It is also safe from the evening of the fourth day after the peak day, to the beginning of the next menstruation. Once a woman has ovulated, her cervical mucus will begin to dry up, so the **peak day** is the last day of cervical or vaginal wetness.

Advantages

The advantages of this method are similar to those associated with the use of the basal body temperature method.

Disadvantages

CMM has a high failure rate because it needs several days of abstinence and a lot of experience in using the method to be effective. It is also difficult to use this method in the case of vaginal infections, as the cervical mucus secretions may be misleading.

Method of CMM

Instruct women to be able to:
- Use a chart to record their mucus pattern.
- Look at their cervical mucus in the morning, and every time after using the toilet, using a clean cloth or tissue paper to determine the cooler and consistency of the mucus.
- Touch the secretion to determine its stretchiness and slipperiness
- Feel how wet the sensation is in their genitalia when they are walking.
- Abstain from sexual intercourse on the day when mucus appears, regardless of its consistency, until the third evening after the 'peak day'.

LACTATIONAL AMENORRHEA METHOD

- The lactational amenorrhea method (LAM) is the use of breastfeeding as a contraceptive method.
- Lactational means breastfeeding and amenorrhea means not having monthly bleeding.
- In this case, there is a delay in ovulation caused by the action of prolactin hormone from the effect of lactation or breastfeeding.
- An infant's suckling of the nipple sends neural signals to the mother's hypothalamus (part of the brain), which influences the anterior pituitary gland to secrete prolactin to stimulate the breast for milk production.
- This, in turn, inhibits the secretion of follicle stimulating hormone (FSH) and luteinizing hormone (LH), and as a result ovulation does not occur. While women are exclusively breastfeeding, prolactin continues to be secreted and pregnancy is unlikely.
- When prolactin levels decrease, the woman's monthly bleeding may return, and if she continues to have unprotected sexual intercourse she may get pregnant.

Factors Affecting LAM

Any factor that causes a decrease in suckling can result in the return of ovulation and decreased milk production. These factors include supplemental feeding of the infant, reduction in the number of breastfeeds or long intervals between breastfeeds, maternal stress and maternal/child illness. In these cases, the client should not rely on LAM.

Advantages

- Effectively prevents pregnancy for at least six months.
- Encourages the best breastfeeding pattern.
- Can be used immediately after birth.
- Does not interfere with sexual intercourse.
- No hormonal side-effects.

Disadvantages

- Not a suitable method if the mother is working outside the home.
- No protection against STIs including HIV.
- If the mother has HIV, there is a small chance she may pass it to her baby in breast milk.
- Not effective after six months.

Important Points about LAM

Women should use both breasts to breastfeed their babies on demand, with no more than a four hour interval between breastfeeds during the daytime, and no more than a six hour interval between breastfeeds during the night-time. If they are unable to fulfil these conditions, you should advise and provide them with a complementary family planning method. If a woman has any risk of STI/HIV infection, you should advise her to use condoms.

COITUS INTERRUPTUS (WITHDRAWAL OR PULLING OUT) METHOD

Coitus interruptus or withdrawal is a traditional family planning method in which the man withdraws or pulls out his penis from his partner's vagina and ejaculates outside, keeping his semen away from her genitalia.

Mechanism of Action of Withdrawal Method

Coitus interruptus prevents fertilization by stopping contact between spermatozoa in the sperm and the ovum or egg.

Advantages

- It is important for you to teach this method as part of natural family planning methods.
- It costs nothing and requires no devices or chemicals. It is available in any situation and can be used as a back-up method of contraception.

Disadvantages

- It has several disadvantages. Interruption of the excitement of sexual intercourse may result in the incorrect or inconsistent use of this method, as well as decreasing sexual pleasure for both partners.
- A high failure rate may be due to a lack of self-control, and semen containing sperm may leak into the vagina before the person ejaculates.
- There is a further possibility of premature ejaculation by the man. In addition, the couple is not protected from STIs, including HIV.

Effectiveness of Withdrawal Method

This is the least effective method because it depends on the man's ability to withdraw before he ejaculates. However, it is about 73% effective if used correctly.

CONDOM

Male Condom

The latex condom is the classic barrier method. It prevents sperm from entering the woman's body, protecting against pregnancy and STDs. Of couples who rely only on male condoms, 15% get pregnant in a year.

- **Pros:** Widely available, protects against STDs, inexpensive.
- **Cons:** Only effective if used correctly every time. Can't be reused.

Female Condom

The female condom is a thin plastic pouch that lines the vagina and can be put in place up to 8 hours before sex. Users grasp a flexible, plastic ring at the closed end to guide it into position. It's somewhat less effective than the male condom.

- **Pros:** Widely available, some protection against STDs, conducts body heat better than a male condom.
- **Cons:** Can be noisy, 21% of users get pregnant, not reusable. Should not be used with a male condom, to avoid breakage.

Benefits of Condom

The female condom provides an opportunity for women to share responsibility for the use of condoms with their partners.

- A woman can use the female condom if her partner refuses to use condoms.
- The polyurethane is less likely to cause an allergic reaction than a male latex condom. It also tears less often.

  The female condom is available over the counter without a prescription. Unlike a diaphragm, it does not need to be fitted by a medical provider (one size fits all).
- The female condom will protect against most STIs if it is used correctly. It also covers much of the vulva for additional protection in that area.
- The outer ring of the female condom stimulates the clitoris during intercourse.
- The female condom can be used for protection against STIs during oral sex. Its design allows tongue insertion and fingering of the vagina or anus. If using the female condom in the anus, remove the inner ring before insertion.
- It can be inserted up to 8 hours before sex so it does not interfere with "the moment."
- The polyurethane is thin and conducts heat well so sensation is preserved.

Disadvantages of Condom

- The outer ring is visible outside the vagina, which makes some women self-conscious in front of their partners.
- It makes crackling and popping noises during intercourse. Extralubricant may help this problem.
- It has a higher failure rate than non-barrier methods such as oral contraceptive pills.
- It is somewhat cumbersome to insert.
- Each female condom can be used just once and is relatively expensive.

BIOLOGICAL, CHEMICAL AND MECHANICAL METHODS

Spermicide

Spermicidal contains a chemical that kills sperm. It comes in the form of foam, jelly, cream, or film that is placed inside the vagina before sex. Some types must be put in place 30 minutes ahead of time. Frequent use may cause tissue irritation, increasing the risk of infections and STDs. Spermicides are most often used along with other birth control methods.

- **Pros:** Easy to use, inexpensive.
- **Cons:** May increase the risk of STDs, 29% get pregnant.

Diaphragm

The diaphragm is a rubber dome that is placed over the cervix before sex. It is used with a spermicidal. Effectiveness

compares to the male condom—16% of average users get pregnant, including those who don't use the device correctly every time.
- **Pros:** Inexpensive
- **Cons:** Must be fitted by a doctor, no STD protection. Can't be used during the period due to a risk of toxic shock syndrome.

Cervical Cap

A cervical cap is similar to a diaphragm, but smaller. The FemCap slips into place over the cervix, blocking entry into the uterus. It is used with spermicide. The failure rate for the cervical cap is 15% for women who have never had children and 30% for those who have.
- **Pros:** Can stay in place for 48 hours, inexpensive
- **Cons:** Must be fitted by a doctor, no protection.

Birth Control Sponge

The birth control sponge, sold as the Today Sponge, is made of foam and contains spermicide. It is placed against the cervix up to 24 hours before sex. The sponge is about as effective as the cervical cap, with a failure rate of 16% for women who have never had children and 32% for those who have. But unlike the diaphragm or cervical cap, no fitting by a doctor is required.
- **Pros:** No prescription, effective immediately.
- **Cons:** Difficult to insert correctly, no STD protection. Can't be used during the period.

Birth Control Pill

The most common type of birth control pill uses the hormones estrogen and progestin to prevent ovulation. When taken on schedule, the pill is highly effective. About 8% of typical users get pregnant, including those who miss doses. Like all hormonal contraceptives, the pill requires a prescription **(Fig. 16.12)**.
- **Pros:** More regular, lighter periods, or no periods, depending on the type of pill. Less cramping.
- **Cons:** Cost, no STD protection. May cause side effects, including breast tenderness, spotting, serious blood clots, and raised blood pressure. Some women should not use birth control pills.

Birth Control Patch

Women who have trouble remembering a daily pill may want to consider the birth control patch. The Ortho Evra patch is worn on the skin and changed only once a week for three weeks with a fourth week that is patch-free. The patch releases the same types of hormones as the birth control pill and is just as effective.
- **Pros:** More regular, lighter periods with less cramping, no need to remember a daily pill.
- **Cons:** Cost, may cause skin irritation or other side effects similar to birth control pills. Does not protect against STDs.

Vaginal Ring

The NuvaRing is a soft plastic ring that is worn inside the vagina. The ring releases the same hormones as the pill and patch and is just as effective. But it only needs to be replaced once a month.
- **Pros:** Lighter, more regular periods, only replaced once per month.
- **Cons:** Cost, may cause vaginal irritation or other side effects similar to pills and the patch. Does not protect against STDs.

Birth Control Shot

The birth control shot, known as Depo-Provera, is a hormonal injection that protects against pregnancy for three months. For the typical couple, it is more effective than the birth control pill-only 3% of users get pregnant in a year.
- **Pros:** Only injected four times per year, highly effective.
- **Cons:** Cost, may cause spotting and other side effects. Does not protect against STDs.

Birth Control Implant

The birth control implant (Implanon) is a matchstick-sized rod that is placed under the skin of the upper arm. It releases the same hormone that's in the birth control shot, but the implant protects against pregnancy for 3 years. The failure rate is less than 1%.
- **Pros:** Lasts three years, highly effective.
- **Cons:** More expensive upfront, may cause side effects, including irregular bleeding. Does not protect against STDs.

IUD

IUD stands for intrauterine device, a T-shaped piece of plastic that is placed inside the uterus by a doctor. The copper IUD, ParaGard, works for as long as 12 years. The hormonal IUD, Mirena, must be replaced after 5 years. Both types make it more difficult for sperm to fertilize the egg. Fewer than eight in 1,000 women get pregnant.
- **Pros:** Long-lasting, low-maintenance.
- **Cons:** Irregular or heavier periods. More expensive upfront, may slip out, may cause side effects.

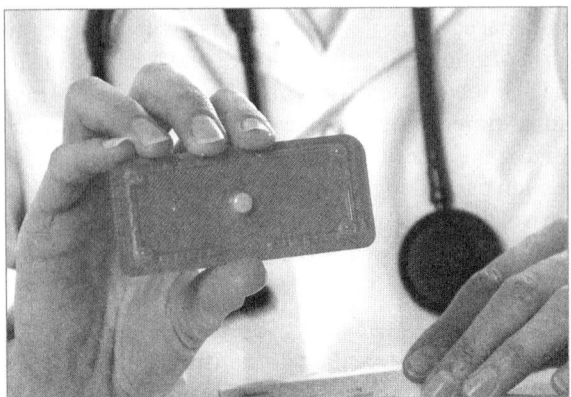

Fig. 16.12: Oral pill method of contraceptive.

Tubal Implant

A newer procedure makes it possible to block the fallopian tubes without surgery. Small implants of metal or silicone are placed inside each tube. Scar tissue eventually grows around the implants and blocks the tubes. Once an X-ray confirms the tubes are blocked, no other form of birth control is needed.
- **Pros:** Permanent, no surgery, almost 100% effective.
- **Cons:** Takes a few months to become effective. May raise the risk of pelvic infections, irreversible, expensive.

TERMINAL METHODS (TUBECTOMY, VASECTOMY)

Sterilization is the most effective, and one of the most widely used contraceptive methods available worldwide. It is often the best contraceptive choice when desired family size has been achieved. Both tubal ligation in women, and vasectomy in men, are one-time procedures that are safe, inexpensive and relatively straightforward to do for a trained person. Sterilization does not require constant use of a contraceptive method, regular visits to health facilities or repeated expenditure on contraceptive supplies. Although sterilization procedures usually demand a greater investment in skill, training and equipment than temporary methods of contraception, they provide lifelong protection against pregnancy, and are therefore more cost-effective.

Enumerate the Guidelines for Case Selection Fit for Sterilization

- Male clients should be at least 22 years old and ideally be below the age of 60 years.
- Female clients should be below the age of 49 years and above the age of 22 years.
- The couple should have at least one child whose age is above 1 year unless the sterilization is medically indicated.
- Clients or their spouses/partners must not have undergone sterilization in the past (not applicable in the cases of failure of previous sterilization).
- Clients must be in a sound state of mind so as to understand the full implications of sterilization.
- Mentally ill clients must be certified by a psychiatrist, and a statement should be given by the legal guardian/spouse regarding the soundness of the client's state of mind.
- A relevant medical history, physical examination and laboratory investigations need to be completed to ascertain eligibility for surgery.

Advantages of Terminal Methods of Sterilization

- Does not require sustained motivation.
- It is the most effective method of contraception.
- Low rate of complications if the surgery is correctly performed.
- Does not require any action at the time of intercourse.

Disadvantages of the Terminal Methods of Sterilization

- Need for a trained doctor for performing the surgery.
- Need for facilities for the surgery.
- Reversibility is difficult.
- Does not protect against STD/HIV.

Vasectomy (Male Sterilization)

Besides condoms, a vasectomy is the only birth control option available to men. It involves surgically closing the vas deferens—the tubes that carry sperm from the testes, through the reproductive system. This prevents the release of sperm but doesn't interfere with ejaculation. Terminal methods of sterilization for male is depicted in **Figure 16.13**.

Steps of the Procedure of Vasectomy

- Vas is clamped at two points.
- A piece of approximately 1 cm is resected from the segment between the two clamps.
- The cut ends are ligated.
- The ends are folded onto themselves and sutured in that position.
- The removed section is gently squeezed onto a glass slide, stained with Wright's stain, and examined under the microscope to confirm that the removed part is the Vas only and not any other structure.

Postoperative Advice to be Given after Vasectomy

Warn the client that he is not immediately rendered sterile after vasectomy.
- He should use another method of contraception till azoospermia is established. This takes approximately 30 ejaculations.
- Avoid bathing for next 24 hours at least.

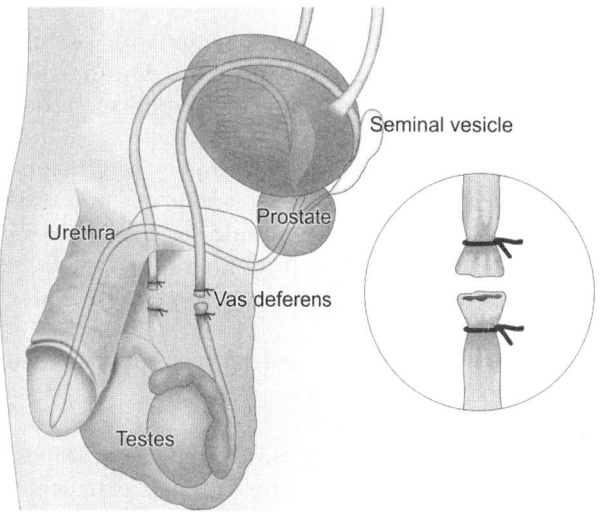

Fig. 16.13: Terminal methods of sterilization for male.

- He should wear a T-bandage or scrotal support (Langot) for 15 days after surgery. This bandage should be kept clean and dry.
- Avoid cycling and lifting heavy weight for next 15 days.
- To report back for stitch removal on the 5th postoperative day.
- The client should be warned that there is a small possibility of recanalization of the vas, which may result in failure of contraception. His written consent should include the acknowledgement of having received this information.
- He should report for semen analysis after 3 months.

Failure Rate of Vasectomy

Failure rate for vasectomy: 0.15 pregnancies per HWY
Mention some causes of failure of vasectomy.
- Mistaken identity of the vas at the time of surgery
- Spontaneous recanalization of the vas
- Occurrence of more than one vas on one side
- Sexual intercourse before total disappearance of sperms from the reproductive tract

Complications of Vasectomy

Early Postoperative
- Pain
- Scrotal hematoma
- Local infection

Late Postoperative
- Sperm granules
- Spontaneous recanalization

Psychological
- Decreased sexual performance
- Impotence
- Fatigue
- Headache

Contraindications to Male Sterilization Surgery

There are no absolute contraindications for performing vasectomy. However, there are certain relative contraindications where one needs to apply the criteria of 'caution', 'delay' or 'special'.

Caution: The procedure is normally conducted in a routine setting, but with extra preparation and precautions.
- Young age—young men should be counseled about the permanency of sterilization and the availability of alternative, long-term and highly effective methods
- Depressive disorders
- Diabetes mellitus—increased risk of postoperative wound infections
- Previous scrotal injury
- Large varicocele—the vas may be difficult or impossible to locate; a single procedure to repair varicocele and perform a vasectomy is advocated
- Large hydrocele—the vas may be difficult or impossible to locate; a single procedure to repair hydrocele and perform a vasectomy is advocated
- Cryptorchidism—if unilateral; if bilateral along with demonstrated fertility the surgery will be more complicated and will be assigned to 'special' category.

Advantages
- Permanent birth control
- Requires no daily attention
- Does not affect sexual pleasure
- Less complicated than female sterilization.

Disadvantages
- Not immediately effective
- Requires minor surgery in a hospital
- May not be reversible
- Possible regret
- Possible rejoining of the vas deferens.
- Does not protect against STIs, including HIV/AIDS.

Tubal Ligation

The traditional method for women is called tubal ligation or "having your tubes tied." A surgeon closes off the fallopian tubes, preventing eggs from making their journey out of the ovaries. Terminal methods of sterilization for female is depicted in **Figure 16.14**.

Procedure

Tubal ligation (TL) is a surgical sterilization technique for women, where the fallopian tubes are cut, or blocked with rings, bands or clips. This procedure closes the fallopian tubes, and stops the egg from travelling to the fallopian tubes where fertilization takes place. It also prevents sperm from travelling up the fallopian tube to fertilize an egg. Sterilization is effective immediately after the procedure. Tubal ligations are 99.5% effective as a birth control method.

Advantages
- Permanent birth control
- Immediately effective
- Requires no daily attention

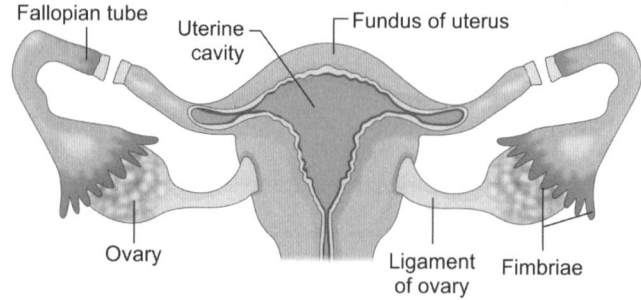
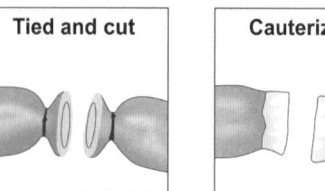
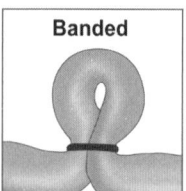

Fig. 16.14: Terminal methods of sterilization for female.

- Cost-effective in the long term
- Does not affect sexual pleasure.

Disadvantages
- Requires surgery and has risks associated with surgery
- More complicated than male sterilization
- May not be reversible, resulting in possible regret
- Does not protect against sexually-transmitted infections (STIs), including HIV/AIDS.

Emergency Contraception

Emergency contraception refers to methods of contraception that can be used to prevent pregnancy after sexual intercourse. These are recommended for use within 5 days but are more effective the sooner they are used after the act of intercourse.

Key Facts
- Emergency contraception (EC) can prevent up to over 95% of pregnancies when taken within 5 days after intercourse.
- EC can be used in the following situations: unprotected intercourse, concerns about possible contraceptive failure, incorrect use of contraceptives, and sexual assault if without contraception coverage.
- Methods of emergency contraception are the copper-bearing intrauterine devices (IUDs) and the emergency contraceptive pills (ECPs).
- A copper-bearing IUD is the most effective form of emergency contraception available.
- The emergency contraceptive pill regimens recommended by WHO are ulipristal acetate, levonorgestrel, or combined oral contraceptives (COCs) consisting of ethinyl estradiol plus levonorgestrel.

Mode of Action
- Emergency contraceptive pills prevent pregnancy by preventing or delaying ovulation and they do not induce an abortion.
- The copper-bearing IUD prevents fertilization by causing a chemical change in sperm and egg before they meet.
- Emergency contraception cannot interrupt an established pregnancy or harm a developing embryo.

Who Can Use Emergency Contraception?
- Any woman or girl of reproductive age may need emergency contraception to avoid an unwanted pregnancy.
- There are no absolute medical contraindications to the use of emergency contraception.
- There are no age limits for the use of emergency contraception.
- Eligibility criteria for general use of a copper IUD also apply for use of a copper IUD for emergency purposes.

Situation

Emergency contraception can be used in a number of situations following sexual intercourse. These include:
- When no contraceptive has been used.
- Sexual assault when the woman was not protected by an effective contraceptive method.
- When there is concern of possible contraceptive failure, from improper or incorrect use, such as:
  - Condom breakage, slippage, or incorrect use;
  - 3 or more consecutively missed combined oral contraceptive pills;
  - More than 3 hours late from the usual time of intake of the progestogen-only pill (minipill), or more than 27 hours after the previous pill;
  - More than 12 hours late from the usual time of intake of the desogestrel-containing pill (0.75 mg) or more than 36 hours after the previous pill;
  - More than 2 weeks late for the norethisterone enanthate (NET-EN) progestogen-only injection;
  - More than 4 weeks late for the depot-medroxyprogesterone acetate (DMPA) progestogen-only injection;
  - More than 7 days late for the combined injectable contraceptive (CIC);
  - Dislodgment, breakage, tearing, or early removal of a diaphragm or cervical cap;
  - Failed withdrawal (e.g. ejaculation in the vagina or on external genitalia);
  - Failure of a spermicide tablet or film to melt before intercourse;
  - Miscalculation of the abstinence period, or failure to abstain or use a barrier method on the fertile days of the cycle when using fertility awareness based methods; or
  - Expulsion of an intrauterine contraceptive device (IUD) or hormonal contraceptive implant.

COUNSELING IN REPRODUCTIVE, SEXUAL HEALTH INCLUDING PROBLEMS OF ADOLESCENTS

Counseling is a skilled process which enables clients to explore concerns, difficulties and problematic areas. Counseling provides the opportunity to share thoughts and feelings, concerns, difficulties and problematic areas with a qualified professional. Clients are respected for who they are, with unconditional, positive regard and acceptance in a non-judgmental environment.

Purposes of Counseling

The purpose of counseling young people on reproductive health issues is to help them to:
- Make rational decisions
- Cope with their existing situation.

The more a young person can be made comfortable, the more likely they are to express their sexual and reproductive health problems. This enables you to effectively counsel and serve them so that they can achieve control over their own behavior, understand them, anticipate the consequences of their actions, and making long-term plans. In counseling there are two actors: you the counselor and the young person.

The behavior as well as the characteristics of the young person can affect the counseling process.

Counseling is a person-to-person, two-way communication during which you:
- Provide adequate information to help the young person make an informed decision.
- Help the young person evaluate their feelings and opinions regarding the problem for which help was sought.
- Act as emotional support for them.

Counseling is not:
- A method of providing solutions to the young person's problems
- A method of giving instructions
- The promotion of a life plan that has been successful for you.

Roles

R = Relax the client by using facial expressions that show interest
O = Open up the client by using a warm and caring tone of voice, i.e. help them to talk
L = Lean towards the client, not away from them
E = Establish and maintain eye contact with the client
S = Smile.

Counseling for Approaches

- Be genuinely open to their questions or needs for information
- Avoid judgmental words or body language that suggests disapproval of the young person or their questions and needs
- Understand that the young person has various feelings of discomfort and uncertainty. Be reassuring in responding to the young person, making them feel more comfortable and confident
- Demonstrate sincerity and willingness to help
- Reinforce their decision to seek counseling and/or healthcare; do not give them the impression that you think their visit was unnecessary
- Exhibit honesty and forthrightness, including an ability to admit when you do not know the answer
- Demonstrate responsibility in fulfilling your professional role
- Exhibit confidence and professional competence in addressing adolescent and youth reproductive health issues.

Behavior Likely to Promote Trust: Practical Arrangements

Here are some practical tips to create a good, friendly first impression.
- Start on time.
- Smile and warmly greet the client.
- Introduce yourself and explain what you do.

It will help to establish rapport during the first session if you:

- Face the young person, sitting in similar chairs
- Use the young person's name during the session
- Begin the session by allowing the young person to talk freely before you ask questions
- Congratulate the young person for seeking help.

Counseling Challenges

- Silence
- Crying
- Threat of suicide
- Need to talk.

Need for Counseling Adolescents

Adolescence is a phase during which tremendous physical and psychological changes occur, along with changes in social perceptions and expectations. Some of the public health challenges for adolescents include pregnancy, excess risk of maternal and infant mortality, sexually transmitted infections and reproductive tract infections, and the rapidly rising incidence of HIV in this age group. Thus, it is important to influence the health-seeking behavior of adolescents as their situation will be central in determining India's health, mortality and morbidity; and the population growth scenario. Investment in adolescent reproductive and sexual health will positively influence maternal mortality rate, infant mortality rate reducing incidence of teenage pregnancy, meeting unmet contraceptive needs, reducing the incidence of sexually transmitted infections (STIs) and reducing the proportion of HIV positive cases.

MEDICAL TERMINATION OF PREGNANCY AND MTP ACT

- The medical termination of pregnancy Act was passed by the Indian Parliament in 1971 and came into force from April 1, 1972.
- The medical termination of pregnancy Act was passed by the measure which helps to reduce maternal morbidity and mortality resulting from illegal abortions (**Fig. 16.15**).

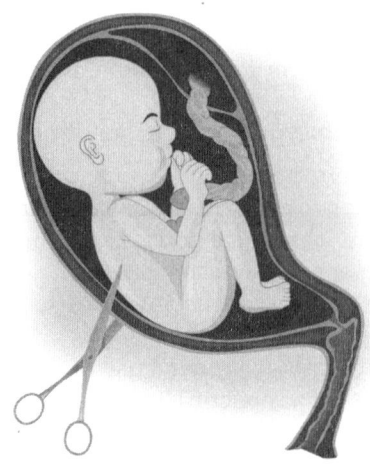

Fig. 16.15: Medical termination of pregnancy.

Reason for MTP

- **Medical:** Where the continuation of the pregnancy might endanger the mother's life or cause grave injury to her physical or mental health.
- **Eugene:** Where there is substantial risk of the child being born with serious handicaps due to physical or mental abnormalities.
- **Humanitarian:** Where pregnancy is the result of rape.
- **Socioeconomic:** If there is any risk of injury to the health of mother or any foreseeable environments.
- **Failure of contraceptive devices:** Unwanted pregnancy resulting from a failure of IUD or oral pills.

Proposed Features of the Bill

- The bill seeks to amend medical termination of pregnancy (MTP) Act 1971
- The Bill proposes the requirement of the opinion of **one** registered medical practitioner (instead of two or more) for termination of pregnancy up to 20 weeks of gestation (fetal development period from the time of conception until birth).
- It introduces the requirement of the opinion of two registered medical practitioners for termination of pregnancy of 20–24 weeks of gestation.
- It has also enhanced the gestation limit for 'special categories' of women which includes survivors of rape, victims of incest and other vulnerable women like differently-abled women and minors.
- It also states that the "name and other particulars of a woman whose pregnancy has been terminated shall not be revealed", except to a person authorized in any law that is currently in force.

Medical Termination of Pregnancy (Amendment) Bill, 2020

Recently, the Union Cabinet has approved the Medical Termination of Pregnancy (MTP) (Amendment) Bill, 2020. The Bill seeks to extend the termination of pregnancy period from 20 weeks to 24 weeks, making it easier for women to safely and legally terminate an unwanted pregnancy (**Fig. 16.16**).

The Medical Termination of Pregnancy (Amendment) Bill, 2020 was introduced in Lok Sabha by the Minister of Health and Family Welfare, Dr. Harsh Vardhan on March 2, 2020. The Bill amends the Medical Termination of Pregnancy Act, 1971 which provides for the termination of certain pregnancies by registered medical practitioners. The Bill adds the definition of termination of pregnancy to mean a procedure undertaken to terminate a pregnancy by using medical or surgical methods.

Termination of pregnancy: Under the Act, a pregnancy may be terminated within 12 weeks, if a registered medical practitioner is of the opinion that:

- Continuation of the pregnancy may risk the life of the mother, or cause grave injury to her health, or
- There is a substantial risk that the child, if born, would suffer physical or mental abnormalities. For termination of a pregnancy between 12 to 20 weeks, two medical practitioners are required to give their opinion.

Bill Amends

- The Bill amends this provision to state that a pregnancy may be terminated within 20 weeks, with the opinion of a registered medical practitioner.
- Approval of two registered medical practitioners will be required for termination of pregnancies between 20 to 24 weeks.
- The termination of pregnancies up to 24 weeks will only apply to specific categories of women, as may be prescribed by the central government.
- Further, the central government will notify the norms for the medical practitioner whose opinion is required for termination of the pregnancy.
- Under the Act, if any pregnancy occurs as a result of failure of any device or method used by a married woman or her husband to limit the number of children, such an unwanted pregnancy may constitute a grave injury to the mental health of the pregnant woman.

MTP Act 1971	MTP amendment bill 2020
One registered and recognized medical practitioner in opinion to terminate the pregnancy along with the consent of the mother is required to terminate the pregnancy **till 12th week**	One registered and recognized medical practitioner in opinion to terminate the pregnancy along with the consent of the mother is required to terminate the pregnancy **till 20th week**
Two or more registered and recognized medical practitioner in opinion to terminate the pregnancy along with the consent of the mother is required to terminate the pregnancy **12th to 20th week** (in case of vulnerable women)	Two or more registered and recognized medical practitioner in opinion to terminate the pregnancy along with the consent of the mother is required to terminate the pregnancy **20th to 24th week** (in case of vulnerable women)
It does not mention clearly about the confidentiality and privacy of the women and the case	This amendment emphasizes to **protect the women's privacy and confidentiality** of the data related to termination of pregnancy

Fig. 16.16: MTP amendments.

- The Bill amends this provision to replace 'married woman or her husband' with 'woman or her partner'.

Constitution of a Medical Board

The Bill states that the upper limit of termination of pregnancy will not apply in cases where such termination is necessary due to the diagnosis of substantial fetal abnormalities. These abnormalities will be diagnosed by a Medical Board. Under the Bill, every state government is required to constitute a Medical Board. These Medical Boards will consist of the following members: (i) a gynecologist, (ii) a pediatrician, (iii) a radiologist or sonologist, and (iv) any other number of members, as may be notified by the state government. Note that, the central government will notify the powers and functions of these Medical Boards.

Protection of Privacy of a Woman

The Bill states that no registered medical practitioner will be allowed to reveal the name and other particulars of a woman whose pregnancy has been terminated, except to a person authorized by any law. Anyone who contravenes this provision will be punishable with imprisonment of up to one year, or with a fine, or both.

NATIONAL FAMILY WELFARE PROGRAMME

India launched the National Family Welfare Programme in 1951 with the objective of "reducing the birth rate to the extent necessary to stabilize the population at a level consistent with the requirement of the National economy. The Family Welfare Program in India is recognized as a priority area, and is being implemented as a 100% centrally sponsored program **(Fig. 16.17)**.

Family welfare programs include:
- Family planning information, counseling and services to women for healthy reproduction.
- Education about safe delivery and post-delivery of the mother and the baby and the treatment of women before pregnancy.
- Healthcare for infant's immunization against preventable diseases.
- Prevention and treatment of sexually and Reproductive Tract infection.

History

- It was started in the year 1951.
- In 1977, the Government of India redesignated the "national family planning program" as the "national family welfare program", and also changed the name of the ministry of health and family planning to ministry of health and family welfare.
- It is a reflection of the government's anxiety to promote family planning through the total welfare of the family.
- It is aimed at achieving a higher end, i.e., to improve the quality of life of the people.
- India is the first country in the world that implemented the family welfare program at government level.
- Health is a part of concurrent list but center provides 100% assistance to states for this program.
- Government has concentrated on this program in various five-year plans though higher priority was accorded to it after 4th five year plan.
- Due to bad effects of emergency and faulty propaganda, family planning suffered major setback, during 1977–1979.
- It was decided in national health policy 1983, that net reproduction rate (NRR) should be 1 by the year 2000.
- The 7th five year plan placed more emphasis on the use of spacing methods between the births of two children.
- Family welfare program has been remained the important aspects of each five year plan, national health.

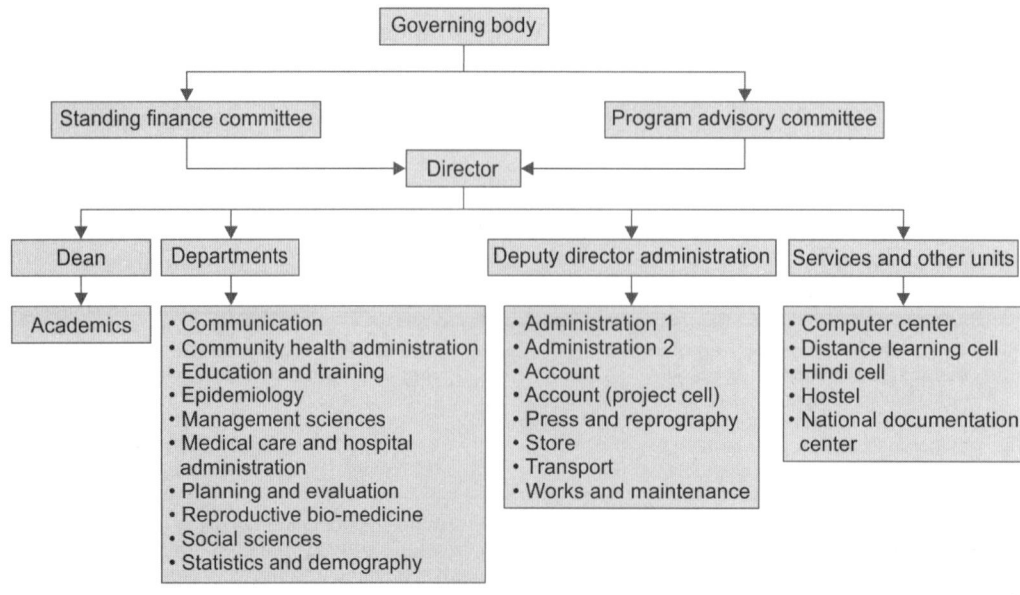

Fig. 16.17: Family welfare program organizing committee.

Early Development

- The second five year plan (1956 to 1961) the "clinic approach" was adopted. Large no-of family planning clinic were opened.
- The 3rd year plan (1961 to 1966) emphatic recognition was given to family planning.
- In 1960 the NFWP entered a new technological era with introduction of the Lippi's loop later replaced by copper T.

Later Development

- Target bound program.
- IUD insertion at the rate of 20/1,000 urban and 10/1,000 rural.
- Integration with maternal and child welfare, immunization, nutrition and non formal education.
- Medical termination of Pregnancy Act.

Objective: To destabilize the population at the level of some 130 million by the year 2050 AD through small family norms.

Aim: To achieve a higher end that is to improve the quality of the life of the people.

Vision and Mission

Vision: NIHFW is to be seen as an Institute of global repute in public health and family welfare management.

Mission: To act as think tank, catalyst and innovator for management of public health and related health and family welfare programs by pursuing multiple functions of education and training, research and evaluation, consultancy and advisory services as well as provision of specialized services through inter-disciplinary teams.

Organization Chart

Goals of the Family Welfare Programme

- Reduction of birth rate from 29 per 1000 (in 1992) to 21 by 2000 AD.
- Reduction of death rate from 10 (in 1992) to 9 per 1000.
- Raising couple protection rate from 43.3 (in 1990) to 60%.
- Reduction in average family size from 4.2 (in 1990) to 2.3.
- Decrease in infant mortality rate from 79 (in 1992) to less than 60 per 1,000 live births.
- Reduction of net reproduction rate from 1.48 (in 1981) to 1.

Impact of Family Welfare Activities

- Nearly 98% of women and 99% of men in the age group of 15 and 49 have a good knowledge about one or more methods of contraception. Adolescents seem to be well aware of the modern methods of contraception.
- Over 97% of women and 95% of men are knowledgeable about female sterilization, which is the most popular modern permanent method of family planning. While only 79% of women and 80% of men have heard about male sterilization.
- 93% of men have awareness about the usage of condoms while only 74% of women are aware of the same.
- Around 80% of men and women have a fair knowledge about contraceptive pills.

Importance of Family Welfare Programme

- The year 2010–11 ended with 34.9 million family planning acceptors at national level comprising of 5.0 million Sterilizations, 5.6 million IUD insertions, 16.0 million condom users and 8.3 million O.P (oral pills). users as against 35.6 million family planning acceptors in 2009–10.
- Over the decades, there has been a substantial increase in contraceptive use in India.
- IUD Insertions: During the year 2010–11, 5.6 million IUD insertions were reported as against 5.7 million in 2009–10. Assam, Bihar, Gujarat, Jharkhand, Uttar Pradesh, Arunachal Pradesh, Delhi, Goa, Meghalaya, Mizoram, Sikkim, D and N Haveli reported better performance in 2010–11.
- Condom Users and O.P. (Oral Pills) Users: Based on the distribution figures reported, there were 16.0 million equivalent users of Condoms and 83.07 million equivalent users of Oral Pills during 2010–11.
- Number of Births Prevented: Implementation of various Family Planning measures prevented 16.335 million births in the country during 2010–11 as compared to 16.605 million in 2009–10. The cumulative total of births avoided in the country up to 2010–11 was 442.75 million.

Strategies of Family Welfare Program (FWP)

- **Integration with health services:** Family welfare program (FWP) has been integrated with other health services instead of being a separate service.
- **Integration with maternity and child health:** FWP has been integrated with maternity and child health (MCH). Public are motivated for postdelivery sterilization, abortion and use of contraceptives.
- **Concentration in rural areas:** FWP are concentrated more in rural areas at the level of subentries and primary health centers. This is in addition to hospitals at district, state and central levels.
- **Literacy:** There is a direct correlation between illiteracy and fertility. So stress and priority is given for girl's education. Fertility rate among educated females is low.
- **Breastfeeding:** Breastfeeding is encouraged. It is estimated that about 5 million births per annum can be prevented through breastfeeding.
- **Raising the age for marriage:** Under the child marriage restraint bill (1978), the age of marriage has been raised to 21 years for males and 18 years for females. This has some impact on fertility
- **Minimum needs program:** It was launched in the Fifth Five Year Plan with an aim to raise the economical standards. Fertility is low in higher income groups. So fertility rate can be lowered by increasing economical standards.

- **Incentives:** Monetary incentives have been given in family planning programs, especially for poor classes. But these incentives have not been very effective. So the program must be on voluntary basis.
- **Mass media:** Motivation through radio, television, cinemas, news papers, puppet shows and folk dances is an important aspect of this program.

Components of National Family Welfare Programme

- **Administration and organization:** This includes appointing the employee and arranging the resources.
- **Training:** Training the medical, nursing and paramedical staff.
- **Social and health education.**
- **Supplies and services:**
  - The scope of activities carried out under family welfare program.
  - Mother and child health
  - Small family norm
  - School health.

Program Conducted by National Family Welfare Programme

- The universal immunization program aimed at reduction in mortality and morbidity among infants and younger children due to vaccine preventable disease was started in 1985–86.
- The oral rehydration therapy was also started in view of the fact that diarrhea was a leading cause of death among children.
- The other various programs under MCH were also implemented during the seventh five year plan.
- Child survival and safe other motherhood program (CSSM) in 1992–8th five year plan.
- Reproductive and child health program (RCH) in 9th five year plan.

Objectives of the Above Programs

- The program was convergent and aimed at improving the health of the mother and young children.
- To improve the facilities for prevention and treatment of major diseases.
- The separate identity for each program was causing problem in its effective managements and somewhat reducing the outcomes.
- The population of the country should be stabilized at the level of consistent with the equipment of national development.

Main Objectives of NFWP

- Reduction in population growth rate.
- To assess need for reproductive and child health at PHC level.
- To provide need based demand high quality integrated reproductive child healthcare.
- Reducing infant and maternal morbidity and mortality rate.

Family Planning Programme: Under the Family Planning Programme services like sterilization, IUCD, Oral pills and supply of Nirodh are made available to eligible couples on a cafeteria approach. The aim is to achieve 60% couple protection rate, birth rate of 21 and net reproductive rate of one. The Family Planning Program is implemented all over India.

Immunization against vaccine preventable diseases Under the immunization activities, coverage of children against killer disease like Polio. Diphteria, Pertussis, Tetanus, Tuberculosis and Measles are undertaken through routine immunization program. The program also aims at immunizing 100% pregnant women against tetanus.

Medical Termination of Pregnancy Act: Medical Termination of Pregnancy Act was introduced in 1971 in order to improve health of mother and as a first resort to avoid unwanted pregnancies.

RCH

The reproductive and child health program was formally launched by Government of India on 15th October 1997. As per recommendation of International Conference on Population and development held in Cario in 1994.

- In ICPD at Cairo, fathallah defined RCH as "A state of complete, physical, mental, and social well-being and merely the absence of disease or infirmity in all matters relating to reproductive system and its function and process."
- "A state in which people have the ability to reproduce and regulate their fertility are able to go through pregnancy and child birth, the outcome of pregnancy is successful in terms of maternal and infant survival and well-being, and couples are able to have sexual relation free of the fear of pregnancy and of contracting diseases."

Objectives

- To promote the health of the mothers and children to ensure safe motherhood and child survival.
- The intermediate objective is to reduce IMR and MMR.
- The ultimate objective is population stabilization, through responsible reproductive behavior.

Components of RCH

Following services are included in the reproductive health area as proposed by Government of India.

Main Components

- Family planning.
- Child survival and safe motherhood program.
- Prevention/management of RTI/STD AND AIDS.
- Client approach to healthcare.
- Providing counseling, information and communication services on health, sexuality and gender difference.
- Referral services for all above intervention.
- Growth monitoring, nutrition education, reproductive health services for adolescents, etc.

Other Activities

- **For maternal services (safe motherhood):** The service components are obstetric care, infection control and nutrition promotion.
- **For child services (child survival):** The essential care of the newborn, including care of the at risk newborn by prompt referral service: Infection control measures. Nutritional Promotions. RCH package for various services.
- **Reproductive health:** Fertility control-MTP services (for prevention and management of unwanted Pregnancies. Adolescent-HIV/AIDS.

Under the RCH Program Phase-1, various provisions were made to improve the status of maternal and child health.

These include:
- Provision of essential and emergency and essential care.
- Provision of equipment and drug kits to selected PHCs and selected FRUs in all districts.
- Provision for additional ANM, Staff nurse, and Laboratory technicians for selected districts.
- Provision for 24 hours delivery services at PHCs and CHCs.
- Referral transport in case of obstetric complication.
- Immunization and oral rehydration therapy.
- Prevention and control of vitamin A deficiency in children.
- Integrated management of childhood illness (IMCI).
- District surveys for focused intervention to reduce IMR and MMR.
- New initiative undertaken during phase 1 of RCH is: Setting up of blood storage units at FRUs.

Training of MBBS doctors in anesthetic skills for emergency obstetric care at FRU. They were as follows:
- The outreach services were not available to the vulnerable and needy population.
- The management of financial resources was inadequate.
- The human resources such as doctors, nurse, health worker, etc. were deficient.
- The management information and evaluation system was lacking.
- The effective network of first referral units was lacking.
- Quality of services in PHCs and CHCs was poor.
- Lack of community participation.

ROLE OF A NURSE IN FAMILY WELFARE PROGRAM

The main role of a nurse is to assist the doctor in various types of surgeries. According to the three tier constitution of health centers in India, in the primary centers—the nurses act as the primary guide for different types of treatment. There are certain types of nurses which are known as assistant nurse midwifery or ANM nurse who does simple type of obstetric care and referral services in subcenters. The nurses are the first line of Healthcare provider in the rural areas **(Fig. 16.18)**. Community health nurse has a vast role to play in family welfare services.
- Survey work.
- Collecting demographic facts.
- Making list of homes and finding out housing location.
- Collecting information about pregnant mothers, eligible couples, infants and children below the school going.

Survey Work
- Collecting demographic facts.
- Making list of homes and finding out housing location.
- Collecting information about pregnant mother, eligible couples, and infants.

Educational Functions and Motivation
- Explaining the importance and necessity of family planning to masses.

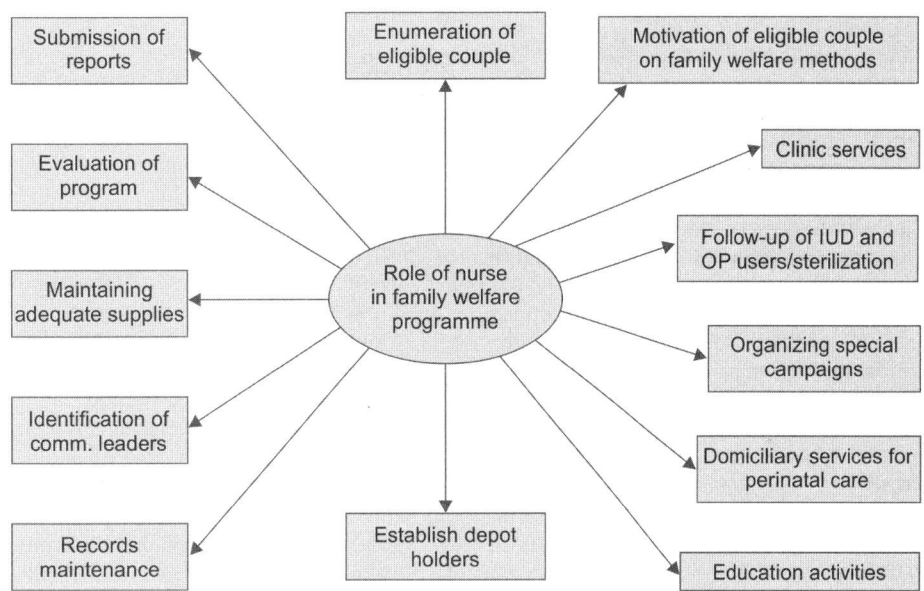

Fig. 16.18: Role of nurse in family welfare program.

- Using various techniques of teaching and communication to propagate the message of family planning to common man.
- Motivating the eligible couple to use contraceptives and educating them about its uses.
- Motivating people for family planning operation or permanent contraception.

Managerial Functions

- Conducting clinics.
- Deciding the date and place of clinics.
- Arranging equipment and other resources at clinics.
- Arrangements and distribution of contraceptives.
- Insertion and removal of IUDs.

Organizing Family Planning Camps

- Arranging family planning operations (sterilization male/female) through special camps.
- Making arrangements at the camps and following aseptic techniques.
- Motivating eligible couples and preparing them for the operation.
- Assisting the doctor in operation.

Maintaining the Records

- Keeping the eligible couple register update.
- Maintaining the register of sterilization cases, contraceptives users, and pregnant mothers.
- Maintaining other records related to family planning.

Liaison work: Soliciting the cooperation of NGOs/voluntary organization.

BIBLIOGRAPHY

1. Boivin J, Bunting L, Collins JA, et al. International estimates of infertility prevalence and treatment-seeking: potential need and demand for infertility medical care. Human reproduction (Oxford, England) 2007;22(6):1506–12. doi: 10.1093/humrep/dem046 [published Online First: 2007/03/23]
2. Cheng D, Schwarz E, Douglas E, et al. Unintended pregnancy and associated maternal preconception, prenatal and postpartum behaviors. Contraception. 2009; 79(3):194–8.
3. D'Angelo D, Gilbert BC, Rochat R, et al. Differences between mistimed and unwanted pregnancies among women who have live births. Perspect Sex Reprod Health. 2004;36(5):192–7.
4. Gavin L, Moskosky S, Carter M, et al. Providing quality family planning services: recommendations of CDC and the US Office of Population Affairs. MMWR Recomm Rep. 2014;63 (No. RR-04).
5. Gipson J, Koenig M, Hindin M. The effects of unintended pregnancy on infant, child and parental health: A review of the literature. Studies in Family Planning. 2008;39(1):18–38.
6. Gore AC, Chappell VA, Fenton SE, et al. EDC-2: The Endocrine Society's Second Scientific Statement on Endocrine-Disrupting Chemicals. Endocrine Reviews 2015; 36(6):E1-E150. doi: 10.1210/er.2015-1010
7. Government of India, November 2014. Reference Manual for Female Sterilization, Family Planning Division, Ministry of Health and Family Welfare, New Delhi.
8. Government of India, October 2013. Reference Manual for Male Sterilization, Family Planning Division, Ministry of Health and Family Welfare, New Delhi.
9. Kost K, Landry D, Darroch J. Predicting maternal behaviors during pregnancy: Does intention status matter? Fam Plann Perspect. 1998;30(2):79–88.
10. Mascarenhas MN, Flaxman SR, Boerma T, et al. National, regional, and global trends in infertility prevalence since 1990: A systematic analysis of 277 health surveys. PLoS Med 2012;9(12):e1001356. doi: 10.1371/journal.pmed.1001356 [published Online First: 2012/12/29]
11. Park K. Demography and family planning. In: Park K. Park's Textbook of Preventive and Social Medicine, 24th edition. Jabalpur, India: Banarsidas Bhanot Publishers, 2017; pp. 525–52.
12. Rutstein SO, Shah IH. Infecundity infertility and childlessness in developing countries. Geneva: World Health Organization 2004.
13. Segal TR, Giudice LC. Before the beginning: environmental exposures and reproductive and obstetrical outcomes. Fertility and Sterility 2019;112(4):613–21.
14. Sonfield A, Hasstedt K, Gold RB. Moving Forward: Family Planning in the Era of Health Reform, New York: Guttmacher Institute, 2014.
15. World Health Organization (WHO). International Classification of Diseases, 11th Revision (ICD-11) Geneva: WHO 2018.
16. Zegers-Hochschild F, Dickens BM, Dughman-Manzur S. Human rights to in vitro fertilization. International Journal of Gynecology and Obstetrics 2013;123(1):86–89.

REVIEW QUESTIONS

Long Essays

1. Define demography. Explain the uses and importance of demography.
2. Define demographic cycle. Describe the stages of demographic cycle
3. Define family planning. Explain the objectives and importance of family planning in India.
4. Describe the types of family planning methods.
5. Define family planning programme. Explain the objectives and history of family planning in India.
6. Describe counseling in reproductive, sexual health including problems of adolescents.

Short Essays

1. Scope of demography.
2. World population trends.
3. Concept of fertility and infertility.
4. Small family norm.
5. Effects of family size.
6. Hazards of large and unplanned family.
7. Advantages of adopting small family norm.
8. Scope of family planning services.
9. Advantages of family planning.
10. Importance of family planning in india.
11. Natural methods of space methods.
12. Biological, chemical and mechanical methods.
13. Medical termination of pregnancy and MTP ACT.
14. National Family Welfare Program.
15. Strategies of Family Welfare Program (FWP).
16. Importance of Family Welfare Programme.
17. Role of a nurse in family welfare program.

Chapter 16: Demography and Family Welfare

Short Answers
1. Demographic factors.
2. Demographic trends.
3. Infertility.
4. Causes of infertility.
5. Factors involve small family.
6. Benefits of family planning/contraception.
7. Intrauterine devices.
8. Emergency contraception.
9. Health aspects of family planning.
10. Benefits of using family planning.
11. Birth control pills.
12. Calendar or rhythm method.
13. Cervical mucus method.
14. Lactational amenorrhea method.
15. Cervical cap.
16. Benefits of condom.
17. Vaginal ring.
18. Tubal implant.
19. Components of National Family Welfare Programme.

Multiple Choice Questions
1. Demography includes study of:
    a. Fertility
    b. Mortality
    c. Social morbidity
    d. All of the above.
2. Which of the following is not a copper-releasing IUD?
    a. LNG 20
    b. CuT
    c. Lippes Loop
    d. a and c
3. Which of the following is not the characteristic of an ideal contraceptive?
    a. Irreversible
    b. Easily available
    c. User-friendly
    d. Effective with least side effects
4. What is the expansion for MTP?
    a. Medical Termination of Parturition
    b. Mechanical Transfer of Pollen
    c. Medical Termination of Pregnancy
    d. Maternally Transmitted Pathogens
5. Amniocentesis is a process used to:
    a. Grow cells on culture media
    b. Know about brain disease
    c. Determine mutations
    d. Determine a disease of the embryo
6. The function of Copper-T is:
    a. Stop gastrulation
    b. Stop cleavage
    c. Check mutation
    d. Stop fertilization
7. By which name is family planning currently known?
    a. Reproductive and child care
    b. Family and child care
    c. Reproductive and child health
    d. Reproductive and child health care
8. What problems in reproductive health care require a doctor's help?
    a. STDs
    b. Conception, parturition and abortion
    c. Contraception, infertility, menstruation problem
    d. All
9. In the IVF technique zygote or early embryo is transferred into:
    a. Cervical canal
    b. Uterus
    c. Fallopian tube
    d. Vagina
10. The programs to get total reproductive health as a social goal at the national level are called:
    a. Family organization
    b. Family planning
    c. Family care
    d. Reproductive care
11. Test tube baby implies which of the following techniques?
    a. IUI
    b. ICSI
    c. GIFT
    d. ZIFT
12. Which technique is used to detect AIDS?
    a. Northern blot and ELISA
    b. Immunoblot and ELISA
    c. Western blot and ELISA
    d. Southern blot and ELISA.

ANSWERS

1. d	2. d	3. a	4. c	5. d	6. d	7. d	8. d	9. c	10. b	11. d	12. c

Health Team

LEARNING OBJECTIVES

Health Team
1. Concept
2. Composition
3. Functions

Role of nursing personnel at various levels
4. District public health nursing officer
5. Block health nurse
6. Public health nurse
7. Lady health visitor/health supervisor
8. Health worker female/ANM

INTRODUCTION

Health workers including community health nurse who can also involve personnel from these sectors at community level to promote health activities, e.g., agricultural workers can promote production of appropriate foodstuff and their consumption by families; teachers in schools can promote good sanitation, encourage healthful behavior in students, conduct courses on nutrition and first aid; mass media personnel can popularize various primary healthcare services by disseminating authentic in different communities, etc. Evidence-based practice (EBP) entails making decisions about how to promote health or provide care by integrating the best available evidence with practitioner expertise and other resources, and with the characteristics, state, needs, values and preferences of those who will be affected. This is done in a manner that is compatible with the environmental and organizational context. Evidence is comprised of research findings derived from the systematic collection of data through observation and experiment and the formulation of questions and testing of hypotheses.

DEFINITIONS

- A health team is a group of persons who work together to promote better health in the community.
- The health team members function according to the rules laid down by the Ministry of Health and Family Welfare, Government of India in consonance with their policies.
- A team is defined as group of persons with different levels of knowledge, abilities and personalities who must complement each other and who share a common goal.
- A team of health personnel together can provide better health services than when they are functioning alone.

BUILDING UP OF A TEAM

Effective team does not just happen. Team is formed based on tasks. Team building requires specific knowledge, skill and work. The following are the steps of team building:

- **Select team members:** Ability to contribute to the work of the team (task) and to work as a member of a team (relationship), is an important consideration for selection of team members.
- **Set goals:** The purposes and objectives or goals of the team should be clearly stated.
- **Define roles:** The role of individual team members should be clearly defined. Ambiguity in the individual's roles can cause conflicts among team members. These conflicts can immobilize the team and even contribute to its demise.
- **Develop team identity and cohesiveness:** The team members should know about their team and its functions. The more the team members know about their team and its functions the more they can identify and affiliate themselves with the team.
  - The team needs an ideal place to meet especially, one that is sufficiently quite comfortable and private so that team matters can be discussed freely. The team also needs to acquire functional and psychological spheres in the organization or community within which it functions. Other healthcare providers must also recognize and accept the function and purpose of the team.
  - The team members should meet at regular intervals or whenever required. The members should share their experiences with each other.
  - The team leader should ask other team members to offer help when someone in the team needs help in solving a problem.

- When a job is done well by the team, the leader must appreciate the members to enhance their morale and increase team cohesiveness.
- **Guide decision-making:** The leader should select appropriate method for decision-making, which may include majority vote, unanimous consent, etc. At times decision by authority may be necessary.
- **Influence group norms:** Norms are unwritten rules that prescribe acceptable behavior in the group. The group leader should be alert to the development of norms within the team; she should reinforce those norms that support effective working relationships and challenge those that reduce effectiveness preferably before they become well established.
- **Encourage open communication within the team:** Open communication leads to a kind of understanding that promotes positive relationship. It is the means by which purposes and objectives are clarified, roles defined and negotiated, conflicts dealt with and decisions made. The team needs to know what type of work is being done by other teams, to prevent duplication of effort.
- **Manage conflicts:** As a general rule conflicts are neither to be avoided nor stimulated but managed. Conflicts can stimulate creativity and provide opportunity to improve interpersonal and leadership skills and to develop deeper understanding of people.

CHARACTERISTICS OF AN EFFECTIVE TEAM

The following are the characteristics of an effective team:
- **Clarity of purpose:** The purpose of the team should be clear.
- **Harmony:** The team members should have harmonious relationship with each other.
- **Optimum use of resources:** For proper functioning of the team, resources of man, money and material should be utilized effectively.
- **Process oriented:** Team members should be work oriented and must possess positive attitude towards the work.
- **Listening and discussion:** The members must listen to each other. There should be open discussion among the team members to arrive at unanimous decision so that every member is actively involved in the work.
- **Cohesiveness:** Have trust and empathy, accommodate each other and be sincere towards the group and the job.
- **Negotiation and initiative:** The team members must take initiative.
- **Constructive criticism:** Constructive criticism helps to improve the team functioning.
- **Informal and relaxed atmosphere:** It helps to promote and improve the work efficiency of the team members.

ADVANTAGES AND DISADVANTAGES OF TEAM FUNCTIONING

Advantages
- The team functioning helps to provide comprehensive healthcare services.
- It helps the team members to contribute their own expertise or skills in caring for patients or family.
- It promotes higher job satisfaction among the team members.
- Coordination between the team members reduces duplication and omission of work. It also reduces conflicting advices by different team members, e.g., if there is no coordination while taking care of a client, one member may advise the client to take more rest and the other may advise more exercise.
- The team functioning stimulates each team member to work and reinforce the other. This helps to improve the quality of work.
- The team members are able to help one another and to substitute for each other in an emergency. Hence, the team is more flexible and responsive than the individual worker.
- Team functioning provides emotional support to its members. Effective teams can help manage anxieties and tensions within.
- When team members have been involved in setting the team's objectives and in deciding how they will be met, they are usually most committed to the achievement of these objectives.
- In a team, the team members work closely together and share their experiences. Team members have better scope to expand their knowledge and skills.

Disadvantages
- Effective teamwork requires a considerable amount of interpersonal relationship and skills from team members as well as from the leader. Without this skill teamwork can be a frustrating, discouraging and energy consuming experience.
- If team goals are not well defined or when roles and responsibilities of individual members are not clearly differentiated it may cause conflicts.
- Team functioning becomes time consuming if it takes more time to bring team members together to ask for their inputs or decisions.
- It reduces autonomy of the members: Some team members may find it difficult to compromise or to get along with the team's decision when it is not in agreement with their own.
- Authoritarian team leader may prohibit disagreement and pressurize its members to adhere to group norms. Thus giving rise to jealousy on complexes.
- It becomes difficult to hide mistakes and inadequacy while working in a team.
- When responsibility for patient care outcome is shared by all the team members, each member should be able to trust the skill and judgement of other team members.

AIMS OF HEALTH TEAM

The major aims of health team are:
- **Promoting wellness:** The activities carried out to promote wellness involve health education to individual

and community, e.g., periodic health check up and need based health education.
- **Preventing illness:** The objective of illness prevention activities is to reduce the risk of illness, to promote good health habits and to maintain individual's optimal functioning, e.g., encouraging immunization against various diseases.
- **Restoring health:** This area focuses on the individual with an illness, but ranges from early detection of disease to rehabilitation and teaching during recovery, e.g., teaching colostomy care to a patient with cancer colon, who is to undergo surgery.
- **Facilitating coping mechanisms:** Health team facilitates client and family, in coping with altered function and death. Altered function results in a decrease in an individual's ability to carry out activities of daily living, e.g., modification of lifestyle for amputated patient. Health team also provides care to both patient and families during the terminal illness.

ROLE OF NURSE IN TEAM FUNCTIONING

- **Nurse as a leader:** Leadership is the ability to direct or motivate others towards the achievement of predetermined goals; and the leader may work towards influencing an individual or a group. The nurse can use the dynamics of leadership for growth or change in many areas, including their client's healthcare pattern, healthcare agency, community and the healthcare system in general.
- **Nurse as a communicator:** Nurses role as a communicator is very important in healthcare agency whether it may be between nurse to nurse, nurse to client, nurse to physician or other healthcare workers or nurse to family. Both as a team member and a team leader nurse must develop one of the most important skills of effective communication. It helps in improving personal relationship and better understanding towards patient client care.
- **Nurse as teacher and counselor:** In a health team, the nurse assumes the role of a teacher and a counselor, when clients have identifiable health needs. As a teacher she helps to identify higher own health needs and how to overcome them. As a Counselor she counsels and guides the client and the family to accept and cope up with the illness and lead a normal life without being overpowered by the limitation laid down by the illness. In an academic setting, a nurse teacher educates and guides her subordinates and students to attain professional expertise. Whatever the situation may be, a nurse, teacher and counselor need to possess interpersonal skills of warmth, friendliness, openness and empathy for successful teaching and counseling.
- **Nurse as a researcher:** Research provides an important step towards expanding and updating the professional role of nursing and acquiring new knowledge to improve client care and being competent as a member of the interdisciplinary health team. This helps the professional members to place themselves at par with the other disciplines.
- **Nurse as an advocate:** In the healthcare team, the nurse adopts the role of an advocate by informing the clients of their rights and by supporting decisions concerning healthcare 'choices'. Moreover, the nurse also advises the ways and means to the right type of treatment and diagnostic procedures.

ROLES AND RESPONSIBILITIES OF COMMUNITY HEALTH NURSING PERSONNEL IN FAMILY HEALTH SERVICES

All members of the health team work together collaboratively and collectively and cooperatively to achieve the desired health outcome of the people. With the changes in healthcare delivery system the public health team also has to change. The following members of the Health Team deliver the healthcare to the community with cooperation and collaboration:
- DPHN (supervisor/director): District Level
- Public health nurse: Primary Health Centre/Community Health Centre Level LHVI
- Health Supervisor (Male and female): Primary Health Centre Level
- ANM/Health Worker: Subcenter Level
- TBAs and Community Health Volunteers: Community level

DISTRICT PUBLIC HEALTH NURSE

- The district public health nurse (DPHN) is responsible for planning, organizing and directing the public health programs of jurisdiction where she is appointed. 'Participates in policy-making activities in regard to healthcare.
- She needs to learn and understand the policy of organization and administration of the state where she works.
- Evaluation of nursing service is done by DPHN. She plans for continuously improving the quality of client care.
- The district community health nurse is attached to the district health office.
- She is directly responsible to the district health officer and delegates the responsibilities to all nursing personnel in the district community health field, i.e., PHC, SC, family planning and all national health programs.
- She is supervised by nursing' officer at directorate level.

Responsibilities of District Public Health Nurses

Administrator

Responsible for efficient implementation of policies and programs relating to nursing in public health. Will make recommendations to district health officer on:
- Requirements of nursing staff in primary health field.
- Staff development programs for educational and promotional avenues.
- Maintain discipline among the health team members.
- Field visits at least four times a month to supervise each staff member in subcenters and PHCs and ensure the quality care.

- Submit annual complete report for all PHC and SC visits paid and recommendations for improvement of PH. services.

As Supervisor

- Conduct regular meetings and solving official as well as personal problems in best possible way.
- Encourage, initiative and help in promoting professional growth of staff.
- Interpretations of policies, plans and rules to the staff so as to regulate and develop the services.
- Advise on organizing and planning of work, helping the individual staff member to evaluate the needs of their particular areas and to select priority for her work.
- Guidance of staff regarding use of records, reports and on collection of statistical data and record keeping system.

As Educator

- Organize the in-service education program for all nursing staff.
- Initiate and assist in planning and organizing the orientation program for new staff.
- Participate in community health field experience organized for nursing students of schools or colleges of nursing.
- Suggest in selection of areas for practical experience. Provide facilities and resources to students and staff.
- Guide students during field experience.

COMMUNITY HEALTH NURSE

Community health nurse represents the most professional workers in the public health field and nursing services are employed to implement or support virtually all of the services offered to community.

- Participate in program planning, development and evaluation of the agency program as a whole and advising of other administrative staff in nursing matters.
- The special competencies and technical knowledge of nursing have a big contribution in determining the care and content of public health program.
- Use administrative as well as clinical skills in organizing clinics and recruiting and training volunteers.
- Provide family healthcare. She plans her work and evaluates its effectiveness in terms of community as a whole.
- Provides direct nursing care to non-hospitalized sick or teaches the family member to give care to the sick.

Planner/Program

- Identifies needs, priorities, and problems of individuals, families, and communities.
- Formulates municipal health plan in the absence of a medical doctor.
- Interprets and implements nursing plan, program policies, and circular for the concerned staff personnel.
- Provides technical assistance to rural health midwives in health matters.

Provider of Nursing Care

- Provides direct nursing care to sick or disabled in the home, clinic, school, or workplace.
- Develops the family's capability to take care of the sick, disabled, or dependent member.

Community Organizer

- Motivates and enhances community participation in terms of planning, organizing, implementing, and evaluating health services.
- Initiates and participates in community development activities.

Coordinator of Services

- Coordinates with individuals, families, and groups for health related services provided by various members of the health team.
- Coordinates nursing program with other health programs like environmental sanitation, health education, dental health, and mental health.

Trainer/Health Educator

- Identifies and interprets training needs of the RHMs, Barangay Health Workers (BHW), and hilots.
- Conducts training for RHMs and hilots on promotion and disease prevention.
- Conducts pre and postconsultation conferences for clinic clients; acts as a resource speaker on health and health related services.
- Initiates the use of tri-media (radio/TV, cinema plugs, and print ads) for health education purposes.
- Conducts premarital counseling.

Health monitor: Detects deviation from health of individuals, families, groups, and communities through contacts/visits with them.

Role model: Provides good example of healthful living to the members of the community.

Change agent: Motivates changes in health behavior in individuals, families, groups, and communities that also include lifestyle in order to promote and maintain health.

Recorder/Reporter/Statistician

- Prepares and submits required reports and records.
- Maintain adequate, accurate, and complete recording and reporting.
- Reviews, validates, consolidates, analyzes, and interprets all records and reports.
- Prepares statistical data/chart and other data presentation.

Researcher

- Participates in the conduct of survey studies and researches on nursing and health-related subjects.

- Coordinates with government and nongovernment organization in the implementation of studies/research.

HEALTH ASSISTANT SUPERVISOR (FEMALE)

They have been trained to provide specified healthcare in community health nursing: The multipurpose worker's health scheme has designated LHVs as health supervisors (F). They have been given a special training of 6 months to promote as health supervisor and perform the activities to supervise the health workers. The health supervisors are usually placed in PHCs. Their job responsibilities have been listed below:

Job Responsibilities of Health Assistant/Supervisor (Female)

- Under the Multipurpose Workers Scheme a health assistant female is expected to cover a population of 30,000 (20,000 in tribal and hilly areas).
- Supervise and guide the Health Worker (F), Dais and Female Health guides in the delivery of healthcare services to the community.
- Strengthen the knowledge and skills of the Health Worker Female.
- Help the Health Worker (F) in improving her skills in working in the community.
- Help and guide the Health Worker (F) in planning and organizing her program of activities.
- Assess fortnightly the progress of work of the Health Worker (F) and submit an assessment report to the Medical Officer of the Primary Health Program.
- Carry out supervisory home visits in the area of the Health Worker (F) with respect to their duties under various National Health Programmes.
- Supervise referral of all pregnant women for VDRL testing to CHCI Sub-Divisional Hospital.

Responsibilities

General

- Responsible for organizing and conducting the health clinics, e.g., well baby clinic, family welfare and general clinics, etc.
- Supervising, organizing and planning home visits for subordinate nurses and give suggestions for improvement.
- Organize and encourage the educational activities for improving quality care.
- Will interpret the need of the nursing and health services to medical officer.

Supervisory

- Will aim to promote harmony and efficiency within the team to improve the quality of work.
- Seek to promote the professional growth of other staff and encourage initiative.
- Will interpret the staff policies, plans and rules laid down for developing and regulating the service.
- Review the use of records, reports and collection of statistical data and advise where necessary.
- Home visit as per schedule to supervise the staff.
- Arrange orientation program of all new staff posted to training unit area and to acquaint them with the geography of the area, setup, policies, duties of different staff and channels of communication.
- Plans and carry out continuous and effective in-service training program, arranging monthly meetings for all nursing staff.
- Coordinate her activities with those of the Health Assistant (M) and other health personnel including the Dais and Health Guides.
- Maintain the prescribed record and prepare the necessary reports. Conduct weekly MCH clinics at each subcenter with the assistance of the Health Worker (F) and Dais.
- Supervise the immunization of all pregnant women and children (zero to six years).
- Ensure that all cases of malnutrition among infants and young children (0–6 years) are given the necessary treatment and advice and refer serious cases to the Primary Health Center.
- Conduct weekly family planning clinics (along with the MCH Clinics) at each subcenter with the assistance of the Health Worker (F).
- Help the Medical Officers in School Health Services. Carry out educational activities for MCH, family planning, nutrition and immunization, control of blindness, dental care and other National Health Programmes like leprosy and tuberculosis with the assistance of the Health Worker Female.

HEALTH WORKER (FEMALE AND MALE HEALTH WORKER)

Under the Multipurpose Workers Scheme, one Health Worker (F) and one Health Worker (M) are posted at each subcenter and are expected ultimately to cover a population of 5,000 (3,000 in tribal and hilly areas).

She will carry out the following duties:

- Register and provide care to pregnant women throughout the period of pregnancy.
- Assist Medical Officer and Health Assistant (F) in conducting antenatal and postnatal clinics at the subcenter.
- Educate mother individually and in groups in better family health including maternal and child health, family planning, nutrition, immunization, control of communicable diseases, personal and environmental hygiene.
- Spread the message of family planning to the couples and motivate them for family planning individually and in groups.
- Distribute conventional contraceptives and oral contraceptives to the couples, provide facilities and to help prospective acceptors in getting family planning services, if necessary, by accompanying them or arranging for the Dai to accompany them to hospital.

- Identify the women requiring help for medical termination of pregnancy and refer them to nearest approved institution.
- Educate community of the consequences of septic abortion and inform them about the availability of services for medical termination of pregnancy.
- Identify cases of malnutrition among infants and young children (0–6 years), give the necessary treatment and advice and refer serious cases to the PHC.
- Distribute Iron and Folic Acid tablets as prescribed to pregnant and nursing mothers, infants and young children (0–6 years), adolescent girls and family planning acceptors.
- Immunize pregnant women with tetanus toxoid. Roles and Responsibilities of Community Health Nursing Personnel Administer DPT vaccine, oral polio vaccine, measles vaccine and BCG vaccine to all infants and children.

Community Health Nursing Services Administration

- Notify the MO PHC immediately about any abnormal increase in cases of diarrheal dysentery, poliomyelitis, neonatal tetanus, fever with rigors, fever with rash, and fever with jaundice or fever with unconsciousness which she comes across during her home visits, take the necessary measures to prevent their spread, and inform the Health Worker Male to enable him to take further action.
- Record births and deaths occurring in her Aka in the births and deaths register and report them to the Health Worker (M).
- Maintain the prenatal and maternity records and child care records. Provide treatment for minor ailments, provide first aid for accidents and emergencies and refer cases beyond her competence to the Primary Health Center or nearest hospital.
- Attend and participate in staff meetings at Primary Health, Center/Community Development Block or both.

COMMUNITY HEALTH VOLUNTEERS

They are non-government personnel, providing comprehensive healthcare to the defined community. They voluntarily work for three months and get a stipend of ₹ 120/- month during the three months training. At the end of the training, they are given a kit with emergency equipment for minor ailments and wounds and ₹ 60/- every month. CHV is responsible to provide immediate first aid in emergency, treatment of minor ailments, health education on immunization, nutrition, family planning, etc.

TRADITIONAL BIRTH ATTENDANTS (TBAs)

These are the indigenous trained dais, who conducts 70% of rural deliveries. They don't receive any special training, but they learn by virtue of their practice in the field or by elders or seniors who practice in their homes. Due to their unscientific knowledge, the maternal and infant mortality is very high. Hence, the need was felt to train the TBAs of all community; at least one TBA for 1,000 of population should prove safe and scientific deliveries to community. They are provided one month training and id a kit at the end of training to use safe equipment for delivery. The TBAs already in the field of practice are selected for the training.

PRINCIPLES AND TECHNIQUES OF COUNSELING

Counseling is a process, as well as a relationship, between persons. Contrary to what some people believe, counseling is not concentrated advice-giving. The aim of the counselor is usually to assist the person or persons (client or clients) in realizing a change in behavior or attitude, or to seek achievement of goals. Often there are varieties of problems for which the counselee may seek to find help.

Meaning of Counseling

- Counseling is not a process of giving advice, but it is a process of helping your patient who is genuinely in need.
- It aims to help an individual to help himself to overcome his problem.
- Counseling is different from a casual conversation as it builds a professional relationship with the patient.
- It is totally focused, specific and purposeful.
- Counseling is a long-term process and consists of professional communication.

Skills and Techniques of Counseling

- **Listening skills:** You should always listen carefully and not question the patient too frequently. Allow him to ventilate through your listening.
- **Attending skill:** Your proper attention should be given to the patient to show interest and concern-verbal and non-verbal.
- **Feedback:** Expressing the meaning of patient's feelings and summarizing his problems.
- **Probing:** Focusing in depth on particular aspects of the situation.
- **Confronting:** Help the patient to realize his problems or help him to become aware of what he is suffering from, by making proper statements.
- **Interpreting:** Presenting the alternative ways or angles to look at his situation.
- **Self-disclosure:** Share your attitude, opinions and experiences.
- **Non-dependence:** Do not make the patient dependent rather make him self sufficient to solve his problems independently.
- **Questioning:** Ask open ended questions so that the patients gets the clue to open up with you. Do not ask too many close-ended questions.
- **Incomplete sentence:** Encourage the patient to complete the sentence if he is not able to do so.

- **Refocusing:** If the patient is going off track or talking in circles get him back to maintain the theme without hurting any of his feelings.
- **Silence:** Be with the patient's feelings while he is crying and do not prevent him from crying. Let him cry and ventilate himself.
- **Connecting:** Show connection between thought, behavior and result or effect of what has gone before.

Principles of Counseling

- **Principle of acceptance:** Accept the patient with his physical, psychological, social, economical and cultural conditions.
- **Principle of communication:** Communication should be verbal as well as non-verbal and should be skillful.
- **Principle of empathy:** Instead of showing sympathy put yourself in patients shoes and then give reflections accordingly (Empathy is ability to identify with a person).
- **Principle of nonjudge:** Mental attitude-do not criticize or comment negatively regarding patient's complaints.
- **Principle of confidentiality:** Always keep the patient's name, and the problem strictly secretes and assures the patient about the same.
- **Principle of individuality:** Treat each and every patient as unique and respect his problem as well.
- **Principles of nonemotional involvement:** Not getting emotionally involved with the patient and avoid getting carried away with his feelings.

Goals of Counseling

- Listening keenly to the patient is the main goal.
- Identify the need of the patient, e.g., parents need counseling for their children's behavior problems.
- To make the patient to ventilate his emotions properly and help him to be aware of his own emotions and encourage him to be independent.
- Main problem should be focused so that the sub-problems should be identified by the patient himself.
- Make the patient to accept himself with his problem and help him to adjust with it till it gets over.
- To focus on his strengths by studying the case and produce positive attitude in him and ultimately help him to reduce his negativity.

Role of Community Health Nurse in Counseling and Teaching

- CHN is involved in family health counseling and teaching in all aspects of family care.
- Health counseling is the action taken to assist individual to make and carry out his own plans to meet health problems.
- Teaching may be a part of counseling and involves provision of information in such a way that family or individual learns how to apply this information in his own situation and gains a desired healthcare.
- Control of environmental health hazard is an integral part of public health nursing.
- Observation and teaching in this respect help to control the accidents, hazards at home, school, and industries and also to prevent unnecessary exposure to injury or infection.
- Participating in development of the total public health program, the public health nurse plans with medical and administrative personnel within the agency regarding nursing participation and carries out the nursing activities.
- She participates in planning, conducting and evaluating educational program.

CONCLUSION

Community health nursing is a synthesis of nursing practice applied in promoting and preserving the health of the population. Community health implies integration of curative, preventive and promotional health services. The aim of community diagnosis is the identification of community health problems. Remarkable development in public health was successful control of many communicable diseases. Nursing and medical services were strengthened to promote positive health. Nowadays more emphasis is focused on the sick to the well person, from the individual to the community. To attain Health For All through Primary Healthcare led to the restructuring of the rural health services. At present Public health nurses are called as Community health nurses who are registered nurses (RN) trained to work in public health settings. It includes nursing services in all phase of health services which is organized for the welfare of the community. In 1958, Indian Nursing Council has integrated community health into basic curriculum in nursing.

BIBLIOGRAPHY

1. Adams-Skinner J, Exner T, Pili C, et al. The development and validation of a tool to assess nurse performance in dual protection counseling. Patient Educ Couns. 2009;76:265–71.
2. Brindis CD, Geierstanger SP, Wilcox N, et al. Evaluation of a peer provider reproductive health service model for adolescents. Perspect Sex Reprod Health. 2005;37:85–91.
3. Lambert M. Implications of outcome research for psychotherapy integration. In: Norcross J, Goldfind M, (Eds) Handbook of Psychotherapy Integration. New York, NY: Basic Books; 1992:pp.94–129.
4. Nobili MP, Piergrossi S, Brusati V, Moja EA. The effect of patient-centered contraceptive counseling in women who undergo a voluntary termination of pregnancy. Patient Educ Couns. 2007; 65:361–68.
5. Proctor A, Jenkins TR, Loeb T, et al. Patient satisfaction with 3 methods of postpartum contraceptive counseling: A randomized, prospective trial. J Reprod Med. 2006;51:377–82.

Chapter 17: Health Team

REVIEW QUESTIONS

Long Essays
1. Define health team. Describe the characteristics of an effective team.
2. Enumerate the job responsibilities of health assistant/supervisor (female).
3. Describe the principles and techniques of counseling.
4. Enlist the role of community health nurse in counseling and teaching.

Short Essays
1. Advantages and disadvantages of team functioning.
2. Role of nurse in team functioning.
3. Roles and responsibilities of community health nursing personnel in family health services.
4. District public health nurse.
5. Health worker (Female and male health worker).
6. Community health nursing services administration.
7. Skills and techniques of counseling.
8. Principles of counseling.

Short Answers
1. Aims of health team.
2. Community health nurse.
3. Traditional birth attendants.
4. Goals of counseling.
5. Meaning of counseling.

Multiple Choice Questions

1. Team building requires specific:
    a. Knowledge
    b. Skill
    c. Work.
    d. All of the above
2. Characteristics of an Effective Team include all, *except*:
    a. Clarity of purpose
    b. Authoritative
    c. Listening and discussion
    d. Constructive criticism
3. The major aims of health team are:
    a. Promoting wellness
    b. Preventing illness
    c. Restoring health and
    d. All of the above.
4. Who is the chief technical advisor to the government on all matters relating to medical case and public health at the center?
    a. Health secretary
    b. Health minister
    c. Director of health services
    d. Director general of health services.
5. Who is the ex-officio secretary of Panchayat Samiti?
    a. Block development officer
    b. Block medical officer
    c. Collector
    d. District medical officer.
6. The government of India set up "Multipurpose Workers Committee" in which year?
    a. 1948
    b. 1950
    c. 1970
    d. 1972.

ANSWERS

| 1. d | 2. b | 3. d | 4. d | 5. a | 6. d | | | | | |

Health Information System/Health Management Information System

LEARNING OBJECTIVES

1. Concepts, components, uses, sources
2. Statistics
3. Important rates and indicators
4. Vital health records and their uses
5. Basic statistical methods
6. Descriptive statistics

INTRODUCTION

Health management information system (HMIS) is a system whereby health data are recorded, stored, retrieved and processed to improve decision-making. HMIS data quality should be monitored routinely as production of high quality statistics depends on assessment of data quality and actions taken to improve it. Thus, this study assessed accuracy of the routine HMIS data. The objective of the HMIS would be to record information on health events and check the quality of services at different levels of health care. The importance of patient assessment is a part of the concept of giving importance to patient's views in improving the quality of health services. Expected benefits include enhancing patient satisfaction through improved communication; greater provider sensitivity towards patients; enhanced community awareness about the quality of services; and overall better use of services in the health system.

CONCEPT OF HMIS

Health management information systems are one of the six building blocks essential for health system strengthening. HMIS is a data collection system specifically designed to support planning, management, and decision-making in health facilities and organizations.

Definition

Health information system is that system in which collection, utilization, analysis and transmission of information is done for conducting health services, training and research (**Fig. 18.1**).

Objectives

- To provide reliable, latest and useful health information to all levels of health officers and administrators.
- To amend health policies and working system on the basis of feedback, received from health information system.
- To provide information about periodically and time bound programs and for mid-term evaluation.
- To contribute towards achievement of objectives of health policies and programs.
- To increase efficiency and quality in health management.

Characteristics According to WHO

- The information should be problem oriented.
- Information should be population based.
- Functional and directorial wording should be used.
- Information should be expressed in short and in imaginative form (graphs, chart, table, etc.).
- Facility for data feedback must be present in health information system.

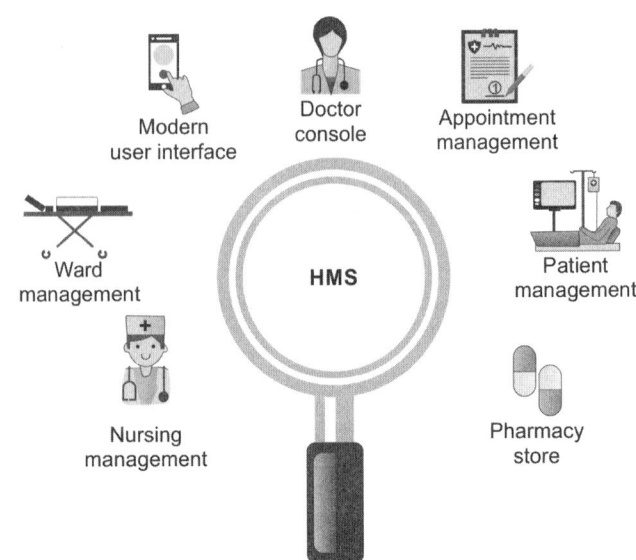

Fig. 18.1: Health management systems.

- Latest technology should be used in health information system.
- Unnecessary figures or data should not be present in information system.
- For information management, organizational structure must be present.

Sources of HMIS

- Census
- Registration of vital events (birth, death, marriage, etc.)
- Notification of diseases and disease registers
- Records and reports of hospitals
- Statistics regarding environmental health
- Statistics regarding health resources and services
- Sample survey (national sample survey organization)
- Population survey
- Statistics regarding efforts to check epidemiological diseases and researches in this field
- School record
- Economic planning
- Plans of social security

Components of Health Information System

Health information systems consist of six key components, including:

1. **Resources:** The legislative, regulatory, and planning frameworks required for system functionality. This includes personnel, financing, logistics support, information and communications technology (ICT), and mechanisms for coordinating both within and between the six components.
2. **Indicators:** A complete set of indicators and relevant targets, including inputs, outputs, and outcomes, determinants of health, and health status indicators.
3. **Data sources:** Including both population-based and institution-based data sources.
4. **Data management:** Collection and storage, QA, processing and flow, and compilation and analysis.
5. **Information products:** Data which has been analyzed and presented as actionable information.
6. **Dissemination and use:** The process of making data available to decision-makers and facilitating the use of that information.

Benefits of Health Information Systems

The healthcare industry relies on a massive amount of data to make decisions about patient care, facilitate the delivery of care, and handle the many complex administrative tasks that go on behind the scenes. Health information systems are valuable tools that aid clinicians and administrative personnel in ensuring a seamless patient experience from end-to-end. Other benefits include:

- **Data analytics:** HIS helps to gather and analyze data to manage population health and reduce healthcare costs.
- **Supports collaborative care:** HIS facilitates the sharing of PHI between providers and organizations, making it possible for patients to receive coordinated care from multiple providers while improving care delivery and patient outcomes.
- **Cost control:** By sharing information, HIS can eliminate duplicate testing and procedures, reduce time demands on staff (such as for sending paper copies of patient records), and reduce costly human errors.
- **Population health management:** Aggregating patient data can help to identify patterns and trends, predict or prevent outbreaks, identify at-risk populations, and more.
- **Clinical decision support:** Integrating a patient's individual data and medical history with broader population data and research improves both diagnostics and treatment.

Problems or Constraints of HMIS in India

Structural

- Multiplicity of institutions and departments
- Fragmentation of data.
- Lack of infrastructural facilities for storage and maintenance of records.

Procedural

- Excessive information
- Encryption/hidden issues
- Exhaustive information, seldom used.
- Overburden of collection and recording of data along with general health care.
- Incomplete, unreliable and intentionally managed information.
- Repetition of general information
- Inappropriate forms/cards/reports
- Less interest of users in information
- Time consuming procedure
- Confusing coding, long list of indices
- Absence of feedback to information suppliers.

Related to Content

- Mostly service utilization statistics.
- Only summarized information reaches at higher level.
- Less emphasis on socioeconomic information.
- No user-friendly.

Related to Human Resource

- Absence or lack of skilled medical record professionals.
- Lack of opportunity for in service training for the staff.
- Healthcare providers/nurses/biomedical trained persons are collecting and preparing data.
- Lack of motivation/extra incentives.

Technological

- Much manual paper-based system.
- Absence or lack of computerized data base system.

Subsystems/Subcomponents of HMIS

- Epidemiological surveillance
- Routine service reporting
- Specific program reporting

- Administrative systems
- Vital registration.

Challenges for HMIS

- Low levels of public will, about vital registration system
- Inadequate government's capacity and lack of firm political decision
- Gender issues in vital events registration
- Fragmentation of health information
- Establishing a unified information system within country.

TYPES OF HEALTHCARE INFORMATION SYSTEMS

Health information systems are available to, and accessed by, healthcare professionals. These include those who deal directly with patients, clinicians, and public health officials (**Fig. 18.2**). Healthcare professionals collect data and compile it for use in making healthcare decisions for individual clients, client groups, and the general public. Health information systems include:

- **Electronic medical record (EMR) and electronic health record (EHR):**
  - Electronic medical records replace paper patient records. Several companies provide such information systems.
  - Medical information on each patient must now be collected and stored electronically.
  - These records would include patient health information, test results, doctor and specialist visits, and healthcare treatments.
- **Practice management software:**
  - Such information systems assist healthcare facilities and personnel with the management of daily operations of the facility.
  - This would include things like scheduling of patients and medical services billing. Regardless of their size from single practice doctors to huge multi-center hospitals, all healthcare providers utilize practice management systems.
  - The goal is to automate administrative tasks carried out as part of doing business in the facility.
- **Master patient index (MPI):**
  - The software of this healthcare information system is aimed at connecting patient records more than one databases.
  - The MPI contains records for any patient registered at a healthcare organization. MPI, as the name suggests, creates an index all the records for that patient.
  - The intent of MPIs is to reduce duplicate patient records and avoid inaccurate patient information that could result in patient claim denials.
- **Patient portals:**
  - This information system lets patients be aware of their health data.
  - They are able to access appointment information, medications they may be receiving, and their lab results via the internet.
  - Some of these patient portals also facilitate patients to have active communication with healthcare professionals including physicians, pharmacists regarding their prescription refill requests, and scheduling of appointments.
- **Remote patient monitoring (RPM):**
  - This is also termed-telehealth. RPM provides medical sensors that have the ability to transmit patient data to healthcare professionals who might very well be halfway around the world.
  - RPM can monitor blood glucose levels and blood pressure. It is particularly helpful for patients with chronic conditions such as type 2 diabetes, hypertension, or cardiac disease.
  - Data collected and transmitted via PRM can be used by a healthcare professional or a healthcare team to detect medical events such as stroke or heart attack that require immediate and aggressive medical intervention.
  - Data collected may be used as part of a research project or health study.
  - RPM is a life-saving system for patients in remote areas who cannot access face-to-face health care.
- **Clinical decision support (CDS):**
  - CDS analyzes data from clinical and administrative systems. The aim is to assist healthcare providers in making informed clinical decisions.
  - Data available can provide information to medical professions who are preparing diagnoses or predicting medical conditions like drug interactions and reactions.

HEALTH INFORMATION SYSTEM (HIS)

Definition

Health information is defined as a mechanism for the collection, processing, analysis and transmission of information required for organizing and operating health services and also for research and training.

Objectives of HIS

- To provide reliable, latest and useful health information to all levels of health officers and administrators.
- To contribute towards achievement of objectives of health policies and programs.

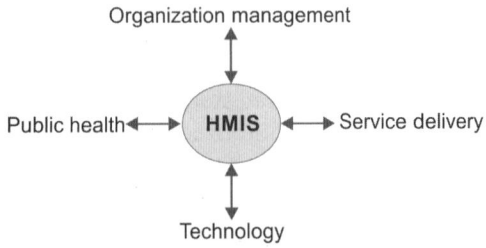

Fig. 18.2: Multiple perspective on HMIS.

- To increase efficiency and quality in health management.
- To provide information about periodically and time bound programs.
- To amend health policies and working system on the basis of feedback.

WHO Expert Committee Criteria

- Health information system should be population based.
- Health information system should be problem oriented.
- Health information system should employ functional and operational terms (e.g., episodes of illness, treatment regimens, laboratory tests).
- The health information system should avoid the unnecessary agglomeration of data.
- The health information system should express information briefly and imaginatively (e.g., tables, charts, percentages).
- The information system should make provision for the feedback of data.

Components of Health Information System

- Demography and vital events.
- Environmental health statistics.
- Health status—morality, morbidity, disability and quality of life.
- Health resources—facilities, beds, manpower.
- Utilization and non-utilization of health services attendance, admission, waiting lists.
- Financial statistics (cost, expenditure) related to the particular objective.
- Indices of outcome of medical care.

Uses of Health Information System

- To measure the health status of the people
- To quantify health problems, medical and healthcare needs.
- To compare local, national and international health status of the people.
- To plan effective management of health services and programs.
- To assess the effectiveness and efficiency of accomplishing their objectives of health services.
- To assess the attitudes and degree of satisfaction of the beneficiaries with the health system.
- To conduct research on particular problems of health and disease.

Sources of Health Information System (Fig. 18.3)

- **Census:** The total process of collecting, compiling and publishing demographic, economic and social data pertaining at a specific time or times, to all persons in a country or delimited territory.
- **Registration of vital events:** It is a legal registration, statistical recording and reporting of the occurrence of statistics and the collection, compilation, presentation, analysis and distribution of statistics pertaining to vital events, i.e., live births, deaths, fetal deaths, marriages,

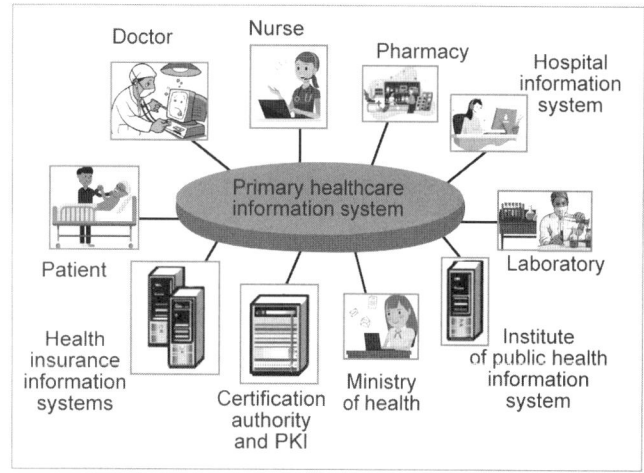

Fig. 18.3: Sources of health information system.

divorces, adoptions, legitimations, recognitions, annulments and legal separations.
- **Sample registration system:** It is used to provide reliable estimates of birth and death rates at the national and state level. It is also a dual records system, consisting of continuous enumeration of births and deaths by an enumerator and an independent survey every 6 months by an investigator-supervisor.
- **Notification of disease:** Notification provides valuable information about fluctuations in disease frequency. It also provides early warning about new occurrence or outbreaks or disease.
- **Hospital records:** The hospital records provides information about age, sex, diagnosis, time interval between occurrence and hospital admission and distribution of patients according to different social and biological characteristics.
- **Disease register:** Morbidity register exist only certain disease and conditions. It also provides information about duration of illness, case fatality and survival. These register allow follow-up of patients and provide a continuous account of the frequency of disease in the community.
- **Record linkage:** Medical record linkage implies the assembly and maintained for each individual in a population, of a file of the more important records relating to his health. The events commonly recorded are birth, marriage, death, hospital admission and discharge.
- **Epidemiological surveillance:** It is a system used to report on the occurrence of new cases and on efforts to control diseases.
- **Other health service records:** It includes outpatient departments, primary health centers, sub-centers, polyclinics, private practitioners, MCH center, school health records, diabetic and hypertensive clinics, etc.
- **Environmental health data:** It is helpful in the identification and quantification of causative factors of disease. Collection of environmental data plays an essential role to remain a major problems for the future.
- **Manpower statistics:** It is an information about physicians, dentists, pharmacists, veterinarians, hospital

nurses, medical technicians, etc. Their records are maintained by the state medical/dental/nursing councils and the directorates of medical education.

NURSING MANAGEMENT INFORMATION SYSTEM (NIMS)

Nursing information systems (NIS) are computer systems that manage clinical data from a variety of healthcare environments, and made available in a timely and orderly fashion to aid nurses in improving patient care.

Fiscal Resource Management

- The information generated can be used to monitor past performance or to predict future performance.
- Accumulated data can be analyzed for the development of trends that can be used to project future expenditures.
- Necessary reallocations and budgetary adjustments can then be made on the basis of these projections.

Workload Measurement and Staffing Requirements

- It helps to store, manipulate and retrieve large volumes of data.
- The information generated assists nursing managers in planning, monitoring and evaluating use of nursing resources on a daily basis and in the longer time frame.
- It is used to generate staff schedules with conjunction with personnel management.

Staff Scheduling

- Nursing managers are able to plan schedules in advance with considerable time savings.
- Staffs are informed well ahead of time.
- Staffing records, if maintained properly, provide useful information for monitoring absenteeism, scheduled time off, and turn over.

Personnel Management

- An employee with a special mix of skills can be located.
- Records are readily accessible needed for accreditation purposes or to monitor contract compliance.
- The information may be retrieved on a daily basis for use in conjunction with workload measurement and contract requirements to plan staffing assignments.

Advantages of NIS

Nursing Administration

- Evaluate quality assurance programs
- Defend resource allocation to nursing
- Demonstrate the contribution nursing, makes to the care of the patient.
- Identify outcomes of nursing care

Nursing Practice

- Enhance documentation by nurses
- Provide data to enable research directed at examining the inter-relationships between data elements and nursing outcomes.
- Facilitate development of the nursing process.

Nursing Research

- To assess variables on multilevels including institutional, local, regional, and national.
- Identify trends to build information and to further synthesize to develop nursing knowledge.

Nursing Education

- To develop body of knowledge with focus on nursing process
- To enable staff educational needs based on follow-up care and outcomes.
- To enhance student nurses accurate documentation

National Health Systems Resource Center (NHSRC) has been set up under the National Health Mission (NHM) as an autonomous registered society, to channelize technical assistance and capacity building support to the states for strengthening the public health system. The NHSRC is also mandated to contribute towards National strategic health planning and program design. Work at NHSRC is organized around multiple divisions, namely—Community Processes, Quality Improvement, Public Health Planning, Public Health Administration, Healthcare Financing and Healthcare Technology, HMIS and Human Resources for Health.

VITAL STATISTICS

Vital statistics has been used to denote acts systematically collected and compiled in numerical form relating to or derived from records of vital events namely, live birth, death, fetal death, marriage, divorce, adoption, legitimating, recognition, annulment or legal separation. Vital statistics provide a tool for measuring the dynamics of change which continuously occur in population. Vital statistics are derived from legally registrable events without including population data or morbidity statistics.

Definitions

- Vital statistics are conventionally numerical records of marriage, births, sickness and deaths by which the health and growth of community may be studied.
- Vital statistics is a part of demography and collective study of mankind. It deals with the data related to vital events.
- It is a branch of biometry deals with data and law of human mortality, morbidity and demography.
- Vital statistics is the numerical description of birth, death, absorption, marriage, divorce, adoption and judicial separation-UNO. Types of vital statistics are explained in **Figure 18.4**.

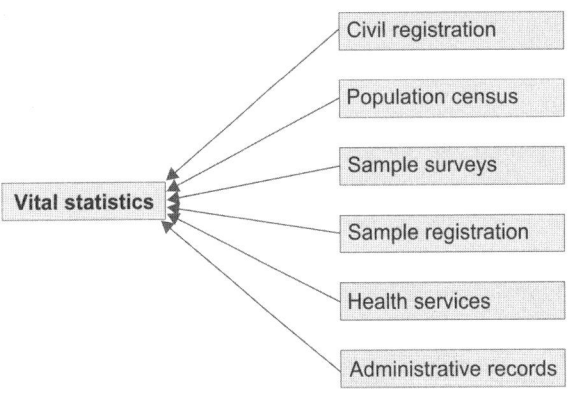

Fig. 18.4: Types of vital statistics.

Source	Apartheid era	Postapartheid
Births register	Occurrence-based births statistics	
Marriage register	Occurrence-based marriage statistics	
Death notification form	Death statistics (after lengthy period of microfilming and verification)	Death statistics (speedily printed from microfilmed images—later terminated in 2003)
Population register (for the production of legal documents)	Identity document with race identifier Birth certificate Death certificate Marriage certificate Certificate of citizenship	Identity document without race identifier Birth certificate Death certificate Marriage certificate Certificate of citizenship
Population register (for the production of vital statistics)	None	Cumulative statistics on births Advance release of deaths statistics (later terminated)

Methods of Obtaining Vital Statistics

- **Census:** It is a simultaneous recording demographic, social and economic data of individuals. It is an important method of collecting vital statistics. Census is conducted every 10 years.
- **Registration**: Registration of vital events (e.g., births, deaths). Keep a continuous check on demographic changes. If registration of vital events is complete and accurate, it can serve as a reliable source of health information.
- **Ad-hoc survey:** Surveys for evaluating the health status of a population, that is community diagnosis of problems of health and disease. It is information about the distribution of these problems over time and space that provides the functional basis for planning and developing needed services.

Purposes

- **Community health:** To describe the level of community health, to diagnose community illness and to discover solutions to health problems.
- **Administrative purpose:** It provides clues for administrative action to create administrative standards of health activities.
- **Health program organization:** To determine success or failure of specific health program or undertake overall evaluation of public health work.
- **Legislation purpose:** To promote health legislation at local, state, and national level.
- **Government purpose:** To develop, policies, procedure at state and central level.

Uses of Vital Statistics

Vital statistics are of much importance for the people and nation.

For the Individual

- Vital statistics are of much use for an individual. A birth certificate issued by the registering authority is an important document which records the date, time, place and parentage of the person.
- It establishes his identity as the citizen of the country.
- It is a legal document which is used for admission to a school, for getting a passport to travel abroad and even to migrate to another country, etc. Similarly, a marriage certificate records the marital status of a couple and legalizes the birth of children from that marriage.

Legal Use

- Vital statistics are legally very useful. Certificates relating to birth, death, marriage, divorce, etc. have legal importance.
- For instance, a death certificate is an important legal document for the settlement of property of the deceased person, the claim of his/her insurance policy, etc.

Health and Family Planning Programs

- Vital statistics relating to births and deaths can be used in health and family planning programs of the government.
- The causes of deaths, and the mortality rates of different categories help in assessing the health condition of the people.
- Accordingly, the state can formulate such health programs as malaria eradication, polio and smallpox immunization, tuberculosis, etc.
- In keeping with the requirements of the population, the government can open hospitals, maternity and child welfare centers, etc.

Study of social conditions: Vital statistics like birth and death rates, divorce rate, widow remarriage, widowhood, etc. throw light on the social conditions of a society, as also its customs and traditions.

For administrators and planners: Data provided by vital statistics relating to trend and growth of population in the various age groups and on the whole, help planners and administrators to plan and formulate policies for public health, education, housing, transport and communications, food supplies, etc.

For the Nation

- Vital statistics are of much importance for the nation. They help in analyzing the population trends at any given point of time.

- They try to fill the gap between two censuses. They relate to the composition, size, distribution and growth of population.
- It is on their basis that population projections can be made. Vital statistics help in formulating policies for providing social security to the people.
- Even the rules for immigration and emigration can be framed on the basis of population growth data.
- Vital statistics are also used for updating electoral rolls and demarcation of constituencies.

VITAL STATISTICS MEASUREMENTS

The vital statistics system provides counts of the number of times specified vital events have occurred. These counts are useful in themselves. For example, the numbers of births and deaths are used in the estimation of population size. For most purposes, however, other statistical measures are needed. For example, comparisons of births in one place with those in another require information on the population size of each area. The simplest and cleanest method of making such comparisons is to compute rates that relate the events to the population exposed to the risk of the event (e.g., the number of births to the number of women of child-bearing age).

- **Crude rates:** The number of events in a given time period divided by the population at risk produces crude rates. The result is multiplied by a constant (typically 1,000 or 100,000) for ease of presentation. Common crude rates include birth, death, marriage, and divorce.
- **Specific rates:** Crude rates may be limited to a specific group, such as deaths from a specified cause or in a specific age group, or births to unmarried women.
- **Age-adjusted rates:** Age-adjustment is a technique used to eliminate the effect of the age distribution of the population on mortality rates. Since the frequency of death varies with age, a measure free of the influences of population composition is needed to make comparisons between areas or over time.
- **Infant mortality rates:** Infant mortality rates reflect the risk of deaths to infants under the age of one year. For infant deaths, the most commonly used estimate of the population at risk (denominator) is the number of live births during the period.
- **Life tables and life expectancy:** A life table is used to measure the effect of mortality on longevity. It shows the mortality experience of a hypothetical group of infants born at the same time and subject to the mortality rates of a specific population group. A life table provides numerous statistics; perhaps the most widely used is life expectancy at birth.

Types of Vital Statistics

- Crude birth rate = $\dfrac{\text{No. of live birth during the year}}{\text{Estimated midyear population}} \times 1{,}000$
- Crude death rate = $\dfrac{\text{No. of death during the year}}{\text{Estimated midyear population in the same year}} \times 1{,}000$
- Infant mortality rate = $\dfrac{\text{No. of deaths of infant in a year}}{\text{No. of total live births in the same year}} \times 1{,}000$
- Neonatal mortality rate = $\dfrac{\text{No. of death of children} < 28 \text{ days of age in a year}}{\text{Total live births in the same year}} \times 1{,}000$
- Maternal mortality rate = $\dfrac{\begin{array}{c}\text{Total No. of female deaths due to complications,}\\ \text{complicating of pregnancy, child birth, or within}\\ \text{42 days of delivery from puerperal causes during,}\\ \text{the given year}\end{array}}{\text{Total No. of live births in the same area and year}} \times 1{,}000$
- General fertility rate = $\dfrac{\begin{array}{c}\text{No. of births in an area during}\\ \text{female population age 15–49}\end{array}}{\text{The same area and year}} \times 1{,}000$

SOURCES OF VITAL STATISTICS

Census

Census is one of the popular approaches that statisticians use in collecting primary data. A census is a collection of information from all units in the population or a 'complete enumeration' of the population. We use a census when we want accurate information for many subdivisions of the population. Such a survey usually requires a very large sample size and often a census offers the best solution.

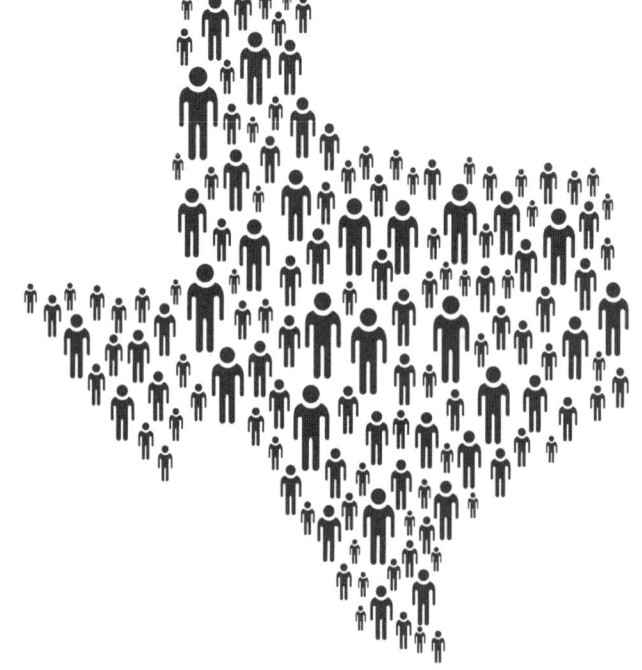

Census Definition

Under the census or complete enumeration method, the statistician collects the data for each and every unit of the population or universe. This universe is a complete set of items which are of interest in any situation.

Merits of a Census Investigation

Now that the census definition is clear, let's look at the merits of a census investigation.
- **Intensive study:** Under census investigation, the obtain data from each and every unit of the population. Further, it enables the statistician to study more than one aspect of all items of the population. For example, the Indian Government conducts a census investigation once every 10 years. The authorities collect the data regarding the population size, males, and females, education levels, sources of income, religion, etc.
- **Reliable data:** The data that a statistician collects through a census investigation is more reliable, representative, and accurate. This is because, in a census, the statistician observes every item personally.
- **Suitable choice:** It is a great choice in situations where the different items of the population are not homogeneous.
- **Basis of various surveys:** Data from a census investigation is used as a basis in various surveys.

Demerits of a Census Investigation

A census investigation also has certain demerits. Some of these demerits are:
- **Costs:** Since the statistician closely observes each and every item of the population before collecting the data, it makes a census investigation a very costly method of investigation. Usually, government organizations adopt this method to collect detailed data like the population census or agricultural census or the census of industrial protection, etc.
- **Time-consuming:** A census investigation is time-consuming and also requires manpower to collect original data.
- **Possibilities of errors:** There are many possibilities of errors in the census investigation method due to nonresponse, measurement, lack of preciseness of the definition of statistical units or even the personal bias of the investigators.

CIVIL REGISTRATION SYSTEM

- Civil registration is the continuous, permanent, compulsory and universal recording of the occurrence and characteristics of vital events **(Fig. 18.5)**.

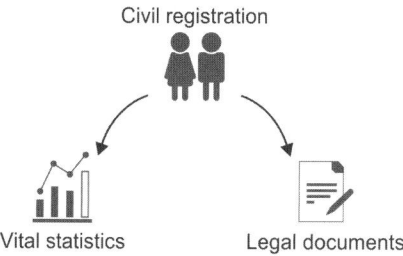

Fig. 18.5: Civil registration system.

- Civil registration is carried out primarily for the purpose of establishing the legal documents provided for by law.
- Civil registration records provide the most effective and efficient source of vital statistics for the whole population.

"Registration of vital events" maintains a continuous record of demographic trends.

Definition (UN)

Legal registration, statistical recording and reporting of the occurrence of and the collection, compilation, presentation, analysis and distribution of statistics pertaining to vital events.

Vital events include:
- Live births
- Deaths
- Fetal deaths
- Marriage
- Divorce
- Adoptions
- Legitimations
- Recognitions
- Annulments
- Legal separations

If registration of vital events is complete and accurate, it can serve as a reliable source of health information. In India, the civil registration system mandates registration of births, deaths and stillbirths.

Vital Events Registration in India

In 1873, GOI passed the "Births, Deaths and Marriages Registration Act". This provided only for voluntary registration. Subsequently, individual States like Tamil Nadu, Karnataka and Assam passed their own **Acts**.

The vital event registration in India is unreliable. It lacks:
- Accuracy
- Timeliness
- Completeness
- Coverage

Also there is lack of uniformity in the collection, compilation and transmission of data, which is different for rural and urban areas and multiple registration agencies (e.g., health agency, panchayat agency, police agency and revenue agency) In 1960, vital statistics was transferred to the office of the Registrar General, India from the Director General of Health services. Thus, population census and vital statistics, including civil registration, came under one office.

Characteristics of Civil Registration Systems

- Legal framework
- Full coverage of population
- Continuous and permanent
- Confidentiality of personal information

The Central Births and Deaths Registration Act, 1969

- This was promulgated with a goal to improve the civil registration system.
- The Act is in force since 1st April, 1970. The Act provides for compulsory registration of births and deaths throughout the country.
- Compilation of vital statistics in the States so as to ensure uniformity and comparability of data.
- The Act fixes the responsibility for reporting births and deaths.
- While the heads of the households have the responsibility to report events occurring in their households, the heads of hospitals, nursing homes, hotels, jails or dharamshalas are to report events occurring in such institutions to the concerning Registrar.
- The time limit for registering the event of births and that of deaths is 21 days uniformly all over India.
- In case of default, a late fee can be levied. The Chief Registrars of Births and Deaths guide in the States and Union Territories, whereas the central authority is the Registrar General of India.

Lay Reporting

- In order to complement the progress in the development of a comprehensive vital registration system, some countries have attempted to employ first line health workers, e.g., village health guides, to record births and deaths in the community.
- In fact, one of the important functions of a primary health worker is to collect and record data on vital events in his or her community.
- Definition of Lay Reporting: 'The collection of information' its use, and its transmission to other levels of the health system by nonprofessional health workers.
- Many countries have adopted this approach to obtain information on vital statistics.
- Demographic survey is another approach but not a satisfactory one. It is best regarded as a temporary substitute for some kind of vital events registration system.

Functions of a Civil Registration System

Birth Registration Outputs Legal

Proving and in establishing, implementing and realizing human rights embodied in international declarations and conventions.

Birth Register

- Basic official document recording the fact of birth of a child, its date and place of birth. It also records the name of the biological parents.
- Complementary events recorded in the same register-like adoption, change of name, etc.
- Required for resolution of judicial disputes.

Administrative

Information compiled using the registration method provides essential data for national or regional planning in health, education and other sectors; for electoral registers. Birth registration records can be the starting point for identifying population needing intervention at individual basis such as
- Infants needing immunizations or health care.
- New mothers requiring postpartum care Birth event records (or certificates) can be (and necessarily needs to be) linked to national ID database.

Statistical

- Provides statistical data for planning, administration and research at whatever geographic or administrative level.
- Basic data on number of births (by place of occurrence and place of usual residence of mother).
- Data on fertility indicators by various characteristics (for example order of birth by age of mother at birth).
- Data on characteristics of birth (e.g., birth weight) Only source that provides data on a continuous basis at the lowest geographical level.

AD-HOC SURVEY

Surveys for evaluating the health status of a population that is community diagnosis of problems of health and disease. It is information about the distribution of these problems over time and space that provides the functional basis for planning and developing needed services.

The meaning of word Ad-hoc is something which is not in order or not organized or unstructured. In the similar note the Ad-hoc testing is nothing but a type of black box testing or behavioral testing.

Characteristics of Ad-Hoc Testing

- Ad-hoc testing is done after the completion of the formal testing on the application or product.
- This testing is performed with the aim to break the application without following any process.
- The testers executing the ad-hoc testing should have thorough knowledge on the product.
- The bugs found during ad-hoc testing exposes the loopholes of the testing process followed.
- Ad-hoc testing can be executed only once until and unless a defect is found which requires **retesting**.

Advantages or Benefits of Ad-Hoc Testing

Below are few of the advantages or benefits related to the Ad-hoc testing:
- Ad-hoc testing gives freedom to the tester to apply their own new ways of testing the application which helps them to find out more number of defects compared to the formal testing process.
- This type of testing can be done at anytime anywhere in the software development life cycle (SDLC) without following any formal process.

- This type of testing is not only limited to the testing team but this can also be done by the developer while developing their module which helps them to code in a better way.
- Ad-hoc testing proves to be very beneficial when there is less time and in-depth testing of the feature is required. This helps in delivering the feature with quality and on time.
- Ad-hoc testing can be simultaneously executed with the other types of testing which helps in finding more bugs in lesser time.
- In this type of testing, the documentation is not necessary which helps the tester to do the focused testing of the feature or application without worrying about the formal documentation.

Disadvantages of Ad-Hoc Testing

- Since ad-hoc testing is done without any planning and in unstructured way so recreation of bugs sometime becomes a big trouble.
- The test scenarios executed during the ad-hoc testing are not documented so the tester has to keep all the scenarios in their mind which he/she might not be able to recollect in future.
- Ad-hoc testing is very much dependent on the skilled tester who has thorough knowledge of the product it cannot be done by any new joiner of the team.

VITAL REGISTRATION

Vital registration includes births, deaths, marriages, divorce, adoption, legitimations, legal separations, recognitions and annulments. These are vital events that need recording and are helpful in day-to-day civilian affair regulations. Such recordings were seen in Egypt long before 1250 BC. Baptism, marriage and deaths used to be recorded in Churches long before the civilized activities. In India voluntary registration existed since 1873, and a compulsory Act came into existence in 1970. Time limit is prescribed in the Central Births and Deaths Registration Act **(Fig. 18.6)**.

- **Disease notifications:** This regulation and policy as a part of disease control and prevention came into existence. It is a valuable morbidity data. Public Health Act and Epidemic Disease Act synchronize the action of disease notification. International modifiable diseases like cholera, plague, yellow fever, National notifiable diseases like polio, influenza, malaria, cholera, plague, typhoid, hepatitis, District notifiable diseases according to local epidemic and public health problems decide the data enunciation. Underreporting and lack of accuracy marks the loophole in disease surveillance.
- **Diseases registry:** Little extension of notification is the permanent recording of specified diseases like cancer, stroke, blindness, birth defects, tuberculosis and leprosy help in planning and implementation of control measures.
- **Medical records:** Cumulative health record system in different placements like school, college, industry, working place gives cumulative data for required action in health policy.
- **Hospital records:** This is century old basic and primary data from hospitals where curative services are provided. This is extended to health centers where both curative and preventive services are provided. Only drawback is that this cannot be generalized since population covered (denominator) is not specific.
- **Environmental health data:** This is a new area of inclusion since morbidity and mortality are closely related to environmental influences.

Nonroutine

- **Sample registration system:** It is an ad-hoc system to get quick required data for policy making and measures to be taken.
- **Disease surveillance:** Surveillance system is built upon diseases of public health problem. Major examples are AIDS surveillance, Polio surveillance and malaria surveillance. It is a valuable data in control, prevention and eradication.

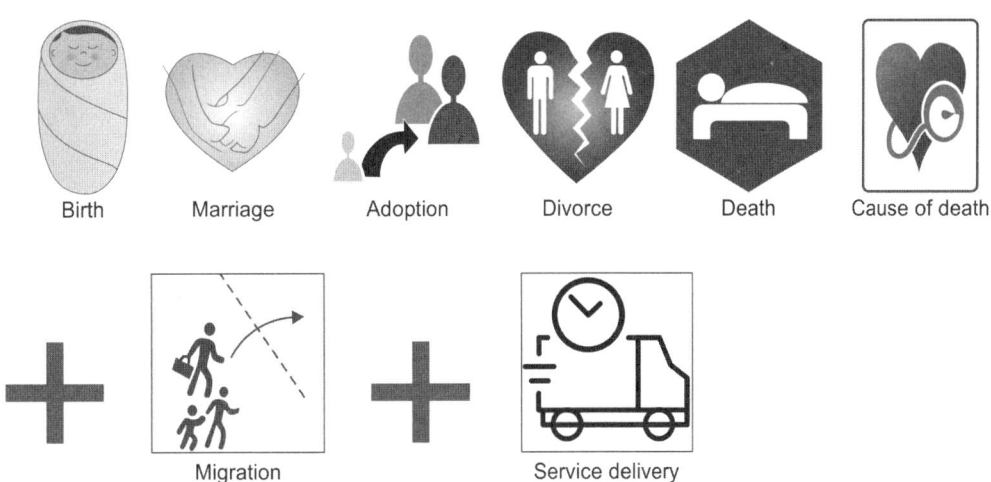

Fig. 18.6: Vital registration.

- **Manpower statistics:** Health information of India, health information of states, health information of district are made available as annual reports which are incredible tool in the hands of administrators.
- **Surveys:** Importance is given to population based surveys. This recognizes mortality, morbidity, fertility, nutritional status and any required data from time to time. National health survey has given us good guidelines in action on local health problems. The methodology adopted could be interview based, examination based, record based or postal enquiry based.
- **Additional ad-hoc demographic data:** Apart from census we need situation analysis on population movement, natural calamity, major epidemics, awareness, practice, etc., which form demographic tool to epidemiologists.
- **Economic and fiscal data:** Consumption of goods, export and import, drugs and employments have been collected from time to time which help Planning Commission for formulation of health policies.
- **Security schemes and social schemes:** Medical insurance, sickness absenteeism, disability benefits and welfare schemes are examples of this type of data.

COMMON SAMPLING TECHNIQUES

There are several different sampling techniques available, and they can be subdivided into two groups: probability sampling and non-probability sampling. In probability (random) sampling, a complete sampling frame of all eligible individuals from which select the sample. In this way, all eligible individuals have a chance of being chosen for the sample, and will be more able to generalize the results from the study **(Fig. 18.7)**.

Probability sampling methods tend to be more time-consuming and expensive than non-probability sampling. In non-probability (nonrandom) sampling, do not start with a complete sampling frame, so some individuals have no chance of being selected. Consequently, the investigator cannot estimate the effect of sampling error and there is a significant risk of ending up with a nonrepresentative sample which produces nongeneralizable results. However, nonprobability sampling methods tend to be cheaper and more convenient, and they are useful for exploratory research and hypothesis generation.

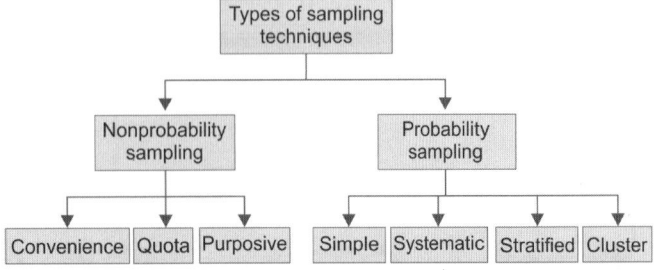

Fig. 18.7: Types of sampling techniques.

Probability Sampling Methods

Probability Sampling

This sampling technique uses randomization to make sure that every element of the population gets an equal chance to be part of the selected sample. It is alternatively known as random sampling.

Simple Random Sampling

Every element has an equal chance of getting selected to be the part sample **(Fig. 18.8)**. It is used when we don't have any kind of prior information about the target population. For example, random selection of 20 students from class of 50 student. Each student has equal chance of getting selected. Here probability of selection is $\frac{1}{50}$.

Stratified Sampling

This technique divides the elements of the population into small subgroups (strata) based on the similarity in such a way that the elements within the group are homogeneous and heterogeneous among the other subgroups formed. And then the elements are randomly selected from each of these strata. We need to have prior information about the population to create subgroups **(Fig. 18.9)**.

Cluster Sampling

Our entire population is divided into clusters or sections and then the clusters are randomly selected. All the elements of the cluster are used for sampling.

Clusters are identified using details such as age, sex, location, etc.

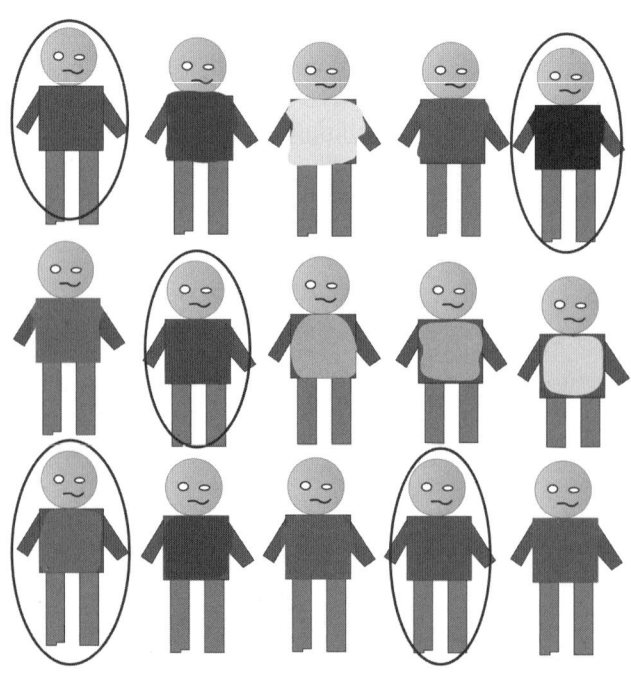

Fig. 18.8: Simple random sampling.

Cluster sampling can be done in following ways:
- **Single stage cluster sampling:** Entire cluster is selected randomly for sampling (**Fig. 18.10**).
- **Two stage cluster sampling:** Here first we randomly select clusters and then from those selected clusters we randomly select elements for sampling (**Fig. 18.11**).

Systematic Clustering

Here the selection of elements is systematic and not random except the first element. Elements of a sample are chosen at regular intervals of population. All the elements are put together in a sequence first where each element has the equal chance of being selected. For a sample of size n, we divide our population of size N into subgroups of k elements (**Fig. 18.12**).

We select our first element randomly from the first subgroup of k elements.

To select other elements of sample, perform following:
- We know number of elements in each group is k i.e., N/n
- So if our first element is n1 then
- Second element is n1 + k, i.e., n2
- Third element n2 + k, i.e., n3 and so on.
- Taking an example of N = 20, n = 5
- No of elements in each of the subgroups is N/n, i.e., 20/5 = 4 = k
- Now, randomly select first element from the first subgroup.
- If we select:
  n1 = 3
  n2 = n1 + k = 3 + 4 = 7
  n3 = n2 + k = 7 + 4 = 11

Multi-stage Sampling

It is the combination of one or more methods described above. Population is divided into multiple clusters and then these clusters are further divided and grouped into various subgroups (strata) based on similarity (**Fig. 18.13**).

One or more clusters can be randomly selected from each stratum. This process continues until the cluster can't be divided anymore. For example, country can be divided into states, cities, urban and rural and all the areas with similar characteristics can be merged together to form a strata.

Nonprobability Sampling

It does not rely on randomization. This technique is more reliant on the researcher's ability to select elements for a sample. Outcome of sampling might be biased and makes

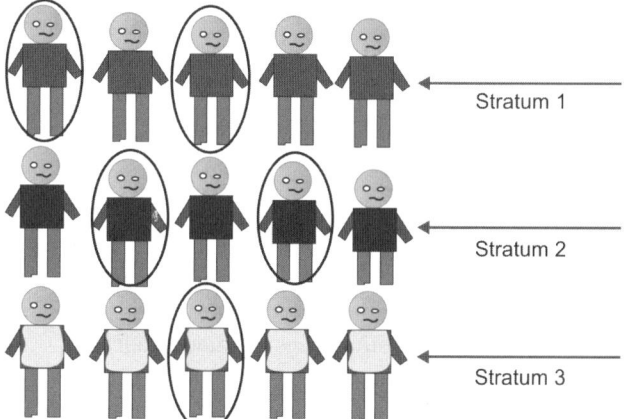

Fig. 18.9: Stratified sampling.

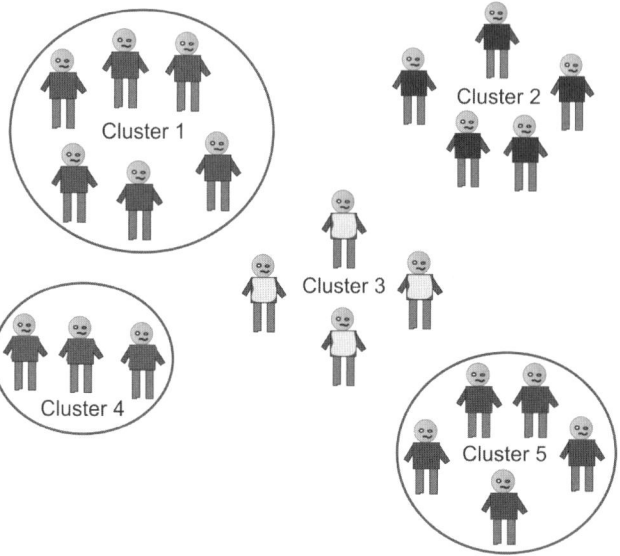

Fig. 18.10: Single stage cluster sampling.

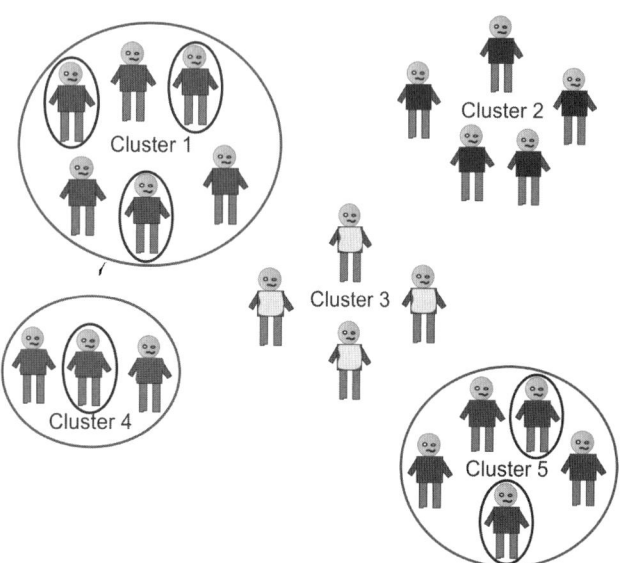

Fig. 18.11: Two stage cluster sampling.

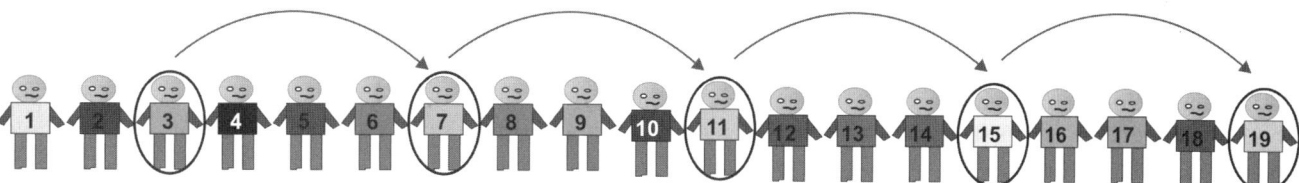

Fig. 18.12: Systematic cluster sampling.

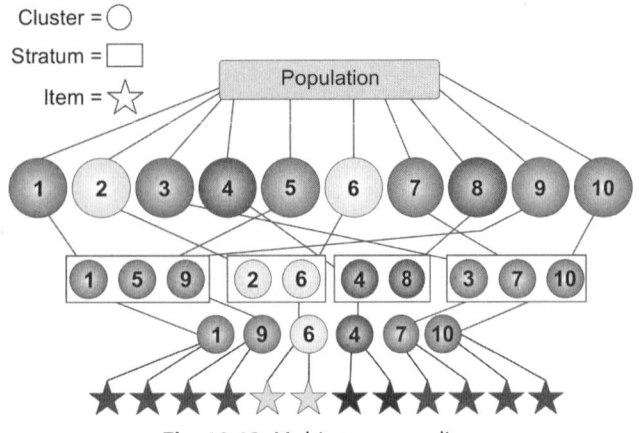

Fig. 18.13: Multi-stage sampling.

difficult for all the elements of population to be part of the sample equally. This type of sampling is also known as non-random sampling.

Convenience Sampling

Here the samples are selected based on the availability. This method is used when the availability of sample is rare and also costly. So based on the convenience samples are selected. For example, researchers prefer this during the initial stages of survey research, as it is quick and easy to deliver results.

Purposive Sampling

This is based on the intention or the purpose of study. Only those elements will be selected from the population which suits the best for the purpose of our study. For example, if we want to understand the thought process of the people who are interested in pursuing master's degree then the selection criteria would be "Are you interested for Masters in…?"

All the people who respond with a "No" will be excluded from our sample.

Quota Sampling

This type of sampling depends of some pre-set standard. It selects the representative sample from the population. Proportion of characteristics/trait in sample should be same as population. Elements are selected until exact proportions of certain types of data are obtained or sufficient data in different categories is collected. For example, if our population has 45% females and 55% males then our sample should reflect the same percentage of males and females.

Referral/Snowball Sampling

This technique is used in the situations where the population is completely unknown and rare. Therefore, we will take the help from the first element which we select for the population and ask him to recommend other elements who will fit the description of the sample needed. So this referral technique goes on, increasing the size of population like a snowball **(Fig. 18.14)**.

For example, it is used in situations of highly sensitive topics like HIV Aids where people will not openly discuss and participate in surveys to share information about HIV Aids.

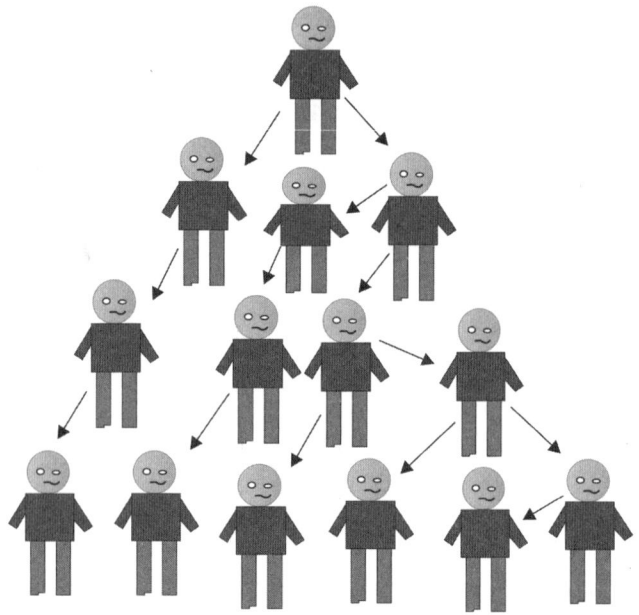

Fig. 18.14: Snowball sampling.

Bias in Sampling

There are five important potential sources of bias that should be considered when selecting a sample, irrespective of the method used. Sampling bias may be introduced when:
- Any preagreed sampling rules are deviated from
- People in hard-to-reach groups are omitted
- Selected individuals are replaced with others, for example if they are difficult to contact
- There are low response rates
- An out-of-date list is used as the sample frame (e.g., if it excludes people who have recently moved to an area).

Determining Sample Size

Knowing the target population, you have to decide the number of the participants in a sample, which is termed as the "sample size". Aside from the estimated number of people in the target population, the sample size can be influenced by other factors such as budget, time available, and the target degree of precision. The sample size can be calculated using the formula:

$$n = \frac{t^2 \times p(1-p)}{m^2}$$

Where:
n = required sample size
t = confidence level at 95% (standard value of 1.96)
p = estimated prevalence of the variable of interest (e.g. 20% or 0.2 of the population are smokers)
m = margin of error at 5% (standard value of 0.05)

FREQUENCY DISTRIBUTION

Frequency distribution is a representation, either in a graphical or tabular format that displays the number of observations within a given interval. The interval size depends on the data being analyzed and the goals of the analyst.

Types of Frequency Distribution Tables

Regular Frequency Distribution	Grouped Frequency Distribution
• Lists all of the individual categories (X values) 	X	f	 	1	2	 	2	5	 	3	4	 	4	2	 	5	1	 		Σf = 14		• When listing all of the individual categories is not possible/helpful/reasonable, e.g., Test scores 0–100

The intervals must be mutually exclusive and exhaustive. Frequency distributions are typically used within a statistical context. Generally, frequency distribution can be associated with the charting of a normal distribution.

Definitions

- The frequency is the number of oscillation per unit time. It is used for defining the cyclic process like rotation, oscillation, wave, etc. The completion of the cyclic process at particular interval of time is known as the frequency.
- A frequency distribution table is a chart that summarizes values and their frequency. It is a useful way to organize data if you have a list of numbers that represent the frequency of a certain outcome in a sample. A frequency distribution table has two columns. The first column lists all the various outcomes that occur in the data, and the second column lists the frequency of each outcome. Putting this kind of data into a table helps make it simpler to understand and analyze.

Characteristics of Frequency Distribution

There are four important characteristics of frequency distribution. They are as follows:
1. Measures of central tendency and location (mean, median, mode)
2. Measures of dispersion (range, variance, standard deviation)
3. The extent of symmetry/asymmetry (skewness)
4. The flatness or peakedness (kurtosis).

Importance

It has great importance in statistics. Also, a well-structured frequency distribution makes possible a detailed analysis of the structure of the population with respect to given characteristics. Therefore, the groups into which the population breaks down can be determined.

Components of Frequency Distribution

The various components of the frequency distribution are: Class interval, types of class interval, class boundaries, midpoint or class mark, width or size of class interval, class frequency, frequency density = class frequency/class width, relative frequency = class frequency/total frequency, etc.

Uses of Frequency Distribution

- It is quite useful for data analysis.
- It assists in estimating the frequencies of the population on the basis of the ample.
- It facilitates the computation of different statistical measures.

Frequency Distribution Table

Frequency distribution table (also known as frequency table) consists of various components (**Fig. 18.15**).
- **Classes:** A large number of observations varying in a wide range are usually classified in several groups according to the size of their values. Each of these groups is defined by an interval called class interval. The class interval between 10 and 20 is defined as 10–20.
- **Class limits:** The smallest and largest possible values in each class of a frequency distribution table are known as class limits. For the class 10–20, the class limits are 10 and 20. 10 is called the lower class limit and 20 is called the upper class limit.
- **Class limit:** Class limit is the midmost value of the class interval. It is also known as the mid value. Mid value of each class = (lower limit + Upper limit)/2.
- **Magnitude of a class interval:** The difference between the upper and lower limit of a class is called the magnitude of a class interval.
- **Class frequency:** The number of observation falling within a class interval is called class frequency of that class interval.

Types of Frequency Distribution

- **Relative frequency distribution:** It is a distribution where we mention relative frequencies against each class interval.. Relative frequency of a class is the frequency obtained by dividing frequency by the total frequency. Relative frequency is the proportion of the total frequency that is in any given class interval in the frequency distribution.

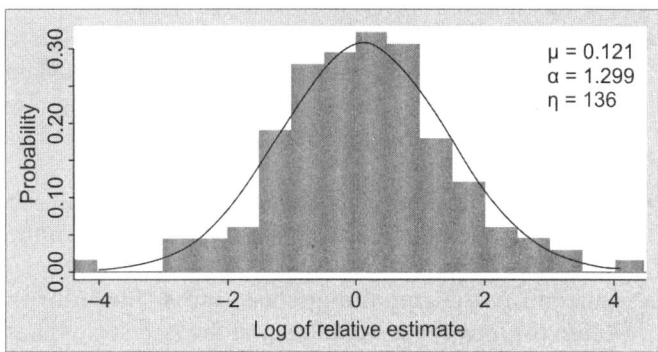

Fig. 18.15: Frequency distribution graph.

- **Cumulative frequency distribution:** One of the important types of frequency distribution is Cumulative frequency distribution. In cumulative frequency distribution, the frequencies are shown in the cumulative manner. The cumulative frequency for each class interval is the frequency for that class interval added to the preceding cumulative total. Cumulative frequency can also be defined as be the sum of all previous frequencies up to the current point.
- **Simple frequency distribution:** Simple frequency distribution is used to organize the larger data sets in an orderly fashion. When there are several cases to be studied, it is a good idea to list them separately, or else there will be a lengthy list to use. A simple frequency distribution shows the number of times each score occurs in a set of data. To find the frequency for score count how many times the score occurs.
- **Grouped frequency distribution:** A grouped frequency distribution is an ordered listed of a variable X, into groups in one column with a listing in a second column, which is called the frequency column. A grouped frequency distribution is an arrangement class intervals and corresponding frequencies in a table.
- **Ungrouped frequency distribution:** A frequency distribution with an interval width of 1 is called ungrouped frequency distribution. Ungrouped frequency distribution is an arrangement of the observed values in ascending order. The ungrouped frequency distribution is those data, which are not arranged in groups. They are known as individual series.
- **Mean of frequency distribution:** Mean of frequency distribution can be found by multiplying each midpoint by its frequency, and then dividing by the total number of values in the frequency distribution.

Mean = $\sum = f \times xn \sum = f \times xn$ where, f = frequency in each class n = sum of the frequencies.

Method to Draw the Frequency Distribution Table

- **Find the range of the data:** The range is the difference between the largest and the smallest values. In our example it is 44–18 = 26.
- **Decide the approximate number of classes:** Which the data are to be grouped. In the case of Thomas, the data size was small so only 3 intervals were selected.
- **Determine the approximate class interval size:** The size of class interval is obtained by dividing the range of data by number of classes. In the case of fractional results, the next higher whole number is taken as the size of the class interval.
- **Decide the starting point:** The lower class limits or class boundary should cover the smallest value in the raw data.
- **Determine the remaining class limits (boundary):** When the lowest class boundary of the lowest class has been decided, then by adding the class interval size to the lower class boundary, compute the upper class boundary. The remaining lower and upper class limits may be determined by adding the class interval size repeatedly till the largest value of the data is observed in the class.
- **Distribute the data into respective classes:** All the observations are marked into respective classes by using Tally Bars (Tally Marks) methods which is suitable for tabulating the observations into respective classes.

Simple Case Study

Mr. X obtained the following marks in his 10 Statistics tests during the semester: 24, 26, 18, 21, 27, 27, 30, 44, 32, 38.

First step is to summarize and see what the data has to say. So how would you organize, classify this data, form the table and present it in the form of a picture? Simplest is to put it in a tabular form (Frequency Distribution):

Class	Frequency
15–25	3
25–35	5
35–45	2

Here the total number of classes is 3. And we can clearly see that most of the marks secured in the mid range. Small number of times very low and very high marks are secured.

COLLECTION OF DATA

The word 'data' is a plural form of the word 'datum' which means information that is systematically collected in the course of a study. The word 'method' refers to the means of gathering data that are common to all sciences including nursing. Questionnaires and interviews are probably the most frequently used data-collection methods in nursing research. Observation is also an important method of testing research hypothesis and seeking answers to research questions.

Data collection is defined as the procedure of collecting, measuring and analyzing accurate insights for research using standard validated techniques. A researcher can evaluate their hypothesis on the basis of collected data. In most cases, data collection is the primary and most important step for research, irrespective of the field of research. The approach of data collection is different for different fields of study, depending on the required information.

DATA COLLECTION PROCESS

There are five important questions to ask when the researcher is in the process of collecting data: What? How? Who? Where? When **(Fig. 18.16)**?
- **What data will be collected?** This question calls for a decision to be made about the type of data that is being sought. The type of data needed to answer the research questions or to test the research hypothesis should be the main consideration in data collection.
- **How will the data be collected?** Some types of research instrument will be needed to gather the data. This can vary from a self-report questionnaire to the most sophisticated

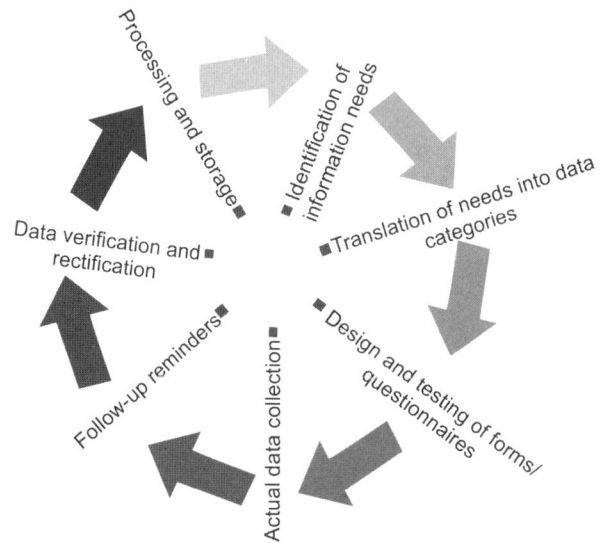

Fig. 18.16: Data collection process.

interest. When several types of data collection methods produce similar results, greater confidence in the study findings will occur.
- Data collection instruments also called research instruments or research tools are the devices used to collect data. The type of instruments used in a study will be determined by the data-collection methods selected.
- Developing an instrument if no instrument can be discovered that is appropriate for a particular study, the researcher is faced with developing a new instrument. It may be possible to revise an existing instrument. Causation must be exercised when this approach to instrument developing is used.
- Pilot study—a pilot study is a small-scale, trial run of the actual research project. A pilot study should be conducted whenever a new instrument is being developed or when a pre-existing instrument is being used with people who have different characteristics from those for whom the instrument was originally developed.

of physiological instruments. Choosing a data collection instrument is a major decision that should be made only after careful consideration of the possible alternatives.
- **Who will collect the data?** If the researcher is going to collect all the data, this question is easy to answer. The people outside the research team may also be used in the data-collection phase. But training will be needed for the data collections and checks should be made on the reliability of the collected data.
- **Where will the data be collected?** The setting for data collection must be carefully determined. Optimum conditions should be sought. If the questionnaires are being used, a researcher might ask respondents to complete the questionnaires while the researcher remains in the same immediate or general area.
- **When will the data be collected?** The determination will need to be made of the month, day and sometimes even one hour, for data collection. Also, how long will data collection take? if questionnaires will be used, they should be protested with people similar to the potential research subjects to determines the length of time for completion of the instruments.

DATA COLLECTION METHODS AND INSTRUMENTS

- There are many alternatives to choose from when selecting a data-collection method. These methods include questionnaires, interviews, physiological measures, attitude scales, psychological tests and observational measures.
- The data collection methods are governed by several factors including the research questions or hypothesis, the design of the study and the amount of knowledge available about the variable of interest.
- Many studies use more than one data-collection method; in fact, nursing studies are increasingly reporting the use of more than one method of measuring the variables of

SELECTION CRITERIA FOR DATA COLLECTION METHOD

There are several criteria to be considered when deciding on a data-collection instrument; these include the practicality, reliability and validity of the instrument.
- **Practicality of the instrument:** The practicality of the instrument concerns its cost and appropriateness for the population.
- **Reliability of the instrument:** The reliability of an instrument determines its consistency and stability.
    - *Stability reliability:* The consistency of a research instrument over time, test-retest procedures and repeated observation are methods to test the stability of an instrument.
    - *Equivalence reliability:* The degree of an instrument to which two forms of an instrument obtain the same results or two or more observers obtain the same results when using single instruments to measure a variable.
    - *Internal consistency reliability:* (scale homogeneity) The extent to which all items of an instrument measure the same variable.
- **Validity:** The validity refers to how well the results among the study participants represent true findings among similar individuals outside the study. The types of validity are face, content, criterion and construct.
    - *Face validity:* It measures the degree to which an instrument appears, on the surface, to measure the variable of interest.
    - *Content validity:* It is concerned with the scope or range of items used to measure the variable.
    - *Criterion validity:* It considers the degree to which an instrument correlates with some criterion measure on the variable of interest. Two types of criterion validity are concurrent and predictive.
        i. **Concurrent validity:** Compares an instrument's measurement of a variable with a criterion measure of the same variable.

ii. **Predictive validity:** It examines the ability of an instrument to predict behavior of subjects in the future.
- **Construct validity:** It concerns the measurement of a variable that is not directly observable but rather is closely associated.

QUESTIONNAIRES

Questionnaires is a paper-pencil, self-report instrument. It contains questions that respondents are asked to answer in writing. Questionnaires can be used to measure knowledge levels, opinions, attitudes, beliefs, ideas, feelings and perceptions, as well as to gather factual information about the respondents **(Fig. 18.17)**.

Factors to consider in constructing questionnaires are overall appearance, language and reading level, length of questionnaires and questions, wording of questions, types of questions and placement of questions.

Types of Question

- **Ambiguous questions** contain word that has more than meaning.
- **Double barreled questions**—ask two questions in one.
- **Demographic questions**—it concerns subject characteristics.
- **Open ended questions**—it allows respondents to answer questions in their own words.
- **Closed ended questions** are very structured and respondents are asked to choose from given alternatives.
- **Contingency questions** are items that are relevant for some respondents and not for others.
- **Filler questions** are items in which the researcher has no direct interest but are included on a question to reduce the emphasis on the specific purpose of other question.

Advantages of Questionnaires

- It is a quick and generally in expensive means of obtaining data from a large number of respondents.
- It is one of the earliest research instruments to test for reliability and validity.
- The administration of questionnaires is less time consuming than interviews or observation research.
- Data can be obtained from respondents in wide-spread geographical area.
- Respondents can remain anonymous.
- If anonymity is assured, respondents are more likely to provide honest answers.

Disadvantages of Questionnaires

- Mailing of questionnaires may be costly
- Response rate may be low.
- Respondents may provide socially acceptable answers.
- Respondents may fail to answer some of the items.
- There is no opportunity to clarify items that may be misunderstood by respondents.
- Respondents must be literate.
- The respondents may not be representative of the population.

INTERVIEWS

An interview is a data-collection method in which an interviewer obtains responses from a subject in a face to face meeting or from telephone interviews. Interviews are frequently used in descriptive research studies and qualitative studies. Interviews are used to obtain factual data about people as well as to measure their opinions, attitudes, and beliefs about certain topics **(Fig. 18.18)**.

Definitions

- Interview is a method of data collection in which one person asks questions of another person. Interviews are conducted either face to face or by telephones.
- The interview constitutes a social situation between two persons, the psychological process involved requiring both individuals mutually respond though the social research purpose of the interview calls for a varied response from the two parties concerned.

Types of Interviews

- **Unstructured interviews:** It contains open-ended questions and is appropriate for exploratory studies where the researcher possess little knowledge of the study topic.

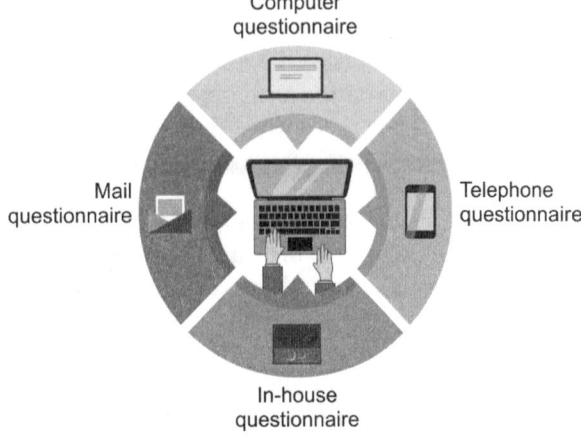

Fig. 18.17: Types of questioning technique.

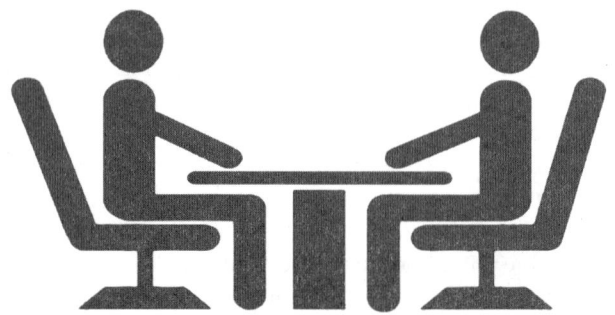

Fig. 18.18: Interview techniques.

- **Structured interviews:** It uses closed-ended questions and are generally used to obtain straight forward, factual information.
- **Semi-structured interviews:** It contains both open-ended and close-ended questions. The majority of interviews are of the semi structured type.

Aims of Interview

- **Direct contact:** The first and the foremost aim of the interview method is to bring the interviewer and the interviewer into direct contact so that both may know each other and understand the respective need of each other.
- **Eliciting intimate facts:** There are many facts of personal life, which a person does not like to reveal. An interviewer concentrates on knowing the unique facts about a person.
- **Establishing hypothesis:** Sometimes the interviewer reveals such facts about the background of his peculiar attitudes, outlooks, aspirations and behaviors as are not already in the comprehension of the interviewer.

Advantages of Interviews

- Responses can be obtained from a wide range of subjects.
- Response rate is high.
- Most of the data obtained are usable.
- In-depth responses can be obtained.
- Nonverbal behavior and verbal mannerisms can be observed.

Disadvantages of Interviews

- Training programs are needed for interviewers.
- Interviews are time consuming and expensive.
- Arrangements for interviews may be difficult to make.
- Subject may provide socially acceptable responses.
- Subject may be anxious because answers are being recorded.
- Subject may be influenced by interviewer's characteristics,
- Interviewer may misinterpret non-verbal behavior.

OBSERVATION METHODS

Observation research is concerned with gathering data through visual observation. Nurses are well qualified to conduct observation research because observations of clients in healthcare setting are an everyday experience. The researcher must decide what behaviors will be observed, who will observe the behavior, what observational procedure will be used and what type of relationship will exist between the observer and the subjects. Few types pf observational methods are depicted in **Figure 18.19**.

Types of Observation Procedures

- **Structured observations** are carried out when the researcher has prior knowledge about the phenomenon of interest. The data collection tool is usually some kind of checklist. The expected behavior or interest has been identified on the checklist. The observer only needs to indicate the frequency of occurrence of these behaviors.
- **Unstructured observations:** The researcher attempts to describe events or behaviors as they occur, with no preconceived ideas of what will be seen. This requires a high degree of concentration and attention by the observer.

Relationship between Observer and Subjects

- **Nonparticipant observer-overt:** The observer openly identifies the research is being conducted.
- **Nonparticipant observer-covert:** Does not identify herself as a researcher. This type of observation is quite likely to be unethical.
- **Participant observer-overt:** Involves with subjects openly and with the full awareness of those people who will be observed in their natural settings.
- **Participant observer-covert:** Interacts with subject's observers their behavior without their knowledge.

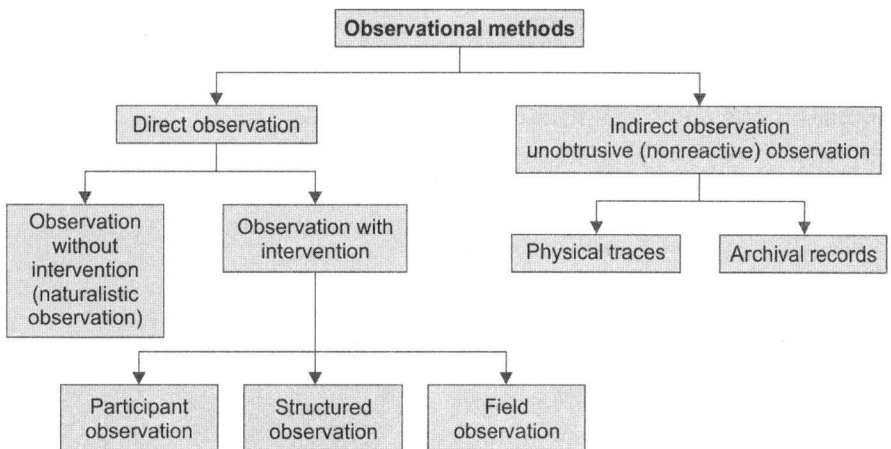

Fig. 18.19: Types of observation method.

OTHER OBSERVATIONAL METHODS

- **Physiological measures:** Measures involve the collection of physical data from subjects. These measures are generally quite accurate. Many physiological data-collection devices are available to nurses, such as thermometers, sphygmomanometers and stethoscopes. Results of electrocardiograms, electroencephalograms and other tests are also readily available to nurse researcher. One of the greatest disadvantages is that special expertise may be necessary to use some of these devices.
- **Attitude scale:** Attitude scales are self-report data collection instrument that ask respondents to report their attitudes or feelings on a continuum. The attitude scales are composed of a number of related items, and respondents are given a score after the item responses are totaled.

Types of Attitude Scale

- **Likert scale:** The Likert scale was named after its developer, Rensis Likert. These scales usually contain five or seven responses for each item, ranging from strongly agree to strongly disagree. An approximately equal number of positively and negatively worded items should be included on a Likert instrument.
- **Semantic differential scale:** This technique was developed by Osgood, Suci and Tannenbaum (1957) to measure the psychological meaning of concepts. They used the term semantic differential to indicate that the difference in subject's attitudes could be compared by examining their responses in "semantic space" or attitudinal space. This technique also may be used to evaluate a setting a person, a group or an educational course.

PSYCHOLOGICAL TESTS

- **Personality inventories:** They are self-report measures used to assess the differences in personality traits, needs or values of people. These inventories seek information about a person by asking questions or requesting responses to statements that are presented. Scores are then derived for each person for the trait being measured. Some of the commonly used personality inventories are the Minnesota multiphasic personality inventory (MMPI) and Edwards personal preference schedule (EPPS).
- **Projective techniques:** A data-collection method that is believed to be more accurate in gathering psychological data is the projective method. In the various projective techniques, a subject is presented with stimuli that are designed to be ambiguous or to have no definite meaning. Then the person is asked to describe the stimuli or to tell what the stimuli appear to represent. The response reflects the internal feelings of the subjects that are projected onto the external stimuli. The commonly used projective test is the thematic appearance test.

Other Methods

- **Q-methodology:** Also called Q-sort, is a means of obtaining data in which subjects sort statements into categories, according to their attitudes forward or rating of the statements. The statements are written on card or pieces of paper and respondents are asked to arrange the items in piles according to the intensity of their attitudes or beliefs about the items.
- **Delphi technique:** It uses several rounds of questionnaires to seek consensus on a particular topic from a group of experts. This procedure is appropriate for examining the opinions, beliefs or future predictions of knowledgeable people on a topic of interest.
- **Visual analog scale (VAS):** Represents subjects with a straight line drawn on a piece of paper, and subjects are asked to make a mark on the line at the point that corresponds to their experience of pain, for example.
- **Pre-existing data:** Are data from records of agencies such as hospitals, the governments and public health departments that have not been collected for research purposes.

LIKERT SCALES

The Likert Scale is an ordinal psychometric measurement of attitudes, beliefs and opinions. In each question, a statement is presented in which a respondent must indicate a degree of agreement or disagreement in a multiple choice type format.

The advantageous side of the Likert Scale is that they are the most universal method for survey collection, therefore they are easily understood. The responses are easily quantifiable and subjective to computation of some mathematical analysis. Since it does not require the participant to provide a simple and concrete yes or no answer, it does not force the participant to take a stand on a particular topic, but allows them to respond in a degree of agreement; this makes question answering easier on the respondent (**Fig. 18.20**).

Advantages

- They are quick and economical to administer and score.
- They are easily adapted to most attitude measurement situations.
- They provide direct and reliable assessment of attitudes when scales are well constructed.
- They lend themselves well to item analysis procedures.

Disadvantages

- Results are easily faked where individuals want to present a false impression of their attitudes (this can be offset

Fig. 18.20: Likert scales.

somewhat by developing a good level of rapport with the respondents and convincing them that honest responses are in their best interests).
- Intervals between points on the scale do not present equal changes in attitude for all individuals (i.e., the differences between "strongly agree" and "agree" may be slight for one individual and great for another).
- Internal consistency of the scale may be difficult to achieve (care must be taken to have unidimensional items aimed at a single person, group, event or method).
- Good attitude statements take time to construct (it is usually best to begin by constructing several times as many attitude statements as you will actually need, then selecting only those that best assess the attitude in question).

DATA PRESENTATION

Presentation of data is generally done by either of these two methods: a. Tabular presentation, b. Graphical presentation. Tabulated data will give some information and also allow for further analysis. The columns and rows in a table make eye strain and there are chances of poor visual impression of data presented in a tabular form. In such circumstances data can be presented in the form of picture, diagram or figure which will help in good comparison through good visual impression. Hence, graphs and diagrams are of utmost importance in creating interest from the observational data. One should take care to select major data presentable in graph or diagram. The presentation of data by diagram proves a very considerable aid and has much to commend it, if certain basic principles are not forgotten. Main objective of diagram is to help the eye to grasp series of numbers and to grasp the meaning of series of data and also to assist the intelligence.

Need Data Presentation

Raw data should be presented in a correct manner so that it:
- Arouses interest in the reader.
- Makes the data sufficiently concise without losing important details.
- Enables the readers to form quick impression and to draw some conclusion directly or indirectly.
- Facilitates further statistical analysis.
- It facilitates good communication.

Quantitative Data Presentation

- **Tabulation:** Tabulation is the first step before the data is used for analysis of interpretation. A table can be simple or complex. Both qualitative and quantitative data may be presented in numerical form through tables.
- **Tabular presentation:** Frequency distribution table: It is the method by which data of a long series of observations are systematically organized and recorded. Each one of the observations should fall into one and only one of the categories and there should be at least one category for each observation, i.e., categories should mutually exclusive and exhaustive.

Steps for Presentation of a Frequency Distribution Table

- Determine the range between the highest and lowest observation.
- Settle upon either number or size of the groupings (class intervals) for making classification. Estimate the other (number of classes or size! width) by using the relationship. $W = R/K$; where W is width or size of the class K is no. of class intervals R range (difference between the smallest and the largest observation).
- A commonly followed rule of thumb states that there should be no fewer than six intervals and no more than 15. Those who wish to have more specific guidance in the matter of deciding how many class intervals are needed may use the formula which gives $K = 1 + 3.322 \log(N)$; where, K stands for the no. of class intervals and N is the no. of values in the data set under consideration. Class intervals generally should be of the same width, this is essential for comparison of different class frequencies.
- Tally the observations in their proper class. (Give four straight and one oblique line to make a bundle of five.)
- Count tallies and present the classification in tabular form with a suitable heading.

DIAGRAMMATIC/GRAPHICAL PRESENTATION OF DATA

Charts and diagrams are useful methods of presenting simple statistical data. Diagrams are better retained in the memory than statistical tables. Diagrams are attractive and easy to understand, at the same time they free us from the burden of figures, comparison is made easy, time and energy is saved and they become more effective and useful in research.

General Principles

- It should be simple and attractive
- It should be of proper size
- Minimum use of words and figures
- It should present the reality
- Symbolic presentation and its explanation are essential
- The facts should be clearly classified in the diagram
- Every diagram or chart should have a heading
- The diagram should be absolutely neat and clean.

General Rules of Constructing Diagrams

The following general rules should be followed while constructing diagrams:
- **Title:** Every diagram must be given a suitable title. The title should convey in as few words as possible the main idea that the diagrams intend to portray.
- **Proportion between width and height:** A proper proportion between the height and width of the diagram should be maintained. If the height and width is too short or too long in proportion, the diagram would give an ugly look.
- **Selection of scale:** The scale showing the values should be in even numbers or in multiplies of five or ten, e.g., 25, 50, 75 or 20, 40. 60. Odd values like 1, 3, 5, 7 should be avoided.

- **Footnotes:** In order to clarify certain points about the diagram, footnotes may be given at the bottom of the diagram.
- **Index:** An index illustrating different types of lines or different shades. Colors should be given so that the reader can easily make out the meaning of the diagram.
- **Neatness and cleanliness:** Diagram should be absolutely neat and clean.
- **Simplicity:** Diagram should be as simple as possible so that the reader can understand their meaning clearly and easily.

Advantages of Diagrammatic Presentation

The most important advantages of diagrammatic presentation of data is that diagrams are very attractive and interesting so far as the common man is concerned. Since no efforts are necessary in understanding diagrams they may save time which is otherwise needed in drawing inferences from set of figures.
- To compare two or more numbers (bar, pictogram).
- To express the distribution of individual objects or measurements into different categories (histogram and pie chart).
- To express the change in some quantity over a period of time (line graph).
- To express the relationship between two measurements in it situation where they occur in pairs (scatter diagram).

Presentation of Quantitative, Continuous or Measured Data is Through Graphs

Histogram

It is a pictorial diagram of frequency distribution. It consists of a series of blocks. The class intervals are given along the horizontal axis and the frequencies along the vertical axis. They are of each block or rectangle is proportion to the frequency.
- It is a graphical presentation of frequency distribution. Variable characters of the different groups are indicated on the horizontal line (X-axis) called abscissa while frequency, i.e., number of observations is marked on the vertical line (Y-axis) called ordinate. Frequency of each group will form a column or rectangle.
- If the class intervals are different in certain groups then area of the rectangle alone indicates the frequency, e.g. the frequency of the persons in group with size of Mantoux reaction from 16 to 24 mm may be presented as one rectangle only. In this case to plot the frequency for this group, divide the total frequency by 4 (40 ÷ 4).
- Now the horizontal line will start opposite 10 on the vertical line. It would have given an erroneous idea if the horizontal line would start opposite 40 on the vertical line, instead of 10.

Frequency Polygon

A frequency distribution may also be represented diagrammatically by the frequency polygon. It is obtained by joining the mid-point of the histogram blocks. It has more than four sides. It is particularly effective comparing two more frequency distribution (**Fig. 18.21**).

It is again an area diagram of frequency distribution developed over a histogram. Join the mid-points of class intervals at the height of frequencies by straight lines. It gives a polygon, i.e., a figure with many angles. In this diagram also, the last frequencies in percentages may be grouped into one and the average of 4 groups in percentage may be plotted. The end of the polygon will now be a straight line parallel to the baseline extending from 16 to 24 mm corresponding to the average frequency of this group on the vertical line. It is used when sets of data are to be illustrated on the same diagram such as birth and death rates, birth of diabetics and nonlinear, etc.

Types

There are two ways in which a frequency polygon may be constructed:
1. Draw a histogram of the give data and then join by straight lines the mid pints of the upper horizontal side of each rectangle with the adjacent ones. The figure formed is called frequency polygon.
2. Another method is to take the mid-points of the various class intervals and then plot the frequency corresponding to each point and to join all these points by straight lines. Here there will be no histogram.

Steps in Drawing Frequency Polygon

- First take the first group with the lowest class interval, then take the midpoint of these class interval. So place a point corresponding to OX-axis and on OY-axis.
- The same way all the frequencies are marked.
- Then connect the points with straight line.
- Rather than leaving the graph incomplete assumes that there is another interval above or below which is having frequencies of zero. So correct the curve to this zero line. The graph is allowed to meet X-axis on both ends.

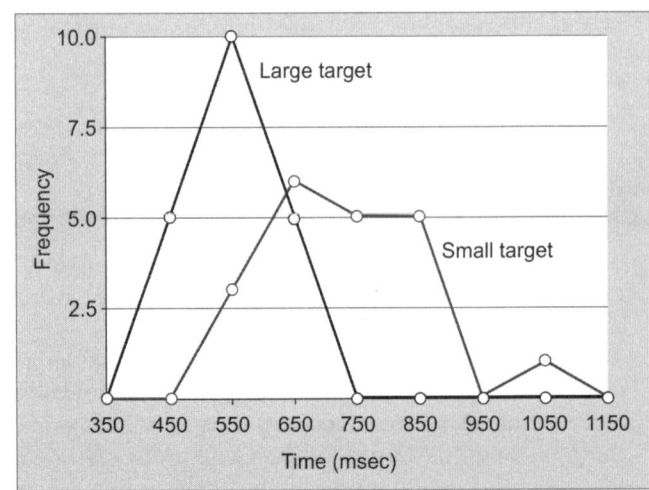

Fig. 18.21: Frequency polygon graph.

Advantages

- Easy to construct and interpret.
- Useful in portaging more than two distributions on same graph with different colors.
- Useful to compare two or more distributions.

Frequency Curve

When the number of observations is very large and group interval is reduced, the frequency polygon tends to lose its angulation giving place to a smooth curve known as frequency curve. This provides continuous graph giving the relative frequency for each value of an attribute such as that of height of a normal curve. Such a curve is obtained in normal distribution of individuals in a large sample or of means in population or of differences in pairs of sample means.

Line Chain or Graph

Line diagrams are used to show the trend of events with the passage of time. The data is presented with the help of horizontal line and the paths of line show the trend of incidents. This is a frequency polygon presenting variations by line. It shows the trend of an event occurring over a period of time rising, falling or showing fluctuations such as of cancer deaths, infant mortality rate, birth rate, death rate, etc., say from year 1900 to 1960. The class interval may be a month, a year, 5 years or 10 years. Deteriorating or improving trend before and after a public health measure, such as fall of malaria cases each year after DDT spray can be seen at a glance from such a figure. Vertical axis may not start from zero but at some point above when frequencies start at high level indicating the population trend in India. The shape of line chart may alter with change of scale on the vertical or horizontal axis but the trend indicated, remains the same. The proportional change may be there when scales are changed.

Cumulative Frequency Diagram or Ogive

Ogive is a graph of the cumulative relative frequency distribution. To draw this, an ordinary frequency distribution table in a quantitative data has to be converted into a relative cumulative frequency table **(Fig. 18.22)**.

Cumulative frequency is the total number of persons in each particular range from lowest value of the characteristic up to and including any higher group value. It is obtained by cumulating the frequency of previous classes including the class in question. The reader is familiar with the cumulative cricket score recorded in a cricket test match after each player, simultaneously with the serial record of the number of runs scored by each individual player. The cumulative frequencies are plotted corresponding to the group limits of the characteristic. On joining the points by a smooth free hand curve, the diagram made is called ogive. Now one can locate any percentile that divides the series into two parts, e.g., first decile divides the total frequency into 10% and 90%.

Instead of frequencies, cumulative frequencies (successive class frequencies are added) are used to draw

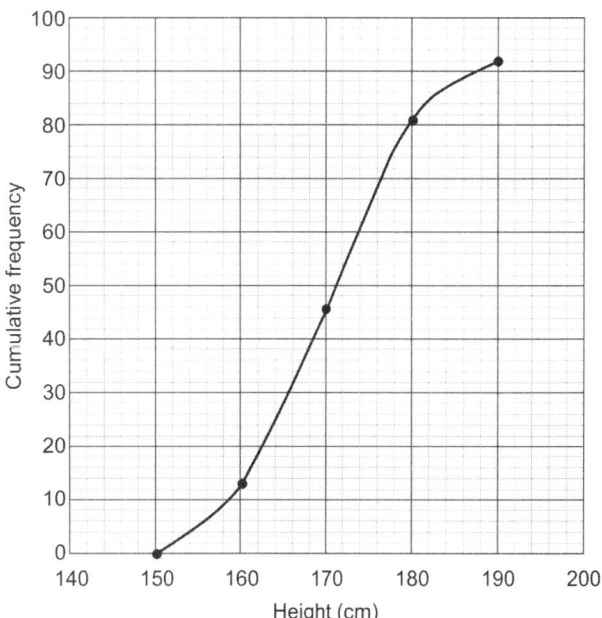

Fig. 18.22: Cumulative frequency diagram.

frequency polygon, similar to frequency polygon. Number or percent of observations falling below or above a specific value can be presented in this graph. Any point below which there are certain percent of observations is called as percentile. For example, 90th percentile is such an observation below which there are 90% observations. Graph drawn out of such points is called a percentile graph.

Methods of Constructing Ogive

There are two methods of constructing ogive, namely:
1. **Less than method:** In the less than method, we start with the upper limits of the classes and go on adding the frequencies. When these frequencies are plotted we get a rising curve.
2. **More than method:** In more than method, we start with the lower limit of the classes and from the frequencies we subtract the frequencies of each class. When these frequencies are plotted we get a declining curve.

Application of Ogive

- By using Ogive, we can locate any percentile that will divide the series into two parts.
- Comparison of one percentile values of a variables of one sample with that of another sample drawn from some population or different population.
- To study growth in children.
- As a measure of dispersion (interquartile range of semi-quartile range) it is also useful.

Scatter or Dot Diagram

Scattered or dot design otherwise called statistical maps. When statistical data refer to geographical or administrative areas; it is presented either as shaded maps or dot maps.

- Scatter diagram shows the relationship between two variables. It is also a simple way of diagrammatic representation of a bivariate distribution by which we can ascertain the correlation between the two variables.
- It is prepared after tabulation in which frequencies of at least two variables have been cross classified.
- It is a graphic presentation, made to show the nature of correlation between two variable characters X and 'Y in the same persons (s) of group(s) such as height and weight in men aged 20 years, hence it is also called correlation diagram. The characters are read on the base (height) and vertical (weight) axes and the perpendiculars drawn from these readings meet to give one scatter point.
- Varying frequencies of the characters give a number of such points or dots that show a scatter.
- This is the best suitable graphical technique to find any possible relationship that may exist between two quantitative variables. When observations for two variables are made/available on the subject to study the possible relationship, values are plotted on the two axes of the graph paper.
- The characters (variables) are read on the horizontal (X-axis) and vertical (Y-axis) axes and the perpendicular drawn from these readings meet to give one scatter point.
- After plotting all the points, when they are viewed collectively the trend of the points will suggest any possible relationship (strength as well as type) that may exist between the variables.

Types of Scatter Diagram

They cover almost all types of scatter diagrams used in project management **(Fig. 18.23)**.

According to the correlation, you can divide scatter diagrams into the following categories:
- Scatter diagram with no correlation
- Scatter diagram with moderate correlation
- Scatter diagram with strong correlation

Limitations of a Scatter Diagram

The following are a few limitations of a scatter diagram:
- Scatter diagrams cannot give you the exact extent of correlation.
- A scatter diagram does not show you the quantitative measurement of the relationship between the variables. It only shows the quantitative expression of quantitative change.
- This chart does not show you the relationship for more than two variables.

Benefits of a Scatter Diagram

The following are a few advantages of a scatter diagram:
- It shows the relationship between two variables.
- It is the best method to show you a non-linear pattern.
- The range of data flow, i.e., maximum and minimum value, can be determined.
- Observation and reading are straightforward.
- Plotting the diagram is easy.

QUALITATIVE DATA PRESENTATION

Charts and diagrams are useful methods of presenting simple statistical data. Diagrams are better retained in the memory than statistical tables. Diagrams are attractive and easy to understand, at the same time they free us from the burden of figures, comparison is made easy, time and energy is saved and they become more effective and useful in research.

General Principles

- It should be simple and attractive
- It should be of proper size
- Minimum use of words and figures
- It should present the reality
- Symbolic presentation and its explanation are essential
- The facts should be clearly classified in the diagram
- Every diagram or chart should have a heading
- The diagram should be absolutely neat and clean.

Presentation of Qualitative, Discrete or Counted Data is through Diagrams

The common diagrams in use are:
- Bar diagram
- Pie or sector diagram
- Pictogram or picture diagram
- Map diagram or spot map.

Uses of graphical presentation:
- Easy for comparison.
- Trends in the observation can be noticed with respect of time.

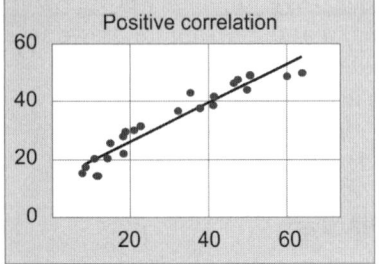 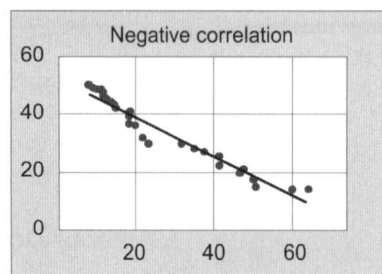 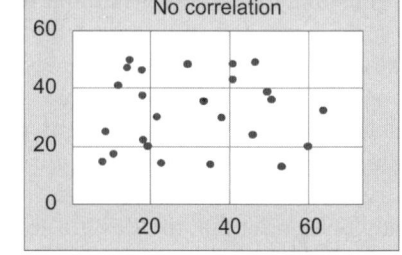

Fig. 18.23: Types of scatter diagram.

- Lay people can understand it.
- Median, percentile, quartile, etc. can be calculated.
- When lot of fluctuations is seen, then semi log or double log graphs can be good representations. Here, by double log graphs, irregularities (that are seen in arithmetic scale) is smoothened out.

Bar Diagram

Bar charts are merely a way of presenting a set of numbers by the length of a bar-the length of the bar is proportional to the magnitude to be represented. Bar charts are a popular media of presenting stationary data because they are easy to prepare and enable values to be compared visually **(Fig. 18.24)**.

- The types of bar charts are simple bar chart, multiple bar charts and component bar chart. From frequency table, data on variable is represented on "X" axis and the frequency on "Y" axis.
- The rectangles drawn are called bars. In the case of qualitative data, bar represents the frequency of a group. In the case of quantitative data, bar represents frequencies of a class interval.
- Breadth of bar represents characteristic group in case of qualitative data and represents length of class interval in case of quantitative data.
- The base will have equal width. Height of bar itself will tell us the comparison.
- The bar can be represented vertically or horizontally which give vertical simple bar diagram or horizontal simple bar diagram.
- In the case of multiple bar diagram, study of sub-classification of data can be done by using more than one bar and are separately indexed to make the graph clearly understandable.
- In the case of component bar chart, the proportion of subgroups between two major categories are represented with a bar giving proportion to each of them within the bar.
- It is also advisable to make one bar as 100% and each subcategory is given proportion within the bar.

Types of Bar Charts

The bar graphs can be vertical or horizontal. The primary feature of any bar graph is its length or height. If the length of the bar graph is more, then the values are greater of any given data. Bar graphs normally show categorical and numeric variables arranged in class intervals. They consist of an axis and a series of labeled horizontal or vertical bars.

Vertical bar graphs: When the grouped data are represented vertically in a graph or chart with the help of bars, where the bars denote the measure of data, such graphs are called vertical bar graphs. The data is represented along the Y-axis of the graph and the height of the bars shows the values.

Horizontal bar graphs: When the grouped data are represented horizontally in a chart with the help of bars, then such graphs are called horizontal bar graphs, where the bars shows the measure of data. The data is depicted here along the X-axis of the graph and the length of the bars denotes the values **(Fig. 18.25)**.

Uses of Bar Graphs

- Bar graphs are used to match things between different groups or to trace changes over time. Yet, when trying to estimate change over time, bar graphs are most suitable when the changes are bigger.
- Bar charts possess a discrete domain of divisions and are normally scaled so that all the data can fit on the graph. When there is no regular order of the divisions being matched, bars on the chart may be organized in any order.
- Bar charts organized from the highest to the lowest number are called Pareto charts.

Advantages of Bar Graph

- Show each data category in a frequency distribution
- Display relative numbers/proportions of multiple categories
- Summarize a large amount of data in a visual, easily interpretable form
- Make trends easier to highlight than tables do

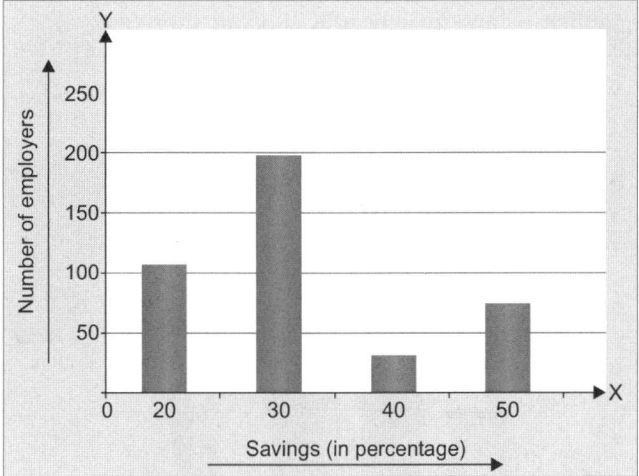

Fig. 18.24: Bar diagram.

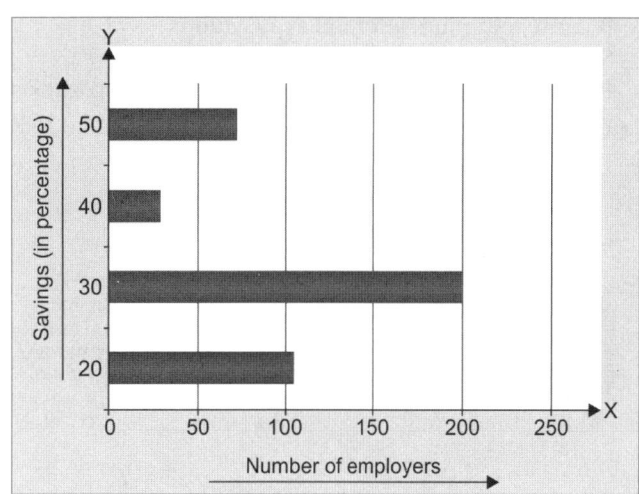

Fig. 18.25: Horizontal bar graphs.

- Estimates can be made quickly and accurately
- Permit visual guidance on accuracy and reasonableness of calculations
- Accessible to a wide audience.

Disadvantages of Bar Graph
- Often require additional explanation
- Fail to expose key assumptions, causes, impacts and patterns
- Can be easily manipulated to give false impressions

Pie Diagram

Pie charts are extremely popular with the laity, but not with statistician who considers them inferior to bar charts. It is often necessary to indicate the percentages in the segments. The pie chart can be made more attractive by giving three dimensional effects to it. The pie diagrams are useful for depicting the relative frequency of disease by system or part of the body affected by place or by season of occurrence (**Fig. 18.26**).

- This is another way of presenting discrete data of qualitative characters such as blood groups, Rh groups, age groups, sex groups, causes of mortality or social groups in a population.
- The frequencies of the groups are shown in a circle. Degrees of angle denote the frequency and area of the sector.
- It gives comparative difference at a glance. Accordingly, the size of angle for blood groups A, B, AB and 0 gives frequency of the groups such as 26.5%, 34.5%, 17.4% and 21.6%, (total 100), respectively can be drawn, in which pie diagram percentage mortality in the world is indicated by 4 major causes of death.

Definition

A pie chart or circle chart is circular statistical chart graph, which is divided into slices to illustrate numerical proportions. While it is named for its similarity to a pie which have been sliced, there are variation on the way it can be presented.

Advantages of Pie Chart
- Display relative proportions of multiple classes of data.
- Require minimum addition explanations
- Summarize a large data set into visual form
- Pie charts are easily understood due to its widespread use in business and media
- Pie charts permit a visual check of the reasonableness or accuracy of calculation.
- Pie charts are visually simpler than other types of graphs.
- Size of the circle can be made proportional to the quantity it represents.

Disadvantages of Pie Chart
- It does not easily reveal exact values
- Pie chart does not easily show changes over time
- Pie charts fail to reveal key assumptions, causes, effects or patterns
- Pie charts can easily be manipulated to yield false impression.

Pictogram or Picture Diagram

Pictogram, the data are made clear with the help of pictures or symbols. Pictograms are a popular method of presenting data to the "man in the street" and to those who cannot understand orthodox charts. The fractions of the picture can be used to represent numbers smaller than the value of a whole symbol. It is a popular method to impress the frequency of the occurrence of events to common man such as attacks, deaths, and number operated, admitted, discharged, accidents, etc. in a population (**Fig. 18.27**).

Advantages of a Pictograph
- Express a large amount of information or data in a simple form.
- Since they make the use of symbols, pictographs attract attention, i.e., it is an attractive way to represent data.
- Pictographs are easy to read since all the information is available at one glance.
- And since pictographs are universally used they do not require a lot of explanation.

Effective Use of Pictograms

There are a number of guidelines to be followed when developing or applying a pictogram to consumer safety information:
- There are no strict rules on what makes a good pictogram. It depends on the product, the hazard, and the consumer audience, and must be fully consumer tested.

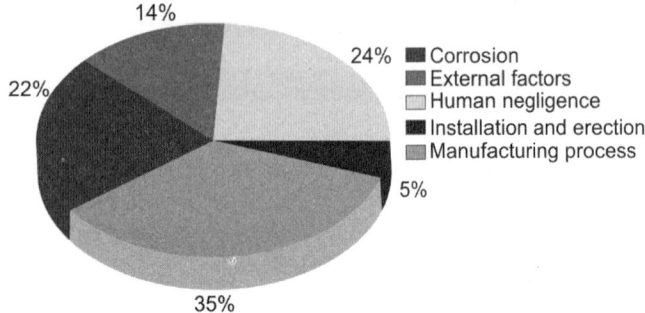

Fig. 18.26: Pie diagram.

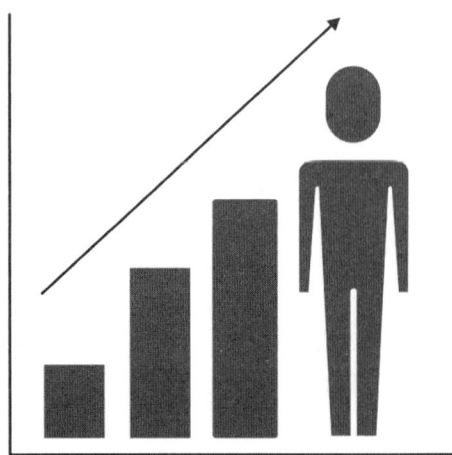

Fig. 18.27: Pictograms.

- There is evidence to suggest that it is more difficult to design pictograms to convey complex safety messages. Care should be taken particularly with the use of pictograms to describe complex prescriptive or proscriptive messages.
- There may be two possible functions for pictograms: as a reminder/attention grabber for an established message, or to stand alone to convey a message. These different functions require different treatment.
- No pictogram will be instantly effective. The longer a pictogram is in circulation the better known it will be.
- Needless differences in the design of pictograms will work only to undermine their effectiveness.

Map Diagram or Spot Map

These maps are prepared to show geographical distribution of frequencies of characteristic. The in the statewise map of India indicates the IMR in the state which is lowest of 23 in Kerala and highest of 126 in Orissa (Fig. 18.28).

Definition

Dot maps are used to visualize distributions and densities of a big number of discrete distributed single objects whereas, in contrast to location maps, not every single object is depicted but one symbol represents a constant number of objects. For this visualization simple or pictorial point symbols can be used. Widely used are points which lead to the name of this map type. Population density maps are often dot maps.

Advantages of Dot Maps

- If well constructed it shows distribution and comparative densities.
- It is easier to show variation in distribution of wide variety of commodities if it is presented using different colors.
- Dot maps are used to represent wide range of items like population, value of minerals, crops and so forth.
- They are very easy to construct compared to proportional circles.
- It is very easy to compare the distribution of items considering the concentration of dots.

Disadvantages of Dot Maps

- It is time consuming especially when marking dots on maps.
- When the scale is small many dots are drawn which cause overcrowding and present difficult in counting them to get the actual value.
- In case even distribution of dots is displayed on the map, false impression that the distribution is the same in represented area is perceived. This perception may be false.
- Locating dots on map is to the certain extent a personal and subjective decision and two dot maps donc by two people using the same data will rarely be identical.
- Construction of dot maps involves tedious calculation especially when determining number of dots.

ANALYSIS OF DATA

Data analysis comprises of a collection of methods to deal with data/information obtained through observations, measurements, surveys or experiments about a phenomenon of interest. The aim and purpose of data analysis is to extract as much information as possible that is pertinent to the subject under consideration (Fig. 18.29).

The nature of the subject and also the purpose of analysis may vary greatly. The subject could be physical, social or economic and the purpose of the analysis could be purely academic or practical. Due to the great diversity of statistical data, the methods of analysis and the manner of application differ significantly from situation to situation. One cannot possibly expect a single unified system of techniques to be applicable to all cases. However, we have several formal methods of analysis are more or less mutually related and have been successfully applied to most, if not all statistical data.

Steps of Data Preparation for Analysis

Firstly, before any analysis is carried out, data is entered into a computer system (if not done already) and has to be checked, updated and validated. Next, it is crucial to read and

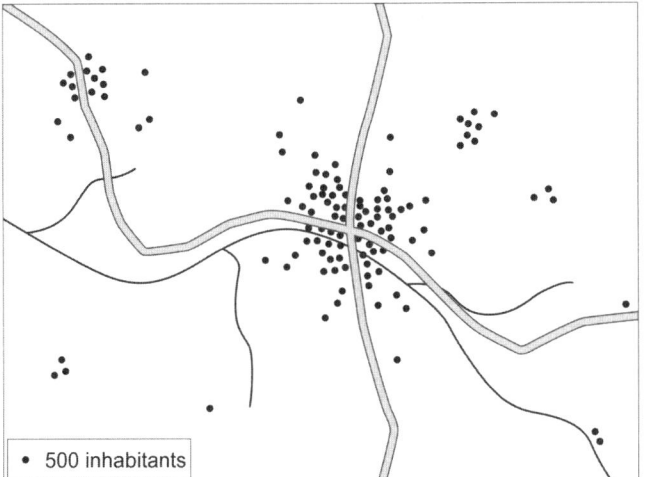

Fig. 18.28: Map diagram or spot map.

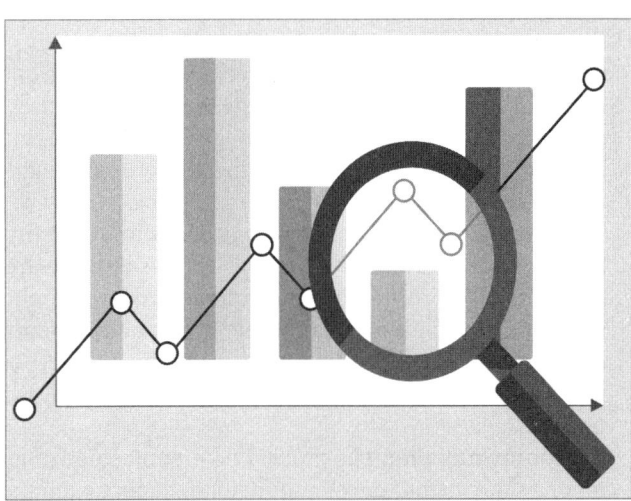

Fig. 18.29: Data analysis.

re-read the data in order to know it inside-out. Get completely familiar with your data before start of any analysis.

Secondly, there follows data manipulation into a structural form suitable for analysis and which the software to be used in the analysis can upload easily. This could involve copying, selecting subsets of the data, transforming and merging the data at various levels. Transforming and deriving new variables from existing ones. This might involve coding and categorizing existing variables. Coding can simply be defined as a process.

Thirdly, it is crucial to identify the data structure, sometimes known as data layers of the data/information to be analyzed. For example, you may have farms, plots within farms or farms, animals within farms or forests, species within forests, etc.

Fourthly, the unit of measurement has to be clearly defined. For example, in a survey that involves farms, information taken will be at individual or at farm level. At the farm level, we may record number of trees, number of persons, and size of the farm in acres and at persons level we could record their ages. Further, we should consider which of our data are quantitative and which are qualitative.

Analysis Styles

- **Quasi-statistical style:** That begins with a pre-established code book of themes or words and that tends itself to basic descriptive statistical analysis.
- **Template analysis style:** That involves the development of an analysis guide used to sort the data.
- **Editing analysis style:** That involves an interpretation of the data on which a categorization scheme is based.
- **Immersion/crystallization style:** That involves the analyst's total immersion in and reflection of text materials. Use a strategy that is best characterized as an editing synthesizing theorizing and re-contextualizing.

Qualitative Analysis Process

- **Comprehending:** The research is able to prepare a thorough and rich description of the phenomenon under study, and new data do not add much to that description. In other words, comprehension is completed when saturation has been attained.
- **Synthesizing:** Synthesizing involves a "sifting" of the data and putting pieces together. At the end of the synthesis process, the researcher can begin to make some, generalized statements about the phenomenon and about the study participants.
- **Theorizing:** Another important process in qualitative analysis is theorizing which involves a systemic sorting of the data. During the theorizing process, the researcher develops alternative explanations of the phenomenon under study. The theorizing process continues to evolve until the best and most parsimonious explanation is obtained.
- **Re-contextualizing:** The process of re-contextualization involves the further development of the theory such that its applicability to other setting or groups is explored.

Analytic Procedures

- The actual analysis of data begins with search for themes. The search for themes involves not only the discovery of commonalities across subjects but also of natural variation in the data.
- The next step generally involves a validation of the thematic analysis.
- Some researchers use quasi-statistics, which involves a tabulation of the frequency with which certain themes or relations are supported by the data.
- In a final step, the analyst tries to weave the thematic strands together into an integrated picture of the phenomenon under investigation.

Ground Theory Analysis

Analytic induction refers to an approach in which the researcher alternates back and forth between tentative definition of emerging hypothesis and tentative explanation.

- **Open coding (level I coding):** The development of a categorization scheme and subsequent initial coding of the data.
- **Axial coding (level II coding):** Is a reconstructive process that puts data back together in new ways by connecting categories and subcategories. The analyst begins the process of integration by reviewing and sorting the memos that have been used to document conceptual ideas throughout the data collection and data analysis process.
- **Selective coding (level III coding):** The ground theory analyst searches for the core category—the central phenomenon used to integrate all others. This phase results in an emergency theory of a basic social process that is grounded in the data.

INTERPRETATION OF DATA

The interpretation of research findings, an activity in which both producers and consumers of research engage, basically is a search of the broader meaning and implications of the results of an investigation. The results of the data analysis need to scrutinized and reflected on with consideration to the conceptual framework, the specific questions that were addressed or the hypothesis that were tested, prior research findings and the short comings of the methods used to answer the research questions. Data analysis and interpretation is the process of assigning meaning to the collected information and determining the conclusions, significance, and implications of the findings (**Fig. 18.30**).

Objectives of Interpretation

- Analyzing the accuracy and believability of the results.
- Searching for the underlying meaning of the results.
- Considering the importance of the findings.
- Analyzing the generalizability and transferability of the finds.
- Assessing the implications of the study in regard of theory, nursing practice and future research.

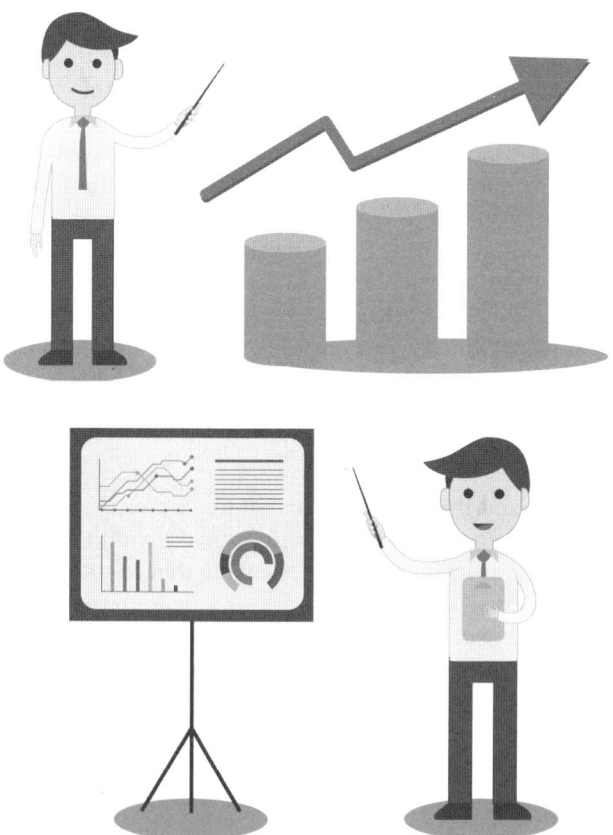

Fig. 18.30: Interpretation of data.

Common Errors of Interpretation

- Failure to see the problem in proper perspective.
- Failure to appreciate the relevance of various elements.
- Failure to recognize limitations in the research evidence.
- Misinterpretation due to unstudied factors.
- Ignoring selective factors.
- Inadequate attention to individual cases.

Numerical Data Interpretation

The analysis of numerical (quantitative) data is represented in mathematical terms. The most common statistical terms include:

- **Mean:** The mean score represents a numerical average for a set of responses.
- **Standard deviation:** The standard deviation represents the distribution of the responses around the mean. It indicates the degree of consistency among the responses. The standard deviation, in conjunction with the mean, provides a better understanding of the data. For example, if the mean is 3.3 with a standard deviation (StD) of 0.4, then two thirds of the responses lie between 2.9 (3.3−0.4) and 3.7 (3.3 + 0.4).
- **Frequency distribution:** Frequency distribution indicates the frequency of each response. For example, if respondents answer a question using an agree/disagree scale, the percentage of respondents who selected each response on the scale would be indicated. The frequency distribution provides additional information beyond the mean, since it allows for examining the level of consensus among the data. Higher levels of statistical analysis (e.g., t-test, factor analysis, regression, ANOVA) can be conducted on the data, but these are not frequently used in most program/project assessments.

Qualitative Data Presentation

- Qualitative data interpretation tends to be more subjective in nature and many times can be influenced by the researcher's biases.
- Effort must be put into the data collection process to eliminate bias including collecting more than one kind of data, get many different kinds of perspectives on the events being studied, purposely look for contradicting information, and acknowledging your biases that relate to the research report.
- Qualitative data analysis is time consuming and complex because a lot of data can be created that is both useful and not useful.
- There is no "correct way" to analyze qualitative data. Efforts can be made to make the data presentation and interpretation more credible and less biased by using the above methods.
- The analysis of narrative (qualitative) data is conducted by organizing the data into common themes or categories. It is often more difficult to interpret narrative data since it lacks the built-in structure found in numerical data.
- Initially, the narrative data appears to be a collection of random, unconnected statements.
- The assessment purpose and questions can help direct the focus of the data organization. The following strategies may also be helpful when analyzing narrative data.

Focus Groups and Interviews

- Read and organize the data from each question separately. This approach permits focusing on one question at a time (e.g., experiences with tutoring services, characteristics of tutor, student responsibility in the tutoring process).
- Group the comments by themes, topics, or categories. This approach allows for focusing on one area at a time (e.g., characteristics of tutor-level of preparation, knowledge of content area, availability).

Documents: Code content and characteristics of documents into various categories (e.g., training manual—policies and procedures, communication, responsibilities).

Observations: Code patterns from the focus of the observation (e.g., behavioral patterns—amount of time engaged/not engaged in activity, type of engagement, communication, interpersonal skills).

The analysis of the data via statistical measures and/or narrative themes should provide answers to the assessment questions. Interpreting the analyzed data from the appropriate perspective allows for determination of the significance and implications of the assessment.

Data Interpretation Method

Descriptive statistics provide a description of what the data look like. They provide a means to describe the points of central tendency (mean, mode, median, etc.) and dispersion (standard deviation, variance, interquartile range, etc.).

Inferential statistics allow the researcher to make inferences about populations from smaller samples of the population. Statistics of the sample are used to estimate parameters of the population. A parameter is a constant value.

Representative of the population (such as population mean and standard deviation) while a statistic is any calculation performed on the sample being tested.

Inferential statistics also allow the researcher to test their research hypotheses. Some measures used in inferential statistics include the standard error of the mean, estimators, and the p-value. The way that the data is interpreted can have varying effects on your conclusions. Absolute honesty in recording and interpreting data is required to maintain the credibility of research. All of the conditions of a situation should be considered and that we make inferences in strict accordance with the data obtained. Using statistics to determine relationships is paramount to the success of good research. Using tools such as ANOVA, correlations, Fisher Exact Tests, regression, etc. can predict whether or not your research hypothesis is satisfied.

Basic Principles in Interpreting the Data

Methods of statistical inference (statistical tests, confidence intervals) are sometimes misused or interpreted incorrectly in practice. Also, the methods should be used consistently with statistical assumptions (including independence assumptions).

Statistical Significance

In general, a statistical test has the following components:
- A **null hypothesis** is formulated. This is usually a probability model that assumes no effect of interest, any apparent effects being attributable to chance.
- A **test statistic** is chosen, which will be computed from results of the experiment to quantify how strongly the results contradict the null hypothesis.
- Once the study has been conducted, the p-value is the probability of any result that contradicts the null hypothesis as strongly as the results actually obtained, based on the value of the test statistic. The p-value from a test is not the probability of truth or untruth of a hypothesis. It is the probability of data that contradict the null hypothesis as strongly as the data actually obtained, if the null hypothesis is true.

Statistical Tests and Randomized Experiments

- Although causal assessments may be based largely on observational data, some consideration of perspectives during planning of a randomized experiment may be helpful in understanding statistical testing concepts.
- At the planning stage, a test statistic is tentatively identified that will be computed from results of the experiment and used in deciding what outcome to report for the experiment.
- In our example, the number of cups that the subject will classify correctly is used to accept or reject the subject's claim.
- A cutoff (critical) value of the test statistic is identified, such that the chance of some erroneous conclusions is acceptably low. Indeed, the experimenter hopes for a low chance of finding an effect, if there really is no effect, i.e., a low chance of a false positive.
- According to the null hypothesis, the treatments may be viewed simply as random labeling of experimental units.
- If the experimenter has decided to enforce a 5% chance of a false positive, use of the critical p-value of 0.05 is justified as just a matter of checking that results satisfy a prespecified criterion, before claiming to have observed something of interest.
- In addition, the experimenter hopes that if there are substantial effects of the treatment, there will be a substantial probability of finding statistical significance, i.e., that the test will have good power.

Confidence Intervals

A 95% confidence interval has the following interpretations:
- There is a 95% chance of the true value of the parameter falling within the interval.
- Values outside the interval can be rejected on the basis of a two-sided statistical test with alpha 5%. Confidence intervals are likely to be more easily interpreted than statistical tests in some situations.
- A large p-value, by itself, is ambiguous, as previously noted. A confidence interval may be more informative, displaying an estimated effect along with a measure of statistical uncertainty (which will be large in case of few or variable data).
- Unlike statistical tests, confidence intervals are neutral regarding the relative "burden of proof" to be associated with various hypotheses about effect sizes.

General Recommendations for the Use of Statistical Tests and Confidence Intervals

- Methods that assume normality should not be applied to data that contain outliers or have heavy-tailed distributions. Rank-based or other outlier-resistant methods may be applied, without needing to exclude putative outliers from the analysis.
- Methods that assume normality may be applied to data with skew distributions if the data are transformed to correct skewness.
- Assessment of distributional assumptions should be based in part on graphical evaluation of distributions and familiarity and experience with particular types of variables, and not only on statistical tests of assumptions. It is often of interest to know in what way a distribution

deviates from normality, e.g., because of outliers or skewness. The normal distribution should not be treated as a default in cases where experience indicates that, say, a particular type of variable is more likely to have a lognormal distribution.
- Possible effects of and remedies for autocorrelation or pseudoreplication should be considered.
- When focusing on effects of one variable, possible effects of other variables should be taken into account. It is desirable to consider methods that minimize confounding. Some standard methods for evaluating the effects of a single variable on a response, while ignoring others may not be suitable for ecological data.
- In a regression context, tests of assumptions are generally applied to regression residuals (differences between observed values of the Y variable, and values predicted by the model).
- Correct use of statistical tests and confidence intervals requires that the appropriate interpretation be kept in mind. In particular, statistical significance (a low p-value) is conceptually distinct from practical significance, i.e., from the issue of whether biological effects observed in a situation are large enough in magnitude to be of practical importance.

COMMUNICATION OF NURSING RESEARCH FINDINGS

There are many different ways for researchers to communicate the results of their studies. They might begin by presenting the results to peers in school or in the agency where they work. Next they might attend a research conference at which they present their study results in an oral presentation or in a poster session. As a next step, they might publish their results in a journal article.

The researchers have the first responsibility of communicating the findings of their studies, other nurses and nursing organizations also bear the responsibility of seeing that research findings are distributed inside the nursing profession to other healthcare disciplines and even to general public.

Methods of Communication

- **The oral presentation** of a research report at a conference is referred to as a paper presentation.
- **Journal articles:** Research is generally published in journal articles. A referred journal is one that uses subject experts to review manuscripts. Non-referred journals use editorial staff members or consultants to review manuscripts.
- **Peers review:** The process involves the review of a manuscript by professional colleagues who have content and methodological expertise in the area of the study discussed in the manuscript.
- **Thesis and dissertations:** They are a means of communicating results of research studies that are conducted in conjunction with educations requirement.

CONCLUSION

The health management information system (HMIS) is a set of integrated components and procedures organized with an objective of generating information which will improve healthcare management decisions at all levels of the health system. It is also a routine monitoring system that plays a specific role in the monitoring and evaluation process which is intended to provide warning signals through the use of indicators.

BIBLIOGRAPHY

1. Health Metrics Network. Version 4.00. Framework and standards for country health information systems: Assessing national HIS information dissemination and use. Geneva, World Health Organization; 2008.
2. Lippeveld, Theo, Sauerborn R and Bodart C. Design and Implementation of Health Information Systems. Health Information System Module. Geneva: WHO; 2000.
3. Park K. Essentials of Community Health Nursing, 4th edition. Jabalpur: Banarasidas Bhanot Publisher; 2004.
4. Swarnkar K. Community Health Nursing, 2nd edition. Indore: N.R. Brother; 2008.
5. World Health Organisation. Components of a strong health information system. A guide to the health metrics network framework. Geneva, World Health Organization; 2008.

REVIEW QUESTIONS

Long Essays

1. Define health management information system (HMIS). Explain the objectives and characteristics.
2. Define health information system (HIS). Explain the objectives, components and uses of health information system.
3. Define vital statistics. Explain the methods of obtaining vital statistics.

Short Essays

1. Components of health information system.
2. Problems or constraints of HMIS in India.
3. Types of healthcare information systems.
4. Sources of health information system.
5. Nursing management information system (NIMS).
6. Health and family planning programs.
7. Vital statistics measurements.
8. Civil registration system.
9. Functions of a civil registration system.
10. Characteristics and advantages of Ad-Hoc testing.
11. Vital registration.
12. Probability sampling methods.
13. Frequency distribution.
14. Types of frequency distribution tables.
15. Selection criteria for data collection method.
16. Data collection methods and instruments.
17. Questionnaires: types and advantages.
18. Types of attitude scale.
19. Likert scales: advantages and disadvantages.
20. Diagrammatic/graphical presentation of data.
21. Steps of data preparation for analysis.
22. Numerical data interpretation.
23. Basic principles in interpreting the data.
24. Communication of nursing research findings.

Chapter 18: Health Information System/Health Management Information System

Short Answers

1. Sources of HMIS.
2. Benefits of health information systems.
3. Challenges for HMIS.
4. Remote patient monitoring.
5. Electronic medical record.
6. Census.
7. Registration of vital events.
8. Sample registration system.
9. Notification of disease.
10. Hospital records.
11. Epidemiological surveillance.
12. Advantages of NIS.
13. Crude rates.
14. Infant mortality rates.
15. Types of vital statistics.
16. Merits of a census investigation.
17. Vital events registration in India.
18. Characteristics of civil registration systems.
19. Birth register.
20. Common sampling techniques.
21. Cluster sampling.
22. Nonprobability sampling.
23. Convenience sampling.
24. Uses of frequency distribution.
25. Data collection process.
26. General rules of constructing diagrams.
27. Frequency polygon.
28. Line chain or graph.
29. Methods of constructing ogive.
30. Scatter or dot diagram.
31. Bar diagram.
32. Pie diagram.
33. Pictogram or picture diagram.

Multiple Choice Questions

1. Health information system is that system in:
   a. Collection
   b. Utilization
   c. Analysis and transmission of information
   d. All of the above.
2. The information of MIS comes from the boot _____ source.
   a. Internal
   b. External
   c. Superficial
   d. Internal and external
3. MIS is normally found in _____ sector.
   a. Service
   b. Education
   c. Manufacturing
   d. Marketing
4. Sources of HMIS includes:
   a. Census
   b. Registration of vital events (birth, death, marriage, etc.)
   c. Records and reports of hospitals
   d. All of the above
5. Which of the following is a branch of statistics?
   a. Descriptive statistics
   b. Inferential statistics
   c. Industry statistics
   d. Both a and b
6. The control charts and procedures of descriptive statistics which are used to enhance a procedure can be classified into which of these categories?
   a. Behavioral tools
   b. Serial tools
   c. Industry statistics
   d. Statistical tools
7. Which of the following can also be represented as sample statistics?
   a. Lowercase Greek letters
   b. Roman letters
   c. Associated roman alphabets
   d. Uppercase Greek letters.
8. To which of the following options do individual respondents, focus groups, and panels of respondents belong?
   a. Primary data sources
   b. Secondary data sources
   c. Itemized data sources
   d. Pointed data sources
9. What are the variables whose calculation is done according to the weight, height, and length known as?
   a. Flowchart variables
   b. Discrete variables
   c. Continuous variables
   d. Measuring variables
10. Which method used to examine inflation rate anticipation, unemployment rate, and capacity utilization to produce products?
    a. Data exporting technique
    b. Data importing technique
    c. Forecasting technique
    d. Data supplying technique
11. Specialized processes such as graphical and numerical methods are utilized in which of the following?
    a. Education statistics
    b. Descriptive statistics
    c. Business statistics
    d. Social statistics
12. What is the scale applied in statistics, which imparts a difference of magnitude and proportions, is considered as?
    a. Exponential scale
    b. Goodness scale
    c. Ratio scale
    d. Satisfactory scale.

ANSWERS

| 1. d | 2. d | 3. c | 4. d | 5. d | 6. d | 7. b | 8. a | 9. c | 10. c | 11. b | 12. c |

19 CHAPTER

Health Agencies

LEARNING OBJECTIVES

International
1. WHO
2. UNFPA
3. UNDP
4. World Bank
5. FAO
6. UNICEF
7. DANIDA
8. European Commission (EU)
9. Red Cross
10. USAID
11. UNESCO
12. ILO
13. CARE

National
14. Indian Red Cross
15. Indian Council for Child Welfare
16. Family Planning Association of India
17. Other NGOs

INTRODUCTION

International health organizations are usually divided into three groups: multilateral organizations, bilateral organizations, and nongovernmental organizations (NGOs). The term multilateral means that funding comes from multiple governments (as well as from nongovernmental sources) and is distributed to many different countries. The major multilateral organizations are all part of the United Nations. The World Health Organization (WHO) is the premier international health organization. Technically it is an "intergovernmental agency related to the United Nations." WHO and other such intergovernmental agencies are "separate, autonomous organizations which, by special agreements, work with the UN and each other through the coordinating machinery of the Economic and Social Council." According to its constitution (1948) its principal goal is "the attainment by all peoples of the highest possible level of health" **(Fig. 19.1)**.

TYPES OF INTERNATIONAL HEALTH AGENCIES

Health services in developing countries mostly reflect their own widely varying capacities. The international system plays an ancillary role, comprising four types of agency: multilateral, bilateral, nongovernmental, and other.

Multilateral Agencies

The term multilateral means that funding comes from multiple governments (as well as from nongovernmental sources) and is distributed to many different countries. Multilateral organizations obtain their funding from multiple governments and spend it on projects in various countries. They normally require job-seekers to have specialized training in relevant fields such as public health, economics, business and social or behavioral sciences, as well as prior experience. The major multilateral organizations are all part of the United Nations.

- The United Nations is made up of 192 countries from around the world. It is often called the UN.
- It was set up in 1945, after the Second World War, as a way of bringing people together and to avoid further wars.
- It started with 51 countries. The United Kingdom is one of the original members. Germany did not join until 1973.

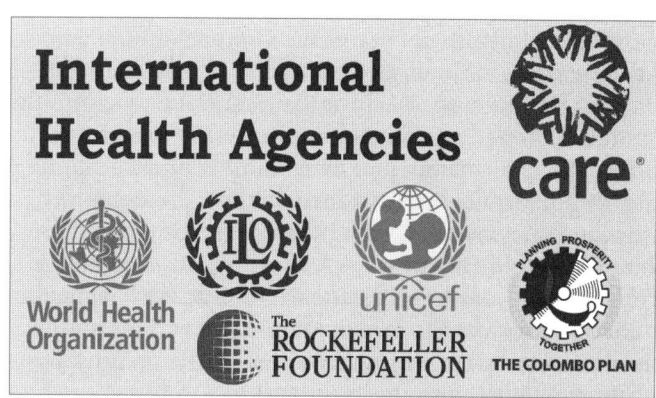

Fig. 19.1: Logo of international health agencies.

The UN has four main purposes:
1. To keep peace throughout the world;
2. To develop friendly relations among nations;
3. To help nations work together to improve the lives of poor people, to conquer hunger, disease and illiteracy, and to encourage respect for each other's rights and freedoms;
4. To be a center for harmonizing the actions of nations to achieve these goals.

Bilateral Agencies

Bilateral organizations receive funding from the government in their home countries, and use the funding to aid developing countries. Job requirements are similar to those of international organizations, though there are more opportunities for internships and entry-level positions:

- Bilateral agencies are governmental agencies in a single country which provide aid to developing countries.
- The largest of these is the United States Agency for International Development (USAID).
- Most of the industrialized nations have a similar governmental agency.
- Political and historical reasons often determine which countries receive donations from bilateral agencies and how much they receive.

Nongovernmental Organizations (NGOs)

- Nongovernmental organizations, also known as private voluntary organizations (PVOs), provide approximately 20% of all external health aid to developing countries.
- Most of these organizations are quite small; many are church-affiliated. In the very poorest countries, hospitals and clinics run by missionary societies are especially important.
- Data from Uganda indicates that church mission hospitals are much more efficient than government health facilities, with mission doctors treating five times as many patients as their counterparts in government facilities and mission nurses attending twice the number of patients that government nurses do. Role of NGOs are depicted in **Figure 19.2**.

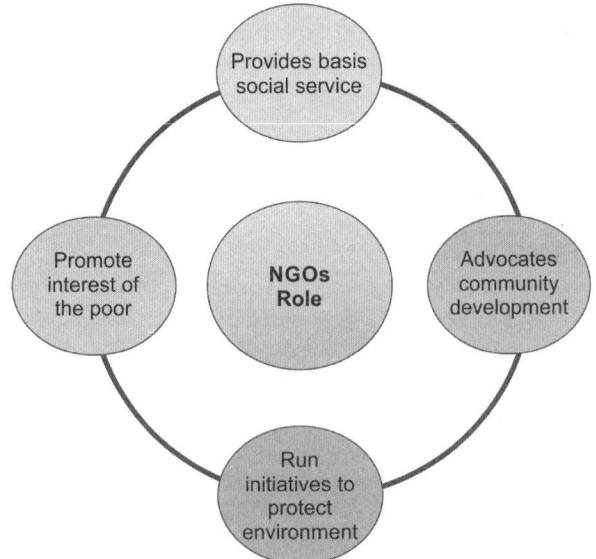

Fig. 19.2: Role of NGOs.

	Governmental organizations	*Nongovernmental organizations*
1.	Public need	Personal initiative
2.	State interest	Group interest
3.	Serves mass needs	Serves individual and group needs
4.	Standard services for all	Flexible and customized services
5.	Administrative apparatus and complex structure	Small functional structures
6.	Financial security	Financial risk
7.	Standard level of professionalism	High level of professionalism
8.	Standard employment contracts	Civil contracts and voluntary work
9.	Standard prices for services	Flexible prices for services
10.	Strict adherence to regulatory requirements	Nonstandard ideas and experience
11.	Institutionalization	Autonomy
12.	Rationality and efficiency	Spontaneity and imagination

WORLD HEALTH ORGANIZATION

The World Health Organization (WHO) is specified nonpolitical health agency of the United Nations with its head quarters at Geneva. WHO had its origin in April 1945 during the conference held at San Francisco to set up the United Nations. The constitution for WHO was drawn up under the chairmanship of Rene Sand at an international health conference in New York in 1946. The constitution came into action on 7th April 1948 which is celebrated every year as "World Health Day". A world health day theme is chosen each year to focus attention on specific aspect of public health. After an examination of the various methods used by countries throughout the world in producing healthcare. WHO introduces primary health center concept in 1975.

Objectives

The main objective is attainment of health for all people. The current objective is to attain health by all people of the world by the year 2000 AD. The level of health which will permit the people to lead a socially and economically produce life known as "Health for All by 2000 AD".

- Complete state of physical, mental and social well-being
- No discrimination in path of attainment of highest standard of health.
- Good health is for attainment of peace and security.
- Good health is valued to all equal development in promotion and control of disease in all the countries.
- Extension to all people of the benefits of medical, psychological and related knowledge.
- Informed opinion and active cooperation.

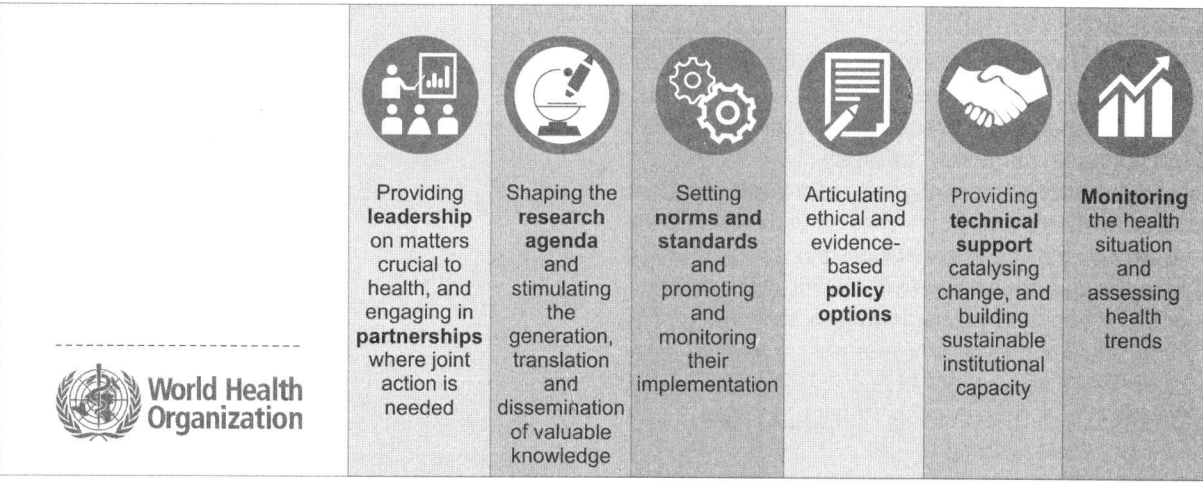

Fig. 19.3: Core functions of WHO.

Functions of WHO

WHO is the World's directing and authority on International health aspect **(Fig. 19.3)**.

- It provides cooperation with other organizations collaborates with UN and with the other specialized agencies and maintains various degrees of working relationships.
- In the aspects of health statistics, it concentrates on morbidity and mortality statistics relating to health problems.
- Regarding environmental health, it advises governments on countries to do the same.
- It carries out various research studies and also motivates informations.
- Acts as a World library issuing health literature and informations.
- Its work extends for prevention and control of specific disease, e.g., global eradication of smallpox, communicable diseases and non-communicable diseases as cancer, cardiovascular diseases, genetic disorders, mental disorders, drug addiction and dental diseases.
- WHO aimed for the development of comprehensive health services like developing primary health centers for the whole population and development of health man power utilization?

Organizational Structure

- **World health assembly:** The World Health Assembly is the highest body of the organization, representing the entire member states, each member state can send three delegates to the assembly and each delegate has the right of one vote. The assembly meets once a year, usually in the month of May, mostly in Geneva and rarely elsewhere. The assembly lays down the policy and the program of the organization approves the budget and appoints the Director General, nominated by Executive Boards.
- **Executive board:** It is a body of technically qualified health experts. The executive board meets twice a year. This board implements the policy decisions of the assembly and formulates the annual budget.
- **Secretariat:** The secretariat is the administrative organ of the WHO, which extends technical and administrative support to the member's states in planning, programming and implementing their national health programs. It is under the Director General, who is the chief technical advisor and administrative officer of WHO.
- **Regional organizations:** WHO had divided the world into six regions, the regional offices came into existence between 1948 and 1952 The regions in order of their establishment are: (i) South East Asia-New Delhi, India (ii) East Mediterranean Alexandria, Egypt (iii) Americans-Washington, USA (iv) Western pacific-Manila-Philippines (v) Africa-Brazzaville, Congo (vi) Europe-Copenhagen, Denmark.

Specific Global Targets of WHO

- Every one in every country will have at least ready access to essential healthcare and to first level referral facilities.
- Everyone will be actively involved in caring for themselves and their families as far as they can in community action for health.
- Communities throughout the world will share with Governments the responsibility for the healthcare of their members for the health of their people.
- All governments will have assumed overall responsibilities to all people.
- Safe drinking water and sanitation will be available to all people.
- All people will be adequately nourished.
- All children will be immunized against the major infectious diseases of childhood.
- Communicable diseases in the developing countries will be of no greater public health significance in the year 2000 than they are in developed countries in the year 1980.
- All possible ways will be applied to prevent and control communicable diseases and promote mental health through influencing lifestyle and controlling the physical and psychological environment.
- Essential drugs will be available to all.

Health Contribution to India

- The control of communicable diseases such as smallpox, leprosy, cholera, malaria, and tuberculosis.
- Assists in biomedical research program in India, including research in family planning methods.
- Education and training of all types of professional and auxiliary health workers. For example, postcertificate BSc Nursing Programs at College of Nursing, Chennai and at Chandigarh were initiated by WHO.
- Strengthening the public health administration.
- Improving environmental sanitation.

UNITED NATIONS FUND FOR POPULATION ACTIVITIES

United Nations Fund for Population Activities (UNFPA), the United Nations Population Fund, is an international development agency that promotes the right of every woman, man and child to enjoy a life of health and equal opportunity. There are close links between sustainable development, reproductive health and gender equality. Within the framework of the International Conference on Population and Development, 179 countries agreed that meeting needs for education and health is a prerequisite for sustainable development over the longer term. They also agreed on a roadmap for progress with the following goals:

Goals

- Universal access to reproductive health services by 2015.
- Universal primary education and closing the gender gap in education by 2015.
- Reducing maternal mortality by 75% by 2015.
- Reducing infant mortality.
- Increasing life expectancy.
- Reducing HIV infection rates.

Origin

The agency began operations in 1969 as the UNFPA under the administration of the United Nations Development Fund. In 1971, it was placed under the authority of the United Nations General Assembly. Its name was changed into United Nations Population Fund in 1987. However, the shortened term of UNFPA has been retained.

Main Activities

UNFPA supports countries in using population data for policies and program to reduce poverty and to ensure that every pregnancy is wanted, every birth is safe, every young person is free of HIV/AIDS, and every girl and woman is treated with dignity and respect. UNFPA helps governments, at their request, to formulate policies and strategies to support sustainable development and gender equality. UNFPA assists in health emergencies and protects human rights. They have celebrity sponsors and key corporations promote causes and raise money for increased aid **(Fig. 19.4)**.

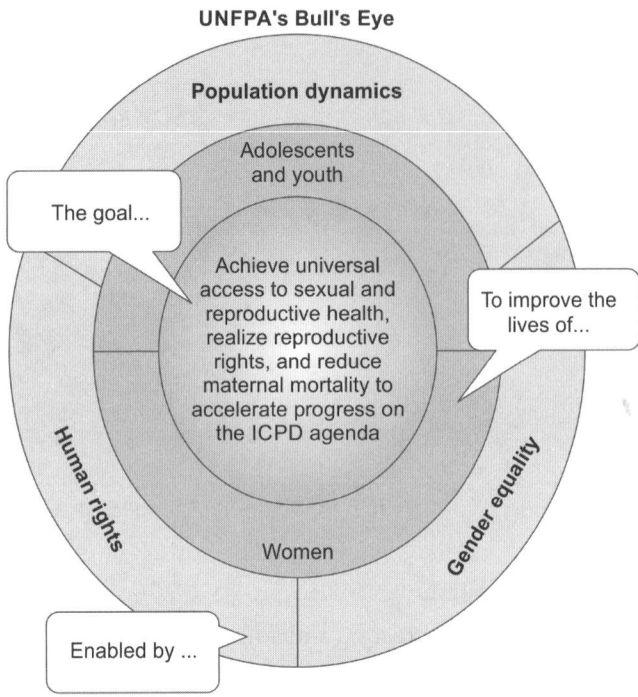

Fig. 19.4: United nations fund for population activities.

UNFPA Supports

- Reproductive healthcare for women and youth in more than 150 countries—which are home to more than 80% of the world's population.
- The health of pregnant women, especially the 1 million who face life-threatening complications each month.
- Reliable access to modern contraceptives sufficient to benefit 20 million women a year.
- Training of thousands of health workers to help ensure at least 90% of all childbirths are supervised by skilled attendants.
- Prevention of gender-based violence, which affects 1 in 3 women.
- Abandonment of female genital mutilation, which harms 3 million girls annually.
- Prevention of teen pregnancies, complications of which are the leading cause of death for girls 15–19 years old.
- Efforts to end child marriage, which could affect an estimated 70 million girls over the next 5 years.
- Delivery of safe birth supplies, dignity kits and other life-saving materials to survivors of conflict and natural disaster.
- Censuses, data collection and analyses, which are essential for development planning.

UNFPA Activities in India

- Providing assistance to India since 1974.
- Funding national level schemes, area projects for intensive development of health and family welfare infrastructure and improvement in the availability of services in the rural areas.
- To develop national capability for the manufacture of contraceptives.

- To develop population education programs.
- To undertake organized sector projects.
- To strengthen program management as well as to improve output of grass-root level health workers.
- Introduction of innovative approaches to family planning and MCH care.

UNITED NATIONS DEVELOPMENT PROGRAMME

The United Nations Development Programme (UNDP) is the United Nations' global development network. It advocates for change and connects countries to knowledge, experience and resources to help people build a better life for them. It provides expert advice, training and grants support to developing countries, with increasing emphasis on assistance to the least developed countries. It promotes technical and investment cooperation among nations.

- The United Nations Development Programme was established in 1966 contributes towards increasing the pace of development in the third world countries.
- Headquartered in New York City, the status of UNDP is that of an executive board within the United Nations General Assembly.
- The UNDP Administrator is the third highest-ranking official of the United Nations after the United Nations Secretary-General and Deputy Secretary-General.
- It supports all phases of socioeconomic development including agriculture, industry, education, health and social welfare.
- It is the main source of funds for technical assistance. The basics objective of the UNDP is to help poorer nations develop their human and natural resources more fully.

Key areas of UNDP rule of law and human rights work include:

- Improving access to justice and remedies, and helping people enforce their rights.
- Assisting governments to establish capable justice systems, including the rapid restoration of justice services and dispute resolution mechanisms following crisis or conflict (targeting, in particular, previously marginalized communities).
- Increasing community security and reducing armed violence, including through curbing the proliferation of small arms and light weapons.
- Addressing sexual and gender-based violence and increasing women's participation and leadership in justice and security institutions, particularly in peace building and recovery contexts.
- Supporting the promotion and protection of human rights, including strengthening the work of National Human Rights Institutions, supporting engagement with the international human rights machinery and promoting the application of the human rights-based approach to development programming and national planning processes.
- Supporting transitional justice to promote redress for past violence and human rights violations and to enable societies to recover from the legacy of violence.

The UNDP projects cover virtually every economic and social sector—agriculture, industry, education and science, health, social welfare, etc. The member countries—rich and poor—of the United Nations meet annually and submitting proposal to the UNDP. Focused areas.

- Poverty Reduction and Millennium Development Goals
- Democratic Governance
- Environment and Energy for Sustain Development
- Crisis Prevention and Recovery
- UNDP is at the center of the UN's efforts to reduce global poverty.
- Chairs the United Nations Development Group (UNDG), which includes the UN's key players in international development.
- UNDP's network links and coordinates global and national efforts to achieve the Millennium Development Goals (MDGs).
- At the country level, UNDP plays two important roles, one as a partner for development work and the other as manager of the Resident Coordinator system.
- UNDP helps developing countries attract and use aid effectively.
- It encourages the protection of human rights and the empowerment of women.
- Coordinates the development activities of the United Nations.
- Plays a key role in helping to reform the UN as part of the United Nations Development Group (UNDG).

WORLD BANK

The World Bank was established in December 1945 at the United Nations Monetary and Financial Conference in Bretton Woods, New Hampshire. It opened for business in June 1946 and helped in the reconstruction of nations devastated by World War II. Since 1960s the World Bank has shifted its focus from the advanced industrialized nations to developing third-world countries.

Organization and Structure

- The organization of the bank consists of the Board of Governors, the Board of Executive Directors and the Advisory Committee, the Loan Committee and the president and other staff members.
- All the powers of the bank are vested in the Board of Governors which the supreme policy is making body of the bank.
- The board consists of one Governor and one Alternative Governor appointed for five years by each member country.
- Each Governor has the voting power which is related to the financial contribution of the Government which he represents.
- The Board of Executive Directors consists of 21 members, 6 of them are appointed by the six largest shareholders,

namely the USA, the UK, West Germany, France, Japan and India. The rest of the 15 members are elected by the remaining countries.
- Each Executive Director holds voting power in proportion to the shares held by his government. The board of Executive Directors meets regularly once a month to carry on the routine working of the bank.
- The president of the bank is appointed by the Board of Executive Directors. He is the Chief Executive of the Bank and he is responsible for the conduct of the day-to-day business of the bank. The Advisory committees appointed by the Board of Directors.
- It consists of 7 members who are in different branches of banking. There is also another body known as the Loan Committee. This committee is consulted by the bank before any loan is extended to a member country.

Capital Resources of World Bank

The initial authorized capital of the World Bank was $ 10,000 million, which was divided in 1 lakh shares of $ 1 lakh each. The authorized capital of the Bank has been increased from time to time with the approval of member countries. On June 30, 1996, the authorized capital of the Bank was $ 188 billion out of which $ 180.6 billion (96% of total authorized capital) was issued to member countries in the form of shares.

Member countries repay the share amount to the world bank in the following ways:
- 2% of allotted share are repaid in gold, US dollar or Special Drawing Rights (SDR).
- Every member country is free to repay 18% of its capital share in its own currency.
- The remaining 80% share deposited by the member country only on demand by the World Bank.

Objectives

The following objectives are assigned by the World Bank:
- To provide long-run capital to member countries for economic reconstruction and development.
- To induce long-run capital investment for assuring Balance of Payments (BoP) equilibrium and balanced development of international trade.
- To provide guarantee for loans granted to small and large units and other projects of member countries.
- To ensure the implementation of development projects so as to bring about a smooth transference from a war-time to peace economy.
- To promote capital investment in member countries by the following ways:
  - To provide guarantee on private loans or capital investment.
  - If private capital is not available even after providing guarantee, then IBRD provides loans for productive activities on considerate conditions.

Functions

World Bank is playing main role of providing loans for development works to member countries, especially to underdeveloped countries. The World Bank provides long-term loans for various development projects of 5 to 20 years duration.

The main functions can be explained with the help of the following points:
- World Bank provides various technical services to the member countries. For this purpose, the Bank has established "The Economic Development Institute" and a Staff College in Washington.
- Bank can grant loans to a member country up to 20% of its share in the paid-up capital.
- The quantities of loans, interest rate and terms and conditions are determined by the Bank itself.
- Generally, Bank grants loans for a particular project duly submitted to the Bank by the member country.
- The debtor nation has to repay either in reserve currencies or in the currency in which the loan was sanctioned.
- Bank also provides loan to private investors belonging to member countries on its own guarantee, but for this loan private investors have to seek prior permission from those counties where this amount will be collected.

FOOD AND AGRICULTURE ORGANIZATION

The Food and Agriculture Organization (FAO) was formed in 1945 with headquarters in Rome. It was the first United Nations organization specialized agency created to look after several areas of world cooperation. FAO's primary aim is to increase agriculture production to keep pace with growing population in the world.

Origin

- The idea of an international organization for food and agriculture emerged in the late 19th and early 20th century, advanced primarily by Polish-born American agriculturalist and activist David Lubin.
- In May–June 1905, an international conference was held in Rome, Italy, which led to the creation of the International Institute of Agriculture (IIA) by the King of Italy, Victor Emmanuel III.
- The IIA was the first intergovernmental organization to deal with the problems and challenges of agriculture on a global scale.
- It worked primarily to collect, compile, and publish data on agriculture, ranging from output statistics to a catalog of crop diseases. Among its achievements was the publication of the first agricultural census in 1930.

Definition

The Food and Agriculture Organization (FAO) is an agency of the United Nations (UN). The FAO contributes to international efforts to defeat hunger and improve local economies by helping its member countries modernize and improve agriculture, forestry, and fisheries practices.

Aims of FAO

The aims of FAO are as follows:
- To help nations raise living standards.
- To improve the nutritional status of people of all countries.
- To increase the efficiency of farming, forestry and fisheries.
- To better the condition of rural people and better the opportunity of productive work.

The objectives are:
- To increase the efficiency of farming, fisheries and forestry.
- To improve the condition of rural people.
- To ensure that the food is consumed by the people who need it in sufficient quantities and in right proportions.
- To develop and maintain a better state of nutrition throughout the world.
- To help nations raise their living standards.

Structure

FAO has a staff with more than 3600 units and its internal structure is composed by: Conference of the Member Nations, Council of the Organization, the Director-General, Departments, Regional Offices, Sub-Regional Offices and Country Offices.
- **Conference of the member nations:** Meets every two years to analyze the activities and approve the work program; decrees the general policy and approves the budget; exudes the Rules of Procedure and the Financial Regulations of the Organization; may make recommendations to Member States on issues related to food and agriculture and elects the Council.
- **Council of the organization:** It is the governing body of FAO and consists of 49 Member States with only one vote each and a prime minister appointed by the conference. In carrying out its functions, the board is assisted by a Program Committee, a Finance Committee, a Committee of the Constitutional and Legal Matters, by a Committee of the Products, a Committee of the Fish Ponds, a Committee of the Forest, which a committee of agriculture and a Committee on World Food Security.
- **Director-general of the organization:** Appointed by the conference for a term of 6 years and is re-elected, and has full power and authority to direct the work of the organization; participate without vote in all meetings of the conference and of the council and shall them to examine the proposals for appropriate action in the field of problems within their competence.
- **Departments:** Department of Agriculture and Consumer Protection, Department of Economic and Social Development, Department of Natural Resources Management and Environment, Fisheries and Aquaculture Department, Forestry Department, Department of Technical Cooperation, Knowledge and Communication Department and the Department of Human Resources, Financial and Physical.
- **Regional offices:** The principal function of the regional offices is the overall identification, planning and implementation of FAO's priority activities in the region.
- **Sub-regional offices:** Monitoring the level of program implementation.
- **Country offices:** Serve as the channel of FAO's services to governments and other partners (donors, NGOs, CSOs, research institutions, etc.).

FAO is Composed of Seven Departments

- The Agriculture and Consumer Protection Department promotes agriculture to eradicate human poverty while also protecting the environment and ensuring safe food practices and standards.
- The Climate, Biodiversity, Land, and Water Department promotes sustainable management practices for land, soils, energy, water, biodiversity, and genetic resources.
- The Corporate Services, Human Resources, and Finance Department support the entire FAO organization.
- The economic and Social Development Department promotes economic development through internal production and trade.
- The Fisheries and Aquaculture Department promotes the management of aquaculture and fishing.
- The Forestry Department promotes the management of resources through forestry.
- The Technical Cooperation Department supports member countries in their programs and responds to food and agriculture-related threats and crises.

Budget

Projects of the FAO field program have two main funding sources:
- The organization's core budget (also known as the regular program which is funded by contributions from FAO member nations).
- Extra-budgetary resources received from multilateral (e.g., mainly United Nations Development Program—UNDP and other UN funds) and bilateral donors.

Each FAO Member State pays annually its contribution to the budget organization. The total FAO budget for 2012–13 is $ 2.4 billion. The 42% of the budget comes from contributions of member countries, while 58% through voluntary contributions from members and other partners. As for the research programs funded by FAO are more than 4,000, and include coordinated actions in different sectors: Agriculture (60%), Environment (12%), Nutrition and Feeding (11%), Services (7%), Fisheries and Aquaculture (7%), Social (2%) and Forestry (1%).

Objectives of FAO

The FAO has organized a World Freedom from Hunger Campaign (FFHC) in 1960. The primary objective of FAO is towards ensuring that the food is consumed by the

people who need it in sufficient quantities and in right proportions to develop and maintain a better state of nutrition throughout the world. The FAO's official strategic objectives include:
- Help eliminate hunger, food insecurity, and malnutrition.
- Make agriculture, forestry, and fisheries more productive and sustainable.
- Reduce rural poverty.
- Enable inclusive and efficient agricultural and food systems.
- Increase the resilience of livelihoods to threats and crises.
- Establish technical quality, statistics, and cross-cutting themes.

Priority Work Areas

FAO has outlined the following priorities in its fight against hunger:
- **Help eliminate hunger, food insecurity and malnutrition:** Contribute to the eradication of hunger by facilitating policies and political commitments to support food security and by making sure that up-to-date information about hunger and nutrition challenges and solutions is available and accessible.
- **Make agriculture, forestry and fisheries more productive and sustainable:** Promote evidence-based policies and practices to support highly productive agricultural sectors (crops, livestock, forestry and fisheries), while ensuring that the natural resource base does not suffer in the process.
- **Reduce rural poverty:** Help the rural poor gain access to the resources and services they need—including rural employment and social protection—to forge a path out of poverty.
- **Enable inclusive and efficient agricultural and food systems:** Help to build safe and efficient food systems that support smallholder agriculture and reduce poverty and hunger in rural areas.
- **Increase the resilience of livelihoods to threats and crises**: Help countries to prepare for natural and human-caused disasters by reducing their risk and enhancing the resilience of their food and agricultural systems.

Functions of FAO

The main functions of FAO are:
- The organization shall collect, analyze, interpret and disseminate information relating to nutrition, food and agriculture. FAO serves as a knowledge network. It uses the expertise of its staff, agronomists, foresters, fisheries and livestock specialists, nutritionists, social scientists, economists, statisticians and other professionals, to collect, analyze and disseminate data. FAO also publishes hundreds of newsletters, reports and books, distributes several magazines, and creates numerous electronic fora.
- The organization shall promote and, where appropriate, shall recommend national and international action with respect to:
  - Scientific, technological, social and economic research relating to nutrition, food and agriculture;
  - The improvement of education and administration relating to nutrition, food and agriculture, and the spread of public knowledge of nutritional and agricultural science and practice;
  - The conservation of natural resources and the adoption of improved methods of agricultural production;
  - The improvement of the processing, marketing and distribution of food and agricultural products;
  - The adoption of policies for the provision of adequate agricultural credit, national and international;
  - The adoption of international policies with respect to agricultural commodity arrangements.
- It shall also be the function of the organization:
  - To furnish such technical assistance as governments may request. FAO lends its years of experience to member countries in devising agricultural policy, supporting planning, drafting effective legislation and creating national strategies to achieve rural development and hunger alleviation goals.
  - To organize, in cooperation with the governments concerned, such missions as may be needed to assist them to fulfil the obligation arising from their acceptance of the recommendations of the United Nations Conference on Food and Agriculture and of this Constitution. Policy-makers and experts from around the globe convene at headquarters or in the field offices to forge agreements on major food and agriculture issues. As a neutral forum, FAO provides the setting where rich and poor nations can come together to build common understanding.

UNITED NATIONS INTERNATIONAL CHILDREN'S EMERGENCY FUND

The United Nations International Children's Emergency Fund (UNICEF) was created by the United Nations in 1946 to provide food, clothing, and healthcare to the children of post-World War II Europe. In 1953, UNICEF became a permanent part of the United Nations. While its name was shortened to United Nations Children Fund at that time, it is still referred to as UNICEF.
- UNICEF expanded the scope of its activities in the 1960s to include advocating for and advancing children's rights to education, healthcare, and nutrition. UNICEF won the Nobel Peace Prize in 1965.
- UNICEF eventually expanded its scope to the struggle of women, especially mothers, in the developing world. For example, it launched its 'Women in Development Programme' in 1980.
- In 1982, UNICEF commenced a new children's health program that focused on monitoring growth, oral rehydration therapy, advocating breastfeeding, and immunization. In 1989, the UN General Assembly adopted the convention on the rights of the child, which UNICEF uses as guidance for its programs.

Structure

- UNICEF is governed by an Executive Board consisting of 36 members that are elected to terms of three years by the United Nations' Economic and Social Council.
- Each region that UNICEF serves is allocated a number of seats on the Executive Board, so all regions are represented. UNICEF is headquartered in New York City in the United States.
- There are also 36 national committees across the globe, which are nongovernmental organizations that help promote the rights of children and fundraise.
- While UNICEF is headquartered in the United States, it is active in at least 190 countries around the world.
- Its activities are divided by region and include Central and Eastern Europe and the Commonwealth of Independent States, East Asia and the Pacific, Eastern and Southern Africa, Latin America and Caribbean, Middle East and North Africa, South Asia, West and Central Africa. A regional office is located within each region.

Functions

UNICEF provides services in primary healthcare, nutrition, basic education, sanitation and women's development in developing countries. The main functions of UNICEF are broadly divided into the following categories:

- UNICEF works for the protection of children in respect of their survival, health, and well-being. This is done in cooperation with individuals, civic groups, governments and the private sector.
- It provides funds for training the personnel, including health and sanitation workers, teachers and nutritionists. Universal Child Immunizations against preventable diseases by 1990 was one of the leading goals of UNICEF.
- It provides technical supplies, equipment and other aids, ranging from paper for textbooks, to equipment and medicines to health clinics, to pipes and pumps for bringing clean water to villages.
- It assists governments to plan, develop and extend community-based services in the fields of maternal and child health's, nutrition, clean water and sanitation.
- It provides help to children and mothers in emergencies arising from natural calamities, civil strafes and epidemics.
- It makes effort to prevent diseases like TB, malaria, eye diseases, skin diseases, etc.
- UNICEF performs various other functions. As the sole agency for children, it speaks on behalf of children and upholds the Convention on the Rights of the Child and works for its implementation. UNICEF was awarded the Nobel Prize for peace in the year 1965 and the Indira Gandhi Prize for peace in 1989.

Funding Sources

- Beginning in 1946 with a modest residue of funds from the UN Relief and Rehabilitation Agency, UNICEF has grown to be a sizable development and humanitarian organization with an annual budget of around $1 billion.
- It operates entirely on voluntary contributions from both governmental and private sources.
- In addition to regular contributions, many governments also make special contributions for specific purposes, especially during emergencies.
- A network of thirty-seven national committees, registered as nonprofit entities in the industrialized countries, inform the public about the needs and rights of the child and raise funds to support UNICEF.

GOBI Strategy by UNICEF

Currently, UNICEF is engaged in affecting child health revolution through GOBI strategy promoting growth monitoring.
G : Oral rehydration therapy
O : Breastfeeding
B : Universal immunization
I : Universal immunization program and ICDS programs.

Regional Organizations of UNICEF

UNICEF has a decentralized organizational structure with its headquarters in New York and separate regional offices for Eastern and Southern Africa, Central and West Africa, and North Africa, South Central Asia, Australia and New Zealand and Japan. UNICEF also maintains a Geneva office. The south Central Asia region includes India, Mongolia, Afghanistan, Sri Lanka, Nepal and Maldives.

UNICEF in India

UNICEF is assisting India with the collaboration to UNESCO. In the expansion of educational institutions and improvement of teaching sciences, science laboratories, equipment, working tools, libraries, audio visual aids, helping training programs for nurses, midwives and health auxiliary personnel, etc.

Rural Health Aspects

- Provided equipment and drugs to primary health centers BCG vaccination program.
- Assist in field of medical education and training.
- Assist in development of rural health services.
- Provided equipment for daily plants in various parts of India, e.g., Bombay, Gujarat, Karnataka, Uttar Pradesh, West Bengal, Andhra Pradesh and Tamil Nadu.

EUROPEAN COMMISSION

The European Commission (EC) is the executive branch of the European Union, responsible for proposing legislation, implementing decisions, upholding the EU treaties and managing the day-to-day business of the EU. Commissioners swear an oath at the European Court of Justice in Luxembourg City, pledging to respect the treaties and to be completely independent in carrying out their duties during their mandate. The Commissioners are proposed by the Council of the European Union, on the basis of suggestions made by the national governments, and then appointed by the European Council after the approval of the European Parliament. It is common, although not a formal requirement, that the commissioners have previously held senior political positions, such as being a member of the European Parliament or a government minister.

Definition

The European Union is an economic and political organization which is constantly evolving and which, because of its intrinsic and unique features, prompts lively doctrinal debate as to its legal nature. Because its institutional structure and decision-making procedures are so complex, it cannot be readily be assigned to any one specific category of international organization.

Goals

The goals of the European Union are:
- Promote peace, its values and the well-being of its citizens.
- Offer freedom, security and justice without internal borders.
- Sustainable development based on balanced economic growth and price stability, a highly competitive market economy with full employment and social progress, and environmental protection.
- Combat social exclusion and discrimination.
- Promote scientific and technological progress.
- Enhance economic, social and territorial cohesion and solidarity among EU countries.
- Respect its rich cultural and linguistic diversity.
- Establish an economic and monetary union whose currency is the euro.

Values

The EU values are common to the EU countries in a society in which inclusion, tolerance, justice, solidarity and non-discrimination prevail. These values are an integral part of our European way of life:
- **Human dignity:** Human dignity is inviolable. It must be respected, protected and constitutes the real basis of fundamental rights.
- **Freedom:** Freedom of movement gives citizens the right to move and reside freely within the Union. Individual freedoms such as respect for private life, freedom of thought, religion, assembly, expression and information are protected by the EU Charter of Fundamental Rights.
- **Democracy:** The functioning of the EU is founded on representative democracy. Being a European citizen also means enjoying political rights. Every adult EU citizen has the right to stand as a candidate and to vote in elections to the European Parliament. EU citizens have the right to stand as candidate and to vote in their country of residence, or in their country of origin.
- **Equality:** Equality is about equal rights for all citizens before the law. The principle of equality between women and men underpins all European policies and is the basis for European integration. It applies in all areas. The principle of equal pay for equal work became part of the Treaty of Rome in 1957. Although inequalities still exist, the EU has made significant progress.
- **Rule of law:** The EU is based on the rule of law. Everything the EU does is founded on treaties, voluntarily and democratically agreed by its EU countries. Law and justice are upheld by an independent judiciary. The EU countries gave final jurisdiction to the European Court of Justice which judgements have to be respected by all.
- **Human rights:** Human rights are protected by the EU Charter of Fundamental Rights. These cover the right to be free from discrimination on the basis of sex, racial or ethnic origin, religion or belief, disability, age or sexual orientation, the right to the protection of your personal data, and/or the right to get access to justice.

Objectives

The European Union's main objective is to promote peace, follow the EU's values and improve the well-being of nations. The European Parliament and other institutions see to it that these objectives are achieved.

The main objectives are:
- **A common European area without borders:** The objective is to create a free and safe Europe with no internal borders. The citizens living in the area enjoy the rights granted by the European Union.
- **Internal market:** The objective is to ensure smooth and efficient trade within Europe. Competition between companies is free and fair.
- **Stable and sustainable development:** The objective is to ensure Europe's sustainable and steady development. It means balanced economic growth and stable prices. The European Union seeks to create a competitive market economy which takes into account people's well-being and social needs. An important issue is environmental protection. Efforts are made to protect the environment and repair any damage made.
- **Scientific and technological development:** The European Union supports the advancement of science and technology and invests in education. Another objective is to achieve a skilled workforce and a high standard of technological production.
- **Prevention of social exclusion:** The European Union works hard to prevent social exclusion. It seeks to prevent people from drifting outside the labour market and society. Efforts are made to eliminate poverty. The Union works for equality. Minority rights are protected. Social security is improved. Men and women must be treated equally. Children's rights must be protected and children given a happy childhood. Old people must be looked after and respected.
- **Solidarity:** Solidarity between countries and people is promoted in the field of the economy, social equality and regions. The member states must be loyal to one another. It means that states must take responsibility for and be understanding of one another.

- **Respect for languages and cultures:** The European Union respects the languages and cultures of the individual countries. National cultures and the common European culture are cherished and developed.
- **Common foreign and security policy:** The European Union seeks to promote peace not only in Europe but also elsewhere in the world. It seeks to ensure that peace is maintained in Europe and that people have security. With the common foreign policy, the European Union wants to make sure that the resources of the planet are used sensibly and that the environment is not destroyed.

Functions

- EU's law and regulation is meant to create a cohesive economic entity of its countries, so that goods can flow freely across the borders of its member nations, without tariffs, with the ease of one currency, and the creation of one enlarged labor pool, which creates a more efficient distribution and use of labor.
- There is a pooling of financial resources, so that member nations can be "bailed out" or lent money for investment.
- Union's expectations in areas such as human rights and the environment have political implications for member countries. Union can exact a heavy political cost such as severe cutbacks and an austerity budget on its members as a condition of giving aid.
- This is a great experiment, really, in cooperation amongst nations, who wish to be economically unified, ceding as little political and national power as possible.
- Trade:
  - Free trade among its members was one of the EU's founding principles. This is possible thanks to the single market. Beyond its borders, the EU is also committed to liberalizing world trade.
  - The European Union is the largest trade block in the world. It is the world's biggest exporter of manufactured goods and services, and the biggest import market for over 100 countries.
- Humanitarian aid:
  - The EU is committed to helping victims of man-made and natural disasters worldwide and supports over 120 million people each year.
  - EU and its constituent countries is the world's leading donor of humanitarian aid.
- Diplomacy and security: The EU plays an important role in diplomacy and works to foster stability, security and prosperity, democracy, fundamental freedoms and the rule of law at international level.

Challenges and Reforms

- It is no longer self-evident that all old member states will stay in the Union. The Treaty of Lisbon gave the members the right to leave the EU. The financial crisis has hit Greece so hard that many people have predicted for a long time that the country will exit from the Union.
- Layoffs, redundancies and migration of jobs to countries where labor is cheap affect the daily lives of European citizens. The EU is expected to find solutions to economic problems and employment.
- There is also demand for standard labor agreements on terms of employment and working conditions that would apply across Europe and even worldwide. As a member of the World Trade Organization, the European Union is in a position to influence developments worldwide.
- EU is a global leader in the development of Key Enabling Technologies (KETs). However, EU's record in translating this knowledge advantage into marketable products and services does not match this. KETs-related manufacturing is decreasing in the EU and patents are increasingly being exploited outside the EU.
- Europe is experiencing a renaissance of national sovereignty supported by a nationalistic turn of public opinion and represented by parties on both ends of the political spectrum. Popular disaffection toward EU membership is fuelled by the contemporaneous occurrence of two shocks, the economic and the migration crises.
- USA, by withdrawing from the Paris climate change deal, by pulling out of the Joint Comprehensive Plan of Action (JCPOA) on Iran's nuclear program, and by attacking the integrity of the international trading system through the unilateral imposition of tariffs, has called into question Europeans' formerly unshakeable faith in diplomacy as a way to resolve disagreements and to protect Europe.
- European leaders now fear that the transatlantic security guarantee will center not on alliances and common interests but purchases of American technology and material.
- Like the United States, the EU has been forced to reconsider its relationship with a more assertive Russia with implications for European security and stability. The EU has sought to support Ukraine's political transition, condemned Russia's annexation of Crimea in March 2014, and strongly urged Russia to stop backing separatist forces in eastern Ukraine.
- Democratic regression in Ukraine combined with a hardening attitude in Moscow imposes constraints on the Ukrainian government's freedom of maneuver in pursuing its European Union membership.
- Brexit: EU has imposed too many rules on business and charged billions of pounds a year in membership fees for little in return.
  - The EU added Eight eastern European Countries in 2004, triggering a wave of immigration that strained public services. In England and Wales, the share of foreign-born residents had swelled to 13.4% of the population by 2011, roughly double the level in 1991.
  - Brexit supporters wanted Britain to take back full control of its borders and reduce the number of people coming here to live and/or work.
  - They argued that the EU is morphing into a super-state that increasingly impinges on national sovereignty.

Britain has global clout without the bloc, they said, and can negotiate better trade treaties on its own.
- Withdrawal from the EU is governed by Article 50 of the Treaty on European Union.
- A deal between UK and EU that gives it control over immigration and also preferential access to the EU's tariff-free single market of 500 million people (UK), the economic backbone of the world's largest trading bloc is rejected by Germany and other EU leaders.

EU and India

- The EU works closely with India to promote peace, create jobs, boost economic growth and enhance sustainable development across the country.
- As India graduated from low to medium income country (OECD 2014), the EU-India cooperation also evolved from a traditional financial assistance type towards a partnership with a focus on common priorities.
- At the 2017 EU-India Summit, leaders reiterated their intention to strengthen cooperation on the implementation of the 2030 Agenda for Sustainable Development and agreed to explore the continuation of the EU-India Development Dialogue.
- The EU is India's largest trading partner, accounting for €85 billion (95 billion USD) worth of trade in goods in 2017 or 13.1% of total India trade, ahead of China (11.4%) and the USA (9.5%).
- The EU's share in foreign investment inflows to India has more than doubled from 8% to 18% in the last decade, making the EU the first foreign investor in India.
- EU foreign direct investment stocks in India amounted to €73 billion in 2016, which is significant but way below EU foreign investment stocks in China (€178 billion).
- INDIA-EU Bilateral Trade and Investment Agreement (BTIA): It is a Free Trade Agreement between India and EU, which was initiated in 2007. Even after a decade of negotiations, India and EU have failed to resolve certain issues which have led to a deadlock.
  - "Data Secure" status not granted by EU affecting prospects of India's IT-enabled exports.
  - Presence of nontariff barriers on Indian agricultural products in the form of sanitary and phyto-sanitary (SPS) measures which are too stringent and enable the EU to bar many Indian agricultural products from entering its markets.
  - EU wants India to liberalize accountancy and legal services. India denies on the ground of already shortage of jobs.
  - EU demands tax reduction on wines and spirits but in India these are regarded as 'sin goods' and the states which derive huge revenue from liquor sales would be reluctant to cut taxes.
  - Reduction of taxes on automobiles not acceptable to India as its own automobile industry would not be able to match the competition from EU automobiles.
  - India has rejected an informal attempt by the European Union (EU) to work towards a global investment agreement at the World Trade Organization (WTO)—level that would incorporate a contentious Investor-State Dispute Settlement (ISDS) mechanism which will allow corporations to take sovereign governments to international arbitration. The ISDS mechanism permits companies to drag governments to international arbitration without exhausting the local remedies and claim huge amounts as compensation losses they suffered due to reasons, including policy changes.
  - The nontariff barriers in pharmaceuticals that EU has imposed include requirement of WTO—Good Manufacturing Practice Certification, import bans, antidumping measures and preshipment inspection among others.
  - India has cancelled most individual bilateral investment agreements with EU member states on grounds that they were outdated. By doing this India is putting pressure on EU to sign BTIA on favoring terms.

INTERNATIONAL RED CROSS

The International Red Cross and Red Crescent Movement is an international humanitarian movement with approximately 97 million volunteers, members and staff worldwide which was founded to protect human life and health, to ensure respect for all human beings, and to prevent and alleviate human suffering. The movement consists of several distinct organizations that are legally independent from each other, but are united within the movement through common basic principles, objectives, symbols, statutes and governing organizations.

Origin

- The Red Cross idea was born in 1859, when Henry Dunant, a young Swiss man, came upon the scene of a bloody battle in Solferino, Italy, between the Armies of Imperial Austria and the Franco-Sardinian alliance. Some 40,000 men lay dead or dying on the battlefield and the wounded were lacking medical attention.
- Dunant organized local people to bind the soldiers' wounds and to feed and comfort them. On his return, he called for the creation of national relief societies to assist those wounded in war, and pointed the way to the future Geneva Conventions.
- "Would there not be some means, during a period of peace and calm, of forming relief societies whose object would be to have the wounded cared for in time of war by enthusiastic, devoted volunteers, fully qualified for the task?" he wrote.
- The Red Cross was born in 1863 when five Geneva men, including Dunant, set up the International Committee for Relief to the Wounded, later to become the International Committee of the Red Cross. Its emblem was a red cross on a white background: the inverse of the Swiss flag. The following year, 12 governments adopted the first Geneva Convention; a milestone in the history of humanity, offering care for the wounded, and defining medical services as "neutral" on the battlefield.

Basic Principles

- **Humanity:** The Red Cross, born of a desire to bring assistance without discrimination to the wounded on the battlefield, endeavors—in its international and national capacity—to prevent and alleviate human suffering wherever it may be found. Its purpose is to protect life and health and to ensure respect for the human being. It promotes mutual understanding, friendship, cooperation and lasting peace amongst all peoples.
- **Impartiality:** It makes no discrimination as to nationality, race, religious beliefs, class or political opinions. It endeavors to relieve the suffering of individuals, being guided solely by their needs, and to give priority to the most urgent cases of distress.
- **Neutrality:** In order to continue to enjoy the confidence of all, the Red Cross may not take sides in hostilities or engage at any time in controversies of a political, racial, religious or ideological nature.
- **Independence:** The Red Cross is independent. The national societies, while auxiliaries in the humanitarian services of their governments and subject to the laws of their respective countries, must always maintain their autonomy so that they may be able at all times to act in accordance with Red Cross principles.
- **Voluntary service:** The Red Cross is a voluntary relief movement not prompted in any manner by desire for gain.
- **Unity:** There can be only one Red Cross society in any one country. It must be open to all. It must carry on its humanitarian work throughout its territory.
- **Universality:** The Red Cross is a worldwide institution in which all societies have equal status and share equal responsibilities and duties in helping each other.

Functions

- Red Cross promotes the humanitarian values, which encourage respect for other human beings and a willingness to work together to find solutions to problems. From the seven fundamental principles, the movement aims to influence the behavior of all the people.
- Disaster response continues to represent the largest portion of IRCS work, with assistance to millions of people annually ranging from refugees to victims of natural disasters.
- Guiding and supporting the development of its Societies is one of the Red Cross's fundamental tasks and runs through these four areas and others.
- Capacity building programs and activities include: management and volunteer training, improving branch structures, planning, fund-raising and gender equality, creating the opportunity for Red Cross Societies to network.
- **Other Major activities includes:** Hospital services, blood bank, HIV/AIDS programs, home for disabled servicemen, vocational training centers, tracing activities, maternity, child and family welfare, nursing, junior red cross activities, preparedness and prevention of communicable and infectious diseases, relief operations in fire, railway and other accidents and events.

Promoting Fundamental Principles and Humanitarian Values

- The International Committees of the Red Cross and National Societies have a consistent and inspirational approach to promoting humanitarian values and the seven Fundamental Principles of the Red Cross and Red Crescent Movement.
- The aim is to influence the behavior of the people we work with, through a better understanding of Fundamental Principles and Humanitarian Values.
- The three main target groups are those working within Red Cross and Red Crescent societies, public and private authorities and members of the communities where we work.

Developing a Better Understanding Internally

- New initiatives are being taken to ensure that Red Cross Red Crescent volunteers and staff understand and act on the basis of the Fundamental Principles in their work with vulnerable people in times of peace, disaster or armed conflict.
- Training includes the legal and ideological basis of the Red Cross Red Crescent, decision-making processes, mandates, as well as communications and relations with others.

Influencing Behavior in the Community

The values that the Movement has formally stated to be of importance for promotion are:
- The protection of life, health and human dignity.
- Respect for the human being.
- Nondiscrimination on the basis of nationality, race, gender, religious beliefs, disability, class or political opinions.
- Mutual understanding, friendship, cooperation and lasting peace among people.
- Service by volunteers.

Disaster Relief

The Indian subcontinent is highly prone to droughts, floods and other natural calamities. Among the states as many as 22 states are said to be multi-disaster-prone regions. Among all the disasters that occur in India, floods are the most devastating. Over 40 million hectare of land has been identified as flood prone. An average of 18.6 million hectare of land is flooded annually.

Disaster Response

Disasters are becoming more complex, with increasingly long-term consequences as they strike countries with economic problems or political instability, and weaken already fragile public services such as health, water and sanitation. Recurrent crises, such as floods year after year, give people and their crops no time to recover.

- The emergency phase of a relief operation aims to provide life-saving assistance; shelter, water, food and basic healthcare are the immediate needs; along with a sense of humanity and a sign that someone cares. Subsequent needs include reconstruction and rehabilitation.
- These needs can continue for several years, particularly in the case of refugees and victims of socioeconomic collapse.
- IRCS approaches to disaster response on these lines and works to improve the quality of humanitarian assistance provided to beneficiaries.
- The Indian Red Cross Society has been equipping itself with its manpower and physical infrastructures for a nation-wide Disaster Preparedness/Disaster Response (DP/DR) Programme.
- The urgent and serious need for substantial disaster preparedness measures in India had been recommended by a number of agencies (including DFID and the UK Disasters Emergency Committee) after major disaster response operations for the 1998. Super Cyclone in Orissa, the 2000 floods in Assam and the massive earthquake in Gujarat in 2001, Tsunami in 2004, Floods and earthquake in 2005. It is proved that the amount spent in prevention pays richly and saves a lot in relief.

Disaster Preparedness

- The Indian Red Cross Society (with Federation support) initiated a nation-wide Community Based Disaster Preparedness (CBDP) training program in 1999 after a series of awareness raising workshops between 1996 and 1998.
- In 2000, the National Society convened a national strategic planning workshop attended by 19 State Branches from which a strategic plan for DP/DR (2004–2007) was formulated and its activities are still continuing.
- The vision of the program is institutional strengthening, training and knowledge sharing through the establishment of a Disaster Management structure, programs for strengthening and expanding community based disaster preparedness (CBDP) in disaster affected areas.

Other Activities

Blood Bank

- The Indian Red Cross is a pioneer in the field of blood services and one of the largest voluntary blood banks in India since 1962.
- IRCS regularly conducts motivational campaigns to organize Voluntary Blood Donation Camps. It has more than 100 blood banks all over the country under different states and district branches.

HIV/AIDS

- The IRCS is very active in the prevention of HIV/AIDS. It trains youth to disseminate information about the prevention of HIV/AIDS through Youth Peer Education Programme.
- It also has programs and projects for children of HIV positive mothers, to provide comprehensive care.

Hospital Services

- IRCS provides service for sick and wounded men of the defence forces.
- Trained IRCS Lady Welfare Officers run welfare services for these people in military Hospitals.
- The officers run and maintain amenity stores and libraries as well as diversionary therapy programs such as teaching handicrafts to convalescing patients encouraging ailing soldiers to participate in recreational activities and to give Psychological support for their disability and sickness.
- **Home for disabled servicemen:** IRCS runs home in Bangalore for servicemen since 1946. The center is provided with an operation theater, physiotherapy department, recreation room, library and diversionary therapy all free of cost.

Vocational Training Center

- The IRCS provides opportunities to increase vocational skills and the earning opportunities of low-income groups and to raise the status of women socially and economically by making them available opportunities for learning and leadership.
- The Vocational Training Centers (VTCs) were started in areas which are dominated by backward classes and tribal population. IRCS in respect for gender equality and to augment the participation of women in economic development process started 2 vocational training centers, one each at Salt Lake, Calcutta (West Bengal) and at Arakkonam (Tamil Nadu) in the years 1989 and 1993.
- These centers besides providing training to the needy women also have developed as nucleus points for promoting women/child development activities.
- These centers also serve as garment production centers for use by the society in its relief operations it helps in supplementing family income, enabling mothers to spend more liberally on the welfare and upbringing of their children, give economic independence and improve the status of women in the community, enhance their decision-making role and improve the quality of life for the family and the communities in which they live.

Tracing Activities

- IRCS helps people trace or send massage to missing loved who have been separated ones through forced, unseen and inevitable circumstances when all other means of locating them have not yielded results.

- It also reunites families who have been separated under similar circumstances.

Maternity and Child Welfare

- Maternity and Child Welfare schemes of National Headquarters were started in 1954 to extend Maternal and Child Development activities for the Weaker Section of the Community.
- The welfare activities are being continued through various Hospitals, Subcenters and Bal Vikas Kendras.

Family Welfare

- These are run by different states and district branches.
- All Red Cross MCW hospitals and centers, as well as family welfare clinics, carry out family welfare work.
- They motivate eligible couples to adopt small family norms and provide them with contraceptives and other family planning devices.
- Many of these centers are equipped to meet motivational and clinical arrangements.

Nursing

The Red Cross MCW units teach home nursing skills to auxiliary nurses, midwives and housewives.

UNITED STATES AGENCY FOR INTERNATIONAL DEVELOPMENT

In 1961, Congress cemented US foreign assistance programs by separating military and non-military aid; The U.S. Agency for International Development (USAID) was born. It became the first US foreign assistance organization whose primary emphasis was on long-range economic and social development assistance efforts. Freed from political and military functions that plagued its predecessor organizations, USAID was able to offer direct support to the developing nations of the world. Its work supports long-term and equitable economic growth and advances foreign policy objectives by supporting: (a) economic growth, (b) agriculture and trade, (c) global health, and (d) democracy, conflict prevention and humanitarian assistance. USAID works in agriculture, democracy and governance, economic growth, the environment, education, health, global partnerships, and humanitarian assistance in more than 100 countries to provide a better future for all.

Main Activities

- USAID's commitment to improving global health includes confronting global health challenges through improving the quality, availability, and use of essential health services.
- USAID's objective is to improve global health, including child, maternal, and reproductive health, and reduce abortion and disease, especially HIV/AIDS, malaria, and tuberculosis.
- USAID's Global Health Bureau supports field health programs and innovation with a portfolio of nearly $4.15 billion. American Schools and Hospitals abroad administers a grant program that expands medical opportunities in developing countries.

Goals

USAID's decentralized network of resident field missions is drawn on to manage US government (USG) programs in low-income countries for a range of purposes.

Disaster Relief

- Some of the US Government's earliest foreign aid programs provided relief in crises created by war. In 1915, USG assistance through the Commission for Relief of Belgium headed by Herbert Hoover Prevented Starvation in Belgium after the German invasion. After 1945, the European Recovery Program championed by Secretary of State George Marshall (the "Marshall Plan") helped rebuild war-torn Western Europe.
- USAID manages relief efforts after wars and natural disasters through its office of US Foreign Disaster Assistance in Washington D.C. Privately funded US NGOs and the US military also play major roles in disaster relief overseas.

Poverty Relief

- After 1945, many newly independent countries needed assistance to relieve the chronic deprivation afflicting their low-income populations.
- USAID and its predecessor agencies have continuously provided poverty relief in many forms, including assistance to public health and education services targeted at the poorest.
- USAID has also helped manage food aid provided by the US Department of Agriculture.
- In addition, USAID provides funding to NGOs to supplement private donations in relieving chronic poverty.

Global Issues

- Technical cooperation between nations is essential for addressing a range of cross-border concerns like communicable diseases, environmental issues, trade and investment cooperation, safety standards for traded products, money laundering, and so forth.
- The USG has specialized agencies dealing with such areas, such as the Centers for Disease Control and the Environmental Protection Agency.
- USAID's special ability to administer programs in low-income countries supports these and other USG agencies' international work on global concerns.

Environment

- Among these global interests, environmental issues attract high attention. USAID assists projects that conserve and protect threatened land, water, forests, and wildlife. USAID also assists projects to reduce greenhouse-gas

emissions and to build resilience to the risks associated with global climate change.
- US environmental regulation laws require that programs sponsored by USAID should be both economically and environmentally sustainable.

US Bilateral Interests

- To support US geopolitical interests, USAID is often called upon to administer exceptional financial grants to allies. Also, when US troops are in the field, USAID can supplement the "Civil Affairs" programs that the U.S. military conducts to win the friendship of local populations.
- In these circumstances, USAID may be directed by specially appointed diplomatic officials of the State Department, as has been done in Afghanistan and Pakistan during operations against al-Qaeda.
- US commercial interests are served by US law's requirement that most goods and services financed by USAID must be sourced from US vendors.
- USAID is also sometimes called upon to support projects of US constituents that have exceptional interest.

Socioeconomic Development

- To help low-income nations achieve self-sustaining socioeconomic development, USAID assists them in improving management of their own resources.
- USAID's assistance for socioeconomic development mainly provides technical advice, training, scholarships, commodities, and financial assistance.
- Through grants and contracts, USAID mobilizes the technical resources of the private sector, other USG agencies, universities, and NGOs to participate in this assistance.
- Programs of the various types above frequently reinforce one another. For example, the Foreign Assistance Act requires USAID to use funds appropriated for geopolitical purposes ("Economic Support Funds") to support socioeconomic development to the maximum extent possible.

Modes of Assistance

USAID delivers both technical assistance and financial assistance.

Technical Assistance

- Technical assistance includes technical advice, training, scholarships, construction, and commodities.
- Technical assistance is contracted or procured by USAID and provided in-kind to recipients.
- For technical advisory services, USAID draws on experts from the private sector, mainly from the assisted country's own pool of expertise, as well as from specialized USG agencies.
- Many host-government leaders have drawn on USAID's technical assistance for development of IT systems and computer hardware procurement to strengthen their institutions.
- To build indigenous expertise and leadership, USAID finances scholarships to US universities and assists the strengthening of developing countries' own universities.
- Local universities' programs in developmentally important sectors are assisted directly and through USAID support for forming partnerships with US universities.

The various forms of technical assistance are frequently coordinated as capacity building packages for development of local institutions.

Financial Assistance

- Financial assistance supplies cash to developing country organizations to supplement their budgets.
- USAID also provides financial assistance to local and international NGOs who in turn give technical assistance in developing countries. Although USAID formerly provided loans, all financial assistance is now provided in the form of nonreimbursable grants.
- In recent years, the USG has increased its emphasis on financial rather than technical assistance.
- In 2004, the Bush Administration created the Millennium Challenge Corporation as a new foreign aid agency that is mainly restricted to providing financial assistance.
- In 2009, the Obama Administration initiated a major realignment of USAID's own programs to emphasize financial assistance, referring to it as "government-to-government" or "G2G" assistance.

USAID on Health in India

- Malaria eradication program
- Medical education
- Nursing education
- Health education
- Water supply and sanitation
- Control of communicable diseases
- Nutrition
- Family planning.

UNITED NATIONS EDUCATIONAL SCIENTIFIC AND CULTURAL ORGANIZATION

- UNESCO is the United Nations Educational Scientific and Cultural Organization (UNESCO). It contributes to peace and security by promoting close collaboration among nations through education, science and culture. It furthers universal respect for justice, rule and law, human rights and fundamental freedoms.
- UNESCO is sometimes believed to have originated from the International Institute of Intellectual cooperation. August 1, 1945, the Government of Britain communicated the revised draft to the Allied and Associated powers and invited them to an International conference in London.

- UNESCO is an intergovernmental organization with membership of 158 countries and 2 associate members (British Virgin Islands and Netherlands Antilles) at present. The first session of the General conference of UNESCO was first conceived as UNECO—without the S. The person who successfully promoted the "S" was the US poet Archibald Macleish.
- UNESCO took possession of its new headquarters at a Place de Fontenoy in Paris in September 1958. As against only 26 members in 1946, the membership at present stands at 158 nations. This has meant considerable increase in the responsibilities and resources of the organization. On November 4, 1986, UNESCO completed 40 years of its existence.

Objectives

The main objective of UNESCO is to contribute to peace and security in the world by promoting collaboration among nations through education, science, culture and communication in order to further universal respect for justice, for the rule of law, and for the human rights and fundamental freedoms which are affirmed for the peoples of the world, without distinction of race, sex, language or religion, by the Charter of the United Nations.

In support of this objective, UNESCO's principal functions are:
- To promote intellectual cooperation and mutual understanding of peoples through all means of mass communication.
- To give fresh impulse to popular education and to the spread of culture.
- To maintain, increase and diffuse knowledge.
- To encourage scientific research and training.
- To apply sciences to ensure human development and the rational management of natural resources.

Responsibilities of the Bureau of Strategic Planning

- Preparation and monitoring of the UNESCO Medium-Term Strategy and the Biennial Program and Budget of the Organization.
- Implementation of the principles of the results-based management and the risk management approaches.
- Monitoring of the implementation of the approved program and its work plans through regular reviews to assess progress towards the expected results, and report thereon periodically to the governing bodies in the context of the statutory reports.
- Leading and coordination of UNESCO's participation in and contribution to United Nations system inter-agency activities, in particular concerning global program issues, and those aiming to enhance system-wide coherence, globally, regionally and at the country levels.
- Integration of a future-oriented approach and foresight in all the fields of competence of the organization.
- Monitoring the implementation of the program activities related to the two global priorities of the Organization, Gender Equality and Africa.
- Promotion of South-South and North-South-South cooperation; support to the least developed countries (LDCs); the small island developing states (SIDS); the most vulnerable segments of society; indigenous peoples; countries in post-conflict and post-disaster situations and to countries in transition as well as middle-income countries.
- Coordination and backstopping for the inter-sectoral platforms.
- Leading the intersectoral and interdisciplinary program of action for a culture of peace and non-violence.
- Monitoring the implementation of the integrated comprehensive strategy for category 2 institutes and centers.
- Management of the System of Information on Strategies, Tasks and the Evaluation of Results (SISTER) and provisions of capacity training programs for staff and permanent delegations.

Governing Bodies of UNESCO

- The General Conference consists of the representatives of UNESCO's Member States.
- It meets every two years, and is attended by Member States and Associate Members, together with observers for non-Member States, intergovernmental organizations and non-governmental organizations (NGOs).
- Each country has one vote, irrespective of its size or the extent of its contribution to the budget.
- It determines the policies and the main lines of work of the organization. Its duty is to set the programs and the budget of UNESCO. It also elects the Members of the Executive Board and appoints, every four years, the Director-General.
- The working languages of the General Conference are Arabic, Chinese, English, French, Russian and Spanish.

Executive Board

- The Executive Board ensures the overall management of UNESCO. It prepares the work of the General Conference and sees that its decisions are properly carried out.
- The functions and responsibilities of the Executive Board are derived primarily from the Constitution and from rules or directives laid down by the General Conference.
- Every two years the General Conference assigns specific tasks to the Board. Other functions stem from agreements concluded between UNESCO and the United Nations, the specialized UN agencies and other intergovernmental organizations.
- The Executive Board's fifty-eight members are elected by the General Conference.
- The choice of these representatives is largely a matter of the diversity of the cultures they represent, as well as their geographic origin.
- Skillful negotiations may be needed before a balance is reached among the different regions of the world in a way that will reflect the universality of the organization. The Executive Board meets twice a year.

UNESCO Activity Planning

The Bureau of Strategic Planning (BSP) is the central focal point of UNESCO for all strategic, programmatic and budgeting issues, as well as for cooperation with extra budgetary funding sources and public-private partnerships (PPPs), and it provides advice to the Director-General on all these matters.

The activities of UNESCO fall under the following broad heads education, natural sciences, social sciences, Human sciences, culture, communication, cooperation with nongovernmental organizations and publications. Typical activities of UNESCO include the organization in various parts of the world of conferences and meeting of experts, coordination of international scientific efforts, standardization of documents and procedures, clearing house services, assistance to nongovernmental organizations a wide range of publications and the establishment of international agreements to which states are invited to adhere or confirm.

Functions

The main functions of the UNESCO are:

Education

- The largest sector of UNESCO's activity is in the field of education. Removal of illiteracy by encouragement to adult education, distance-education and the open school system.
- Emphasis on education of women and girls.
- Financial assistance for the education of disabled children.
- Provision of grants and fellowships to teachers and scholars, organization of library systems, and promotion of international understanding through education.
- Organization of book fairs and festivals at international and national levels. As example, Development of library system is an important component of continuing education. Delhi Public Library established in 1951 with financial assistance from UNESCO has developed into a big metropolitan public library system.
- Encouragement of science education by providing regional training centers.
- Promotion of education as an instrument for international understanding.

Scientific Activities

The scientific activities undertaken by the UNESCO are:
- UNESCO organizes seminars and conferences of scientists of various countries and circulars information through journals, press and exhibitions. 'Courier' is the official monthly magazine of UNESCO.
- It promotes basic research in fields like geology, mathematics, physics and oceanography. As a result, it finances engineering and technology schemes in a number of developing countries.
- It helps in correction the imbalance in scientific and technological manpower that exists, because 90% of trained manpower is concentrated in the industrialized countries.
- It encourages the study of social sciences in order to focus attention on combating all forms of discrimination, improving the status of women and helping the youth in solving their problems.

Communication

UNESCO develops communication for dissemination of information:
- It has set up regional networks, trained technologies and deals with both hardware and software aspects of informatics.
- It improves the quality of the Press, the films and video services.
- It assists developing countries to develop communications.
- It upholds the freedom of the press and independence of the media.

Preservation of Cultural Heritage

- It encourages modernization without the loss of cultural identity and diversity. UNESCO provides technical advice and assistance, equipment and funds for the preservation of monuments and other works of art. It has prepared a World Heritage List to identify the monuments and sites which are to be protected.
- It aims to protect the world inheritance of books, works of art and rare manuscripts.
- It gives encouragement to artistic creations in literature and fine arts.
- It pays attention towards the cultural development through the medium of films.
- It sends cultural missions to different countries so that there would be development of contracts which may promote peace and prosperity. In the past it has provided travel grants to writers and artists under a project named Mutual Appreciation of Eastern and Western Cultural Values. Under this scheme, India's talented exponents of classical music and dance travelled to Europe and America.

Indian National Commission for Cooperation with UNESCO

The main functions of the National commission are to serve as a link between UNESCO and institutions working in this country in the field of education, science and culture to advise the government of India on matters relating to UNESCO and to promote understanding of the aims and policies of UNESCO among the people of India.

International Days Observed at UNESCO

- 27 January: International Day of Commemoration in Memory of the Victims of the Holocaust
- 13 February: World Radio Day
- 21 February: International Mother Language Day
- 8 March: International Women's Day
- 23 April: World Book and Copyright Day
- 30 April: International Jazz Day
- 3 May: World Press Freedom Day

- 21 May: World Day for Cultural Diversity for Dialogue and Development
- 22 May: International Day for Biological Diversity
- 25 May: Africa Day/Africa Week
- 5 June: World Environment Day
- 8 June: World Oceans Day
- 9 August: International Day of the World's Indigenous People
- 12 August: International Youth Day
- 23 August: International Day for the Remembrance of the Slave Trade and its Abolition
- 8 September: International Literacy Day
- 15 September: International Day of Democracy
- 21 September: International Day of Peace
- 5 October: World Teachers' Day Second Wednesday in October: International Day for Disaster Reduction
- 17 October: International Day for the Eradication of Poverty
- 20 October: World Statistics Day
- 27 October: World Day for Audiovisual Heritage
- 10 November: World Science Day for Peace and Development Third Thursday in November: World Philosophy Day
- 16 November: International Day for Tolerance
- 19 November: International Men's Day
- 25 November: International Day for the Elimination of Violence against Women
- 29 November: International Day of Solidarity with the Palestinian People
- 1 December: World AIDS Day
- 10 December: Human Rights Day
- 18 December: International Migrants Day

INTERNATIONAL LABOR ORGANIZATION

The International Labor Organization (ILO) was established in the year 1919. The ILO is a United Nations agency dealing with labor issues, particularly international labor standards and decent work for all. 185 of the 193 UN member states are members of the ILO. In 1969, the organization received the Nobel Peace Prize for improving peace among classes, pursuing justice for workers, and providing technical assistance to other developing nations. Soon after the First World War, it was recognized that problems of industry, like disease, know no frontiers. In 1919, ILO was established as an affiliate of the League of Nations to improve the working and living conditions of the working population all over the world. The headquarters of ILO is in Geneva, Switzerland.

The primary goal of the ILO is to promote opportunities for women and men to obtain decent and productive work, in conditions of freedom, equity, security and human dignity.

Aims

- To promote rights at work
- Encourage decent employment opportunities
- Enhance social protection and
- Strengthen dialogue on work-related issues.

Purposes of ILO

- To contribute to the establishment of lasting peace by promoting social justice.
- To improve, through international action, labor conditions, and living standards.
- To promote economic and social stability.

The ILO has four strategic objectives:
1. To promote and realize standards and fundamental principles and rights at work.
2. To create greater opportunities for women and men to secure decent employment.
3. To enhance the coverage and effectiveness of social protection for all.
4. To strengthen tripartism and social dialogue.

These objectives are realized in a number of ways:
- Formulation of international policies and programs to promote basic human rights, improves working and living conditions, and enhances employment opportunities.
- Creation of international labor standards in the form of conventions and recommendations, backed by a unique system to supervise their application.
- An extensive program of international technical cooperation.
- Training, education, research, and publishing activities to help advance all of these efforts.

Membership

As per the amendments of Constitution in 1945, the membership rules of ILO are as follows:
- Any original member of UNO may become member of ILO by accepting its obligations of its constitutions.
- If a State is not the member of the UNO, the ILO confers on the ILC (Parliamentary Wing of the ILO) the right to admit that state to membership which it had assumed de facto during the period of ILO with League.

The membership of ILO has increased from 45 in 1919 to 151 in 2003.

Functions of the ILO

- Creation of coordinated policies and programs directed at solving social and labor issues.
- Adoption of international labor standards in the form of conventions and recommendations and control over their implementation.
- Assistance to member-states in solving social and labor problems.
- Human rights protection (the right to work, freedom of association, collective negotiations, protection against forced labor, protection against discrimination, etc.).
- Research and publication of works on social and labor issues.

The basis of the ILO is the tripartite principle, i.e., the negotiations within the organization are held between the representatives of governments, trade unions, and member-states' employers.

One hundred and eighty seven (187) conventions and recommendations on social and labor issues have been adopted since 1919.

International Labor Standards

- The ILO sets international labor standards with conventions, which are ratified by member states. These are non-binding.
- Conventions are drawn up with input from governments, workers' and employers' groups at the ILO and are adopted by the International Labor Conference.
- In ratifying an ILO convention, a member state accepts it as a legally binding instrument. Many countries use conventions as a tool to bring national laws in line with international standards.

India and ILO

India is a founding member of the ILO and it has been a permanent member of the ILO Governing Body since 1922. In India, the first ILO Office was started in 1928. The decades of productive partnership between the ILO and its constituents has mutual trust and respect as underlying principles and is grounded in building sustained institutional capacities and strengthening capacities of partners.

COOPERATIVE FOR AMERICAN RELIEF EVERYWHERE

Cooperative for Assistance and Relief Everywhere (CARE) is a nongovernmental organization which was started in 1946. It began working in India in 1950. CARE was found in North America in the wake of the Second World War in the year 1945. It is one of the world's largest independent, non-profit, non-sectarian international relief and development organization.

- One of the world's largest independent, nonprofit, nonsectarian international relief and development organization.
- Provides emergency aid and long-term development assistance.
- Began its operation in India in 1950.
- Till the end of 1980s, primary objective of CARE—India was to provide food for children in the age ground of 6–11 years.
- From mid 1980s, CARE—India focused food support in the ICDS program and in development of programs in the areas of health and income supplementation.
- CARE—India works in partnership with the Government of India, State Governments, and NGOs, etc.

Mission

CARE's mission has evolved over the decades. CARE continues to provide emergency relief during and after disasters, but the organization today focuses on addressing underlying causes of poverty. In such areas such as health, HIV/AIDS, natural resources, education and economic development, CARE works to empower women, because experience has shown that women's gains yield dramatic benefits for families and communities.

It is helping in the following projects:
- Integrated Nutrition and Health Project.
- Better Health and Nutrition Project.
- Anemia Control Project.
- Improving Women's Health Project.
- Improved Healthcare for Adolescent Girl's Project.
- Child Survival Project.
- Improving Women's Reproductive Health and Family Spacing Project.
- Konkan Integrated Development Project, etc.

CARE Campaigns in the Fight Against Global Poverty

- The World Hunger Campaign
- Education (To improve quality and accessibility of basic education)
- HIV/AIDS (Efforts to reduce spread of disease and to aid the affected ones).
- Victories over poverty: (Long-term solutions to poverty)
- CARE for the child.

Objectives of CARE India

The primary objective of CARE: India was to provide food for children in the age group of 6–11 years. From mid 1980s CARE-India focused its food support in the ICDS program and in development of programs in the areas of health and income supplementation.

CARE: India and Projects

CARE India is helping the following projects:
- Integrated Nutrition and Health Project (INHP)
- Promoting Linkages for Urban Sustainable Development (PLUS) Project.
- Better Health and Nutrition Project (BHNP).
- Sustainable Tribal Empowerment Project (STEP).
- Anemia Control Project.
- Credit Rotation for Empowerment and Development through Institution. Building and Training project (CREDIT).
- Maternal and Infant Survival Project (MISP).
- Girls Primary Education (GPE) Project.
- Improving Women's Health Project.
- Improved Healthcare for Adolescent Girls Project.
- Konkan Integrated Development Project.
- Child Survival (CS) Project.
- Improving Women's Reproductive Health and Family Spacing Project.

It has been helping with the school mid-day meal scheme. Apart from this, it also provides help in the fields of medicine, literacy vocational training and agriculture.

CARE-India works in partnership with government of India, state governments, nongovernmental organizations, etc.

In fiscal year 2010, CARE worked in 87 countries around the world, supporting 905 poverty-fighting projects to reach more than 82 million people, over half of whom are women.

CANADIAN INTERNATIONAL DEVELOPMENT AGENCY

The Canadian International Development Agency (CIDA) is Canada's lead agency for development assistance. Its aim is to reduce poverty, promote human rights, and support sustainable development. CIDA was established in 1968 to administer the bulk of Canada's official development assistance program. CIDA works in concert with its development partners, fragile states and countries in crisis, selected countries and regions, and the Canadian population and institutions. The measure of its success lies in its contribution to the achievement of the Millennium Development Goals and Canada's broader international policy objectives.

Origin

- CIDA was formed in 1968 by the Canadian Government under Lester B Pearson. CIDA reported to the Parliament of Canada through the Minister for International Cooperation.
- Its mandate was to "support sustainable development in developing countries" in order to reduce poverty and contribute to a more secure, equitable, and prosperous world.
- CIDA had its headquarters at "200 Promenade du Portage in Gatineau, Quebec".
- CIDA funding was the subject of intense debate, and the conservative government made major revisions to the funding process, including reductions to NGOs described as supporting "left-leaning causes", such as Montreal-based Alternatives.

Main Activities

CIDA has made progress, as follows:
- Worldwide, from 1990 to 2004, the proportion of people living in extreme poverty fell from nearly one third to 19%;
- Progress has been made in getting more children into school in the developing world; and
- Child mortality has declined globally, and it is becoming clear that the right lifesaving interventions are proving effective.

Functions

- **Social development:** CIDA has supported programs relating directly to the treatment of STDs in developing countries. It also cites basic education and child protection as priorities in the social development of countries that it aids.
- **Economic well-being:** Promoted and funded Microfinance and Education for Sustainable Development Programs.
- **Environmental sustainability:** With a focus upon issues such as climate change, land degradation, and water supply, CIDA sought to help developing nations maintain healthy ecosystems. CIDA was a partner in the Canada Iraq Marshlands Initiative. For example, CIDA was a major donor to the International LUBILOSA Program: which developed a biological pesticide for locust control, in support of small-holder farmers in the Sahel.
- **Governance:** CIDA strove for human rights, democracy, and good governance. The agency also supported gender equality.

JHPIEGO

JHPIEGO is an "international on profit health organization affiliated with Johns Hopkins University." The group was founded in 1973 and initially called the Johns Hopkins Program for International Education in Gynecology and Obstetrics, but is now referred to simply as JHPIEGO.

Member Profile

- For 35 years, JHPIEGO has empowered front-line health workers by designing and implementing effective, low-cost, hands-on solutions to strengthen the delivery of healthcare services for women and their families.
- By putting evidence-based health innovations into everyday practice, JHPIEGO works to break down barriers to high-quality healthcare for the world's most vulnerable populations.
- JHPIEGO'S program management strategy recognizes the technical complexity and geographical, cultural, socio-economic and political diversity among our programs.
- It develops global program initiatives and technical interventions that can be adapted to each country.

Our Mission

- JHPIEGO creates and delivers transformative healthcare solutions that save lives.
- In partnership with national governments, health experts and local communities, JHPIEGO builds health providers' skills and develops systems that save lives now and guarantee healthier futures for women and their families.

Our Vision

- Self-reliant countries, healthy families and resilient communities.
- All women and families, regardless of where they live, having equitable access to high-quality, lifesaving healthcare delivered by competent and caring providers.

Current Program Areas

In its early years, JHPIEGO was recognized as an expert in reproductive health and family planning. As the organization has grown and become more field-based, its programming areas have grown and expanded. As of 2015, JHPIEGO's primary program areas are:
- Maternal, newborn, and child health
- Family planning and reproductive health

- HIV/AIDS prevention and care
- Infection prevention and control
- Malaria prevention and treatment
- Cervical cancer prevention and treatment
- Tuberculosis (TB)
- Urban and community health
- Education and training
- Innovations.

Main Activities

- The JHPIEGO model is based on developing strong partnerships with communities, governments and organizations to build sustainable local health systems.
- Through the use of innovative approaches, it puts research to practice for creative solutions to improve the health of women and families throughout the world.
- Its core competencies are: human capacity development; standards and guidelines; education, training and curriculum development; and performance and quality improvement.
- JHPIEGO's work is focused on: maternal and child health; family planning and reproductive health; HIV/AIDS prevention and care; infection prevention and control; malaria prevention and treatment; and cervical cancer prevention and treatment.

JHPIEGO in India

- In the past four years, JHPIEGO has supported the Government of India to save the lives of an estimated 83,000 children and 9,900 women through improved contraceptive services. Averting an estimated 16.4 million unintended pregnancies and 10 million abortions saved an estimated US$549 million (INR 38.5 billion) in direct healthcare spending.
- An independent evaluation of JHPIEGO's initiative in India to implement the World Health Organization's Safe Childbirth Checklist (which addresses the major causes of maternal death, intrapartum-related stillbirths and neonatal deaths) showed an 11% decline in stillbirths and very early neonatal deaths at the 100 healthcare facilities where it was implemented.
- Through its collaboration with the public and private sectors, Jhpiego helped ensure that competent healthcare workers provided high-quality childbirth services for more than 2.8 million deliveries across the country.
- As a result of JHPIEGO's work in India in 2018, 38 national and subnational policies, regulations, guidelines and strategies were approved. Also, JHPIEGO-led advocacy resulted in more than US$49 million mobilized at the national level and more than US$6 million at subnational level.

ROCKEFELLER FOUNDATION

The Rockefeller foundation is a philanthropic organization chartered in 1913 and endowed by Mr John D Rockefeller. Its purpose is to promote the well-being on mankind throughout the world. It is a nongovernmental agency that started functioning in India from 1920. The foundation contributed meaningfully to the implementation of public health programs and the advancement of social and agricultural sciences. The main area of interest has been medical education and research.

Activities of Rockefeller Foundation

- Training of competent teachers and research workers.
- Sponsoring of visits of a large number of medical specialists from the USA.
- Providing grants in aid to selected institutions.
- Development of medical college libraries.
- Population studies.
- Assistance to research projects and institutions.

FORD FOUNDATION

Ford Foundation was started as a contemporary of the Rockefeller Foundation. Ford Foundation is an organization which is dedicated to the field of rural health services and family planning.

Activities of Ford Foundation

- It provides help in short-term training Programs in community health.
- Pilot projects of health services.
- RCA projects and research programs in family planning.

The Ford Foundation has provided help in the water supply and drainage of sewage systems in Kolkata and the establishment of National Health and Family Welfare Institute in Delhi.

- **Orientation Training Centers** at Singur, Poonamallee and Najafgarh. The centers provide training courses in public health for medical and paramedical personnel from all over India.
- **Research-cum-action (RCA) projects:** Aimed at solving some of the basic problems in environmental sanitation, e.g., designing and construction of hand-flushed acceptable sanitary latrines in rural areas.
- **Pilot project in Rural Health Services, Gandhigram (Tamil Nadu):** Among a rural population of 100,000 people, an attempt was made to develop and operate a coordinated type of health service which will provide a useful model for health administrators in the country.
- **Establishment of NIHAE:** has supported the establishment of the National Institute of Health Administration and Education at Delhi. The Institute provides a senior staff-college type training for health administrators.
- **Calcutta Water Supply and Drainage Scheme** has helped in the preparation of a master plan for water

supply, sewerage and drainage for the city of Calcutta in collaboration with other international agencies.
- **Family planning program:** Supporting research in reproductive biology and in the family planning fellowship programs.

COLOMBO PLAN

The Colombo Plan is a regional organization that embodies the concept of collective inter-governmental effort to strengthen economic and social development of member countries in the Asia-Pacific region. The primary focus of all Colombo Plan activities is on human resources development. Colombo plan is a cooperative venture of a unique kind which was inaugurated in 1950 by 20 governments of common wealth countries to provide economic development. In south and South-East Asian countries, e.g., Australia, Canada, Japan, New Zealand, Britain, and America are its members.

Purposes

- The Colombo Plan is not intended as an integrated master plan to which national plans were expected to conform.
- It is, instead, a framework for bilateral arrangements involving foreign aid and technical assistance for the economic and social development of the region.

Objectives

- To promote interest in and support for the economic and social development of Asia and the Pacific.
- To promote technical cooperation and assist in the sharing and transfer of technology among member countries.
- To keep under review relevant information on technical cooperation between the member governments, multilateral and other agencies with a view to accelerating development through cooperative effort.
- To facilitate the transfer and sharing of the developmental experiences among member countries within the region with emphasis on the concept of South-South cooperation.

Present members: The Colombo Plan currently has 27 members, including countries in the Asia-Pacific region, non-Commonwealth countries and countries belonging to regional groupings such as Association of South-East Asian Nations (ASEAN) and South Asian Association for Regional Cooperation (ASEAN).

VOLUNTARY ASSOCIATION

A voluntary group or union (also sometimes called a voluntary organization, common-interest association, or just an association) is a group of individuals who enter into an agreement, usually as volunteers, to form a body (or organization) to accomplish a purpose.

Definition

A voluntary association is a group or organization that people may join or leave freely, that is free of external control, and whose purpose, goals, and methods are up to the members to determine. Sociologically, voluntary associations are often seen as crucial to the functioning of democracy, especially by providing a way for individuals to become involved in public life beyond the privacy of home and family.

Objectives of Voluntary Organizations

Some of these objectives and functions of Voluntary Organizations may be discussed as follows:

- **Man is by nature gregarious.** The urge to act in groups is fundamental in him. People therefore form groups and associations voluntary for their benefit as also of others with a view to lead a full and richer life as is reflected in voluntary associations formed for promotion of recreational and cultural activities, social services, professional interests, etc.
- **A pluralistic society with a democratic system** requires multitude of independent, voluntary nongovernment associations as buffer between the individual and the state preventing the government from developing monopoly in various fields. Voluntary organizations involve citizens in noble affairs and avoid concentration of powers in the hands of government and thus serve as power breakers.
- **They enable the individuals to learn the fundamentals of groups and political** action through participation in the governing of their private organizations.
- **Organized voluntary action helps groups and individuals** with diverse political and other interests, contributes to strengthening of feeling of national solidarity and promotes participative character of democracy.
- **The state does not have the requisite financial resources and manpower** to meet all the needs of its citizens. It can therefore have the responsibility of providing them minimum needs. The voluntary organizations by raising additional resources locally can meet uncovered needs and enrich local life.
- **Voluntary organizations also help the state in the area** which are its exclusive responsibility but for which it has limited sources and perform such functions in much better way as compared to the state organizations.
- **Voluntary organizations thus have not only a role to play** in the field of accepted state responsibilities but they can also venture into new needs, work in new areas, unveil social evils and give attention to hitherto unattended and unmet needs. They can act as sappers and miners of unfolding development revolution. They can function as reconnaissance squads. They can be fore-runners of change and anticipate and take action to make it less painful. They can work for progress development and consequently in course of time they can help the state in extending its activities over wider areas, thus raising the national minimum.
- **They provide avenues for activities to those persons** why do not relish participation in the activities of the state through politics and government, but organize into voluntary groups thus making their talent, experience and spirit of service available to society in bringing about changes in it with a view to meeting the needs

and aspirations of the people concerned and enriching the lives.
- **They act as a stabilizing force by welding together** people with such groups as are not politically motivated and are no concerned about the fortunes of one or the other political party in capturing government power but are above party politics and are interested in other areas of nation building and thus contribute to national integration and concentration on nonpolitical issues.
- **They also perform the functions of educating the members** and the public at large about the policies and programs of the government about their welfare, their right and obligations and also are in a position to offer constructive criticism in respect of wrong policies and activities of governor without any fear and with courage of conviction obliging the government to make necessary adjustments to accommodate the viewpoints of the public likely to be affected by such policies and actions as has been the experience in the case of program concerning scheduled tribes and environment conservation and preservation.
- **The endeavor to meet the special requirements of specialized interests** and special groups such as the aged, the handicapped, women, children, etc. which cannot be adequately met by the state for reasons of financial scarcity. Age-India and Help Age are voluntary organizations engaged in the welfare programs of the aged.
- **They are in a better position to function to their own satisfaction** as also at that of their clientele for the reason that they can identify the needs of individuals, groups and community being close to them and formulate appropriate programs to meet them, make necessary changes and modification in the light of the experiences gained in their implementation processes, involve people's participation, raise necessary funds and win public confidence and cooperation by human touch.

Meaning of Voluntary Association

The term 'Voluntarism' is derived from the Latin word 'voluntas' which means "will" or "freedom". Harold Laski, an eminent British Political Scientist, defined, "Freedom of Association" as a recognized legal right on the part of all persons to combine for the promotion of purposes in which they are interested. Article 19(c) of the Constitution of India confers on the Indian citizens the right 'to form association'. Freedom of association is rightly regarded as taking high rank among the liberties of man.
- It is the liberty of the widest scope for men may wish to associate for any purpose which two or more of them may have in common.
- They may wish to associate to do something together, or to get something done to further their own or other people's interest, to resist oppression or injustice or to pursue great or small, general or public object.
- In the UN terminology voluntary organizations are called nongovernmental organizations (NGOs).

- Norman Johnson in his examination of the various definitions of voluntary social services points out their four main characteristics:
  1. Method of formation, which is voluntary on the part of a group of people;
  2. Method of government, with self-governing organization to decide on its constitution, its servicing, its policy and its clients;
  3. Method of financing, with at least some of its revenues drawn from voluntary sources; and
  4. Motives with the pursuit of profit excluded.

Characteristics of Voluntary Organization

The definitions of a voluntary organization given above bring out its following main characteristics:
- It is registered under the Societies Registration Act, 1880, the Indian Trusts Act, 1882; the Cooperative Societies Act, 1904 or the Joint Stock Companies Act, 1959 depending upon the nature and scope of its activities to give it a legal status.
- It has definite aims and objectives and programs for their fulfillment and achievement.
- It has an administrative structure and a duly constituted management and executive committee.
- It is an organization initiated and governed by its own members on democratic principles without any external control.
- It raises funds for its activities partly from the exchequer in the form of grants-in-aid and partly in the form of the contributions or subscription from the members of the local community and/or the beneficiaries of the programs.

Factors Motivating Voluntary Action

- The factors which motivate people to take to voluntary action or the sources of voluntarism may be identified as religion, government, business, philanthropy and mutual aid.
- The missionary zeal of religious organizations, the commitments of government organization to the public interest, the profit making urge in business, the altruism of the 'social superiors' and the motive of self-help among fellowmen all are reflected in voluntarism.
- At the operational level, the above mentioned components may not differ much from one another but each of them is moved by an impulse with service as the common motivation.
- Bourdillon and William Beveridge viewed mutual aid and philanthropy as two main sources from which voluntary social service organizations would have developed.
- They spring from individual and social conscience respectively. The other factors motivating voluntary action could be cited as personal interest, seeking benefit such as experience, recognition, knowledge and prestige, commitment to certain values, etc.
- Further, impulses of a great variety move men for their grouping or forming voluntary associations to serve

themselves, their fellowmen or the unfortunate lot of the society.
- These are idealistic, educative, psychological and social in character operating separately or on varying combination.
- Idealistically voluntary associations preserve democracy and the individuals' personality and contribute to the general health of the society.
- They are a strong agent of political socialization in a democracy and educate their members about the social norms and values and help combat loneliness.
- Psychological impulses lead people to join voluntary associations for security, self expression and for satisfaction of their interests with the decaying of social institutions like family, church and community.

Functions of Voluntary Health Agencies
- Creating a sense of responsibility through direct involvement.
- Channelize human resources.
- Effective policy formation through interpretation of public opinion.
- Participation of beneficiaries.
- Flexibility and experimentation.
- Initiative and leadership.
- Supplements the efforts of government.
- Help in efficient program implementation.
- Advancing health legislation.

Problems of Voluntary Health Agencies
- Governmental interference in the activities of voluntary organizations.
- Lack of interest among the intellectual elite.
- Lack of effective collaboration among voluntary agencies themselves.
- Lack of competence to develop integrated area plan.
- Poor linkage with the beneficiaries.
- Absence of sound administrative set up to deal with social work.

Significance
- The VHAs share the burden of healthcare of the masses with the government and the private practitioners.
- By doing pioneering work, they draw the attention of the government to the solving of pressing health problems.
- Some of the activities initiated by VHAs are maternal and child welfare, family planning, counseling for the drug addicts, medical insurance, sanitary latrines, welfare of the handicapped, and cancer detection and treatment.

Advantages
- Compared to the official programs, those undertaken by the VHAs are carried out with greater participation by the people and are therefore better accepted by them.
- The programs of VHAs are not governed by the rigid rules as are the official programs. In other words, the former are flexible.
- As bureaucratism and red-tapism do not handicap them, the VHAs work fast and at low operative costs.
- They provide an opportunity to those individuals who have free time to channelize their energy into useful social activities.

Disadvantages
- The programs of VHAs often relate to noncritical health problems.
- Their services are not always targeted to those who are in the greatest need of them; nor are they conducted in areas that need them the most.
- The programs of VHAs are often not run according to the modern principles and techniques of management.

INDIAN RED CROSS SOCIETY

This was set up in 1920 under the Indian Red Cross Society (IRCS), Act. Its President is the President of India. It is affiliated to the International Red Cross. The Managing Committee of IRCS consists of a Chairman, who is appointed by the President, and 12 members who are elected by the state committees. The Managing Committee appoints the Secretary General and the Treasurer.

During peacetime, IRCS supplies milk and medicine to hospitals, dispensaries, and orphanages. It runs the Red Cross Home situated at Bangalore devoted to the care of those who were wounded during World War II. It operates blood-banking services. It runs maternity and child welfare centers and family planning clinics. It imparts training in first aid to school children. In the wake of disasters, IRCS volunteers actively participate in providing rescue and relief to the victims.

Organization
- The IRCS has 35 State/Union Territories Branches with their more than 700 districts and sub-district branches.
- The President of India is the President of the IRCS.
- The Minister of Health and Family Welfare is the Chairman of the Society.
- The National Managing Body consists of 19 members.
- The Chairman and 6 members of the managing body are nominated by the President. The remaining 12 are elected by the state and union territory branches through an electoral college.
- The Vice Chairman is elected by the members of the Managing Body.
- The Managing Body is responsible for governance and supervision of the functions of the society through a number of committees.
- The Secretary General is the Chief Executive of the Society.

Strategic Objectives

Objective 1
Enhance the capacity of Indian Red Cross to deliver its humanitarian message both within and outside the society, and to advocate tolerance and coexistence in the communities.

Action 1:1: Systematically organize, train and share knowledge among Red Cross members, volunteers, governance and management about Red Cross and Red Crescent Movement history and structure, Fundamental Principles and International Humanitarian Law.

Action 1:2: Raise the awareness and strengthen the knowledge, understanding and respect of the public authorities and others to the Fundamental Principles, the Emblem and International Humanitarian Law.

Objective 2
Increase the capacity in disaster preparedness and disaster response in disaster prone branches and National Headquarters and reduce the vulnerability of communities in key disaster prone areas.

Action 2:1: Develop Disaster Management policy, strategy, plans and protocols.

Action 2:2: Develop effective and sustainable disaster management mechanisms guided by sphere standards.

Action 2:3: Enhancing community capacities and creating awareness.

Action 2:4: Improved advocacy, coordination, collaboration and integration.

Objective 3
Increase the capacity in health and care in branches and National Headquarters and improve the health of vulnerable people and communities.

Action 3:1: Develop health policy, strategy, plans and protocols and design and develop health and care programs.

Action 3:2: Strengthen prevention focused volunteer based community healthcare.

Action 3:3: Enhance the Indian Red Cross emergency health Capacity.

Action 3:4: Help and support the vulnerable to handle HIV/AIDS epidemic and respond to public health crisis with particular focus on HIV Aids.

Objective 4
Raise the capacity of the branches and that of National Headquarters in mobilizing, organizing and managing local resources in order to improve the situation of the vulnerable under each strategic objective, one or several actions, which need to be taken to achieve it, are identified and explained. This is followed by a listing of expected results and of concrete implementation measures.

Action 4:1: Develop a national branch development policy and strategy and increase the capacity of the national headquarters and state branches to provide development support to the branches.

Action 4:2: Promote the integrity of the Indian Red Cross ensuring respect and compliance with the Fundamental Principles by reviewing, amending and establishing the constitution organizational structure, rules, policies and procedure in according with the need of the organization and in coherence with the policies of the Red Cross and Red Crescent Movement.

Action 4:3: Develop and establish a national resource development strategy and policy integrating financial, material as well as member and volunteer development, mobilization and maintenance components.

Action 4:4: Improve and upgrade the capacity for information and communication at the district level and at national headquarters.

Action 4:5: Improve and upgrade the capacity for financial planning, management and reporting at the national headquarters and design and establish a finance development project for the branches.

Action 4:6: Develop and establish a community-based volunteer management system including a relief and emergency volunteers.

Action 4:7: A human resource development system and phased training program for governance, volunteers and staff developed and established.

Seven Fundamental Principles of Red Cross

1. **Humanity:** The International Red Cross and Red Crescent Movement, born of a desire to bring assistance without discrimination to the wounded on the battlefield, endeavors, in its international and national capacity, to prevent and alleviate human suffering wherever it may be found. Its purpose is to protect life and health and to ensure respect for the human being. It promotes mutual understanding, friendship, cooperation and lasting peace amongst all peoples.

2. **Impartiality:** It makes no discrimination as to nationally, race, religious beliefs, class or political opinions. It endeavors to relieve the suffering of individuals, being solely by their needs, and to give priority to the most urgent cases of distress.

3. **Neutrality:** In orders to enjoy the confidence of all, the movement may not take sides in hostilities or engage in controversies of a political, racial, religious or ideological nature.

4. **Independence:** The Movement is independent. The National Societies, while auxiliaries in the humanitarian services of their governments and subject to the laws of their respective countries, must always maintain their autonomy so that they may be able at all times to act in accordance with the principles of the Movement.

5. **Voluntary service:** It is voluntary relief movement not prompted in any manner by desire for gain.

Chapter 19: Health Agencies

6. **Unity:** There can be only one Red Cross or Red Crescent in any one country. It must be open to all. It must carry on its humanitarian work throughout its territory.
7. **Universality:** The International Red Cross and Red Crescent Movement, in which all societies have equal status and share equal responsibilities and duties in helping each other, is worldwide.

INDIAN COUNCIL OF CHILD WELFARE

Historically by 1920 the first children's organization has been formed with child membership called "Balkanji Bari" with headquarters in Mumbai. In 1924, the guild of services started its excellent child welfare services in Chennai, spreading to most of South India. The Indian Council for Child Welfare (ICCW) was formed in 1952 which is the first National Organization to mobilize voluntary activity in every state in favor of all aspects of children's needs. In 1953, the Central Social Welfare Board was established.

Child care programs and projects such as rural balwadis, holiday homes have been started ad grants to over 7,000 non-governmental agencies for conducting orphanages, crèches, women's homes, etc., have been sanctioned. Eventually it became part of its program for improving the lives of women and children.

The Indian Council for Child Welfare organized the national consultation in collaboration with UNICEF, brought out sharply the inadequacies in the enforcement of the provision of the UN convention on the "Rights of the Child" contrary to the official claims.

Vision: A society for its children by giving first priority to their needs, rights and protection thereby ensuring opportunities for the fullest development of the innate potential of every child leading to the well-being and happiness of both.

Mission and Objective

- To ensure for the children their basic human right to survival, physical, mental and social development and opportunity to grow to their full potential.
- To work for the protection of children against neglect, abuse and exploitation.
- To initiate, support or undertake any activity for betterment of families and communities, which will ultimately enhance the quality of life for children.
- To initiate, undertake or aid directly or through District Councils or Institutional Members, schemes for furtherance of Child Welfare/Development in Tamil Nadu (TN branch).
- To promote dissemination of knowledge and information and to educate public opinion of Child Welfare/Development programs on a scientific basis.
- To promote enactments of legislation relating to matters concerning children and their welfare and to work towards the implementation of the provisions.

Functions of ICCW

- The "Indian Council for Child Welfare" not only drew up the original syllabus but has continued the balwadis which were consequently set up from the third five year plan onwards and have proved to be the important base for nutrition and immunization programs.
- The Indian council for child welfare, New Delhi is one of the major voluntary organizations.
- The ICCW with other voluntary organizations and ministries of social welfare and community development initiated training of preschool workers.
- Balasevikas were trained in the Balasevika training centers set up by the Central social welfare board through grants-in-aid to voluntary organizations like Indian council for child welfare.
- A guidebook for Balasevika training institution has been prepared by ICCW. It has also drawn up a proposal for a five day refresher course in service training of Balasevikas.
- Regional workshops are also held for the instructors of the Balasevika training centers, so as to provide them orientation in training methodology and new concepts and methods of child development.

FAMILY PLANNING ASSOCIATION OF INDIA

It was established in 1949 with headquarters at Mumbai. Family Planning Association of India (FPAI) runs family welfare clinics in many cities and offers family planning services including MTP and sterilization. It holds mobile camps for the benefit of people in rural areas.

It undertakes training of doctors, paramedics, social workers, rural and urban volunteers, and opinion builders in family planning. It has two Regional Training Centers at Hyderabad and Gwalior.

FPAI imparts community education about population control, family life, sex and prevention of STDs including AIDS. It organizes seminars, workshops, and conferences. It publishes a quarterly journal devoted to family welfare. FPAI gives financial assistance to other NGOs undertaking family welfare activities.

Vision: FPA India envisions sexual and reproductive health for all as a human right, including gender equality leading to alleviation of poverty, population stabilization and sustainable development.

Mission

- FPA India strengthens a voluntary commitment to advocate for SRH and Rights and, choices.
- It promotes access to SRH information and services related to family planning, safe abortions, HIV/AIDS and sexuality to poor, marginalized and vulnerable populations including young people.

Activities

- FPAI runs clinics providing family welfare services including MTP and sterilization.
- It conducts mobile camps in rural areas.

- It conducts training programs for doctors, para-medical workers, volunteers and opinion builders in the area of family planning.
- It has two Regional Training Centers at Hyderabad and Gwalior.

Health Education

- It publishes quarterly journals related to family welfare.
- It gives financial assistance to other NGOs undertaking family welfare services.

Current Programs at Family Planning Association of India

- HIV/AIDS Prevention Program
- Prevention of unsafe abortion and sex selective abortions.
- SALIN + (Youth Project)
- Research, programs and advocacy of adolescents and youth, married couples and work with health service providers.
- Computer skills.
- Provide technical assistance to different stakeholders in sexual and reproductive health programs.
- Target Intervention (HIV/AIDS Project).
- Work with high-risk behavior groups for AIDS control program.
- Clinical services.
- Diagnosis and treatment of reproductive tract infections and sexually transmitted infection and other reproductive healthcare for men and women.

Other Programs

- JIGYASA Youth Center
- Panchsheel Skills Development Center
- Youth HIV Projects
- Twin E-learning Project for Urban Youth.

TUBERCULOSIS ASSOCIATION OF INDIA

The Tuberculosis Association of India (TAI) has been serving the cause of tuberculosis since 1939. It is one of the oldest and largest voluntary organizations having its affiliates all over the country. It was set up in February 1939, as a registered society by incorporating the King Emperor's Anti-Tuberculosis Fund and King George Thanks-giving (Anti-Tuberculosis) Fund. Her Excellency the Marchioness of Linlithgow was the first President of the Association when the Tuberculosis Association of India was established on February 23, 1939.

Aims and Objectives

- The prevention, control, treatment and relief of tuberculosis.
- The encouragement of and assistance in the establishment throughout India of State Associations having objectives similar in whole or in part to those of the Association.
- The affiliation or control of and the rendering of assistance to any institution having objectives similar in whole or in part to the objects of the association.
- The undertaking of the research and investigation on subjects concerning tuberculosis and allied chest diseases.
- The doing of all such things as are incidental or conducive to the attainment of the above objectives.

Present Major Activities of the TAI

- Publication of the prestigious Indian Journal of Tuberculosis quarterly being uninterruptedly published since 1953. It is the only journal in India devoted exclusively to the cause of tuberculosis and chest diseases.
- Organization of the National Conference on Tuberculosis and Chest Diseases (NATCON). Since the year 1939 the association is organizing an annual conference wherein around 500 delegates from all over India assemble and exchange views, research papers and attend seminars on tuberculosis and diseases allied to it. NATCON is organized in collaboration with one or other of the State affiliates of the Association.
- TB Seal Campaign is organized every year. The Honorable President of India who is also the Patron of the Association generally inaugurates the Campaign on 2nd October, the Gandhi Jayanti Day at Rashtrapati Bhawan. The TB Seals Campaign conveys the message that TB is preventable. It also helps to raise funds for promoting voluntary anti-TB work in the country and provides opportunity to every citizen to contribute to the fight against this antihuman disease. The campaign is being organized since 1950.
- Providing quality diagnostic and treatment services through its New Delhi TB Center.

Fund Raising for the Foregoing Activities

- TAI does not receive any Government grants for its activities. A TB Seal Campaign which is inaugurated every year on 2nd October by the President of India who is the Patron of TAI. A TB Seal costs 2 rupees and carries a message about tuberculosis. Last year the Association was able to sell 1.8 crores of TB seals. 93% of the collections are retained in the States for grass-roots activities and TAI receive 7% for its activities. TAI also gets donations from the public.
- Technical education by way of holding national and state level conferences which serve the scientific purpose of updating knowledge of tuberculosis workers besides providing a platform to researchers to interact. It may be mentioned that tuberculosis research in India has provided the basis of national tuberculosis control program the world over.
- The TAI also runs standard training course for Tuberculosis Health Workers, Laboratory Technicians and DTCD/RNTCP orientation seminars for medical officers.
- The Indian Journal of Tuberculosis is published quarterly. It is an authoritative and only journal devoted to tuberculosis, along with other chest diseases.

- Since 1975, the TAI has established a Research Fund from contributions received from the states to provide financial assistance for research proposals forwarded by them, along with technical guidance and to publish the findings in the Indian Journal of Tuberculosis.

CENTRAL SOCIAL WELFARE BOARD

The Central Social Welfare Board (CSWB) is the key organization in the field of social welfare in India. Created in 1953 it comprises of a full-time chairperson and members representing state and union territories. Its general body consists of 51 members headed by the chairperson. She is appointed by the government in consultation with the ministry of social welfare from amongst prominent women social workers.

The general body consists of representatives nominated by state governments, social scientists, representatives from the ministries of finance, rural reconstruction, health education and social welfare and one member from Planning Commission. In addition three members of parliament, social workers, social scientists and social welfare administrators are also included in the general body.

Mission

- As a National Organization, strive to be recognized as the most progressive entity for providing services of unequivocal excellence to women and children for their protection, capacity building and total empowerment.
- To raise awareness about the legal and human rights of women and girl child and to run campaigns against social evils affecting them.

Vision

The Board must:
- Act as a change maker with a humanitarian approach by reinforcing the spirit of voluntarism.
- Create an enabling mechanism to facilitate networking of committed social workers for the empowerment of women and children.
- Develop a cadre of sensitive professionals with a gender centric vision committed to equity, justice and social change.
- Recommend gender specific policy initiatives to meet the new challenges for women and children in emerging areas.
- Strengthen voluntary organizations and expand coverage of 'engendered' schemes in areas where they have not yet reached.
- Initiate and strengthen its monitoring role to act a social audit and guide for the voluntary sector so as to access Government funds as resource.
- Generate awareness about the challenges of a society in transition where negative use of technologies and practices are impacting on the well-being of women and children.

Main Objectives of CSWB

- To study the needs and requirements of social welfare organizations from time to time through surveys, research and evaluation in such manner as may be considered necessary.
- To evaluate the programs and projects of the aided agencies.
- To coordinate assistance extended to social welfare. Activities by various ministries in Central and State Government in the programs entrusted to the Central Social Welfare Board.
- To promote the setting up of social welfare organizations on a voluntary basis in places where no such organizations exist and to promote additional organizations wherever necessary.
- To render technical and financial aid, when necessary to deserving institutions organizations including Panchayat Raj institutions in accordance with schemes/principles approved by Government of India.
- To promote social welfare activities intended of the general welfare of the public such as welfare of the family, women, children and the handicapped.
- To organize or promote programs of training in social work as and when required and also to organize and work pilot projects whenever necessary.
- To organize through its machinery, emergency reliefs in case of calamities, national natural or otherwise whatever deemed fit or necessary.

Activities

- It surveys the needs and requirements of voluntary welfare organizations in the country.
- It promotes the formation of social welfare organizations.
- It provides financial aid to deserving welfare organizations.
- It has started a scheme of "Industrial Cooperatives" under which the women of the lower middle class in urban areas, were employed and given salary, thus releasing their economic status.
- It has initiated "Family and Child Welfare Services" in 1968, in rural areas for the welfare of women and children through various activities such as mother craft, social education, literacy classes, distribution of milk, organization of play centers for children, etc.

Functions of CSWB

- Surveying the needs and requirements of voluntary welfare organizations in the country.
- Promoting and setting up of social welfare organization on a voluntary basis.
- Rendering of financial aid to deserving existing organizations and institutions.

Statutory Functions

- To survey the need and requirements of social welfare organizations.

- To promote the setting up of social welfare institutions in remote areas.
- To promote programs of training and organize pilot projects in social work.
- To subsidies hostels for working women and the blind.
- To give grants-in-aid to voluntary institutions and NGOs providing welfare service to vulnerable sections of society.
- To coordinate assistance extended to welfare agencies by Union and State governments.

Some of these Welfare Activities of the Target Groups

- Running of rehabilitation centers and cooperative societies for destitute, widows, orphans and deserted women and children.
- Educating and training women to acquire vocational skills to become employable.
- Organizing family welfare camps to promote small family norm through opinion leads.
- Providing hostels for working women of low income groups with adequate security.
- Operating urban welfare centers in towns for recreational activities and learning programs for women and children.
- Supplying nutritional supplementary diet and tonics to malnourished mothers and children below 5 years through balwadis and daycare centers.

ALL INDIA WOMEN'S CONFERENCE

The All India Women's Conference (AIWC) is a nongovernmental organization (NGO) based in Delhi. It was founded in 1927 by Margaret Cousins in order to improve educational efforts for women and children and has expanded its scope to also tackle other women's rights issues. The organization is one of the oldest women's groups in India and has branches throughout the country.

Aims and Objectives

- To work for a society based on the principles of social justice, personal integrity and equal rights and opportunities for all.
- To secure recognition of the inherent right of every human being to work and to the essentials of life, such as food, clothing, housing, education, social amenities and security, in the belief that these should not be determined by accident of birth or sex but by planned social distribution.
- To support the claim of every citizen to the right to enjoy basic civil liberties.
- To stand against all separatist tendencies and to promote greater national integration and unity.
- To work actively for the general progress and welfare of women and children and to help women to utilize to the fullest the Fundamental Rights conferred on them by the Constitution of the Indian Union.
- To cooperate with people and organizations of the world for the implementation of those principles which alone can assure permanent international amity and world peace?

Activities of the All India Women's Conference

- Special contribution in the running of maternal and child health clinics.
- Health centers and child health clinics.
- Arranges for adult education and milk centers.
- Teachers mother craft.
- Organize balwadi.

ALL INDIA BLIND RELIEF SOCIETIES

This organization financed by the Government of India, was established in 1946 for the purpose of bringing together the work of mainly different institutions for the care of the blind. Earlier relief work for the blind had been done by private and government agencies, but some of it was discontinued because of lack of funds.

ACTIVITIES

- It organizes eye relief camps and other measures for the relief camps of the blind.
- It also organizes health education and eye relief camps.

School Education

- The Government-aided JPM School is an all-boys residential school providing education and comprehensive range of services free to around 200 students under its care.
- The School is affiliated to the Central Board of Secondary Education. The School also has a Nursery Section, which prepares children for future educational tasks through the play way method.
- The foundation of learning laid here helps build a sound educational edifice in years ahead.
- Special academic and equipment support is also provided to the children with low vision.
- Activities like music, dance, sports, yoga, martial arts, reflexology, trekking are integral to the school program.

Technical Training

- The Center offers vocational training in a wide range of industrial and other occupations to visually impaired adults.
- The training also includes orientation and mobility, communication skills, etc.
- General Mechanic-cum-Machine Operator's Course (1 Year) is for those who have passed Class VIII. Training covers areas of factory work like assembly jobs, inspection work, operating such machines as power press, drilling and tapping machines.
- The Course is recognized by the Board of Technical Education, Government of Delhi as a regular ITI Course.

Massage Training (3 Months)

- The training for visually challenged adults has been designed in collaboration with the famous VLCC Institute covers Swedish, Thai, Aroma and Head Massage.
- For imparting further training to the past trainees special course in Ayurvedic Massage is being conducted under the care and support of Shahnaz Husain International Beauty Institute.
- In addition, visiting experts impart skills in pain-management through reflexology and magneto-therapy. These skills have opened up new avenues for the visually challenged for jobs and self-employment.

Multi-skill Training

- An innovative 1-year training program designed for adult blind (male/female) between the age of 18 to 35 years who have either missed-out school education or are marginally educated to acquire a variety of skills to become useful workers for industry or become self-employed.
- Skills covered are book binding and paper craft, basic massage, chair caning, candle making, packaging etc. The trainees also have supportive sessions on personality development, understanding computer, Braille, music, orientation and mobility.

Electronic Training: The 1-year training prepares low-vision and orthopedically handicapped in the repair and maintenance of household electrical and electronic gadgets.

Candle Making

- The program provides training and remunerative work to the visually impaired. Also, representatives/persons deputed by NGOs/welfare organizations are welcome to undergo training to start such programs in their centers.
- Representatives/persons deputed by NGOs/welfare organizations are welcome to undergo training to start such programs in their centers.
- Wide range of candles produced at BRA has great demand, particularly during Diwali season.

HIND KUSHT NIVARAN SANGH

Hind Kusht Nivaran Sangh (HKNS) (Indian Leprosy Association) is an old and prestigious body of people committed towards treatment, rehabilitation of leprosy patients and elimination of leprosy from India. Abbreviated as HKNS, Hind Kusht Nivaran Sangh was founded on 27th January 1925 with the name of Indian Council of British Empire Leprosy Relief Association (BELRA) with three objectives: (i) to carry out research on various aspects of leprosy; (ii) to provide short courses of training, treatment of leprosy; and (iii) to carry out propaganda. When the Indian Council of BELRA was established by his excellency the earl of reading and; then Viceroy and Governor-General of India, there were two headquarters, one located at Indian Red Cross Society Office, New Delhi (inaugurated by Sardar Bahadur Balwant Singh Puri) functioning as Administrative Office and the other headquarter working as Technical Office situated at the Department of Leprosy, School of Tropical Medicine and Hygiene, Calcutta under the leadership of Dr Ernest Muir.

Activities

- Leprosy Free India.
- Mass awareness campaigns.
- Capacity Building Training (Training of trainers).
- Socio-economic empowerment of leprosy affected persons.
- Publication and distribution of IEC material.
- Rehabilitation of the patients.
- 30th January: Anti-Leprosy Day Activities.

Present Activities of Hind Kusht Nivaran Sangh (Indian Leprosy Association)

- Production and distribution of health education and publicity material on leprosy.
- Publication of quarterly Indian Journal of Leprosy and bi-monthly news bulletin Kusht Vinashak for leprosy workers and the general public.
- Production and distribution of leprosy seals to create awareness about leprosy and help other organizations in raising funds for their work through the sale of these seals.
- Observance of Anti-Leprosy Day on the 30th January every year to create mass awareness about leprosy.
- Conducting training courses of 9 months duration for physiotherapy technicians of at two leprosy training centers (Naini, Allahabad, Uttar Pradesh, Purulia and West Bengal).
- Organizing the All India Leprosy Workers Conference and Regional Leprosy Workers Conferences in collaboration with the state branches and other voluntary organizations.
- Providing assistance to voluntary organizations and leprosy patients.
- Maintaining a house called "Shanthi Illam" at Vellore (Tamil Nadu) where leprosy patients who come for surgical treatment at the Christian Medical College and Hospital, Vellore are provided free boarding and lodging facilities.
- Running of two mobile leprosy treatment units in two districts of Delhi (North-East and West) with funds provided by the Government of India.
- Organizing exhibitions on leprosy in Delhi.

CHILD RELIEF AND YOU

- Late Rippan Kapur, an Air India flight purser, founded CRY in 1981. The aim of Child Relief and You (CRY) is to promote collective action for the welfare of deprived children like street children, bonded children, children of prostitutes, and children in remand homes. It ensures that each such child gets the chance to attend a school, participate in games and sports and attain positive health.

It has set up a materials bank at Delhi where toys, clothes, books, and the like are accepted and given to the needy children. CRY provides support to other agencies involved in child development projects by way of materials, money and training. CRY has instituted Rippen Kapur Fellowship Awards. Every year these are given to persons who have done exemplary work for the upliftment of special children. CRY raises finances by selling selected products of private manufactures at a commission. Additionally, it sells greeting cards, calendars, folders, and the like made for it free of cost by its patrons.

Fundamental Rights of Children

- The right to survival, to life, health, nutrition, including nationality.
- The right to development of education, care, leisure, and recreation.
- The right to protection from exploitation, abuse and neglect.
- The right to participation in expression, information, thought and religion.

CRY works to ensure the above-mentioned rights to all categories of children, who could be street children, children bonded in labor, children of commercial sex workers, physically and mentally challenged children and children in juvenile institutions, or even children from privileged homes.

BHARAT SEVAK SAMAJ

Bharat Sevak Samaj (BSS) is a nonpolitical and nonofficial organization was formed in 1952. The primary objectives of the BSS are to develop help people to achieve health by their own actions and efforts. The BSS has branches in all the states and in nearly all the districts.

Objectives

- To find and develop avenues of voluntary service for the citizens of India.
- To promote national sufficiency and to build up the economic strength of the country.
- To promote national sufficiency and to build up the community and to mitigate the privations and hardships of less favored sections.
- To draw out the available unused time, energy and other resources of the people and direct them into fields of social and economic activity.
- To take all steps which are necessary for the fulfillment of the aforesaid objects.

Five Point Code for BSS Workers

1. Integrity
2. Loyalty to the Nation
3. Selfless Service
4. Peaceful Conduct
5. Economic Living

Activities of BSS

- To promote environmental sanitation in villages in one of their key activities.
- To organize youth camps, teacher training camps, college student's camps, and health publicity.
- Improvement of sanitation in villages.

KASTURBA MEMORIAL FUNDS

The Kasturba Memorial Fund was created in memory of Kasturba Gandhi in 1944 after her death. The trust has nearly a crore of rupees and is actively engaged in various welfare projects in the country. The memorial fund is utilized in many women welfare projects. This trust also carries out antileprosy work.

Aims

Mahatma Gandhi ji set up the objective of providing healthcare, education, and economic welfare of needy rural women and children. The Trust aims at building a social structure based on nonviolent power of the people, through women's empowerment.

Objectives of the Kasturba Memorial Fund

The trust conducts and promotes charitable activities for the welfare of mothers and children through the establishment of hospitals, dispensaries, cottage industries and training campaigns in first aid, home nursing, child welfare, indigenous remedies.

CONCLUSION

Several healthcare agencies around the world working towards the ultimate goal to achieve better health of the community. Primarily established for the control of spread for communicable diseases, attention has now begun to be given to noncommunicable diseases including oral diseases.

BIBLIOGRAPHY

1. Park K. Essentials of Community Health Nursing, 4th Edition. Jabalpur: Banarasidas Bhanot Publisher: 2004.
2. Park K. Park's textbook of preventive and social medicine. 18th edition Banarasidas Bhanot Publishers. Jabalpur, India. 2005.
3. Peter S. Health agencies around the world. In: Peter S. (Ed) Essentials of Preventive and Community Dentistry. 2nd edition Arya (medi) Publishing House. New Delhi: 2003.
4. Swarnkar K. Community Health Nursing, 2nd edition. Indore: N.R. Brother; 2008.

Chapter 19: Health Agencies

REVIEW QUESTIONS

Long Essays
1. Define International Health Organizations. Explain the types of international health agencies.
2. Define World Health Organization. Describe the objectives and functions of World Health Organizations.
3. Define JHPIEGO. Explain aims, objectives and activities.
4. Indian red cross society, seven fundamental principles of red cross.

Short Essays
1. Specific global targets of WHO.
2. United Nations Fund for Population Activities.
3. United Nations Development Programme.
4. World Bank: Organization and Structure.
5. Food and Agriculture Organization.
6. United Nations International Children's Emergency Fund.
7. European Commission (EC): goals and values.
8. International Red Cross.
9. United States Agency for International Development.
10. United Nations Educational Scientific and Cultural Organization.
11. International Labor Organization.
12. Cooperative for American Relief Everywhere.
13. Canadian International Development Agency.
14. Indian Council of Child Welfare: objectives and functions.
15. Colombo Plan: purposes and objectives.
16. Tuberculosis Association of India: objectives and main activities.
17. Central Social Welfare Board.
18. Child Relief and You.

Short Answers
1. Multilateral Agencies.
2. Nongovernmental Organizations.
3. Bilateral Agencies.
4. UNFPA Activities in India.
5. Aims of FAO.
6. Objectives of FAO.
7. GOBI Strategy by UNICEF.
8. UNICEF in India.
9. USAID on Health in India.
10. Functions of the ILO.
11. Objectives of CARE India.
12. Activities of Ford Foundation.
13. Family Planning Program.
14. Objectives of Voluntary Organizations.
15. Characteristics of Voluntary Organization.
16. Functions of Voluntary Health Agencies.
17. Problems of Voluntary Health Agencies.
18. All India Women's Conference.
19. All India Blind Relief Societies.
20. Hind Kusht Nivaran Sangh.
21. Bharat Sevak Samaj.
22. Objectives of the Kasturba Memorial Fund.

Multiple Choice Questions
1. International health organizations are usually divided into:
    a. Multilateral organizations
    b. Bilateral organizations
    c. Nongovernmental organizations (NGOs)
    d. All of the above
2. Headquarter of World Health Organization is located in:
    a. Washington   b. California
    c. Geneva   d. Arizona
3. WHO (World Health Organization) was established in:
    a. 7 October, 1948   b. 7 April, 1948
    c. 7 July, 1948   d. 7 June, 1948
4. A goal of United Nations Fund for Population Activities (UNFPA) is:
    a. Reducing infant mortality.
    b. Increasing life expectancy.
    c. Reducing HIV infection rates.
    d. All of the above
5. Bharat Sevak Samaj (BSS) is a nonpolitical and nonofficial organization was formed in:
    a. 1950   b. 1951
    c. 1952   d. 1953
6. Objectives of the Kasturba Memorial Fund
    The trust conducts and promotes charitable activities for the welfare of mothers and children through the:
    a. Establishment of hospitals, dispensaries
    b. Training campaigns in first aid and home nursing
    c. Child welfare and indigenous remedies
    d. All of the above
7. The All India Women's Conference (AIWC) is a nongovernmental organization (NGO) based in:
    a. Delhi.   b. Mumbai
    c. Bangalore   d. Chennai
8. All India blind relief societies financed by the Government of India, was established in:
    a. 1945   b. 1946
    c. 1947   d. 1948

ANSWERS

| 1. d | 2. c | 3. b | 4. d | 5. c | 6. d | 7. a | 8. b | | | | |

Index

Page numbers followed by *b* refer to box, *f* refer to figure and *t* refer to table

A

Aam Aadmi Bima Yojana 209
Abdomen 40
    circumference 40
    distention 111
    examination 47
Abiotic 282
    environment 268
    resources 270
Abortion 178
Accidentology 179
Accidents 192, 248, 318
    prevention of 87
Accredited Social Health Activist worker 197*f*
Accumulated solid waste, health hazards of 319
Acephate 322
Acetic acid 86
Acid
    mine drainage 278
    rain 272, 292
Acute radiation syndrome 316
Acute respiratory infections
    control programme 325, 326
    prevention of 326
Ad-Hoc testing 394
    advantages of 394
    benefits of 394
    characteristics of 394
    disadvantages of 395
Adolescent Health Programme 346
Advisory body 169
    functions of 169
Aerobic method 320
Aerosols 231
Agent-host-environmental model 9, 9*f*
Aging theory, types of 238*f*
AIDS 264, 430
Air (Prevention and Control of Pollution) Act 300
Air 312
    change 315
    composition of 312
    conditioning 315
    disinfection of 314
    functions of 312
    humidity 317
    movement 317
    pollution 272, 289, 300, 312-314
        causes of 289
        control of 289, 314
        prevention of 314
        sources of 313
    temperature 317
All India Blind Relief Societies 446
All India Leprosy Workers Conference 447
All India Women's Conference 446
    activities of 446
Allergic rhinitis 110
Alpha-particles 316
Altruism 30
Ambiguity 378
Ambivalence 186
Amebiasis 275, 305
Amenorrhea 184
American Academy of Family Physicians 242
American Association of Public Health 1
American Diabetes Association 242
Amidosulfuron 322
Anaerobic method 320
Analytical method, approaches of 60
Anecdotal records 104
Anemia 43, 111, 119, 120*f*, 279
    causes of 119
    nutritional 267
    physiologic 185
Animal bite 117
Antenatal care 78, 186
    aims of 45
    components of 47
Antenatal examination 78, 186
Anthelmintics 86
Anthracosis 230
Anthrax 232
Anthropometric measurement 190*f*
Antimalaria campaign 328
Antimalaria drug policy 328
Antiseptic 66, 86
Antisera 66
Antitoxins 66
Anus 40
Anxiety 186
APGAR score 39, 178, 189
Appropriate health technology 14
Aqua privy 321
Aquatic ecosystem 282
Arm 40
    recoil 41
Arsenic 275
    groundwater contamination 278
Arsine 230
Arthropods 318
Artificial feeding 194
Asbestos contamination 278
Asbestosis 230
Atmosphere 282
Atmospheric pollution, reduction of 273
Atmospheric pressure 317
Atomic Energy Act 300
Attitude scale 404
    types of 404
Audiometric screening 43
Auditing 103
Auditory disability 249
Auscultation 44
Autism 250
Ayushman Bharat Yojana 145, 209, 209*f*
Azimsulfuron 322

B

Bacillus anthracis 232
Back 47
    pain 112
    referral 93
Bacteria, asymptomatic 185
Bag technique 86
    principles of 86
Bagassosis 230
Bajaj Committee 168
Balanced ventilation 315
Bancroftian filariasis 329
Bangalore method 320
Bar charts, types of 409
Bar diagram 409, 409*f*
Bar graph
    advantages of 409
    disadvantages of 410
    uses of 409
Barrier methods 361, 361*f*
    advantages 361
    disadvantages 361
Barrier-free environment 251
Basal body temperature method 363
Basic healthcare services 82
Battered baby syndrome 8
Battered wife syndrome 8
Behavioral changes 11, 244
Benedict's solution 86
Bensulfuron-methyl 322
Beta-particles 316
Bharat Sevak Samaj 448
    activities of 448
    workers, five point code for 448
Bhore Committee 165
    recommendations 212, 226
Biodiversity
    conversation of 288
    Management Committee 288
    productive use value of 287
    significance of 286
Biogas plant supplement 321
Biogeochemical cycles 285, 285*f*
Biological activities, disposal of 293
Biological Diversity Act 300
Biological environment 6, 63
Biological hazards 231
    control of 232
    prevention of 232
Biological methods 365
Biomass
    energy 279
    inverted pyramid of 284
    pyramid of 283
    upright pyramid of 283
Biopesticides 322
Bio-psychosocial model 256*f*
Biosphere 282
Biotic 282
    environment 268
    organism, damage of 293
    resources 270
Birth
    companion during pregnancy 201
    control
        implant 366

patch 366
pills 360, 361, 366
shot 366
sponge 366
preparation for 186
register 394
registration outputs legal 394
weight 40
Bispyribac-sodium 322
Bladder tone 185
Blastomycosis 231
Bleaching powder 307
Blindness 266
causes of 335
reduce backlog of 334
Block panchayat 138f
Blood
bank 430
glucose 37
fasting 43
pressure 37, 39, 47, 185
high 111, 240
Blue baby syndrome 275
Body mass index 43
Boiling water 88
Boric acid 322
Breast 41, 182
changes 47, 184
Breastfeeding 189, 192, 194, 337, 373
position 193f
principles of 194
procedures for 192
technique 189f, 193f
use of 362
Breathing
effort 40
rate 39, 40
Brittle bones 245
Brugian filariasis 329
Bucket latrine 321
Budget 423
Byssinosis 230

C

Caisson 228
Calcium 276, 277
deficiency 267
Calcutta Water Supply and Drainage Scheme 438
Calendar method 363
Canadian International Development Agency 437
activities 437
functions 437
origin 437
Cancer 241, 264, 314
pancreatic 242
Candy's filter 306
Capacity building 77, 158, 220
Carbamate 322
Carbon dioxide 230
exposure 230
Cardiac output 185
Cardiovascular disease 43, 265
Cardiovascular system 44, 111
Care
implementation of 74
integration of 77
plan, disadvantages of 32
Carriers, detection of 329
Case fatality ratio 56
Cataract 248, 316, 335

Census 389, 391, 392
investigation, demerits of 393
report 105
Centers for Disease Control and Prevention 242
Central Births and Deaths Registration Act 394
Central Council of Health 133, 166
functions of 133
Central Government Health Scheme 133, 142, 209
Central Health Education Bureau 133
aims of 212
Central Level Healthcare Administration 131, 131f
Central nervous system 314
Central Social Welfare Board 445
activities 445
functions of 445
mission 445
objectives of 445
vision 445
Central venous system 314
Cerebral palsy 249
Cerebrovascular accident 241
Cervical cap 366
Cervical mucus method 363, 364f
advantages 364
disadvantages 364
mechanism of action of 363
method of 364
Chadah committee 166
Chadwick's sign 184
Chemical 275, 313
agents 63
closet 321
disinfection 88
fertilizers, reduced use of 290
hazards
and health 229
control of 231
prevention of 231
industrial 292
method 307, 365
parameters 307t
Chemotherapy 329
Chest pain 111
Chief Medical and Health Officer 135
Chief Minister's Comprehensive Insurance Scheme 210
Chilblains 228
Child health
problems 191
stages 181
Chiranjeevi Yojana 200
Chloramines 306
Chlordane 322
Chlorimuron-ethyl 322
Chlorinated lime 307
Chlorination 306
methods of 306
principles of 306
Chlorine 67
compounds 67
gas 306
Chlorofluorocarbons 289
Chloromycin eye 115
Cholera 275, 305
Chromium 276, 277
Civic functions 138
Civil Registration System 393, 393f
characteristics of 393
functions of 394
Cleaning 87, 88
Cleanliness 406

Client's care, planning of 74
Climacteric 182
Climate
change 271, 294
causes of 295
concept of 294
control of 273
desert type of 317
elements of 317
influences 317
measurement of 317
monsoon type of 317
tropical type of 317
types of 317
Clinical decision support 387, 388
Clitoris 181
Cluster sampling 396, 397
Coagulation 306
Coal burning 278
Coccidioidomycosis 231
Coitus interruptus method 365
Colombo plan 439
Color blindness 248
Commode toilet 321
Communicable diseases 264
control of 164, 234, 432
prevention of 215, 234
Communication 103, 434
methods of 415
principle of 384
technology 387
Community 1, 429
advantages for 356
approach 105
assessment 26, 27, 28t
bag, importance of 86
clinic services 89
development 127, 149, 174
principles of 150f
diagnosis 28
stages of 28
health 1, 391
assessment 34
concept of 1, 1f
diagnosis 28
history of 3
process 26f
volunteers 383
healthcare plan, process of 31f
level 116
healthcare administration 135
nursing 58
process 26
organizer 381
participation 14
practice 20f
rehabilitation 254
resources 69
standing
management 117-124
orders 117-124
Community Development Block
functions of 150
operation 150
Community Development Programme 150
activities of 174
types of 150f
Community Health Center 148
functions of 135
staffing pattern of 22f
Community health nurse 67, 79, 217, 381
functions of 23, 79, 90, 329

qualities of 23
responsibilities of 78
role of 14, 15f, 23f, 67, 79, 105, 186, 261, 337, 384
skills of 22
Community health nursing 2, 19, 101, 104, 174, 174f
concept of 20
development of 3
diagnosis 29
goal of 20f, 21
history of 3
objectives of 20, 20f
personnel
responsibilities of 380
role of 380
philosophy of 20
principles of 21, 21f
process 19, 25
registers 106
scope of 24
services 23, 24f
administration 383
Community health planning
levels 175
objectives of 175
Community Health Programme 217
importance of 213f
scope of 213, 213f
Community health services 19f, 71
sectors 175f
Community health team 22
members, functions of 22
Community-based rehabilitation 260
objectives of 260
services 253
Comprehensive Antitobacco Programme 341
Comprehensive geriatric assessment 51f, 238f
components of 50
Comprehensive health
assessment 44
care 127
Comprehensiveness 13
Conciseness 102
Condom 365
benefits of 365
disadvantages of 365
female 365
male 365
Conduction deafness 249
Confidence intervals 414
Confidentiality 102, 106
principle of 384
Congenital disorders, treatment of 189
Congenital rubella syndrome 337
Conjunctiva
inflamed 114f
normal 114f
Conservation planning 309
Constipation 117, 117f, 184
Constructional refuse 320
Constructive epidemiology 56
Contraception
benefits of 357, 357f
emergency 358, 369
Contraceptive
methods, long-term 361
oral pill method of 366f
Convulsions 115
first-aid in 115f
Copper 276, 277

Cord
care of 189
cutting technique 189f
Core competencies family health nurse 76
Corneal blindness 335
Coronary heart disease 242
Cost control 387
Cough 110
Counseling 383
goals of 384
principles of 383, 384
purposes of 369
techniques of 383
Coxiella burnetii 232
Crazy consumerism 298
impact of 298
reasons for 298
Creche 234
Cretinism 305
Criterion validity 401
Crops, genetic modification of 272
Cross ventilation 315
Cross-linking theory 239
Crude birth rate 392
Crude death rate 56, 392
Cubic space 315
Cultural heritage, preservation of 434
Cumulative frequency
diagram 407f
distribution 400
Current global warming, causes of 295
Current systemic illness 46
Cyclops 329
Cyclosulfamuron 322

D

Daily living, activities of 50
Data
analysis of 411, 411f
collection 27, 60, 235, 400, 401f
collection methods 27, 74, 401, 402
diagrammatic presentation of 405
find range of 400
graphical presentation of 405
interpretation 412, 413f
method 27, 414
management 387
preparation, steps of 411
presentation 405
selection criteria for 401
principles of 28
sources of 27, 27f
sources 387
Deafness 248
types of 249
Death rate 56
age specific 56
Decomposable refuse 319
Decompression sickness 228
Deep trench latrine 321
Deep wells 305
Deforestation 272, 273, 302
causes of 273
effects of 273
Delirium 34
Delphi technique 404
Democracy 426
Demographic cycle 351
Demographic transition cycle 352f
Demographic trends 352, 352f
Demography 349

concept of 349
importance of 350
scope of 351
uses of 349
Dental
caries 305
diseases, scope of 200
health 215
pain, common type of 122f
Descriptive method 60
objectives of 60
Desertification 280
causes of 280
Determinants 56
De-worming 220
Diabetes mellitus 43, 264
Diaphragm 365
Diarrhea 111, 115
causes of 115f
disease 264
features of 115f
Diazinon 322
Dichotomies 58
Dietary management 186f
Dietary pattern 183
deficiencies syndrome 28
Diffusion 315
Digestive system 111
Dilution 314
Diphtheria 336
Diplomacy 427
Direct pit latrine 321
Disability 179, 246, 260, 261
causes of 261
certificates, issue of 251
indicates 179
limitation 12, 66
prevention of 250
types of 261
Disablement benefit 233
Disaster
preparedness 430
relief 429, 431
response 429
Disease
antecedents 58, 61
bacterial 305
behavior 58, 61
conditions 254
control 164
objectives of 66
correlates 58, 61
cycle 61
free body 38
natural history of 62-64
notification of 389, 395
prevalence, reduction of 161
prevention
levels of 65
strategies 17
register 389
spectrum of 62, 62f
surveillance 395
transmission, modes of 62
viral 305
Disengagement theory 238
Disinfection 66, 67, 87, 88, 306
methods of 67
Disposal, methods of 320
Distillation 307
District Cancer Control Programme 341

District Health Organization, functions of 136
District Health Societies 334
District Health System, functions of 135
District Level Healthcare Administration 134, 134f
District Malaria Control Societies 327
District Mental Health Programme 345
District Public Health Nurse 380
    responsibilities of 380
Documentation 101
Dog bite 117, 117f
    immediate care of 117
Domestic refuse 320
Domiciliary care 24
Domiciliary nursing service 25
Dot diagram 407
Dot maps
    advantages of 411
    disadvantages of 411
Down syndrome 247, 250
Dr YSR Aarogyasri Healthcare Trust 211
Dracunculosis 329
Drainage system 306
Draw frequency distribution table 400
Drinking water 338
    chemical
        quality of 307
        standards of 307
    physical
        quality of 307
        standards of 307
Droplet infection 62
Drought prone area programme 311
Drug standards, control of 132
Dry heat 88
Dursban 322
Dust 230, 313
    control 314
    diseases 313
Dysentery 275, 305
Dyslipidemia 43
    prevalence of 265
Dysmenorrhea 34, 112
Dysphagia 34
Dyspnea 34
Dysuria 34

E

Ear 41, 110
    problems 111
Early neonatal care 188
    objectives of 189
Ecological pyramid 283, 283f
Ecological studies 59
Ecology 270
Economical concept 70
Economical security 70
Economical use supplies 87
Ecosystem 281, 282, 284f
    diversity 286
    functions of 282
    importance of 283
Edema 121, 121f, 185
    causes of 121
Education 42, 354, 434
Educational functions 79
    and motivation 338, 375
Edwards personal preference schedule 404
Effective solid waste management 291
Effective team, characteristics of 256, 379
Elderly abuse 242
    types of 242
Electronic health records 220, 388
Electronic medical record 388

Elevated estrogen levels 184
Emergency ambulance services 207, 207f
    concept of 207
Emergency care, imparting skills of 220
Emotional care 70, 240, 240f
Emotional changes 11, 186
Emotional dimension 6
Empathy, principle of 384
Employee State Insurance 142
    Act 233
        benefits of 233
    Scheme 209
Employment 42
    provision 233
Endocrine 183
Endometrium 183
Energy
    conservation of 280
    flow 284
    pyramid of 284
    resources 279
Enhanced Malaria Control Project
    components of 328
    objectives of 328
Environment
    health hazards of 303
    types of 268
Environmental chemistry 270
Environmental education 290, 301
Environmental health 302, 302f
    and sanitation 301
        concept of 302
    data 395
    hazard, control of 384
    role of 304
Environmental hygiene 165
Environmental origin, diseases of 231
Environmental policy 299
Environmental pollution 288
Environmental problems 269, 277, 280
Environmental Protection Act 299, 300
Environmental sanitation 234, 303
    dimensions of 303
    problems 266
Environmental science, importance of 269
Epidemiological concept 70
Epidemiological methods 60
    principles of 53
Epidemiological surveillance 389
Epidemiological treatment 333
Epidemiological triad 62, 63f
Epidemiology
    advantages of 59
    aims of 55
    components of 55
    concept of 54, 54f
    functions of 55
    history of 53
    importance of 61
    objectives of 55
    principles of 53, 57
    scope of 57
    types of 56
    uses of 55, 58
Epitasis 120
Equipment 88, 89
Ergonomics 179
Estimated tuberculosis burden 326
Estrogen ad progesterone 184
Ethoxysulfuron 322
European commission 425
    functions 427
    values 426

Excreta, disposal of 321
Executive board 433
Exercise 183
Experimental epidemiology 56
Experimental method 60
Ex-situ conservation 288
Extended Pradhan Mantri Surakshit Matritva Abhiyan 199
Extremities, edema of 185
Eye 17, 41, 110
    accidents 110
    care 189
        services, development of 334
    diseases 244
    drops 86, 115
    exams 17
    health services 215
    infections 110
    problems 314

F

Face 40
    validity 401
Factories Act 232, 300
Fallopian tubes 368
Family 70
    advocate 79
    assessment of 75
    budgets, less pressure on 355
    centered nursing 69
    characteristics 74
    concept of 70
    developmental task 69
    dynamics 11, 74
    folder 101
    functions of 69, 70
    health 69, 82, 83
        assessment 74
        determinants of 71
        factors of 71
        nurse, qualities of 83
        practices 75
        records 79, 89
        report 89
        service 77, 79, 380
    lifestyle 75
    medicine 164
    nursing
        care plan 76
        process 73
    planning 25, 356, 432
        services, scope of 357
    practices 2
    process 69, 82
    records 104
    roles, impact of 11
    size
        effects of 354
        larger 354
    structure 69, 74
    system theory 69
    types 70
    violence 8
    Welfare 349, 431
        activities, impact of 337, 373
        Services 337
Family health nursing 72
    advantages of 72
    care 69
    disadvantages of 72
    objectives of 72
    principles of 72
    process 73

Family healthcare 71, 89
    aims of 72
    objectives of 72
    principles of 72
    settings 82
Family Planning Association of India 443, 444
    activities 443
    mission 443
Family planning methods
    natural 361, 362, 362t
    types of 357
Family Planning Programme 354, 359, 374, 391, 439
    impact of 360
    objectives of 359
Family planning
    advantages of 358
    benefits of 357, 357f, 359
    challenges in 363f
    health aspects of 358
    history of 359
    importance of 357, 360
Family Welfare Programme 360, 372, 375, 375f
    aims of 337
    concept of 337
    goals of 337, 373
    importance of 337, 373
    objectives of 337
    organizing committee 372f
    strategies of 337, 373
Family-centered nursing 83
    approach 72
Fecal-borne disease, transmission of 321
Feeding 190
Female health worker, functions of 22
Female infertility treatment 353
Female reproductive system 181
    part of 182f
Fertility
    awareness method 358, 362
    concept of 353
Fetal
    death syndrome 337
    health 358
Fever 113
    causes of 113
    chronic 113
    continuous 113
    intermittent 113
    paratyphoid 275, 321
    remittent 113
    treatment depot 327
    types of 113
Filariasis 264
Filtration 297, 306
Fimbriae 182
Financial assistance 432
Financial support 290
First referral units 148
First-aid 115f, 119f-121f, 234
    aims of 118
    and emergency 215
Fiscal resource management 390
Five year plan 169, 170, 170f, 218, 225
    eighth 172
    eleventh 173
    fifth 171
    first 170
    fourth 171, 218
    ninth 172
    objectives of 170
    second 170
    seventh 172
    sixth 172
    tenth 173
    third 171, 218
    twelfth 170
Flawless skin 37
Flazasulfuron 322
Flocculation 306
    hydroxide 306
Fluorides 275
Fluorine 267, 305
Fluorosis 267
Flupyrsulfuron-methyl-sodium 322
Follicular ovary 183
Food 273
    and nutrition 354
    craving 184
    crops 278
    resources 278
        conservation of 281
    sanitation 303
    security 325
Food and Agriculture Organization 322, 422
    aims of 423
    budget 423
    functions of 424, 425
    objectives of 423
    structure 423
Forces influence the health system 129
Ford foundation 438
    activities of 438
Foreseeable crisis 75
Forest (conservation) Act and Rules 300
Forest
    conservation of 281
    ecosystem 282
    products 273
    resources 273
    significance of 273
Formaldehyde 67
Formative evaluation 30
Foster care services 82
Fracture 118, 119
    compound 119
    first-aid for 119f
    simple 118
    types of 118
Fraud 243
Free radical theory 239
Frequency 56
    curve 407
Frequency distribution 398
    characteristics of 399
    components of 399
    graph 399f
    mean of 400
    table 399
        presentation of 405
    types of 399
    uses of 399
Frequency polygon 406
    graph 406f
Freshwater ecosystem 282, 283
Frost bite 228
Frustrations 232
Fuel minerals 276
Fuel wood 273
Fundal height examination 47
Fundamental rights 448
Funding sources 425
Funeral benefits 233

G

Gamma rays 316
Gas 230
    natural 276
Gastric motility 184
Gastrointestinal changes 184
General hygiene and sanitation 218
Genetic disorders, symptoms of 247
Genitalia, external 181
Geographical data 350
Geoscience 270
Geothermal energy 279
Geriatric care 236f, 237, 253
    goals of 237
Geriatric community health assessment, components of 29f
Geriatric nurse 236, 237
    characteristics of 238
Geriatric nursing 236
    assessment 236f
    care 238f, 241
    goals of 237
    management 241
    process application 244
    services 25, 25f
Gestational assessment 40
Giardiasis 305
Glare, absence of 314
Glaucoma 248, 335
Global environmental problems 294
Global warming 295, 313
    causes of 296, 313
    effects of 296
    human influences of 296
    natural causes of 296
Glutaraldehyde 67
Glyphosate 322
Goiter, endemic 305
Good clinic, criteria for 90
Good intranatal care, aims of 187
Good lighting
    factors essential for 314
    requirements of 314
Good referral system 94b
Goodell's sign 184
Government Health Insurance Schemes 208
    benefits of 209
    features of 209
    types of 209
Graphical presentation, uses of 408
Grassland ecosystem 282
Greater vestibular glands 181
Green stick fracture 119
Greenhouse effect 295
Gross domestic product 146
Ground theory analysis 412
Ground water 305, 308
Grouped frequency distribution 400
Groups, fundamentals of 439
Growing fetus, acceptance of 186
Growth 17
    chart, uses of 191
    monitoring 191
        alternative methods of 191
Guinea worm 329
    disease 330

H

Habitat loss 287
Haemophilus influenzae type B 336
Halosulfuron-methyl 322

Index

Handicap 179, 261
   education of 215
Handwashing 87
Harmony 379
Hazardous waste management 297
   components of 297
Hazards
   control of 232*f*
   prevention of 232*f*
Head 40
   circumference 40
   growth 190
   nurse 31
   to toe examination 44
Headache 112
Health 6, 71, 391
   administration 127, 129
      history of 129
      objectives of 129
   agencies 417
   allied resources 6
   and disease, concept of 2
   appraisal 214
   assessment 34, 35, 35*f*, 36, 38, 41, 42, 45, 48, 50, 51
      components of 50
      concept of 34
      principles of 35
      recording of 51
   assistant, job responsibilities of 382
   belief model 9, 10*f*
   care 128
      levels of 11, 94, 97
      measures 165
      pyramid of level of 95*f*
   concept of 2*t*
   condition 204
   contribution 420
   deficits 75
   determinants of 6, 6*f*
   dimensions of 5, 5*f*
   education 165, 215, 231, 232, 234, 235, 313, 374, 444
   effects 303, 304
   facility 199
   finance 161
   for all 14, 127, 338
      concept of 15*f*
   hazards 319, 321
   illness continuum 9
   indicators 7
      types of 7*f*
   information system 162, 386, 388
      benefits of 387
      components of 387, 389
      concept of 386
      sources of 387, 389, 389*f*
      uses of 389
   infrastructure 162
   insurance system 142
   intelligence 133
   issued 171
   maintenance 16
      components of 17
   organization 136, 137
   planning 160, 175
      constrains of 164
      phases 160*f*
      purposes of 161
      steps in 162, 162*f*
      strategies of 165
   policy, elements of 168
   prevention, levels of 64*f*
   problems 214, 227, 266*f*
      assessment of 75
   programme organization 391
   promotion 12, 16, 17*f*, 65, 87, 216
      components of 17
      model 10, 10*f*
      strategies 17*f*
   record 75
      informations 223*f*
      need of 223
   related services 7
   research 164
   risk families, assessment of 75
   screening 190, 220
   secretariat 133
   service 6, 116, 165
      coverage of 161
      delivery of 146-148
      provision 219
      records 389
   situation, analysis of 163
   status 64, 74, 161
      assessment 75
   survey 61, 166, 235
   systems 94, 127, 128, 144
      administration of 131
      aims of 128
      determinants of 128
      goals of 128
      organization of 131
      performance 161
      purposes of 94
      strengthening 161
   teacher 79
   team 31, 378
      aims of 379
   wellness model 9
   worker 229*f*, 382
      goals of 356
Healthcare
   delivery
      model 131*f*
      system 130, 141, 141*f*, 144
      types of 141
   entity 82
   information systems, types of 388
   interventions 331
   organization, levels of 143*f*
   pathways 93
   plan 82
   programme 164
   quality, domains of 247*f*
   services 25, 82
   setting 82, 83, 94
      concept of 83
   structure 144
   system 99, 127, 130*f*, 144
      levels of 128*f*
   team 83, 248*f*
   worker 82, 136*f*
Healthful housing
   criteria for 318
   objectives of 318
   principles of 318
Healthful school environment 215
Healthy eyes 37
Healthy hair 37
Healthy individual, characteristics of 36, 36*b*
Hearing
   assessment 249*f*
   disability 261
   impairment 246, 248
   screening 43
Heart
   burn 184
   disease 240
   failure, prevalence of 265
   rate 40, 185
   sounds 40
Heartbeat 39
Heat
   cramps 228
   exhaustion 228
   stroke 120
      first-aid in 121*f*
Hegar's sign 184
Height 47, 190
   measurement of 88
Helminthic disease 305
Hemoglobin 43
Hemorrhage, secondary 188
Hemorrhoids 111
Hepatitis
   A 305
   B 336
   E 305
High grade minerals, rapid depletion of 276
High temperature 228
High-density lipoprotein cholesterol, high level of 38
Hind Kusht Nivaran Sangh 447
   activities 447
Histogram 406
Histoplasmosis 231
Hog feeding 320
Holistic care 241*f*
Home care 25
   services 82
Home health nurse, responsibilities of 247
Home healthcare services 82
   types of 84
Home visiting 69, 85
   advantages of 86
   concept of 85
   principles of 85
   purposes of 85
   steps in 85
Horizontal bar graphs 409, 409*f*
Hospice care 179
Hospital
   records 389, 395
   refuses 320
   services 430
Host 61
   defences 66
   factors 63
Housing 318
   sanitation 303
   standards 318
Human dignity 426
Human environment 295
Human excreta 321
Human immunodeficiency virus 362 430
Human resource 14, 162, 335
Humanity 429, 442
Hydrogen peroxide 67
Hydropower 279
Hydrosphere 282
Hygiene and environmental health, components of 303
Hymen 181
Hyperemia 184
Hyperlipidemia 43

I

Hyperventilation 186
Hypotension 241

Illness 313
   behaviour, stages of 10, 10*f*
   causes of 64*f*
   impact of 11*t*
   prevention, levels of 12
Illumination 315
Imazosulfuron 322
Immunity
   active 66
   cellular 66
   humoral 66
Immunization 66, 219, 374
   expanded programme of 336
   passive 66
   record 39
Impairment 179, 260
Implementation 220, 330
In vitro fertilization 354
Incentives 374
Incidental reports 105
Incineration 321
Inclusion 78
Indian Council of Child Welfare 443
   functions of 443
Indian Fisheries Act 300
Indian Forest Act and Amendment 300
Indian Leprosy Association 447
Indian National Commission for Cooperation with UNESCO 434
Indian Red Cross Society 441
Industrial health 165
Industrial nursing 23, 234
   services 25
Industrial refuse 320
Industrial units, accountability of 290
Industrial workers, provision of 233
Industrialization 289, 302
Infant care 189, 190
Infant mortality rate 358, 392
Infection 197
   bacterial 114*f*
   prevention of spread of 24
   reservoir of 53
   source of 53, 321
   viral 114*f*
Infectious diseases 192
   control of 66
Infertility 353
   causes of 353
   concept of 353
   male 354
Information products 387
Informed consent 101, 105
Informed referral services 199
Infra red radiation 228
Insecticides 322
In-situ conservation 288
Institutional standing orders 109, 113
Instrument, reliability of 401
Integrated Child Development Service Programme 344
Integrated health service 166
Integrated rural development 151
   program implementation 151
Integration with health service 337, 373
Integration with maternity and child health 337, 373
Integumentary system 44
Intensive study 393

Interconception stage 181
Interfacility transfer 199
Internal consistency reliability 401
International Day of Disabled Person 261
International Health Agencies
   logo 417*f*
   types of 417
International Health Organizations 417
International Health Relations and Quarantine 132
International Labor Organization 325, 435
   functions of 435
   membership 435
   purposes of 435
International labor standards 436
International red cross 428, 442
   functions 429
Interpretation, common errors of 413
Intersectoral coordination 14
Inter-tropical convergence zone 295
Interviews 402
   advantages of 403
   aims of 403
   disadvantages of 403
   techniques 402*f*
   types of 402
Intoxications
   group
      A 231
      B 231
Intracytoplasmic sperm injection 354
Intranatal care 78, 187, 187*f*
   objectives of 187
Intranatal counseling 187
Intranatal education 187
Intrauterine contraceptive device 358, 366
Intrauterine insemination 354
Iodine Deficiency Control Programme 335
Iodine 307
   deficiency disorders 267
Iodized salt, production of 335
Iodophors 67
Iron 276, 277
Irrigation hours ordinance 309
Irritability 40
Irritant gases 230
Isolation 24

J

Janani Shishu Suraksha Karyakram 199
Janani Suraksha Yojana 199, 205, 205*f*, 210
   Benefits 205*f*
   concept of 205
   important features of 207
   objectives of 206, 206*f*
Jaundice 275
Johns Hopkins Program for International Education in Gynecology and Obstetrics, 437, 438
   activities 438
   member profile 437
   mission 437
   vision 437
Joint family 70
Judicial functions 138
Jungalwala Committee 166

K

Kartar Singh Committee 167, 218
Karunya Health Scheme 211
Kasturba Memorial Fund 448
   objectives of 448
Kata thermometer 317

Katadyn process 307
Kayakalp 145
Kwashiorkor 279

L

Labia
   majora 181
   minora 181
Labor 178, 181
   institutes, activities of 234
Lactational amenorrhea 358
   method 362, 364
Lady Chelmsford League 180
Land
   pollution 289, 291
   resources 279
Laser injuries 229
Latrines, types of 321
Lead 275
Leadership 380
Leg cramps 186
Legal issues 243
Legal records 105
Legal registration 393
Legal use 391
Legislation
   approach 290
   important component of 354
   purpose 391
Legislative method 314
Legs 40
   varicose veins of 185
Leprosy 264, 331
   nursing 24
Leptospirosis 231
Leucorrhea 184
Liaison activities 217
Life expectancy 161, 392
Life-span, shortening of 316
Lifestyle 6, 71, 244, 281
Light, color of 314
Lighting 314
   measurement of 314
   types of 314
Likert scales 404, 404*f*
   advantages 404
   disadvantages 404
Listening skills 383
Literacy 337, 373
Lithosphere 282
Livestock 278
Living components 282
Locomotors disability 261
Low birth weight 191, 267
Low resting heart rate 37
Luminance 315
Luminous flux 314
Luminous intensity 314
Lungs 40

M

Magnesium 276, 277
Mahatma Jyotirao Phule Jan Arogya Yojana 210
Major maternity and child health problems 197
Malaria 264, 275, 327
Malaria Control Project 328
Malaria Eradication programme 432
Malaria Voluntary Link Worker Scheme 327
Malathion 322
Male health workers, functions of 22
Male sterilization 367, 368
Malnourishment 279

Index

Malnutrition 424
    problems of 279
Mamata Sakhi 201
Mammary gland 182
Mamta Ghar 200
Managerial function 79, 338, 376
Manganese 276, 277
    fumes 231
Map diagram 411, 411f
Marasmus 279
Marine ecosystem 282, 283
Marine pollution 292
    effects of 292
Mass
    drug administration 329
    level 290
    media 337, 374
Master patient index 388
Maternal and child health 32, 182
    bond 192f
    care, components 181f
    development stages 181
    objectives 196
    programme 196
        activities of 77
        aims of 77
        objectives of 77, 196
    service 178, 180, 180f, 182
        aims of 196
        importance of 197
        programme 77, 78
Maternal care 200
Maternal health 16, 362
Maternal mortality rate 392
Maternity and Child Welfare 431
Maternity
    benefits 233, 234
    care 178
Measles 336
Mechanical ventilation 315
Medical board, constitution of 372
Medical education 133, 432
    programme, reorientation of 147
Medical record 395
    department, functions of 106
    linkage 389
    system of 106
Medical Termination of Pregnancy Act 370, 371, 371f, 374
Medical tourism and telemedicine 143
Medicine, indigenous system of 142
Membrane theory 239
Meningitis 336
Menopause 182
Menstrual cycle 182, 183f
    phases of 183
Menstrual education 183
Menstrual hygiene 182, 183
Menstrual problems 112
Menstrual symptoms 183
Mental dimension 5
Mental disability 249
    levels of 249
    types of 249
Mental handicap 261
Mental health 17, 164, 215, 234
    nursing service 25
Mental healthcare 345
Mental retardation 179, 247
    levels of 249, 250f
        mild 249
        moderate 250
        severe 250
    types of 248, 250
Merchant Shipping Act 300
Mercury 231
Metaldehyde 322
Metallic minerals 276
Meteorological environment 317
Methane 230
Methemoglobinemia 305
Methylated spirit 86
Micro-birth planning and counseling 48
Microorganisms 62
Microwave injuries 229
Mid-Day Meal Programme 344
    salient features of 345
Milk, types of 194
Millennium development goals 15, 16f
Mineral
    contamination 277
    resources 275
        exploitation of 276
        types of 275
    types of 275f
Minimum Need Programme 337, 339, 373
Minnesota Multiphasic Personality Inventory 404
Minor ailments 109-112
    management of 110
Mission Indradhanush 145
Mission
    core strategies of 203
    supplementary strategies of 204
    vision of 202
Mitochondrial decline theory 239
Modern agricultural practices 302
Monetary incentive 337
Monitoring 103, 163
Mood 34
    swings 186
Morbidity
    indicators 7, 8
    measurement of 56
Motivational theories 255
Motor
    development 190
    impairment 246
Motor Vehicles Act 300
Mouth 40
    soreness of 111
Movement, freedom of 426
Mudaliar Committee 165, 166, 218
Mukherjee Committee 166
Mukhyamantri Amrutum Yojana 210
Multilateral agencies 417
Multi-skill training 447
Multi-stage sampling 397, 398f
Multi-stakeholder partnerships 158
Municipal services 319
Muscle
    maturity of 41
    strength 38
    tone 40
Muscular dystrophy 249
Musculoskeletal system 44, 245
Mycobacterium
    leprae 331
    tuberculosis 62

N

Nasal congestion 186
National Acute Respiratory Infection Control Programme 325
National AIDS Control Programme 164, 332
National Antimalaria Programme 327
National Biodiversity Act 288
National Cancer Control Programme 164, 340
National Cancer Registry Programme 341
National Cholesterol Education Programme 242
National Development Council and Health 169
    members of 169
National Development Planning 160
National Diabetes Control Programme 339
National Drinking Water Mission 338
National Family Welfare Programme 336, 372-374
    components of 374
    objectives of 374
National Filaria Control Programme 164, 328
    activities of 329
    strategy 329
National Goiter Control Programme 335
National Guinea Worm Eradication Programme 329
National Health Committees 165
National Health Mission 179, 197, 201, 201f, 202, 390
    types of 202f
National Health Planning 160
National Health Policy 168
    objectives of 168
National Health Programme 133, 142, 170, 171, 325, 436
National Health Survey 396
National Health Systems Resource Center 390
National Iodine Deficiency Disorders Control Programme 164
National Leprosy Control Programme 331
National Leprosy Eradication Programme 164, 330
National Level Research Institutes on Occupational Health 234
National Malaria Control Programme 327
National Medical Library 133
National Mental Health Programme 164, 345
National Nutritional Anemia Prophylaxis Programme 342
    20 point Programme 343
    activities 343
National Planning Committee 165
National Policy for Persons with Disabilities 250
National Prevalence of Childhood Blindness 335
National Programme for Control of Blindness 164, 334
National Rural Health Mission 202
    approaches of 203f
National School Health Scheme 219
National Sexually Transmitted Disease Control Programme 333
National Urban Health Mission 204
    benefits of 205
National Vector-Borne Disease Control Programme 164
National Water Supply and Sanitation Programme 338
National Watershed Development Programme for Rainfed Agriculture 311
Natural calamities 302
Natural ecosystem, types of 282
Natural family planning methods 361, 362, 362t
    types of 362
Neatness 406
Neck 40
Neonatal care 78, 188
Nerve
    deafness 249
    maturity of 41

Index

Neuroendocrine theory 238, 239f
Neurologic system 44
Neuromuscular system 112
Neurosis 250
Neutrality 429, 442
Newborn screening, part of 43
Nicosulfuron 322
Night blindness 248
Nitrates 275
Nitrogen 230
    cycle 272, 285
Nocardiosis 231
Nocturia 34
Noise pollution 289, 290, 303, 312
    control 290
    sources of 290
Non-communicable death rates 265f
Non-communicable diseases 264
    types of 264, 265f
Non-decomposable component 319
Nongovernmental organizations 417, 418
    promotion of 251
    role of 418f
Nonionizing radiation 228
Nonliving components 282
Nonmetallic minerals 276
Nonservice latrines 321
Nose bleeding 120
    first-aid in 120f
Nuclear family 70
Nuclear hazards 293
Nuclear pollution, effects of 294
    sources of 294, 294f
Nuclear waste 292
Numerical data interpretation 413
Nurse 31, 380
    responsibilities of 36, 99, 329
    role of 24, 45, 47, 51, 83, 90, 113, 144, 187,
        188, 190, 191, 216, 217, 221, 312, 329,
        346, 375, 375f, 380
    school health, responsibility of 216
    sheet 104
Nurse-client relationship, phase of 31
Nursing 91, 431
    action, planning for 75
    administration 148, 149, 149f, 390
    approach 105
    clinic 89
    education 390
    homes 25, 253
    implementation 29, 258
    personnel, administration of 148
    practice 390
Nursing care 76, 244
    plan 19, 76
        advantages of 32
        qualities of 76
        types of 29
    provider of 381
Nursing diagnosis 19, 244
    formulation of 75
    steps of 28
    types of 29
Nursing information system 390
    advantages of 390
Nursing process 19, 25, 257
    application, steps of 35f
    components of 28, 29f
    implications of 26
Nursing research 390
    findings, communication of 415
Nutrition 17, 165, 234, 339
Nutritional agents 63

Nutritional anemia 267
    prevalence of 267
Nutritional intervention 244
Nutritional observation 87
Nutritional screening 43
Nutritional services 215
Nyaya Panchayat 138

O

Observation method 403
    types of 403f
Observation procedures, types of 403
Occupational accident 179
Occupational disability 179
Occupational disease 179
Occupational environment 224f, 225
Occupational hazards 228, 229
    administrative measures of 233f
    safety measures 228f
Occupational health 165, 179, 225, 231, 234
    Bhore committee recommendations of 226
    concept of 227
    hazards 228f
        health risks of 229f
        sources of 229f
    legal aspects on 234
    nurse 179, 235, 236
        functions of 235
        role of 235
    nursing 179, 224, 226, 234
        beneficiaries of 235
        components of 235
        history of 234
        tools of 235
    programme 179
    services 24, 226, 226f, 232
        aims of 224, 227
        objectives of 224, 227
        scope of 227
Occupational healthcare team 236
    major activities of 236
    members of 236
Occupational medicine 179
Occupational State Health Policy 234
Ocean acidification 272
Operation, modified plan of 327
Oral health 17
Oral rehydration solution 116f
Oral temperature, measurement of 114f
Orem's self-care-deficit theory 256
Organization 102, 106, 132, 135, 421, 441
    chart 373
    set up 150
Organizational structure 341, 419
Organizing family planning camps 338, 376
Organochlorine insecticides 322
Organophosphate 322
Organs, internal 182
Orthopedic impairment, types of 249f
Ortho-phthalaldehyde 67
Orthopnea 34
Orthotolidine (07) test 307
Orthotolidine-arsenite test 307
Ovaries 182
Overcrowding 319
Oxasulfuron 322
Oxidation 297
Oxygen
    consumption 186
    saturation 39
Ozone depletion 298
    danger of 303
Ozonized air 307

P

Pain
    abdominal 111
    assessment of 123f
    evaluation of 45
Palpation 44, 185
Panchayat Samiti 138
Panchayati Raj 127, 137-139
    functions of 138
Panchayati samiti, principles of 138
Paper 273
Paracetamol 86
Parasitic disease 192
Pasteurella tularensis 232
Paterson's filter 306
Pathogen, transmission of 62
Pellagra 279
Peracetic acid 67
Perchloron 307
Perinatal health assessment 46f
Periodic abstinence 362
    methods 362
Periodic health check-up 18
Periodic medical examination 215f
Peripheral arterial disease 242
Personal information, confidentiality of 393
Personal protection 231, 232
Pertussis 336
Pesticides 275, 322
    benefits of 322
    effects of 322
    major advantage of 322
    pollution 304
    types of 322
Pests, types of 322
Petrochemicals 275
Phosphorus 276, 277
Photosynthesis 284f
Physical abuse 243f
Physical disability 248
Physical environment 6, 63
Physical examination 42, 43, 47, 74, 114, 165
Physical hazards 228
    control of 229
    prevention of 229
Physical health 228, 319
Physical method 307
Pictograms 410, 410f
    advantages of 410
    effective use of 410
Picture diagram 410
Pie chart 410, 410f
    advantages of 410
    disadvantages of 410
Planning care, importance of 76
Planning commission 164, 168, 169
    branches of 169
    functions of 168
    members of 169f
Planning cycle 163
    steps of 163
Planning, steps of 160
Plantar creases 41
Plasmodium parasite 327
Plenum ventilation 315
Pluralistic Society with Democratic System 439
Pneumoconiosis 230
    benign 230
    minor 230
Pneumonia 336
Poisoning 192
Polar ice caps 271

Index

Policy 160, 299
    focus of 250
Polio eradication 339
Poliomyelitis 305, 336
Political system 7
Pollutants
    man-made 289
    natural 289
Polluted water, effects of 275
Pollution 288, 289
    classification of 289
    different types of 289
    prevention 312
        concept of 312
    sources of 274
    types of 289
Polycystic ovarian syndrome 353
Poor housing, effects of 318
Popliteal angle 41
Population 55
    activities 420*f*
    coverage 130*f*
    explosion 297, 302
    growth 272
    health 53
        management 387
    problem 266
Poshan Abhiyaan 344
Posterior capsular opacification 335
Posterior segment disorder 335
Postnatal care 78, 187, 188, 188*f*
Postnatal check-up schedule 48
Postnatal examination 188
Postnatal period, complications of 188
Postpartal care, objectives of 187
Postpartum danger signs 49
Postpartum period 178
Potassium 276, 277
    permanganate 307
Poverty relief 431
Pradhan Mantri Jan Arogya Yojana 145
Pradhan Mantri Suraksha Bima Yojana 209
Pradhan Mantri Surakshit Matritva Abhiyan 198, 199*f*
Pregnancy 183
    biologic fact of 186
    medical termination of 370, 370*f*
    outcome, abnormal 316
    weekly changes of 185*f*
Premenstrual syndrome 183
Pressure headache 112
Pre-symptomatic disease, stage of 64
Preventive care 191
Preventive geriatrics 243
Primary health care 12, 14, 77, 95, 127
    attributes of 13
    basic pillars of 136*f*
    concept of 13*f*
    elements of 13, 13*f*
    functions of 14*f*
    principles of 14, 14*t*
Primary Health Center 127, 147
    functions of 135, 147
    level 135
Primisulfuron-methyl 322
Private healthcare system 130*f*
Profound mental retardation 250
Programme
    components 222
    concept of 329
    planning, steps of 219, 222
Projective techniques 404
Promotive health 325

Proportional mortality rate 56
Prostate cancer 242
Prosthetics 247
Protect soil health 157, 280
Protein energy malnutrition 267
Protocol 101
Protozoal disease 305
Psittacosis 232
Psychological environment 268
Psychological tests 404
Psychomotor skills 45
Psychosis 250
Psychosocial development theories 255
Psychosocial effects 318
Psychosocial hazards 232
Puberty 182
Public education programme 309
Public Health 304
    Accreditation Board 34
    Administration 127
    Association 266
    infrastructure 164
    Programme, evaluation of 58
Public healthcare system 130*f*
Publicity 360
Puerperal sepsis 188
Puerperium stage 181
Pulmonary system 44
Pulse 40
Pyrazosulfuron-ethyl 322
Pyrethroid 322
Pyrithiobac-sodium 322
Pyrosis 184

Q

Q fever 232
Q-methodology 404
Qualitative analysis process 412
Qualitative data presentation 408, 413
Quantitative data presentation 405
Quaternary ammonium compounds 67
Quaternary health care 96
Questionnaires
    advantages of 402
    disadvantages of 402
Quota sampling 398

R

Radiation 304, 316
    control of 316
    prevention of 316
    types of 316
Radioactive pollution 316
    sources of 316
Radioactive substances 302, 316
Radioactive waste, management of 294
Radioactivity 316
Rain sensor device 309
Rainwater 304
    harvesting 310, 312
        importance of 310
        methods of 310
Rajiv Gandhi Drinking Water Mission 338
Rapid sand filter 306
Rat infestation 318
Realistic self-concept 36
Recording
    principles of 104
    purposes of 103
Records 101, 102
    care of 104
    concept of 101
    filling 106

    importance of 80, 102
    keeping 87
        nurses responsibility for 108
    legal implications of 105
    linkage 389
    maintenance 105
    purposes of 79
    relation of 101
    review 74
    types of 104
    uses of 103
    values of 103
Red crescent movement 428, 442
Red cross, seven fundamental principles of 442
Referral 93, 94
    form 98
    importance of 97
    network 93
    protocols 93
    register 93
    transport 199
Referral services 94*f*, 96*f*
    levels of 98*f*
Referral system 14, 93, 97, 99
    benefits of 99
    components of 96, 96*f*
    concept of 96
    need of 97
    nurse's role in 99
    principles of 96
Reflex 40
Refractive error 335
Refuse 319
    collection of 320
    composition of 319
    disposal, sanitary methods of 320
    sources of 320
    storage of 320
Regional Cancer Research and Treatment Centers 341
Regional Leprosy Workers Conferences 447
Regional organizations 419
Registers, types of 105, 223
Regular information, collection of 251
Rehabilitation 12, 66, 179, 244, 252, 255-257, 260, 261
    acute 253
    aims of 261
    approaches 260
    areas of 253, 253*f*
    benefits 233
    care, long-term 253
    centers 25
    Council of India Act 254
    gerontological principles of 254
    goal of 253
    historical perspectives of 254
    hospital associated 255
    initial stage of 254
    institution-based 260
    medical 244
    need of 254
    nurse
        job description 253
        qualifications for 253
        responsibilities of 253, 261
        role of 259, 261
        scope of 259
    nursing 252
        objectives of 258
    post-acute 253
    prevention of 216
    principles of 258, 261

professional, role of 257
psychosocial 244
purpose of 253
services 255
team 257*f*
    aims of 256
    objectives of 256
theories 255
types of 253
Rehabilitative care 254
Rehabilitative healthcare team 256
Rehabilitative nursing 258
    philosophy of 259
Renal system 44
Renewable resources 271
Replacement method 314
Reporting
    nurses responsibility for 106
    principles of 104
    purposes of 103
Reports 102, 103, 105
    concept of 101
    importance of 80, 102
    legal implications of 105
    relation of 101
    types of 105
Reproductive and child health 77, 179
    components of 196
    programme 179
        components of 374
Reproductive health 178, 181, 375
Reproductive system 112, 181
Reproductive tract infection 46
Research 103
    institute activities 225
    instruments 401
    tools 401
Researcher 79, 381
Respiration, normal 38
Respiratory infections 62, 264, 318, 325*f*
Respiratory system 314
Respiratory tract 110
Restoration phase 311
Revised National Tuberculosis Control Programme 164, 326
Rheumatic heart disease 111
Rheumatoid arthritis 241
Rhythm method 363
Rimsulfuron 322
River Boards Act 300
Road transport 319
Rockefeller foundation 438
    activities of 438
Roundworm 305
Rural development programme 151*f*
Rural health 339
    scheme 167
    service 142
Rural sanitation programme 338

S

Safe motherhood 375
Safe water, concept of 304
Safety 318
Sample registration system 389, 395
Sampling techniques, types of 396*f*
Sanitary landfill 320
Sanitary latrines, hygienic requirement of 321
Sanitary napkins, care of 183
Sanitary wells 305
Sanitation 268
Sanitation
    barrier 321

basic 303
ecological 303
environmental 234, 303
facilities 338
practices 303
types of 303
Scabies 121
    causes of 121
    features of 121*f*
Scale homogeneity 401
Scams 243
Scarf sign 41
Scatter diagram
    benefits of 408
    limitations of 408
    types of 408, 408*f*
Schistosoma mansoni, principal reservoir of 231
Schistosomiasis 231
School
    and community health activities, integration of 222, 222*f*
    education 446
    health
        committee 179, 218
        nurse 216, 220, 221, 221*f*
        policies 218, 221
        preventive and promotive services 214, 214*f*
        promotion activities 220
        recommendations 218
        scheme major components 212
        team 179, 217
School Health Programme 179
    components of 42, 212*f*, 219
    nature of 213
    objectives of 213
    principles of 214
School health records 106, 223
    essentials of 223
    maintenance of 223, 224
School Health Services 178, 211, 213, 216
    areas of 218
    components of 214
    development of 211
    objectives 213*f*
    relevance of 211
Security 240, 318, 427
    schemes 396
Sedimentation 297, 306
Selective vector control 328
Selenium 276
Self-concepts, impact of 11
Semantic differential scale 404
Sensory screening 43
Septic tank latrine 321
Septran multivitamin 86
Servicea latrines 321
Severe toxemia paralyzing vasomotor system 123
Sewage 292
    treatment 290
Sexual and reproductive health 346
Sexually Transmitted Diseases Control Programme 333
Sexually transmitted diseases
    control of 333
    objectives of 333
Sexually transmitted infection 46, 362
Shallow trench latrine 321
Shock 122
Shock
    anaphylactic 123

cardiogenic 123
hypovolemic 123
neurogenic 123
pathophysiology of 123*f*
septic 123
types of 123
Shrivastav Committee 167
Sick role, assumption of 10
Sickness benefits 233
Siderosis 230
Silicosis 230
Simple frequency distribution 400
Simple random sampling 396, 396*f*
Sinusitis 110
Skeletal changes 186
Skills 35, 385
Skin 245
    cancer 242
    care of 189
    changes 186
    diseases 245
    infections 318
    textures 40
Slow sand filter, advantages of 306
Small family 354, 354*f*, 356
    norm 354
        advantages of 355, 355*f*
        practices for 356
Smell 244
Snake 118
    bite 118, 118*f*
        immediate care of 118
Snowball sampling 398*f*
Social education 374
Social environment 6, 268
Social exclusion, prevention of 426
Social schemes 396
Social security 251
Sodium 276, 277
Soil
    conservation of 273, 281, 290
    erosion, causes of 291
    pollution 289, 291
        control 291
Solar energy 279
Solid waste 319
    classification of 291
    disposal of 319
    management 291
Somatic effects 294
Sore 112
    eye 114
    throat 110, 114
Space methods, natural methods of 362
Specific death rate 56
Specific infectious agent, presence of 53
Specific synthetic chemical pesticides 322
Spermicide 365
Spinal bifida 249
Spine 47
Spiritual health 17
Spot map 411, 411*f*
Square window 41
Standardized death rate 56
Standing order 101, 109, 112-114
    management 115, 116
    purposes of 112
Stannosis 230
State Level Healthcare Administration 133
    functions of 134
Statistical tests 414
    use of 414

Steadiness 314
Sterile compartment 86
Sterilization 66, 87, 88, 358
    terminal methods of 367, 367f, 368f
Stibine 230
Street refuse 320
Streptococcus pneumoniae 336
Stresses 75
Stroke 241
Subcenter 147
    functions of 136
    level 136
Suicidality 42
Suicide risk 242
Sulfometuron-methyl sulfosulfuron 322
Sulfonylurea herbicides 322
Sulphacetamide 115
Supernatant water 306
Supine hypotension syndrome 186
Supplementary feeding 195
Supports collaborative care 387
Surakshit Matritva Aashwasan 198, 198f
Surface water 305, 308
Surrogate 79
Sustainable development goals 151
Swachh Bharat Mission 327
Swelling assessment 121f
System's theory concept 70
Systematic cluster sampling 397f
Systemic minor ailments 109

T

Tanner sexual maturity rating scale 43, 43t
Taste 244
Tay-Sachs disease 247
Team building, steps of 378
Team functioning
    advantages of 379
    disadvantages of 379
Telangana State Government Employees and Journalists Health Scheme 211
Temperature 39, 40
    inequality of 315
    low 228
Terminal family planning methods 362f
Terrestrial ecosystem 282, 283
Tertiary health care 95
Testicular cancer 242
Tetanus 336
Thermal pollution 292, 293
    harmful effects of 293
    sources of 293
Thermometer techniques 88
Thoroughness 102
Thread worm 305
Three tire system 138f
Thrombophlebitis 186, 188
Thyroid
    cancer 242
    disease 242
Toothache 111, 122, 122f
    causes of 122
Total goiter rate 335
Town planning 319
    elements of 319
    importance of 319
    objectives of 319
Toxaphene 322
Toxic agents 230
Toxic shock syndrome, risk of 366
Trachoma 248
Traditional birth attendants 383
Transfer report 105
Transportation 272
Trauma 179
Trench foot 228
Tubal implant 367
Tubal ligation 368
    procedure 368
Tubectomy 367
Tuberculosis 264
    corpus fund 327
    emergence of 327
    management of 200
    nursing 24
Tuberculosis Association of India 444
Tuberculosis Control Programme, goal of 326
Tubewell water 305
Tularemia 232
Tundra ecosystem 282
Twenty point programme 343
    objectives of 343
Two stage cluster sampling 397f
Typhoid 275, 305, 321

U

Ultra-low-volume plumbing fixtures, installation of 309
Ultraviolet radiation 67, 228
Under five clinics 191
    aims of 191
    objectives of 191
    symbol of 191f
United Nations Development Programme 421
United Nations Educational Scientific and Cultural Organization 432
    activity planning 434
    functions of 434
United Nations Fund for Population Activities supports 420
United Nations International Children's Emergency Fund 424
    functions 425
    regional organizations of 425
    structure 425
United States Agency for International Development 431
Universal Health Insurance Scheme 210
Universal Immunization Programme 164
Unsanitary methods 320
Urban Community Health Centers 204
Urban Health Services 142
Urban Malaria Scheme 328
Urban Primary Health Center 204
Urban Sanitation Programme 338
Urinary system 44, 111
Urine analysis kit 86
Uterine tube 182
Uterus 182, 184
    position of 184
    weight of 184

V

Vaccination 17
    administration of 190f
Vagina 182
Vaginal discharge 112
Vaginal ring 366
Vasectomy 367
    complications of 368
    failure rate of 368
    procedure of 367
Vena cava syndrome 186
Ventilation 315
    effects of 315
    natural 315
    prevention of 315
    standards of 315
    types of 315
Vertical bar graphs 409
Vision 17, 43, 373, 443
    screening 43
Visual analog scale 404
Visual disability 248, 261
Visual impairment 242
Vital registration 395, 395f
Vital signs 39, 47, 113
Vital statistics 165, 390-392
    compilation of 394
    measurements 392
    sources of 392
    types of 391f, 392
    uses of 391
Vitamin
    B complex deficiencies 267
    D deficiency 267
    supplements 242
Vocational training center 430
Voluntary Health Agencies 143
    functions of 441
    problems of 441
Voluntary organization 439
    characteristics of 440
    objectives of 439
Voluntary service 429, 442

W

Waste
    excretion of 186
    production 272
Wastewater 297
    management 297
    treatment 297
Water (Prevention and Control of Pollution) Act 300
Water
    associated disease 305
    bacteriological quality of 308
    borne diseases 275, 305
    coagulated 306
    conservation 281
        concept of 309
    cycle 285, 285f
    flow, control of 273
    household purification of 307
    pollutant of 290
    purification processes 305
    purposes of 304
    reserve of 305
    sources of 304
    supply and sanitation 432
Water pollution 272, 274, 275, 289, 290, 300, 303
    control 290
Water resources 274
    development plan 311
    proper management of 275
    types of 274
Watershed management 310
    objectives of 311
    practices 312

Index

programme 311
   steps in 311
   types of 310
Weaning 190, 195
Weekly death rate 56
Weight 47, 190
   measurement of 88
Welfare
   concept of 337, 357
   provisions 233
Wellness theory 255
West Bengal Health Scheme 210
White blood cells 185
Whooping coughs 336
Wildlife Protection Act and Rules 300
Wind energy 279
Withdrawal method
   effectiveness of 365
   mechanism of action of 365
World bank 421
   capital resources of 422
   functions of 422
World food problems 278
World Health Assembly 419
World Health Organization 418
   expert committee criteria 389
   functions of 419
World Population
   Prospects 353
   Trends 352
World Trade Organization 428
Wounds 122
   types of 122

X

Xeriscape 309
   landscape 309
   principles of 309
Xerophthalmia 267

Y

Yaws Eradication Programme 341
Yeshasvini Health Insurance Scheme 210

Z

Zila Parishad
   functions 139
   members of 139
Zinc 277
   deficiency 267
Zoonotic origin, diseases of 231